# Healthcare Informatics and Analytics:

## Emerging Issues and Trends

Madjid Tavana
*La Salle University, USA*

Amir Hossein Ghapanchi
*Griffith University, Australia*

Amir Talaei-Khoei
*University of Technology, Sydney, Australia*

A volume in the Advances in Healthcare Information Systems and Administration (AHISA) Book Series

Medical Information Science
REFERENCE
An Imprint of IGI Global

Managing Director: Lindsay Johnston
Production Editor: Jennifer Yoder
Development Editor: Erin O'Dea
Acquisitions Editor: Kayla Wolfe
Typesetter: Kaitlyn Kulp
Cover Design: Jason Mull

Published in the United States of America by
Medical Information Science Reference (an imprint of IGI Global)
701 E. Chocolate Avenue
Hershey PA, USA 17033
Tel: 717-533-8845
Fax: 717-533-8661
E-mail: cust@igi-global.com
Web site: http://www.igi-global.com



Library of Congress Cataloging-in-Publication Data

Healthcare informatics and analytics : emerging issues and trends / Madjid Tavana, Amir Hossein Ghapanchi and Amir Talaei-Khoei, editors.
p. ; cm.
Includes bibliographical references and index.
Summary: "This book introduces the latest research concerning the innovative implementation of information technology and data analysis in the healthcare field, highlighting current concerns and recent advances in patient care and healthcare delivery"--Provided by publisher.
ISBN 978-1-4666-6316-9 (hardcover) -- ISBN 978-1-4666-6317-6 (ebook) -- ISBN 978-1-4666-6319-0 (print & perpetual access)
I. Tavana, Madjid, 1957- editor. II. Ghapanchi, Amir Hossein, 1981- editor. III. Talaei-Khoei, Amir, 1982- editor.
[DNLM: 1. Medical Informatics. 2. Computing Methodologies. W 26.5]
R858.A2
610.285--dc23
2014017314

This book is published in the IGI Global book series Advances in Healthcare Information Systems and Administration (AHISA) (ISSN: 2328-1243; eISSN: 2328-126X)

British Cataloguing in Publication Data
A Cataloguing in Publication record for this book is available from the British Library.

# Advances in Healthcare Information Systems and Administration (AHISA) Book Series

Anastasius Moumtzoglou
*Hellenic Society for Quality & Safety in Healthcare and P. & A. Kyriakou Children's Hospital, Greece*
Anastasia N. Kastania
*Athens University of Economics and Business, Greece*

ISSN: 2328-1243
EISSN: 2328-126X

## Mission

The **Advances in Healthcare Information Systems and Administration (AHISA) Book Series** aims to provide a channel for international researchers to progress the field of study on technology and its implications on healthcare and health information systems. With the growing focus on healthcare and the importance of enhancing this industry to tend to the expanding population, the book series seeks to accelerate the awareness of technological advancements of health information systems and expand awareness and implementation.

Driven by advancing technologies and their clinical applications, the emerging field of health information systems and informatics is still searching for coherent directing frameworks to advance health care and clinical practices and research. Conducting research in these areas is both promising and challenging due to a host of factors, including rapidly evolving technologies and their application complexity. At the same time, organizational issues, including technology adoption, diffusion and acceptance as well as cost benefits and cost effectiveness of advancing health information systems and informatics applications as innovative forms of investment in healthcare are gaining attention as well. **AHISA** addresses these concepts and critical issues.

## Coverage

- Virtual Health Technologies
- Measurements and Impact of HISA on Public and Social Policy
- Decision Support Systems
- Role of Informatics Specialists
- Medical Informatics
- Clinical Decision Support Design, Development and Implementation
- IS in Healthcare
- Telemedicine
- Pharmaceutical and Home Healthcare Informatics
- Rehabilitative Technologies

IGI Global is currently accepting manuscripts for publication within this series. To submit a proposal for a volume in this series, please contact our Acquisition Editors at Acquisitions@igi-global.com or visit: http://www.igi-global.com/publish/.

The Advances in Healthcare Information Systems and Administration (AHISA) Book Series (ISSN 2328-1243) is published by IGI Global, 701 E. Chocolate Avenue, Hershey, PA 17033-1240, USA, www.igi-global.com. This series is composed of titles available for purchase individually; each title is edited to be contextually exclusive from any other title within the series. For pricing and ordering information please visit http://www.igi-global.com/book-series/advances-healthcare-information-systems-administration/37156. Postmaster: Send all address changes to above address. 

## Titles in this Series

*For a list of additional titles in this series, please visit: www.igi-global.com*

*Laboratory Management Information Systems Current Requirements and Future Perspectives*
Anastasius Moumtzoglou (Hellenic Society for Quality and Safety in Healthcare, Greece & P. & A. Kyriakou Children's Hospital, Greece) Anastasia Kastania (Athens University of Economics and Business, Greece) and Stavros Archondakis (Military Hospital of Athens, Greece)
Medical Information Science Reference • copyright 2015 • 335pp • H/C (ISBN: 9781466663206) • US $245.00 (our price)

*Cloud Computing Applications for Quality Health Care Delivery*
Anastasius Moumtzoglou (Hellenic Society for Quality and Safety in Healthcare, Greece & P. & A. Kyriakou Children's Hospital, Greece) and Anastasia N. Kastania (Athens University of Economics and Business, Greece)
Medical Information Science Reference • copyright 2014 • 342pp • H/C (ISBN: 9781466661189) • US $245.00 (our price)

*Achieving Effective Integrated E-Care Beyond the Silos*
Ingo Meyer (empirica, Germany) Sonja Müller (empirica, Germany) and Lutz Kubitschke (empirica, Germany)
Medical Information Science Reference • copyright 2014 • 366pp • H/C (ISBN: 9781466661387) • US $245.00 (our price)

*Social Media and Mobile Technologies for Healthcare*
Mowafa Househ (College of Public Health and Health Informatics, King Saud Bin Abdulaziz University for Health Sciences, Saudi Arabia) Elizabeth Borycki (University of Victoria, Canada) and Andre Kushniruk (University of Victoria, Canada)
Medical Information Science Reference • copyright 2014 • 372pp • H/C (ISBN: 9781466661509) • US $245.00 (our price)

*Advancing Medical Practice through Technology Applications for Healthcare Delivery, Management, and Quality*
Joel J.P.C. Rodrigues (Instituto de Telecomunicações, University of Beira Interior, Portugal)
Medical Information Science Reference • copyright 2014 • 361pp • H/C (ISBN: 9781466646193) • US $245.00 (our price)

*Handbook of Research on Patient Safety and Quality Care through Health Informatics*
Vaughan Michell (University of Reading, UK) Deborah J. Rosenorn-Lanng (Royal Berkshire Hospital Foundation Trust Reading, UK) Stephen R. Gulliver (University of Reading, UK) and Wendy Currie (Audencia, Ecole de Management, Nantes, France)
Medical Information Science Reference • copyright 2014 • 486pp • H/C (ISBN: 9781466645462) • US $365.00 (our price)

IGI GLOBAL
DISSEMINATOR OF KNOWLEDGE
www.igi-global.com

701 E. Chocolate Ave., Hershey, PA 17033
Order online at www.igi-global.com or call 717-533-8845 x100
To place a standing order for titles released in this series, contact: cust@igi-global.com
Mon-Fri 8:00 am - 5:00 pm (est) or fax 24 hours a day 717-533-8661

# Editorial Advisory Board



# List of Reviewers

# Table of Contents

# Detailed Table of Contents



The utilization of micro-blog-based systems for the dissemination of health-related information offers a number of potential benefits. In this chapter, the authors describe a study of such micro-blog-based dissemination of health information by Australian health-related organisations through the manual categorization of over 4,700 tweets posted during a defined sample period. These tweets were analysed in relation to the sector of the tweeting organisation, health condition area, type of information in the micro-blog post, and level of retweeting. The particular category of public health-related tweets is also analysed in greater detail. This chapter differs from previous health and Twitter-related studies in that it: 1) seeks to characterize the overall and relative Twitter activity of health-related organisations for the sector across a whole nation, rather than collecting a sample matching a specific keyword or health condition; and 2) carries out a more semantically deep analysis of the content of those tweets, hence the manual analysis-based methodology adopted.



The aim of the chapter is to describe and analyse the conception of ICTs for social services on the basis of previous international and national research and a case study of Finnish experiences. The authors describe the concept of ICTs for social services and identify the main areas of interest and research findings in relation to the paradigm of social services informatics. The data for this part was collected by an integrated literature review of ICT research. Next, the authors review and evaluate the development phases of Finnish social services informatics. On the basis of national and international literature, they compare the similarities and distinguishing elements in the evolution of social care ICT in research and practice. On the basis of these findings on the main issues, challenges, opportunities, and trends, some recommendations for future research as well as for working practices are briefly described.



A patient-centric approach to healthcare leads to an informal social network among medical professionals. This chapter presents a research framework to: (1) identify the collaboration structure among physicians that is effective and efficient for patients; (2) discover effective structural attributes of a collaboration network that evolves during the course of providing care; and (3) explore the impact of socio-demographic characteristics of healthcare professionals, patients, and hospitals on collaboration structures, from the point of view of measurable outcomes such as cost and quality of care. The framework uses illustrative examples drawn from a data set of patients undergoing hip replacement surgery. The practical application of the proposed framework reveals structures of physicians' collaborations that are not favourable to cost and quality of care measures such as readmission rate. The authors believe that such a framework will enable healthcare managers and administrators to evaluate the collaborative work environment within their respective healthcare organisations.



Social media technologies represent an emerging means by which older adults can access health and community information, engage in peer-to-peer information sharing, and also potentially decrease social isolation. Privacy concerns, however, have been consistently identified as a barrier for older adults' use of the Web and social media technologies. The authors conduct a preliminary study involving 150 older adult participants, investigating their use and perceptions of social media technologies. The trial involved first providing the participants with brief training in three common social media technologies: Facebook, Twitter, and Skype. The authors carried out a quantitative and qualitative analysis of the participant's use and privacy perceptions of these technologies. Overall, the results are promising as to the potential to address privacy concerns to enable older adults to further utilize these technologies for improved mental, physical, and social health. Implications for future research and usage within the older adult community are also discussed.

Health institutions invest huge amounts in Information Systems (IS). Despite the huge budgets of investments, it is estimated that nearly 60-70% of Information Technology (IT) implementation projects fail in healthcare. In the literature, success factors and the failure reasons have largely been discussed. One of these, both in failure reasons and success factors, is the User Expectations. Expectation Failure, which can be defined as the gap between expectations of the end users from the system and actual performance of it, is introduced as one of the failure reasons of IS. The expectations of users must be well understood and discreetly worked out to design and implement a successful, acceptable, and useful IS. There is no study about the expectations from Healthcare Information System (HCIS) in the literature. The aim of this chapter is to investigate the end user expectations from HIS and their rankings. Seventeen potential end user expectations in four dimensions are examined and ranked according to the importance of expectations to the users.



Older adults want to live independently in their home for as long as possible, and technologies can support them with this goal. However, solutions to help with living alone are often designed from a technical perspective, ignoring the needs and preferences of older adults. This results in strong attitudes and feelings against, and limited adoption of, these technologies. In this chapter, the authors use ethnographic methods to inform the development of solutions taking into account the emotional needs of end-users. They present a three-staged approach by applying it in the domain of personal emergency alarms. First, the authors identify the shortcomings of current emergency alarm systems as perceived by older adults. Then, they develop a prototype that addresses some of the issues identified, focusing on emotional needs. Finally, the authors conduct a trial with the prototype. The results show that considering emotions during system design can improve user experience.

The healthcare industry is one of the most attractive domains to realize the actionable knowledge discovery objectives. This chapter studies recent researches on knowledge discovery and data mining applications in the healthcare industry and proposes a new classification of these applications. Studies show that knowledge discovery and data mining applications in the healthcare industry can be classified to three major classes, namely patient view, market view, and system view. Patient view includes papers that performed pure data mining on healthcare industry data. Market view includes papers that saw the patients as customers. System view includes papers that developed a decision support system. The goal of this classification is identifying research opportunities and gaps for researchers interested in this context.



Elderly care is of increasing global concern. The aging population is expected to increase two-fold by 2050. It is anticipated that there will not be enough caregivers to assist the elderly very soon, and thus, researchers are looking at various technologies and potential applications that will help alleviate the problem of elderly care. This chapter examines one such assistive technology: conversational agents in the form of avatars or robots as an aid to decrease loneliness and depression among the elderly and increase the cognitive function and quality of life. The authors discuss the state-of-the-science of research prototypes and commercial off-the-shelf systems. They propose a novel concept and design, and the authors discuss the ethical ramifications of senior citizens possibly bonding with inanimate objects as if they were human companions.

Digital healthcare is becoming increasingly important as the ageing population and the number of people diagnosed with chronic diseases is increasing. The face of healthcare delivery has changed radically and at its core is a digital and customer revolution. Connected health is the convergence of medical devices, security devices, and communication technologies. It enables patients to be monitored and treated remotely from their home or primary care facility rather than attend outpatient clinics or be admitted to hospital. This chapter discusses the recent advances in connected health technologies and applications. The authors investigate a reconfigurable supporting connected health solution for people with chronic diseases using reconfigurable hardware and intelligent data interpretation and analysis. In addition, a thorough review of the existing information and communications technologies and challenges in the area of connected health including embedded medical devices, sensors, social networking, knowledge management, data fusion, and cloud computing is presented in this chapter. Finally, future directions and ongoing research in the area of connected health are presented.

# Preface

In the first decade of the 21st century, we experienced exciting technological advancements in computing and decision sciences. As we are approaching the mid-point in the second decade, we are witnessing a radical transformation in healthcare administration and management. Healthcare is embracing computing technologies and decision analytics paradigms to deliver effective services. Remote care using information technologies has become a norm in medical practices. Ubiquitous technologies are facilitating the provision of healthcare services anywhere and anytime. This is causing an exponential proliferation of healthcare information that can be analyzed for effective management in various healthcare settings. As a result, healthcare informatics and analytics has been concerned not only with data management but also with predictive and prescriptive analytics, taking the healthcare sector to a higher degree of intelligence and effective advantages.

Health informatics and analytical methods have provided several advantages in the healthcare context. They have been contributing to the individual's health and have provided comprehensive tools for representing, accessing, and visualizing health data. They have also enabled comprehensive measurement and visualization of the human body and applied formal models for better understanding the functions or workings of the human body. Furthermore, health informatics and analytics has contributed to health knowledge. For example, several data mining algorithms have been applied to analyze data from different perspectives and summarizing it into useful information. The recent advancements in health informatics have enabled individuals to access a wide range of credible health information and knowledge, as well as given patients the ability to monitor and manage their diseases by accessing their own health information. It has also increased the collaboration between patients with chronic illnesses and caregivers by using health informatics tools.

Medical error is one of the primary causes of death in the US. Between 44,000 and 98,000 American deaths are consequences of medical errors in the healthcare industry. The most important causes for these kinds of errors come from communication problems such as unreadable information because of poor handwriting, mislabeled laboratory specimens, loss of medical records, and inaccurate health information in medical records. Investing in computer technologies related to healthcare can radically improve the range and quality of care available to patients and medical specialists such as nurses, doctors, and clinicians. Health informatics can minimize the risk of medical errors and help the early detection of health problems. In-home tele-monitoring of patients with chronic problems such as heart diseases can improve survival rates, reduce hospital days, and save nursing costs. Moreover, e-prescriptions have been reported to decrease errors in drugs dosage.

Healthcare processes are highly collaborative, and professionals from different disciplines must work together to enhance the quality of care. Achievement of this goal has been revolutionized through the use of computerized methods. For instance, Electronic Medical Records (EMRs) are commonly used, replacing paper medical records with digital ones. EMRs can be compared to their paper-based counterparts in three major perspectives: from the viewpoint of patients, General Practitioners (GPs), and health providers. For example, in paper-based systems, patients must physically transfer their health information from one provider to another, but in an electronic system all patient information is stored in the EMR database, and health providers have access to patients' data. Additionally, in paper-based system, patients with chronic diseases cannot update their health progress frequently, but in electronic systems chronic care patients can easily update their medical records and play an active role in their treatment. Furthermore, in paper-based systems, health practitioners may have some difficulties in obtaining relevant patient treatment information, whereas in electronic systems, patient information is stored in an integrated health record database providing for better access, which can lead to improved quality of care. Finally, integrated electronic systems can give healthcare providers access to more reliable and accurate information.

Given these trends, it is obvious that information technologies and analytical methods have played a critical and significant role in enhancing healthcare practices. Despite massive progress in healthcare informatics and analytics research and practice, there is no book that provides a relatively comprehensive set of modern research and practice in the field. Thus, this book aims at providing a big picture of recent advancements in the area of healthcare informatics and analytics.

The principal objective of this book is to provide a collection of recent and state-of-the-art contributions for researchers, academics, healthcare practitioners, and healthcare professionals who are concerned with the novel applications of informatics and analytics in healthcare. The chapters in this book demonstrate cutting-edge scholarly or applied practice methodologies using a wide range of techniques and analytical models including both quantitative and qualitative approaches as well as case studies that describe the significant advances in healthcare informatics and analytics.

The chapters in this book highlight the current state-of-the-art and science of applying informatics and analytics in healthcare. We are beginning to see that these applications are in fact reshaping the daily practices in healthcare settings. In this context, informatics and analytics tools are doing more than simply storing, retrieving, organizing, and analyzing information. The 17 chapters in this book illustrate that healthcare informatics and analytics are transforming delivery as well as the substance practice of healthcare in four different areas, producing the four sections of this book.

## SECTION 1: APPLICATIONS OF ONLINE SOCIAL MEDIA IN HEALTHCARE

This section consists of four chapters and presents the applications of online social media in healthcare. Social scientists have been studying the inter-personal relationships and their impacts in health and health-related settings for a long time. Following the advancements in the Web technology, the past decade has observed a growing interest in how social networks influence healthcare. In recent years, the rapid development of new informatics and tools, such as Web 2.0, has facilitated healthcare participants to utilize social networks. Healthcare organizations can use social media to reach aggregate information and leverage collaboration. As more patients use social networks and Web 2.0 technologies to track their health conditions and care, industry organizations have an opportunity to interact with the members of these online communities and to leverage real world data sets into new treatments and care pathways. This section presents techniques that can be utilized in several healthcare processes.

## Chapter 1

In the first chapter, titled "Twitter and its Role in Health Information Dissemination: Analysis of the Micro-Blog Posts of Health-Related Organisations," Dumbrell and Steele have provided an analysis of the use of a micro-blog system, namely Twitter, in terms of its nationwide use by health-related organizations. This is both novel and challenging as typical Twitter-related studies have concentrated on a more narrowly defined topic given the large volume of micro-blog posts. In addition, a more semantically deep analysis of this content has been carried out considering both the content of the micro-blog posts and the contents of Web pages linked to those micro-blog posts.

## Chapter 2

The aim of the chapter of Kuusisto-Niemi, Saranto, and Rissanen is to describe and analyse the conception of ICTs for social services on the basis of previous international and national research and a case study of Finnish experiences. The theme of their chapter is the development of social services informatics and the importance of special characteristics of it in ICT development. These issues are analysed in the light of national and international research. The chapter also opens a new perspective in ICT research. In the first part, the international research literature is analyzed by a paradigm that has been developed in a Finnish master´s degree program for health and human services informatics for the purposes of directing research and teaching in the most significant areas of informatics. It facilitates the study of previous research and places it in a systematic framework.

## Chapter 3

In the chapter titled "A Social Network Framework to Explore Healthcare Collaboration," Srinivasan and Uddin take a new approach that explores the impact of collaboration among physicians when treating hospital patients admitted for acute care. They utilize principles of two social network theories to offer insights into different types of collaboration patterns among healthcare professionals and explore the impact of different collaboration structures on healthcare cost and quality of care. The proposed collaboration framework is based on network theories of centralization and centrality that can explain how network structure and collaboration patterns affect group and individual performance. This framework is explained using illustrative examples of collaboration that evolves among physicians, while treating hospital patients undergoing hip replacement surgery. This practical application reveals network structures that are not favorable to cost and a quality of care parameter such as readmission rate. Finally, the authors offer some insights into various collaboration models that can provide cost effective and efficient healthcare service to chronic and acute care patients.

## Chapter 4

In their chapter titled "Privacy Perceptions of Older Adults when using Social Media Technologies," Dumbrell and Steele have investigated an important issue in relation to the increasing utilization of social media technologies by older adults for accessing health-related and other types of information. That is, the perceptions of older adults in relation to privacy when using social media. Whilst social media technologies can offer a novel medium for accessing up-to-date and relevant information and such technologies have seen a rapid consumer uptake globally, further understanding of any barriers to adoption particularly for older adults requires better understanding. Dumbrell and Steele have identified privacy concerns as one of the key issues for older adult adoption of social media as has been reported in a number of previous studies. In this chapter, the authors describe that the perceptions of older adults in relation to this issue are multi-faceted and complex. Moreover, Dumbrell and Steele identify and discuss that there were quite different privacy perceptions in relation to the different individual social technologies trialed—Facebook, Twitter, and Skype—and that these perceptions related to the different characteristics of these technologies.

## SECTION 2: USER ACCEPTANCE OF HEALTH INFORMATION SYSTEMS

This section is composed of three chapters and investigates user and usage aspects of health information systems. Complex regulatory concerns and patient-care priorities affect the pace at which technology can be adopted and deployed in the healthcare segment. Poor healthcare outcomes lead to increased levels of morbidity and mortality and obstruct countries' prosperity and business profitability. While there has been considerable interest in healthcare information systems, the uptake and acceptance rates for these systems have not been high enough for healthcare providers to experience the maximum benefits that these system have to offer. Past experiences of health information system adoption have indicated that the low adoption rate could be attributed to both macro-level factors (e.g., supportive policies) from the perspective of the public, healthcare organizations, and the system, and micro-level barriers from the perspective of healthcare providers (e.g., physicians' perception about technological complexity). Overall, uptake of healthcare information systems has been shown to be a very complex issue relating to organizational, people and technological challenges. Section 2 seeks to address these challenges by providing three state-of-the-art chapters.

### Chapter 5

The chapter titled "Perceived Importance of User Expectations from Healthcare Information Systems" by Gürsel is the continuation study of the work "A New Approach in the Evaluation of Hospital Information Systems," which presents an evaluation framework for the Hospital Information Systems (HIS) that evaluates the expectation meeting ratio of the HISs. This chapter represents the next step in this study. In this study, the variables of the framework are rank ordered according to the perceived importance of the users. This study gives important clues for the Healthcare Information System (HCIS) designers and developers. In addition, it gives insight into the research on HCIS, and its success factors and failure reasons. Although the HCIS developing industry is in close contact with the academic developments and studies, the high ratio of failure in health sector Information Technology (IT) projects indicates that they must be more careful in planning and management. Expectation management in an IT project is a critical issue that must be addressed. This item is always ignored in the project management phase of HCISs. Although there is a great deal of work done and remarkable results have already been gained, it seems there are still issues to be resolved and developed further.

## Chapter 6

In their chapter titled "Don't Leave Me Untouched: Considering Emotions in Personal Alarm Use and Development," Pedell, Lopez-Lorca, Miller, and Sterling present a novel approach for including the emotional needs of users in the development of systems and services. The authors illustrate their process with a compelling case study in the area of wellbeing in old age, tackling a truly current problem as the aged population grows as well as aged care costs. Personal alarm systems, usually in the form of a pendant worn around the neck or as a wristband, can be activated if seniors need help. Service providers often bundle the alarms with "check-in" systems, which require the older person to press a button on a daily basis during a specified interval. Pressing this button sends an "I'm OK" signal. If older adults do not press the button, the service provider contacts them and, eventually, their family if the older person cannot be contacted. Despite their technical soundness, these alarm systems often fail in their goal, that is, to provide support in an emergency. In many cases, relatives of older people insist on the installation of these systems, and the result is that the older people reject them. Pedell, Lopez-Lorca, Miller, and Sterling argue that the reasons behind this rejection are in the lack of catering for the non-functional needs of older people. This seems to be a common issue in many assistive systems, where the emotional needs of the intended users are overlooked in favor of specific physical needs dominating the design.

## Chapter 7

The goal of the chapter written by Keikhosrokiani, Mustaffa, Zakaria, and Baharudin is the introduction of the Mobile Healthcare System (MHS) followed by exploring the behavior intention of Smartphone users in Penang, Malaysia to use MHS. For this reason, a survey was conducted by distributing a questionnaire to Smartphone users as respondents in Penang, Malaysia. Partial Least Squares (PLS) was used to analyze the proposed measurement model. The results indicate which factors have significant effect on Smartphone user's behavioral intentions and which factors are not significant. The results assist the researchers in assessing whether MHS is highly demanded by users or not, as well as assist them in the development of the system for the future.

# SECTION 3: EMERGING TECHNOLOGIES FOR HEALTHCARE

This section consists of six chapters and presents emerging technologies for healthcare. New technologies are constantly in development to help people stay healthy, better diagnose disease, treat illness, and provide a better quality of life. While the rapid changes in routines, practices, and regulations push the contemporary healthcare forward, one could argue that nothing is changing the healthcare practices as much as technological advancements. Here, emerging technologies are advancements that can utilize and change the way that healthcare workers conduct their daily duties or the way that patients benefit from healthcare services. Section 3 seeks to address this by providing six interesting chapters.

## Chapter 8

In their chapter titled "Sleep Disorder Diagnosis: An Analytical Approach," Blake and Kerr demonstrate the development and evaluation of online tools to support the diagnosis of a chronic condition, sleep disorders. One of the outputs of this application is the automatic collection of good quality patient history data from every patient that completes the form. Decision analytics has the ability to uncover unknown patterns of patient characteristics, which might be used to develop a low-cost screening tool. To develop targeted instruments that might be used by primary physicians, this chapter proposes to access enough good quality data, which might be analyzed. However, the primary goal of sleep clinics currently is to efficiently diagnose sleep disorders rather than research or the collection of data. This chapter presents a tool that works by collecting the data as a by-product of diagnosis support.

## Chapter 9

In their chapter titled "Supporting Physicians in the Detection of the Interactions between Treatments of Co-Morbid Patients," Piovesan, Molino, and Terenziani address one of the most challenging emerging issues in Healthcare Informatics: the treatment of co-morbid patients (i.e., patients affected by multiple diseases). Nowadays, the number of co-morbid patients is rapidly increasing, due to the aging of population and the increase of chronic diseases (e.g., hypertension, diabetes mellitus, and heart failure). Clinical guidelines are widely used in the clinical practice as a way to implement evidence-based medicine and to provide both the quality and the standardization of healthcare services. However, "clinical practice guidelines provide evidence-based information of interventions, but only on individual pathologies. This sets up the urgent need of developing ways of merging multiple single-disease interventions to provide professionals' assistance to co-morbid patients." In this chapter, Piovesan et al. address such a crucial need by proposing a new computer-assisted methodology to support physicians in the detection of interactions between two or more different guidelines. The central and innovative idea of Piovesan et al.'s approach is that, to provide an adequate support to user-physicians, interaction detection must be interactive, flexible, and more importantly, must consider different levels of abstraction.

## Chapter 10

In their chapter titled "Radio Frequency Identification Technology as an Analytical Lens and Solution in Hospitals: A Novel Approach in BPR/BPM," Unnithan and Fraunholz contribute to the literature by presenting a novel way of using Radio Frequency Identification Technology as not only a technology solution for hospitals but also as an analytical lens to reveal inconsistencies in existing processes. The standard way of deploying a technology by redesigning processes and plugging in the technology may not work with hospitals that are hectic by nature. In the Australian context, while hospitals have discovered the utility value of RFID, there seem to be a certain reluctance in deployment. This chapter is timely in that it explains the way in which RFID can not only be a piece of technology that is useful to enhance processes, but it may also be an analytical tool that helps hospitals reassess their processes and address inconsistencies.

## Chapter 11

Ceruti, Geninatti, and Siliquini present a chapter titled "Use and Reuse of Electronic Health Records: Building Information Systems for Improvement of Health Services" that provides a clear and interesting overview of Electronic Health Records (EHRs), a description of their challenging evolution within the recent expansion of e-health, and of the emerging opportunities through EHR data reuse for the improvement of healthcare services. According to Ceruti, Geninatti, and Siliquini, all professionals in the field of public health should be provided a definition of EHR with respect to the disambiguation of the different health-related electronic records. The authors provide authoritative definitions. However, theoretical explanations are not always translated into practice by clear and distinct means. That is why the authors, while rigorously highlighting such differences among e-health data, direct their efforts to clarify why and how these data are intrinsically linked to each other. Personal Healthcare Records might be increasingly used with the advances in telemedicine, mHealth, and Health 2.0.

### Chapter 12

In their chapter, "The E-Learning Experience in Medical School of Casablanca," Ihssane, Diouny, Serhier, and Othmani bring into focus the current state of medical education, which is facing big advances in knowledge and less time for teaching. The authors point out the role of e-learning in improving the efficiency and effectiveness of educational materials through the description of two projects held by Hassan II University of Casablanca, Morocco, namely (1) the "Digital Environment Work" (DEW), a protected digital space which allows medical students, faculty, and administrators to access information and online services, and (2) "@U-PEL 2010 program," which was launched with a view to supporting holders of a comprehensive strategy for the development of e-learning institutions on the basis of clearly identified projects.

### Chapter 13

The next chapter titled "Knowledge Discovery and Data Mining Applications in the Healthcare Industry: A Comprehensive Study" is presented by Barazandeh and Gholamian. Databases are growing in hospitals, clinics, medical research centers, pharmaceutical companies, and other related businesses. This chapter proposes a well-structured classification that works as a road map for researchers to find their interest areas and conduct their studies in those areas. Research areas and challenges in each area are clearly discussed. The chapter studies recent studies on knowledge discovery and data mining applications in the healthcare industry and proposes a new classification of these applications. This classification is based on main healthcare industry pillars. These pillars includes the patient as the most important pillar, information and knowledge of healthcare activities, practitioners including managers, physicians, nurses, and other personnel, and business issues that cause the industry to survive and establish the relationships between all the pillars.

## SECTION 4: APPLICATIONS OF INFORMATICS FOR AGED CARE AND CHRONIC DISEASES

This section is formed by four chapters and highlights the applications of informatics for aged care and chronic diseases. The world's population is aging rapidly, and the cost of caring for older people is also rising. In 2012, 6.9% of the world population were more than 65 years old, and this is estimated to increase to around 20% by 2050. In addition, the chance for the aged population to suffer from chronic diseases is higher than young ones. This has increased the necessity for innovative approaches in the aged care sector in order to reduce the cost of care. One approach could be the use of technologies to provide efficiencies in patient care and lower costs. There are two main arguments for this. First, seniors traditionally like to live independently and preferably in their own homes. Second, it is commonly believed that the aged care sector will soon face a huge shortage in qualified workers. In addition, remote and regional areas, even basic healthcare services, require patients to travel long distances to get treatment, and this is further exacerbated as the elderly often have transport issues such as restricted movement and an inability to drive. Recent advancements in Information Technology (IT) have resulted in technological products that have potential to assist older people in their daily life activities at their homes. Section 4 addresses these issues through four state-of-the-art chapters.

## Chapter 14

The next chapter is titled "Using Narrative with Avatars and Robots to Enhance Elder Care" and is written by Lundy Lewis. Socialization through narrative and storytelling is important for elder care and quality of life. The elderly enjoy reminiscing and communicating. They enjoy being reminded of past experiences and having conversations with other interested parties such as family and friends about their life history or particular life events. However, there are common reports of frustration, such as caregivers who are around on a daily basis and who do not know the elderly person in the way that families do and thus cannot engage in such meaningful conversation. Lewis's chapter aims to alleviate the common problem of loneliness and depression in the elderly by developing a social companion in the form of an avatar or humanoid robot.

## Chapter 15

The chapter written by Hume, Hume, Johnston, and Whitty is titled "The Role of Knowledge Management (KM) in Aged Care Informatics: Crafting the Knowledge Organization." Aged care is becoming more diverse and complex advancing from residential care to incorporate community-directed care and require practices that enable efficiency and growth. This chapter introduces the concepts of knowledge management, decision support systems, and big data management in aged care, and focuses on the importance of diffusion of knowledge to those in need. This chapter focuses on informing the development of an analytics-driven operational system and advanced KM hub for aged care management and patient care services.

## Chapter 16

In the chapter by Alireza Rahimi and colleagues, they learn current expressions of specification of data quality and the role of ontology-based approaches to develop data quality based on "fitness for purpose" within the health context. They have sighted different mechanisms, including ontologies, to specify DQ in integrated CDM and whether improved DQ will better measure health outcomes. This chapter presents a literature review that suggests that, compared to non-hierarchical data models, there may be more advantages and benefits in the use of ontologies to solve semantic clinical data quality issues and improve the validity and reliability of data retrieval, collection, storage, extraction, and linkage algorithms and tools.

## Chapter 17

The last chapter is titled "A Reconfigurable Supporting Connected Health Environment for People with Chronic Diseases" and is written by Amira, Ramzan, Grecos, Wang, Casaseca-de-la-Higuera, Pervez, Wang, and Luo. The number of elderly and people diagnosed specifically with chronic diseases is increasing dramatically in all regions in the world. This has a huge impact on the cost, quality, and delivery of healthcare services, which are changing from the traditional approach to the connected model. This book chapter discusses the recent advances in connected health technologies and applications. A thorough review of the existing information and communications technologies and challenges in the area of connected health, including embedded medical devices, sensors, social networking, knowledge management, data fusion, and cloud computing, is presented. Finally, future directions and ongoing research in the area of connected health are presented.

All in all, this book will help to simplify the seemingly inexorable complexity involved in development of healthcare informatics and analytics tools, methods, and models that have come to characterize today's world.

*Madjid Tavana*
*La Salle University, USA*

*Amir Hossein Ghapanchi*
*Griffith University, Australia*

*Amir Talaei-Khoei*
*University of Technology, Sydney, Australia*

# Section 1

# Applications of Online Social Media in Healthcare

# Chapter 1
# Twitter and Its Role in Health Information Dissemination:
## Analysis of the Micro-Blog Posts of Health-Related Organisations

**Dan Dumbrell**
*The University of Sydney, Australia*

**Robert Steele**
*The University of Sydney, Australia*

## ABSTRACT

*The utilization of micro-blog-based systems for the dissemination of health-related information offers a number of potential benefits. In this chapter, the authors describe a study of such micro-blog-based dissemination of health information by Australian health-related organisations through the manual categorization of over 4,700 tweets posted during a defined sample period. These tweets were analysed in relation to the sector of the tweeting organisation, health condition area, type of information in the micro-blog post, and level of retweeting. The particular category of public health-related tweets is also analysed in greater detail. This chapter differs from previous health and Twitter-related studies in that it: 1) seeks to characterize the overall and relative Twitter activity of health-related organisations for the sector across a whole nation, rather than collecting a sample matching a specific keyword or health condition; and 2) carries out a more semantically deep analysis of the content of those tweets, hence the manual analysis-based methodology adopted.*

## INTRODUCTION

Health information dissemination has undergone significant changes due to various technological advances. From originally being delivered through the use of posters, bulletin boards and newspaper articles as public health announcements, to dissemination via current traditional mass media (e.g. television, radio) and increasingly now by online means with the rapid uptake of the Internet. Contemporarily, with the introduction and mass-adoption of social networking services (SNSs) by

DOI: 10.4018/978-1-4666-6316-9.ch001

a significant proportion of online users, there are now additional and potentially powerful means of health information dissemination (Steele, 2011).

Twitter, a micro-blogging-based SNS with approximately 240 million active global users, contains useful features and characteristics such as: one-to-many interactions, 'up-to-the-minute' information dissemination, the ability of users to select accounts relevant for them to follow, and the capability of users to generate, receive and share information amongst themselves. This provides an efficient platform for potential Web-based information sharing and retrieval and Twitter can thus potentially aid in achieving the dissemination of health information. Recent reports by social media and marketing-based companies have found that Twitter currently has approximately 2.5 million monthly unique Australian visitors, and this number is rising rapidly (SocialMediaNews.com.au, 2014). The growing proportion of Internet users adopting Twitter, as well as the already widespread uptake of SNSs in Australia, indicates the significance of exploring this medium as a potential tool for health information dissemination.

This chapter will present a detailed overview of how Twitter is currently being used by health-related organisations in Australia, and the health conditions and types of health-related information that are being posted by different organisational sectors. Categorised health information mined from the sample of tweets is also further analysed for the purpose of exploring relationships between the types of disseminators and receivers of health information. The study aims to provide initial empirical data relevant to health organisation utilisation of social media for the health sector on a national scale, rather than necessarily across the entire 'Twittersphere'.

## RELATED WORK

Due to the relatively recent introduction of health information-related micro-blogging, and the recent widespread national and global uptake of Twitter in general, the exploration of health and Twitter is still an emerging area of research. A previous health organisation-related study had found that of those public health department accounts within the US using social media, 86.7% had Twitter accounts (Thackeray, Neiger, Smith & Wagenen, 2012). The researchers of the study categorised tweets based on information presented, however they did not follow any links embedded within the tweets and thus did not analyse the information provided in the linked-to Web pages. This chapter will attempt to provide a deeper semantic analysis whereby micro-blog posts and the specific health conditions and types of information being conveyed will be explored and categorised according to both information presented in the tweet and the linked-to page indicated by any embedded URLs.

The tweeting and sharing of information on specific health conditions has also been explored in a number of works. Sullivan et al. (2012) analysed concussion-related tweets to investigate different themes (e.g. 'news', 'personal situation', 'inferred management') as well as to whom these types of information were being disseminated. Epilepsy-related information dissemination via Twitter has also been studied (Mcneil, Gordon & Brna, 2012), where researchers analysed and coded tweets into specific categories to describe the types of epilepsy-related information that was being tweeted. These studies added support that health information could be effectively disseminated via Twitter, but also found a minority of tweets sampled were actually informative in terms of health information. Other research articles have also examined Twitter and smoking cessation (Prochaska, Pechmann, Kim & Leonhardt, 2011), dental pain (Heaivilin, Gerbert, Page & Gibbs, 2011) and pharmaco-surveillance (Bian, Topaloglu & Yu, 2012) - this again demonstrates that previous studies have tended to focus on specific health condition or health areas.

A previous cross-sectional study of SNS use amongst the Society for Assisted Reproductive Technology highlighted the growing influence of social media in relation to health-related issues and communication (Omurtag, Jimenez, Ratts, Odem & Cooper, 2012). Various clinics within the organisation had their online Websites evaluated and it was found that rather than consumers asking for information, health-related bodies were 'pushing' information through SNSs. This research also demonstrated that in addition to providing clinically relevant health information, SNSs included many other types of information such as 'advertising' (28%), 'support' (19%) and 'irrelevant chatter' (17%). Therefore it would be of interest to carry out similar categorisation and analysis on a more widespread social media platform, such as Twitter, to see if these information types are proportionally consistent.

The idea of influence or scale of dissemination on Twitter can be represented by the measure of how many times a tweet is retweeted, as well as the quantity of audience reached. Cha, Benevenuto and Gummandi (2010) found that Twitter accounts with large numbers of followers had many one-to-one interactions (i.e. mentions and replies), and retweeting was a more suitable way of representing influence of a user beyond a one-to-one interaction domain (i.e. broader community interaction and dissemination). Therefore, they suggested that the most influential users were those who had more of their tweets retweeted and mentioned, rather than judging the influence of an account based on the number of followers.

As mentioned, measuring the reach or dissemination of a micro-blog post or tweet can also involve identifying the retweeting accounts and their numbers of followers. Kwak, Lee, Park and Moon (2010) found from their dataset of 41.7 million user profiles and 106 million tweets, that any retweeted tweet reached an average of 1,000 users – regardless of the number of followers of the original tweeting account.

Whilst some of the studies mentioned have been carried out with non-health-related datasets, or were limited to specific health areas, our work will analyse health-related Twitter usage on a nation-wide basis and across all health topics. This work can be differentiated from previous work in that it analyses the use of micro-blogging across a whole sector (health in this case) for a country rather than selecting a particular narrower health area or topic and retrieving data corresponding to keywords matching that narrower area.

## METHODOLOGY

### Identifying Relevant Accounts

Accounts relevant to the study were found via a three-step method. With each step, identified accounts were examined to see if they met the inclusion criteria for our study (Table 1). First a search was conducted through the search function on the Twitter website (www.twitter.com) utilising health-related and appropriate keywords such as 'health', 'nutrition', 'cancer', 'Australia' etc. to find relevant accounts. The second step involved utilising the search engine Google (www.google.com) to identify additional relevant Twitter accounts that were not found from step one. Searches were performed using a combination of health-related keywords, for example the search 'dementia Australia Twitter' was entered into Google in an attempt to either uncover dementia-related Twitter accounts that were originally overlooked, or

*Table 1. Inclusion criteria*

| Inclusion Criteria | Definition |
|---|---|
| Nationality | Self declared home location is Australia or is a known or deducible to be Australian-based |
| Representativeness | Accounts represent government health bodies or other health organizations (with the link to a relevant website provided in account description) |
| Topic of account | The account pertains to health information, either generically or in relation to a specific condition |
| Content of tweets | Accounts must have at least one health-related tweet or provide links to health articles |
| Activity | Accounts are currently active, as we defined as having tweeted in the month of February 2012 |
| Number of followers | The number of Twitter followers for any given account was set to a minimum of 150 |

to ensure the search for relevant accounts was exhausted. In the third step, already identified accounts had their Twitter feeds and followers examined to uncover further relevant users that met the inclusion criteria.

When considering the various factors required for the identification and inclusion of Twitter accounts, the following factors were considered:

- The specific details of accounts to be identified (according to inclusion criteria),
- Broad topic areas of accounts (i.e. health-related),
- The owner of the account (i.e. what organisational sector they came from).

## Categorising Health Tweets

Individual tweets were grouped and generalized according to similarities for 1) specific health-related conditions (Table 2) and 2) type of tweet identified (Table 3). The first form of categorisation undertaken was in relation to health condition areas - for example, condition-specific tweets about 'skin cancer advice' and 'breast cancer research' were categorised under the umbrella health condition area of 'cancer'. To provide another dimensional view of the collected data, health-related tweets were also categorised according to the type of tweet, independent of health condition area, that the tweet pertained to. Referring to the above example, tweets about 'skin cancer advice' were categorised as 'public health advice' and tweets about 'breast cancer research' were categorised as 'research and project' type tweets.

## Requirement for Manual Tweet Analysis within Methodology

It was deemed that various Twitter analytics tools (e.g. Twitonomy, TweetStats) did not have capabilities that would fulfil the required account identification process (nor the subsequent data collection and deep semantic analysis requirements of collected tweets), and hence a manual approach was adopted throughout the data mining and analysis of this study (Dumbrell & Steele, 2013). The three-step manual methodology provided the process whereby a substantive sample of the current health-related organisational Twitter users meeting these criteria in Australia were identified and compiled.

We identified that current Twitter analytics tools did not provide the capabilities of categorising and semantically-analysing tweets based on complex concepts such as 'public health advice', 'infectious diseases-related' or 'fundraising' and as such, manual categorisation and analysis by a researcher was required. In general, current Twitter analytics tools cannot provide analysis of tweet content based on concepts and semantics within the text of tweets. These analytics tools also do

*Table 2. Proportion of health condition-related areas of sector tweeting*

| | Gov (% of 388 Health Tweets) | FP (% of 1,071 Health Tweets) | NFP (% of 2,331 Health Tweets) | All Sectors (% of 3,790 Health Tweets) |
|---|---|---|---|---|
| Addictive substances | 4.1% | 2.4% | 2.0% | 2.3% |
| Allergies | 0.0% | 0.3% | 0.1% | 0.1% |
| Cancer | 1.3% | 5.0% | 6.2% | 5.4% |
| Children | 0.0% | 0.7% | 0.2% | 0.3% |
| Dental | 0.8% | 1.9% | 0.3% | 0.8% |
| Diabetes | 1.0% | 0.8% | 2.6% | 2.0% |
| Disability | 0.0% | 0.0% | 2.1% | 1.3% |
| Elderly | 0.3% | 1.0% | 0.3% | 0.5% |
| **Gender** | | | | |
| Male | 0.3% | 0.1% | 0.1% | 0.1% |
| Female | 0.0% | 0.3% | 0.0% | 0.1% |
| Heart | 0.3% | 2.1% | 1.2% | 1.3% |
| Indigenous (general) | 0.3% | 0.7% | 3.4% | 2.3% |
| Infectious diseases | 3.1% | 1.0% | 0.4% | 0.8% |
| Injury | 0.8% | 1.1% | 0.0% | 0.4% |
| **Lifestyle** | | | | |
| Fitness | 3.9% | 1.4% | 0.4% | 1.1% |
| Nutrition | 11.6% | 8.5% | 3.7% | 5.9% |
| Maternity | 0.8% | 2.8% | 0.3% | 1.1% |
| Mental health | 7.5% | 6.4% | 9.4% | 8.3% |
| Neurology / Geneology | 0.0% | 0.7% | 0.4% | 0.4% |
| Non-condition specific | 59.5% | 53.3% | 58.1% | 56.9% |
| Obesity | 0.0% | 0.8% | 0.4% | 0.5% |
| Organ donation | 3.6% | 0.5% | 0.5% | 0.8% |
| Osteoporosis / arthritis | 0.0% | 0.1% | 0.9% | 0.6% |
| Pharmaceutical | 0.3% | 4.5% | 0.4% | 1.6% |
| Renal / Kidney | 0.0% | 0.1% | 0.9% | 0.6% |
| Respiratory | 0.0% | 0.1% | 0.3% | 0.2% |
| Sexual | 0.5% | 1.1% | 1.1% | 1.1% |
| Sleep-related health | 0.0% | 0.7% | 0.4% | 0.4% |
| Vaccine | 0.3% | 1.3% | 2.8% | 2.1% |
| Vision | 0.0% | 0.1% | 0.9% | 0.6% |
| **Total** | 100.0% | 100.0% | 100.0% | 100.0% |

*Table 3. Proportion of sector tweeting type*

| | Gov (% of 388 Health Tweets) | FP (% of 1,071 Health Tweets) | NFP (% of 2,331 Health Tweets) | All Sectors (% of 3,790 Health Tweets) |
|---|---|---|---|---|
| Advertising | 0.0% | 1.0% | 0.5% | 0.6% |
| Ambulance updates | 19.3% | 0.0% | 0.0% | 2.0% |
| Awareness | 11.3% | 22.3% | 23.6% | 22.0% |
| Competitions | 4.1% | 0.3% | 2.0% | 1.7% |
| Conferences & events | 3.1% | 3.5% | 7.0% | 5.6% |
| Fundraising | 1.0% | 2.1% | 15.5% | 10.2% |
| Funding | 1.0% | 0.7% | 0.9% | 0.9% |
| Insurance | 0.8% | 2.6% | 1.8% | 1.9% |
| Jobs & Career | 1.8% | 4.5% | 3.6% | 3.6% |
| Medical workforce | 1.3% | 6.1% | 1.7% | 2.9% |
| Motivation & support | 2.1% | 0.8% | 1.8% | 1.6% |
| Organisational news | 6.7% | 21.7% | 17.0% | 17.3% |
| Policy | 3.9% | 3.0% | 0.9% | 1.8% |
| Promotional | 0.5% | 3.5% | 2.4% | 2.5% |
| Public Health Advice | 36.9% | 21.1% | 17.3% | 20.4% |
| Research & Project | 6.2% | 6.6% | 4.0% | 5.0% |
| **Total % contribution** | 10.2% | 28.3% | 61.5% | 100.0% |

not contain the functionality to examine the Web pages linked-to by hyperlinks present in tweets, hence further necessitating the manual approach adopted.

## GENERAL SECTOR CHARACTERISTICS

A total of 114 health-related Australian organisation Twitter accounts, meeting the inclusion criteria, were identified via the three-step process as described above. Three distinguishable organisational sectors were observed during the account identification process: government Twitter accounts, for-profit (FP) organisational accounts, and accounts that represented not-for-profit (NFP) organisations. The 114 identified accounts in the sample were thus categorised into these three sectors - it was found that there were 16 government, 27 FP and 71 NFP Twitter accounts present in the substantiative national sample for this study (Figure 1).

The characteristics of each Twitter account were also collected – such as the number of tweets, accounts followed and following accounts. For comparative purposes, these characteristics were analysed proportionate to the number of Twitter accounts identified for a certain sector (e.g. the mean number of followers for accounts in a sector was the total number of followers divided by the number of accounts identified in that sector). When taking this into consideration, it was found that government health-related accounts had 2,347-followers on average per account, the highest of the three sectors. NFP accounts had on average 1,975 followers per account, which was still a much higher average than compared to

*Figure 1. Proportion of different Australian health-related Twitter accounts identified*

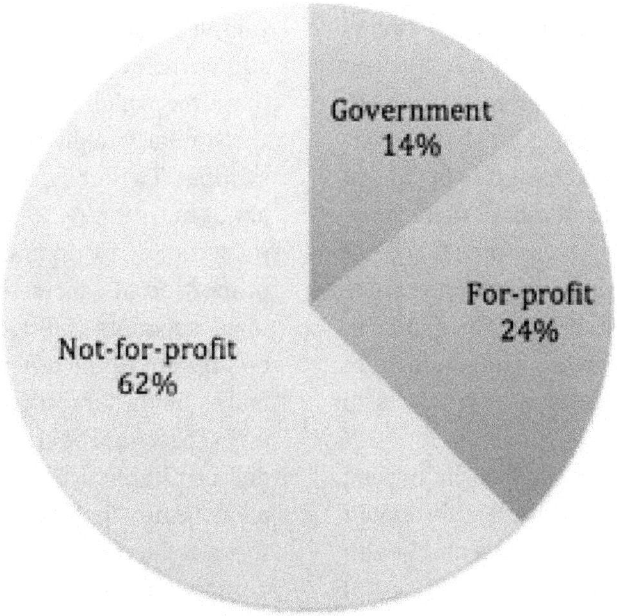


their FP counterparts that had the lowest number of followers on average, with a mean of 1,153 per account.

This low number of followers for FP accounts may be explained by a previous study (Sillence, Briggs, Harris & Fishwick, 2004) that had found Internet users to be more likely to reject sites they considered promotional or sales-based. Therefore, the reputation that FP organisations have (e.g. commercial, product-promotion) may make consumers less trusting of the information on their websites. . This may potentially be why FP Twitter accounts have a lower average number of followers than other sectors. In the sample of the 27 health-related FP organisation accounts, only 4.5% of tweets in the month of February were considered advertising or promotional-related. However, this was still the largest proportion of these tweet types when comparing to the NFP and government subsets

## TWEETING CHARACTERISTICS BY ORGANISATIONAL SECTOR

A total of 4,787 tweets were found to have been posted from across the 114 identified accounts in the month of February 2012. Of these 4,787 tweets, 3,790 (79.2%) were categorised as health-related whilst the remaining 997 (20.8%) were non health-related. This is similar to results found for public health department Twitter accounts in the USA (Thackery et al., 2012). The tables below (Table 2 & 3) represent data that is the proportion of health-related tweets, and thus the analysis does not include the 997 non-health related tweets. As stated in the methodology section, these health-related tweets were looked at according to two separate dimensions and categorised into two separate tables – by health condition area (Table 2) and tweet type (Table 3).

When looking at health condition-related areas identified for the February 2012 sample period, it can be seen that a large proportion of these tweets were categorised under non-condition specific (i.e. developments in the particular health-related sectors without reference to a specific health condition, such as for example the progress of federal health reform). In absolute numbers there were 2,157 identified tweets from the sample that dealt with such health information in a general sense, rather than relating to a specific health condition. Tweets categorised under this group made up more than half (56.9%) of all health-related tweets in the sample.

Outside of the non condition-specific tweets, the top 3 largest contributions to the health-related tweet sample by far were those of mental health (8.3%), nutrition (5.9%) and cancer-related (5.4%) areas. In fact, the next highest represented health-related areas (addictive substances and Indigenous health, both at 2.3% each) were much lower in percentage than these top three health-specific areas.

When comparing the three sectors, we also found that there were differences in the amount of tweeting of certain health areas within each sector. Government accounts tweeted most frequently about lifestyle-related topics (nutrition: 11.6% and fitness: 3.9%), addictive substances (4.1%), organ donation (3.6%) and infectious diseases (3.1%). Interestingly, nutrition-related information was by far the highest specific health area tweeted about by government accounts, and was also the highest proportion when compared to other sectors. The relatively high dissemination of addictive substance-related tweets might be expected as government bodies are frequently rolling out national campaigns for awareness of issues such as binge drinking, drunk driving and the effects of illegal drug use. With regards to the area of infectious diseases, the government also undertakes initiatives to educate and warn people about new or rapidly spreading diseases (e.g. the swine flu pandemics). However in the case of the organ donation-related tweets, the tweet dataset was taken during DonateLife week, which occurs in February. This provides an example of how even samples taken from over a month may potentially still be influenced by specific events occurring at that time which may cause sampling bias.

Similarly to government accounts, FP organisational Twitter accounts tweeted significantly about nutrition (8.5%) and mental health (6.4%) related areas. FP organisations also tweeted a larger proportion of cancer-related tweets than government accounts (5.0%). Also interestingly when comparing to the other two sectors, FP accounts had by far the largest proportion of tweets in health areas that could be considered to have commercial and profitable aspects. One of the most tweeted about health-specific topics from FP accounts were those related to the pharmaceutical area, which comprised 4.5% of total health-related tweets by this sector. This far outweighed the proportion of pharmaceutical-related tweets posted by government (0.3%) and NFP (0.4%) organisations, thus showing that FP organisations may possibly be tweeting about health-related areas more specific to their business goals (e.g. advertising, sales, etc.).

NFP organisations had the highest proportion of mental health and cancer-related tweets, at 9.4% and 6.2% respectively. This sector also tweeted proportionately more about Indigenous health, as 3.4% of their health-related tweets came from this area. This percentage was much higher when compared to FP (0.7%) and government (0.3%) Twitter accounts. These results may suggest that government accounts could tweet more about Indigenous health as government bodies both recognise initiatives and often provide funding in this area. Another significant area of tweeting based around a target group from NFP accounts is the dissemination of disability-related information. This category appears to be under-represented when considering tweets from government and FP accounts (both 0.0%), however when examining NFP organisations it was found that tweets about the disability health-area made up 2.1% of the total health-related tweets from NFP accounts.

There were a relatively small number of tweets for some widespread and significant health conditions affecting Australia. The National Health Priority Areas (NHPAs) is an initiative by the Australian government that aims to identify health areas contributing significantly to the morbidity and mortality rates of the population. Asthma, arthritis and musculoskeletal conditions, injury prevention and control and obesity are four of the nine current NHPAs (Australian Institute of Health and Welfare, 2013) that are under-represented in the identified sample of health-related tweets. Asthma and respiratory disorders ranked as the lowest Twitter communicated NHPA representing only 0.2% of the entire health-related tweet sample, whilst arthritis and musculoskeletal conditions, the most active of these under-represented categories comprised only 0.6% of the total health-related tweets in the sample.

The four mentioned under-represented NHPAs had a total of 65 identified tweets in February 2012. Combined, these conditions contributed to only 1.7% of health-related tweets. Considering that these areas are considered of national importance, these numbers were notably low especially when compared to other NHPAs: cardiovascular health (51 tweets or 1.3%), diabetes (74 or 2.0%), cancer (204 or 5.4%) and dementia and mental health-related tweets (316 or 8.3%). Tweets in these more prominently identified NHPAs accounted for approximately one-sixth (17.0%) of the 3,790 health-related tweets identified in February 2012.

Table 3 was compiled from the same sample of 3,790 health-related tweets collected/analysed for the study (and also used to compile Table 2). This table however provides another dimension to view various proportions of tweet numbers by separating the identified tweets into the type of health information being provided.

FP accounts had 21.7% of their health-related tweets dedicated to providing 'organisational news' (news about the activities of that organisation), whereas NFP organisations tweeted a slightly lower percentage of organisational news as a proportion of their health-related tweets (17.0%). Governmental accounts tweeted significantly lower proportions for organizational news (6.7%) and promotion (0.5%). This suggests that FP accounts are particularly active in promoting developments within their organisations, and suggests an opportunity for government and NFP accounts to provide further organisational news-related tweets to potentially encourage further engagement between their organisations and health consumers.

Fundraising-related tweets alone contributed to approximately 10.2% of the total number of health-related tweets identified in February. Unsurprisingly, many of these tweets (361) came from NFP organisations. Throughout the analysis, Twitter was identified to be a frequent way for NFP accounts to communicate about fundraising, with 15.5% of their health tweets categorised under this type. This medium can potentially be a cost-effective method for NFP organisations to fundraise, especially when considering the costs of developing, promoting and advertising through various traditional media. In addition, the use of Twitter or social media for fundraising has the advantage of potentially reaching a more interested and targeted audience for the specific health area of fundraising.

One of the more interesting findings is that Twitter is already being widely used for 'public health advice' dissemination. Such tweets were defined as health information the consumer could use to potentially change relevant aspects of their current health behaviours. In our sample, 772 or one-fifth (20.4%) of health-related tweets in February fell under this category type. This was an anticipated beneficial function for micro-blog postings. In terms of proportion for a sector, government tweets are most dominated by public health advice with more than one-third (36.9%) of their health-related tweets being categorised under this type, indicating the current frequent use of government Twitter accounts to deliver health advice to consumers. It should be noted that both

FP and NFP accounts also had substantial numbers of public health advice-related posts, with 21.1% and 17.3% respectively. Public health advice tweets were considered an interesting sub-sample of the overall sample to further analyse, given that this was a significant category in terms of number of tweets in addition to the high impact application of micro-blogging in relation to the communication of public health information.

## PUBLIC HEALTH TWEETS AND THEIR DISSEMINATION

The dissemination, or sharing, of micro-blog postings on Twitter is done by a user-driven process referred to as retweeting. Retweeting is the act in which a user shares a tweet posted by another user to their followers, much like somebody forwarding an email to their entire address book. Dissemination of public health information is an interesting concept that has been examined in previous research (Dumbrell & Steele, 2012). The open nature of the medium by which this information is shared, as well as the interface characteristics of Twitter, allows for quantitative measures to be observed. These measures can include how many times a certain type of health information is retweeted, how many end-users this information reaches – and if these factors have any relation to the nature of information being shared or the initial poster of the information. This novel idea and practice of members of the public being involved in health information dissemination allows for users to not only share particular health information with others, but also pass subjective evaluation on that specific piece of information (i.e. is it worth sharing?). Figure 2 shows the frequency with which public health-related tweets from the sample were retweeted, whereas Table 4 compares absolute and proportionate retweeting frequencies throughout the sectors.

A total of 359 of the 772 public health-related tweets identified were retweeted. NFP accounts had more than two-fifths of their public health-related tweets (176 out of 403, or 43.7%) retweeted

*Figure 2. Retweeting frequency*

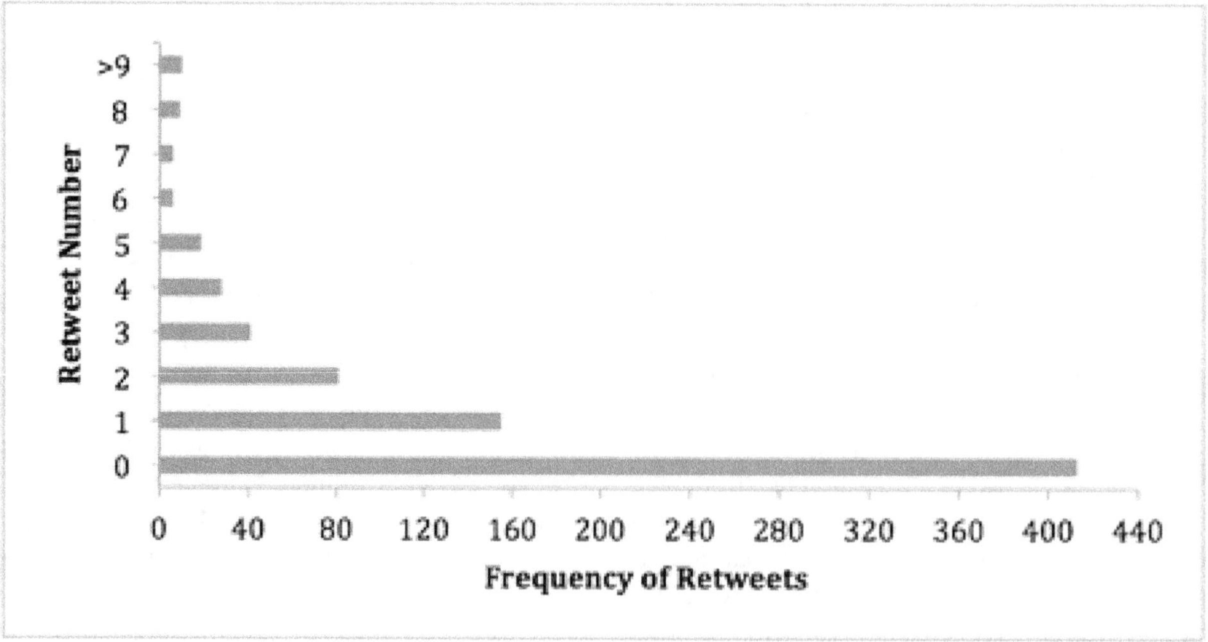

*Table 4. Retweeting frequency between sectors*

| | Government | FP | NFP |
|---|---|---|---|
| Number of Public Health Tweets | 143 | 226 | 403 |
| Proportion of Public Health Tweets in Total Sample (% of 3,790) | 3.7% | 6.0% | 10.6% |
| Proportion of Public Health Tweets within Sector | 36.9% | 21.1% | 17.3% |
| Number of Public Health Tweets Retweeted | 99 | 84 | 176 |
| Percentage of Retweeted Public Health Tweets / Number of Public Health Tweets within Sector | 69.2% | 37.2% | 43.7% |

by other users. FP health-related organisations had the smallest raw number (84) as well as the smallest proportion of retweeted public health advice (37.2%) out of all three sectors, considering 226 of their tweets in February 2012 were public health-related. The government health-related Twitter accounts we identified were found to be the most successful in disseminating health information to the public. Of the 143 government posted public health-related tweets identified in February 2012, 99 were retweeted (approximately 70%). In fact, if taking into consideration the number of Twitter accounts per sector, it could be seen that government accounts had recorded on average a higher reach with their public health information (i.e. due to higher retweet rates and the smaller number of accounts found within this sector).

For this study we also considered the level of dissemination, or the "reach", as an absolute measure of: the number of followers that would receive a certain piece of information, as well as the number of followers of an account that would retweet that piece of information. For example, if an account with 1,000 followers tweeted an article on dementia, and this article was retweeted four times by different accounts, then the reach of this information would be 1,000 plus the sum of followers of the four retweeting accounts (overlap between the followers of accounts not considered).

Table 5 outlines the number of users reached by retweeted public health tweets in our sample. As can be seen, NFP accounts had a larger total reach (283,302) when compared with government (241,320) and FP (223,444) accounts. When taking into account the average reach per account however, it can be seen that retweeted tweets of NFP accounts actually reached approximately three times less users per account (6,555) than both government (20,110) and FP accounts (17,188). Furthermore, when looking at the average number of users reached per retweeted public health-related tweet, it could be seen that FP accounts had a higher number of average users reached per tweet (2,725) with government accounts at the next highest (2,462) and NFP accounts having approximately 1,000 less average users reached per tweet than both the other two sectors at 1,610.

One of the issues found however was that there were a few retweeting accounts with an exceptionally high number of followers that could

*Table 5. Followers reached by retweeted public health tweets*

| | Government | FP | NFP |
|---|---|---|---|
| Total Reach | 241,320 | 223,444 | 283,302 |
| Average Reach per Account | 20,110 | 17,188 | 6,555 |
| Average Reach per Tweet | 2,462 | 2,725 | 1,610 |

impact overall calculations of reach (i.e. outliers). For example, the Twitter account "Dr. Karl" had 147,971 followers at the time of data collection, and even though the account had only retweeted one tweet from a FP account, this increased the reach (total, average per account and average per tweet) of FP accounts by approximately three-fold (as shown in Table 6). Therefore it can be seen how outliers can have a significant impact, as one user with many followers can influence how many users will receive the tweet and the corresponding information presented in this tweet. This also raises the aspect of social media-based information dissemination being influenced by a small set of high-follower accounts and the implications of this for strategies to effectively and widely disseminate public health information via social media.

Table 7 represents the categorisation of accounts that had disseminated any of the 359 retweeted public health advice tweets. Government accounts did the least retweeting of public health advice tweets when compared to other account types with only 44 of the 890 (or 4.9%) retweeting accounts from the government sector. In addition, more than half of the retweets made by government accounts (23) were actually of public health tweets from other health-related government Twitter accounts identified. These numbers show how government accounts have low retweet numbers (potentially due to selectiveness), which may be because they tend to retweet information from other government bodies rather than information from other sectors.

On the other hand, accounts that represented various individual users (i.e. not organisation-based bodies) recorded the highest proportion of the 890 retweeting accounts; with 561 or 63.0% of identified public health information retweets being from individual users. FP organisations had the second highest amount of retweeting activity by organisations at 125 identified accounts, and NFP accounts had retweeted public health tweets only 88 times. The remaining 72 retweeting accounts were ambiguous as to whether they were associated with organisations or individuals, and hence were classified as 'other'. These numbers are interesting, as they show low activity of

*Table 6. Followers reached by retweeted tweets (minus outliers)*

| | FP | FP (Minus Outliers) |
|---|---|---|
| Total Reach | 223,444 | 75,473 |
| Average Reach per Account | 17,188 | 5,806 |
| Average Reach per Tweet | 2,725 | 932 |

*Table 7. Retweeting accounts*

| | Government Tweets | FP Tweets | NFP Tweets | Total |
|---|---|---|---|---|
| **Retweeting Accounts** | | | | |
| Government | 23 | 3 | 18 | 44 |
| FP | 38 | 26 | 61 | 125 |
| NFP | 29 | 4 | 55 | 88 |
| Individual | 146 | 104 | 311 | 561 |
| Other | 23 | 11 | 38 | 72 |
| Total | 259 | 148 | 483 | 890 |

government Twitter accounts when it comes to retweeting public health advice – but illustrate higher proportions of interaction by individual users who disseminate organisation-generated health information.

Table 8 outlines the differences between the number of links (URLs) present in public health-related retweeted and non-retweeted tweets. Government accounts had links present in all their retweeted tweets, however this proportion dropped to 87% when considering the links present in non-retweeted tweets. To a lesser extent, this was also found in NFP organisations, with only a 6.9% difference in link presence when comparing retweeted and non-retweeted public health tweets. FP organisation had links present in every one of their public health-related tweets (both retweeted and non-retweeted). It is also interesting to note that the amount of links present in public health-related tweets is two to three times greater than found in non health-related datasets in previous studies (Poblete, Garcia, Mendoza & Jaimes, 2011).

The authoritativeness of online documents can be quantified to some extent by the Google PageRank function, which is an algorithm that calculates the importance of Web pages by considering both the number of incoming hyperlinks and the importance of the pages from which they are coming from. As can be seen in Table 9, the PageRank of public health-related tweets by Government accounts for both linked-to and the site home Web pages of linked-to pages are the highest when compared to those of FP and NFP organisations. The average PageRank of site home pages of linked-to pages from Government and NFP organisations were similar (6.8 vs. 6.3); with the average of site home Web page PageRank of public health-related FP tweets being the lowest of the three sectors (5.1). FP accounts actually had the lowest average overall PageRank counts of the three sectors, especially when looking at the average PageRank number of their linked-to Web pages (1.5). This may mean that FP organisations tweet links to pages that have generally less authoritative information than government and NFP organisations, and hence may explain why lower proportions of public health tweets are retweeted and to less users (Table 4 & 6). In addition it should be noted that even though FP accounts have links in 100% of their tweets (Table 8), with regards to public health information, this linked-to information is less authoritative than other sectors.

## IMPLICATIONS

Our work found that the information being tweeted by health organisations was largely health-related, with only one-fifth of the data mined categorised as non health-related. On the contrary to the findings by Omurtag et al. (2012), the types of information provided by the sample of organisations identified throughout Twitter were minimally advertising or 'irrelevant chatter'. With regards to influence, it was seen in our sample that government accounts were most influential as they had not only on average more followers, but also more reach (when removing outliers). This also highlights the impact of individuals with large followings on SNSs, as well as the growing role

*Table 8. Percentage of links present in tweets*

| | Government | FP | NFP |
|---|---|---|---|
| Retweeted | 100% | 100% | 91.9% |
| Non-retweeted | 87.0% | 100% | 85.0% |

*Table 9. PageRank of public health tweet web-links by sector*

| | Government | FP | NFP |
|---|---|---|---|
| PageRank of Linked-to Web Page | 4.5 | 1.5 | 4.1 |
| PageRank of Site Home Page of Linked-to Web Page | 6.8 | 5.1 | 6.3 |

of the public in the dissemination and propagation of health information. As the population of online users grows, this also presents a further consideration in relation to privacy issues via the use of this medium for the retrieving and sharing of health information.

There are a number of implications for both government and private health organisations. In relation to government health services that generate online information, this work demonstrates areas where further micro-blog dissemination could occur (e.g. the four underrepresented NHPAs and general Indigenous health). Government organisations could utilise the availability of SNSs to further fill these gaps for health information. In addition, due to the influential and authoritative aspects of government accounts and Web documents, they can be harnessed more so as to act as powerful communicators of high quality health information. The policy implications that arise due to these possible changes will involve actions, such as the reassessment of online responsibilities, quality filters and privacy controls for all entities involved. This is also important due to the greater involvement of the public in public health information dissemination, as appropriate policy procedures would potentially lead to greater community awareness and engagement in the use of SNSs for health information.

In relation to NFP health organisations, the usage for fundraising was demonstrated with our results. The use of SNSs for these purposes would not only be an additional method of raising funds through a more targeted and engaged audience, but also a more cost-effective approach for these organizations. Private health practices can also potentially increase community engagement by mirroring government account strategies, such as disseminating more important (or authoritative) Web documents. Our results also show that the presence of URLs in health-related tweets generally resulted in higher levels of dissemination than tweets without URLs. Health companies and organisations that want to increase their information reach can use this for potential future strategies for effective social media-based dissemination.

This work is also a step towards the further understanding of dissemination for the development of software tools and applications (Steele & Lo, 2009) to improve or optimize the coverage and targeting of public health information sharing and dissemination across a community, nationally or internationally.

## LIMITATIONS

The limitations of such a study come from potential issues in sampling and analysis of Twitter accounts and tweets. Whilst manual methods were utilised to identify relevant accounts according to criteria, some organisation accounts may have been missed. Although our sample is substantive, we cannot claim to have an absolute representation of all Australian health-related bodies and organisations on Twitter, due to the limitations of the search functions themselves. As mentioned in previous sections, there is also a potential risk of bias when collecting tweets over a specific time period when certain health-related campaigns are occurring, thus increasing the prevalence of information related to this area and potentially skewing results. There is also the issue of verification of specific accounts on Twitter, as anybody in the world can create a Twitter account under an available name. Thus other third parties could potentially misrepresent organisations and government bodies that are not verified on Twitter, although this would have been detected during the identification of accounts in our study.

A difficulty in the categorisation of specific health areas was the complexity and factors of various conditions that could relate to more than one category. For example, tweets pertaining to the aged were generally categorized instead under the specific condition they related to (if they were about a specific condition). As shown in Table 2, there were a small proportion of aged-related tweets that were generically health-related (0.5% are classified under 'elderly'). However when taking into account specific categories that may be affected by age (i.e. chronic conditions such as osteoporosis and some cancers) it can be seen that the overall proportion of age-relevant tweets would be substantially higher. Nevertheless, there had to be a distinction within the categorisation process, whereby the information contained in the tweet was categorised according to whether the emphasise was semantically addressing the ageing population, or whether information was provided about the condition in general.

## CONCLUSION

This chapter describes and analyses the Twitter activity of various Australian-based health-related organisation accounts during the month of February 2012. Specific criteria were utilised to identify and include active accounts that represented government, FP and NFP accounts based in Australia. The analysis and categorisation of tweets was carried out in two dimensions, and these were health condition and the type of information that was being tweeted. Further analysis was carried out on the specific sub-sample of public health advice tweets. The analysis in this chapter provides a step to understanding the overall dissemination by health organisations in the Australian context of health information via Twitter.

Future research may examine and analyse further aspects of health information dissemination via social media such as: whether relevant health messages reach the relevant target groups; the number and frequency of such messages; and the nature of dissemination and sharing of these messages by participating members. These issues can be explored throughout various population groups, such as looking at Australia as well as international comparisons to uncover similarities and differences.

## ACKNOWLEDGMENT

The authors would like to thank the anonymous reviewers and the editor for their insightful comments and suggestions.

## REFERENCES

Australian Institute of Health and Welfare. (2013). In National Health Priority Areas. Retrieved May 1, 2013, from http://www.aihw.gov.au/national-health-priority-areas/

Bian, J., Topaloglu, U., & Yu, F. (2012). Towards large-scale twitter mining for drug-related adverse events. In *Proceedings of the International Workshop on Smart Health and Wellbeing*, (pp. 25-32). Hawaii, HI: IEEE. doi:10.1145/2389707.2389713

Cha, M., Haddadi, H., Benevenuto, F., & Gummandi, K. P. (2010). Measuring User Influence in Twitter: The Million Follower Fallacy. In *Proceedings of the 4th International AAAI Conference on Weblogs and Social Media (ICWSM)*, (pp. 10-17). Washington, DC: ICWSM. doi:10.1.1.167.192

Dumbrell, D., & Steele, R. (2012). What are the Characteristics of Highly Disseminated Public Health-related Tweets? In *Proceedings of the 24th Australian Computer-Human Interaction Conference*, (pp. 115-118). Melbourne, Australia: IEEE.

Dumbrell, D., & Steele, R. (2013). Twitter and Health in the Australian Context: What Type of Information are Health-related Organisations Tweeting?. In *Proceedings of the 46th Hawaii International Conference on System Sciences*, (pp. 2666-2675). Hawaii, HI: IEEE.

Heaivilin, N., Gerbert, B., Page, J. E., & Gibbs, J. L. (2011). Public Health Surveillance of Dental Pain via Twitter. *Journal of Dental Research*, *90*(9), 1047–1051. doi:10.1177/0022034511415273 PMID:21768306

Kwak, H., Lee, C., Park, H., & Moon, S. (2010). What is Twitter, a Social Network or a News Media? In *Proceedings of the 19th International Conference on World Wide Web*, (pp. 591-600). Academic Press.

Mcneil, K., Gordon, P. M., & Brna, K. E. (2012). Epilepsy in the Twitter Era: A Need to Re-tweet the Way we Think about Seizures. *Epilepsy & Behavior*, *23*(2), 127–130. doi:10.1016/j.yebeh.2011.10.020 PMID:22134096

Omurtag, K., Jimenez, P. T., Ratts, V., Odem, R., & Cooper, A. R. (2012). The ART of Social Networking: how SART Member Clinics are Connecting with Patients Online. *Fertility and Sterility*, *97*(1), 88–94. doi:10.1016/j.fertnstert.2011.10.001 PMID:22088209

Poblete, B., Garcia, R., Mendoza, G.M. & Jaimes, A. (2011). Do All Birds Tweet the Same? Characterizing Twitter Around the World. In *Proceedings of the 20th ACM International Conference on Information and Knowledge Management*, (pp. 1025-1030). New York, NY: ACM.

Prochaska, J. J., Pechmann, C., Kim, R., & Leonhardt, J. M. (2011). Twitter=Quitter? An Analysis of Twitter Quit Smoking Social Networks. *Tobacco Control*, *21*(4), 447–449. doi:10.1136/tc.2010.042507 PMID:21730101

Sillence, E., Briggs, P., Fishwick, L., & Harris, P. (2004). Trust and Mistrust of Online Health Sites. In *Proceedings of the SIGCHI Conference on Human Factors In Computing Systems*, (pp. 663-670). New York, NY: ACM.

SocialMediaNews.com.au. (2014). Social Media Statistics Australia – December 2013. In *December 2013 Statistics*. Retrieved January 13, 2014, from http://www.socialmedianews.com.au/social-media-statistics-australia-december-2013/

Steele, R. (2011). Social media, mobile devices and sensors: categorizing new techniques for health communication. In *Proceedings of the 5th International Conference on Sensing Technology*, (pp. 187-192). Palmerston North, New Zealand: IEEE.

Steele, R., & Lo, A. (2009). Future personal health records as a foundation for computational health. In Proceedings of Computational Science and Its Applications – ICCSA 2009 (pp. 719-733). Springer.

Sullivan, S. J., Schneiders, A. G., Cheang, C., Kitto, E., Lee, H., & Redhead, J. et al. (2012). 'What's Happening?' A Content Analysis of Concussion-related Traffic on Twitter. *British Journal of Sports Medicine*, *46*(4), 258–263. doi:10.1136/bjsm.2010.080341 PMID:21406451

Thackeray, R., Neiger, B. L., Smith, A. K., & Van Wagenen, S. B. (2012). Adoption and use of social media among public health departments. *BMC Public Health*, *12*(1), 242. doi:10.1186/1471-2458-12-242 PMID:22449137

## KEY TERMS AND DEFINITIONS

**Micro-Blog:** A system with a blog-like nature, where incremental updates are provided over time, but for which the text updates are typically shorter.

**PageRank:** An algorithm introduced by Google that provides a search query-independent quantitative measure of a Web page's 'authority'.

**Public Health Campaign:** A type of media campaign where information which can include educational material is communicated to a population or sub-population to positively affect health behaviours, awareness or preventative actions.

**Social Networking Service (SNS):** A (typically online) service that allows the representation of an individual's profile information and the capturing of the links between individuals and their respective profiles.

**Tweeting:** The act of sending a micro-blog post (limited to 140 characters) within the Twitter system.

**Twitter:** A widely used micro-blogging application.

**Twittersphere:** The overall set of postings and communications within the Twitter micro-blog system.

# Chapter 2
# Informatics in Social Services: Research, Developments, and Outcomes from the Finnish Perspective

**Sirpa Kuusisto-Niemi**
*University of Eastern Finland, Finland*

**Kaija Saranto**
*University of Eastern Finland, Finland*

**Sari Rissanen**
*University of Eastern Finland, Finland*

## ABSTRACT

*The aim of the chapter is to describe and analyse the conception of ICTs for social services on the basis of previous international and national research and a case study of Finnish experiences. The authors describe the concept of ICTs for social services and identify the main areas of interest and research findings in relation to the paradigm of social services informatics. The data for this part was collected by an integrated literature review of ICT research. Next, the authors review and evaluate the development phases of Finnish social services informatics. On the basis of national and international literature, they compare the similarities and distinguishing elements in the evolution of social care ICT in research and practice. On the basis of these findings on the main issues, challenges, opportunities, and trends, some recommendations for future research as well as for working practices are briefly described.*

## INTRODUCTION

The impact of new technology on public-sector service delivery has long been debated by different actors in the Western countries. In particular, political and managerial actors have often mentioned the ICT for public services as a tool for improving the efficiency and quality of services.

DOI: 10.4018/978-1-4666-6316-9.ch002

The European Union has released policy programmes for ICT use since the 1990`s (Growth, Competitiveness, Employment, The Challenge and Ways forward into The 21st Century, 1993), and still promotion of information society is one of the EU's key areas (see, e.g., http://ec.europa.eu/digital-agenda/). The massive research interest in ITC has mainly focused on creating strategies, action plans and projects for health services (Hämäläinen et al., 2008; for Europe, see e.g. https://ec.europa.eu/digital-agenda/en/life-and-work/ehealth-and-ageing), and an influential actor in the field, the International Medical Informatics Association (IMIA, 2014) network has supported the knowledge creation. However, the focus of development has in some instances been on social services ICT (Australian Institute of Health and Welfare, 2005; The Department of Health, 2003), and we consider it a great challenge to combine the social services and health care information domains in the future for the best of people in need of services.

Social services as well as ICT are problematic concepts when conceptualising the overview of ICTs for social services. The concepts social services, social care, social work or broader concepts, such as human services or welfare services, are partly connected to each other. For instance, when comparing different welfare models or regimes, comparative social policy research has used the concepts social services (Kautto, 2002), social care services (Anttonen & Sipilä, 1996) or welfare services (Jensen, 2008), covering partly the same and partly different services. This has affected the research results, and Jensen (2008), for instance, has stated that the production of different welfare services varies and these differences should be taken into account when comparing welfare models. According to this, we adopt social services as a broad concept for the starting point of our chapter. In this sense, these services can include help and services of different kinds for different citizen groups provided by public, private or voluntary organizations. The definition covers both services provided by the public administration and those purchased from business and the third sector.

Even though ICT issues have been extensively discussed, in connection with such areas as child welfare (e.g., Gillingham, 2011; Naccarato, 2010; Tregeagle & Darcy, 2008), mental health (Kapp & Stipp, 2010) and the aged (Blaschke et al., 2009), to name a few, there exist very few proper definitions of what is actually included in social services ICT. The relation of social work and ICT has also been studied in several instances, such as from the viewpoint of social work education (Ahmedani et al., 2011; Burgess, 2004; Fitch, 2005; Youn, 2007), employee attitudes towards ICT (Barcy & Barcy, 2008; Carrilio, 2007), web-based counselling (Mishna et al., 2012; Murphy et al., 2009), online social work (LaMendola, 2010) or Internet advocacy (McNutt, 2000; Moon & DeWeaver, 2005), but even here the definition of ICT is quite labile. During the last few years, the focus of definitions has moved to social work informatics, even though some attempts to describe this area almost beyond reach have been made earlier: Grebel and Steyaert (1995) write about social informatics in the context of social work and education, and Garret (2005) describes the electronic turn in social work, meaning the influence of ICT on work practices, but also pointing out its possibly negative influence on clients' rights.

Parker-Demiris and Oliver have defined social work informatics as a combination of computer science, information science and social work, designed to assist in the management and processing of data, information, and knowledge to support social work practice (Parker-Oliver & Demiris, 2006). This definition looks for models in the definition of nursing informatics, which has the same main elements when defined from the viewpoint of the discipline. It includes computer science, information science and nursing science, and is designed to assist in the management and processing of nursing data, information and knowledge to support the practice and delivery of nursing (Graves & Corcoran 1989). When defined from the viewpoint of professional roles, the definitions highlight the speciality of profession (e.g., American Nurses Association, 2008), and when information technology is highlighted, the focus is on handling, modelling and communicating information through technology (Saba & McCormick, 2002). Naccarato (2010) and Ngyuen (2007) have developed the social work informatics definition further in the context of child welfare informatics, which they specify as a subspecialty in social work, integrating child welfare, computer science and information science to manage and communicate data, information and knowledge in practice in a multi-agent setting. Naccarato (2010) adds information structures, processes and technology to the definition.

Here, we follow loosely the definition of Parker-Oliver and Demiris (2006) and understand social services ICT as the planning, managing, execution and control of information resources in the organization. These elements comprise the substantial and technical entity for ensuring the needs of data, information and knowledge collection specific to social services to satisfy the requirements for the processing of data and information essential for the ethical carrying out of service actions. As the actors in the field, we include both practitioners, clients, management as well as policy-level decision-makers, whose input in ICT development depends on the professional, managerial, financial and technical resources available.

In spite of the above definitions for the main concepts of our chapter, the following factors can be identified as the justification for this chapter. Firstly, the positive future development of practices or research concerning ICT for social services needs research-based information on previous development. When the body of literature develops, it is important to make an inventory of the work done and to identify potential new directions for research. The practical or research history of ICT for social services is not very long, but since it is a very development-intensive branch, there already exists increasingly material for an inventory.

Secondly, it is widely agreed that the best development of actions of different kinds depends on the dialectics between practice and research. This means both the co-operation of different actors (e.g., software developers, researchers and ICT users) and the simultaneous understanding of development practices, as well as of the content of research in the area of ICT for social services. This way of thinking will be summarised more thoroughly in the next section, where the paradigm of health and human services informatics is described, but even this brief justification shows why we have combined previous research in order to analyse one concrete example of ICT development process in one country. Since the 1960s there has been an ongoing development of ICT in social services in Finland, which provides good material for analysis.

Thirdly, ICT for social service continues to face many ethical and educational challenges. For instance, the suitability of ICT for specific social services or service targets is still under debate (Garrett, 2005; Gillingham, 2011). It has also been stated that social services clients have limited possibilities to participate in information collection and interpretation (Askeland & Payne, 1999). For the social services professional, this entails the requirement that they should use ICT and act in the spirit of advocacy for the client (Keegan Eamon et al., 2013; McNutt, 2000). In addition, the need for education in ICT for social services is enormous. This concerns both the professionals' attitudes towards ICT and its concrete use in the workplace (Barcy & Barcy, 2008), as well as data protection and security issues (Congress, 2013; Hayes & Devaney, 2004). In short, the teaching curricula need to be updated for a better understanding of the state of the art in both practise, research and development processes (Fitch, 2005). In the future, on the other hand, there will be less need to focus on the basic ICT skills of future social workers, as they will have been using ICT from their youngest years onwards (Ahmedani et al., 2011).

Based on these arguments, the specific aims of this chapter are 1) to provide an overview of previous research into ICT for social services 2) to describe the national development process of ICT for social services and 3) to combine these results in the form of recommendations for future research as well as for working practices. We will concentrate on organizational issues as our standpoint. In carrying out the review we have taken account of both national strategy and the perspective of the discipline, both of which are essential in the Finnish social services ICT domain.

## PARADIGM OF HEALTH AND HUMAN SERVICES INFORMATICS

The concept of health and human services informatics summarizes our current understanding of the most relevant orientation for research, education and development within ICT for social services as an applied discipline. From the viewpoint of the discipline and its education, social services ICT utilizes systems theory, information systems science and computer science, information science and general social sciences, such as sociology and management science. Methodologically, evaluation research and socio-technical research, together with activity theory research, are considered the most useful instruments. Both clients, carers and professionals are regarded as sources and users of information (Kuusisto-Niemi & Saranto, 2008).

For our study we adopt the concept of paradigm. According to philosopher Thomas S. Kuhn (1970), a paradigm manifests the focal phenomena of the discipline to be observed and researched and the focal research subjects and issues related to it. It also shows how to pose research questions and how to interpret research findings. The paradigm of informatics research (see Figure 1.) with its four basic entities: actors, action, value chain of information, and technology linking these entities, form a sound and interesting, but also a challenging basis for an analysis of how the research has developed. Actors represent persons or communities producing or using services. The value chain of information is understood as a continuum from

*Figure 1. The paradigm of health and human services informatics. Main concepts and research focus.*

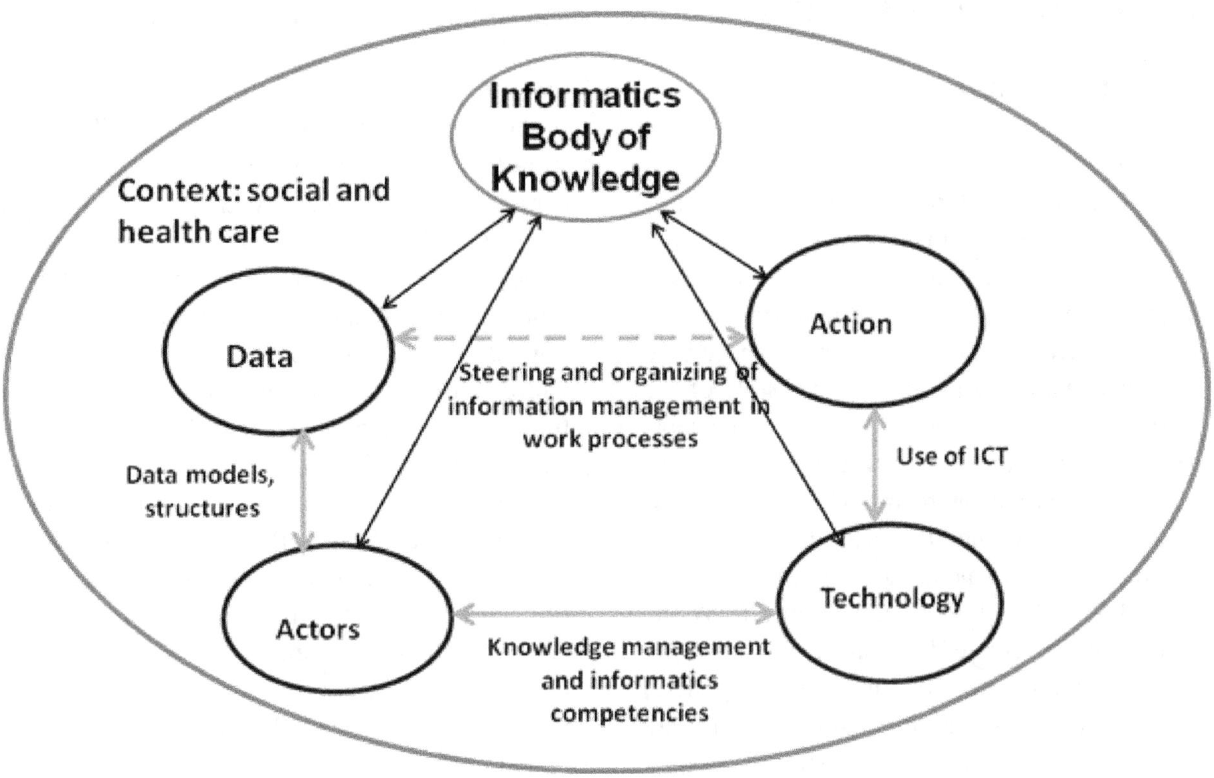

data to wisdom, where complexity and networking increase in the direction of a more highly processed form of information. Action comprises the planning, implementation, use and evaluation of services, and technology stands for the technical and social methods for assessing, using, storing and communicating the information generated in the services (Kuusisto-Niemi & Saranto, 2009; Saranto & Kuusisto-Niemi 2012).

Besides entities, informatics research focuses on the relations between them. Combining the value chain of information with action produces research on information management in service processes. Research on action and technology generates evaluation and development research on ICT. Combining technology and actors generates research on knowledge management, and combining actors and the value chain of information results in development in the body of knowledge (Kuusisto-Niemi & Saranto, 2009; Saranto & Kuusisto-Niemi 2012).

## INTERNATIONAL RESEARCH

### Data and Methods

We have adopted an integrated literature review as the method for the international part of the study. It is a form of research that reviews, critiques, and synthesizes representative literature on a topic in an integrated way, generating new frameworks and perspectives on the topic. The purpose is to trace systematically as much as possible of the literature on the selected topic back to its roots (Hart, 2003).). An integrated review is the most extensive of the various forms of literature review, as it allows the combining of studies employing different research methods in a single review. According to Whittemore and Knalf (2005), the purpose of an integrated literature review is to bring together existing research and present a general summary of many individual studies which are considered to focus on similar or identical research problem formulations. In a situation where the body of literature is in a phase of development, we consider this to be a tenable method for our purposes.

The first literature search was conducted 27 April – 4 May 2011 and the second search 31 January – 10 February 2014 in databases available at the library of the University of Eastern Finland (UEF), with the keywords *social services organization, ICT, information technology, research, education, social work* and *social welfare* and their combinations. The keywords were chosen to reflect both the aim of this article and the entities in the informatics paradigm and their interconnections. The inquiries identified a total of 2,067 citations in the following databases: Arts & Humanities Citation Index (1991–2011), JSTOR Arts & Sciences I Collection (1928–2005), Science Direct (2009–2010), Social Sciences Citation Index (1994-2010), Social Services Abstracts (1979-2010) and Sociological Abstracts (1990-2010). Of these, a total of 724 hits were reviewed by reading the abstracts. The detailed examination of titles and abstracts identified 197 hits specifically addressing the structural issues of the article. After the duplicates were removed, the total number of abstracts was 97. Out of these, 87 full articles were found in the library database, and a further examination of articles, with the exclusion of general policy level papers other than social policy or social services and articles written in other languages than English, produced the final number of 61 articles to be studied for the results and discussion sections of this chapter. Out of these, 26 came from the United Kingdom and 24 from the United States.

The remaining 61 international articles were classified on the basis of the paradigm entities and angles. This division is based on a close reading of the articles and the main issues of the authors discovered in the reading, but the judgement lies entirely with the authors of this chapter. The purpose of the close reading was to illustrate the aptness of paradigmatic thinking and to provide ideas for the further development of paradigm debate. The numbers presented do not match the number of the articles, because one article might contain several themes or ideas presented here.

The limitations of the sample are obvious. Only a part of the vast social services ICT literature can be reached through the UEF library database. In addition in spite of a meticulous search strategy, it is possible that some important publications were overlooked because of the limited key words employed, or misreading abstracts during the sifting process. Grey literature, e.g. reports, was also excluded from the international part of the study. We have taken this into consideration in formulating the results.

The second data set, concerning the Finnish case study, includes development and research project reports, educational articles and legislative documents, mainly in Finnish. These documents were chosen by what is called *utilizing reading,* a term introduced by Luostarinen and Väliverronen (1991) to profile a researcher's proceeding from the hints in known sources of information that lead to new areas of knowledge. This method of data gathering may be likened with what is called snowball sampling, in which one interviewee points to the next one. Using this method requires a fair amount of advance knowledge on the subject. The authors have a long practical experience of social and health care, administration, education and research, which allows data to be gathered with this method. In total, this material includes 20 administrative or non-research reports, excluding legislation, and 5 research reports or articles. For the case study, the most significant milestones of development in 1960–2014 were analysed from four perspectives, which were legislation, project activities, education and research. Content analysis was used as the method for analysing the main content of articles. As Hart (2003) points out, when the focus of interest is language, language as communication and the content of communication, content analysis is the appropriate method, allowing a systematic and objective analysis of documents. This article makes use of deductive content analysis (Miles & Huberman, 1994); in other words, the content analysis is based on entities and their interrelations in the informatics paradigm.

## OVERALL RESULTS OF LITERATURE REVIEW

To clarify the set of themes under each paradigm angle, we present examples of research and educational interests in the following. Concerning the steering and organizing of information management in work processes, the main phenomena of interest are information needs, flow of information and its outcomes. In teaching and researching the use of ICT, we concentrate on information systems and their implementation, in digital services, usability, data security and networks, which form the basic structure of ICT. Knowledge management and information competences also include decision making on all organizational levels. The data is understood as structures of concepts, the forming of classifications, data models and ontologies on a theoretical basis. This angle also includes such actions as standardization and data warehousing, which can be studied on their own, with a low dependency on the everyday life of organizations. Social and health care constitutes the operational environment, where clients, practitioners, administrators and politicians meet. In this structure, ICT is considered a necessary, but not sufficient condition for actions, though ICT simultaneously changes the social milieu of social services (West & Heath, 2011).

To a great extent, the major groups of people in need of social services were covered in this sample. Children as a client group were represented in 23 articles and elderly people in four articles, while clients of mental health services, unemployed people or other needy persons were only discussed in three or four articles. This reflects the emphasis and nature of social services in general. The major focus in this sample is in support to child custody decisions and risk assessment needs, and the primary emphasis was on general and child welfare social work – 32 articles compared to 11 articles focusing primarily on social services ICT.

In relation to the overall paradigm, the largest sample consisted of 23 ICT policy articles. The theme was either presented alone or included in a case study. In these articles, several themes are studied. In the following, we have divided them into four discourses.

The first interesting discourse concerns the administrative or managerial use of ICT. The literature creates a critical picture of ICT development projects and their success. According to Hall et al. (2010), Ince & Griffiths (2011), Pithouse et al. (2012), Shaw et al. (2009) and White et al. (2010), who draw on experiences from UK government programmes for ICT development projects in social care for children, it seems obvious that professional practices are subordinated to the logic of computer systems. Henman and Adler (2003) show in their comparative study on the computerisation of social security systems in 13 OECD countries how information technology has increased management control over personnel and claimants rather than empowered them. The managerial paradigm for public services does not respect professional practice and, at the same time, endangers the work processes, the motivation of professionals and client contacts. As a solution, White et al. (2010) suggest a socio-technical systems design with user participation and optimisation of local autonomy; Jang (2013), too, considers the socio-technical angle to be an important one for developing knowledge management in an organisation.

Secondly, from the client's viewpoint, the threat of a digital divide in its different forms is discussed. Hardey and Loader (2009; also Loader et al., 2008) present that while informatisation may have facilitated the integration of services, older people as inexperienced users of ICT may have been marginalised as participants of increasingly information-led services. The same concerns other disadvantaged groups, such as people with low income or new immigrants (Wong et al., 2009). There is also a demand that social workers should defend the information-deprived clients against the digital divide (Keegan Eamon et al., 2013; Steyaert & Gould, 2009).

The third discourse relates to the position of social workers, both in their attitudes or resistance towards the taking up of ICT (Tregeagle & Darcy, 2008), or the concern about their capacity to make their opinion heard in developing software and other tools for daily use (e.g., Gillingham, 2011; Monnickendam et al., 2004; Parton, 2009). It is also argued that there is a lack of an information-driven culture in the public services in general (Kerslake, 1998; Shah, 2012). Ferguson (2008) describes the liquid nature social work and wonders how the work practices cope with the ever-moving socio-technical changes in society, when the welfare practices are solid and stable.

The fourth theme can be called the impacts of strategy and policy on social services ICT (Berman et al., 1995; McNutt, 1996; West & Heath, 2011), or the tools for collecting and upgrading information (Aarons, 2011; Kum et al., 2009; Pleace, 2011), even though the theme is rather dispersed. Classification and standardization of information involves the danger that both people and instances are simplified (Gillingham, 2011). The concern for the clients' possibility of influencing data collection and aggregation and the complexity of describing any marginalized group have to be taken into account when creating managerial data (Pleace, 2011). Evidence-based practices and self-evaluation are considered rising phenomena in social services (Aarons et al., 2011; Kum et al., 2009), and this links the discussion to the criticism of managerialism described above. In short, these articles create a rather alarming picture of the supremacy of information management in relation to professional knowledge, with no alternatives to the mainstream development (Keymolen & Broeders, 2013).

## Results in the Framework of the Paradigm

Moving to the paradigm angles, we focus firstly on the angle uniting data and action. *Steering and organizing information management in work processes* was the main theme in eight articles. The discussion advances along two directions. On the other hand, the social worker and her attitudes towards ICT are discussed. When systems are properly designed, data can be properly used in multi-actor settings in child welfare (Gillingham, 2011; Shaw et al., 2009; Webster et al., 2002) or elderly care (Loader et al., 2008). This working method demands special skills for monitoring and analysing data, but also cooperation and collaboration skills. The second direction focuses on administrative and policymaking information needs. It is argued that the system dynamics of social services has to be understood before creating databases to help decision-makers (Hovmand et al., 2007; Pithouse et al., 2012). If the input into system design and the implementation of new technologies are not planned properly, tensions between bureaucratic and professional users of ICT sharpen (Burton et al., 2009). In general, there is a strong concern about professional engagement and action in evaluating and choosing data to create confidence in ICT. The problems of child welfare information systems in Britain (Ince & Griffiths, 2011; Pithouse et al., 2012) and Australia (Gillingham, 2011) also provide a broader view of the problems caused by the adoption of systems copied from industry in operating environments of completely different nature.

The second angle of the paradigm, which connects action to technology, stands for the evaluation and development research of ICT. *Use of information and communication technology* was described in 17 articles. Web technologies are a major discussion theme. The web is used in social work in counselling, therapy, client advocacy and the professional creation, management and use of information, for example. It is needed when constructing virtual communities of practice for sharing tacit knowledge and innovations, a new way of professional development which is taking its first steps. (Cook-Craig & Sabah, 2009; Mishna et al., 2012). Menon and Miller-Gribbs (2002) emphasize the difference between the simple provision of information versus the communication and perception of meaning, which is salient for social work. Using the web, it is possible to optimise the targeting of social services to different client groups, so that traditional face-to-face services can still be maintained despite dwindling resources (Askim et al., 2011). Murphy et al. (2009) compared client satisfaction with either face-to-face or online counselling and found that both are equally satisfying and effective when the counsellors have adequate counselling experience and the necessary technological assistance. The authors encourage social workers to familiarize themselves with online ethics, techniques and approaches. On the other hand, Stillman and McGrath (2008) conclude that ICT is not yet well developed for the social welfare sector needs, and that internal information systems and knowledge management should be the first priority of an organisation before engaging in the latest online trends. Web technologies are widely expected to ease the workload, but in practice they are still little used in advocacy, for example (Edwards & Hoefer, 2011). Freddolino and Han (2011) reassemble the findings and list the following elements necessary for web practice implementation: access to resources and services, technology, costs, training, funds and policy support. LaMendola (2010) requires social workers to expand their copresence from physical to networks, where clients also form associations and socialize. The web is used by increasingly young people, and social work should also observe and adopt some of their ways of using it (Ahmedani et al., 2011).

Another theme on this angle of the paradigm is the discussion of the effect of technology on social work practices. There exists a strong concern that the gathering, sharing and monitoring of information and accounting activities will take on a much greater significance compared to direct contacts with clients, because of the growing importance of ICT (Gillingham, 2012). Parton (2009) asks how the nature of the work is changing with this development. When the work focus moves from direct client contacts to administrative work, the form of knowledge in social work changes, too (ibid.). Drawing on the experience in the UK on ICT projects in child welfare, both White et al. (2010), Parton (2009), Peckover and Hall (2009) and Pithouse et al. (2009) demonstrate the domination of computer ontology over professional ontologies, reasserted by the ignorant attitudes of the administration towards the frustrating everyday experiences of front-line workers.

This sample of articles also includes guidelines on ICT use for practical workers. Professional organizations have not always been eager to accept web-based working methods, but since social workers have adopted these instruments in everyday use, ethical and practical discussion is needed to protect both clients and practitioners alike (Menon & Miller-Gribbs, 2002). Legal issues, data security and anonymity are the main themes discussed in addition to ethics and confidentiality (Keegan Eamon et al., 2013; Judd & Johnston, 2012; LaMendola, 2010; Rock, 1999); the need to include ICT education in social work curriculum is identified (Blaschke et al., 2009), and the tasks for professional organizations are defined (Menon et al., 2002). These recommendations are straightforward and practical, to ensure that the social work profession keeps pace with the new and emergent tools of practice (ibid.; Congress, 2012; Keegan Eamon et al., 2013).

The paradigm angle uniting actors and technology, including *knowledge management and informatics competencies*, the education of social workers and the competences of social work teachers, was studied in 19 articles. A fresh viewpoint is the participation of the elderly to assess their own health and well-being through a low-cost information technology system (Manthorpe et al., 2010). Social workers should also teach the clients to use the web when applying for benefits, which requires the practitioners to be trained first (Keegan Eamon et al., 2013). When the assessment tools are sensibly made and include the necessary social inclusion and citizenship elements, both clients and service providers can utilize the system for personalized feedback for clients and resource needs assessment for the authorities. Kunkel and Yowell (2001) describe collaborative case management, which requires information-based decision-making. The evidence shows that once this model of work is spread more widely, information exchange between professionals becomes more open in the form of electronic teamwork and reporting, for example, which promotes virtual communities of practice (see Cook-Craig & Sabah, 2009). Since the web can also be utilized for social support, another question is whether clients are willing to socialise with social workers in the net, even if they use it for other purposes. In a case study, Finn and Kerman (2004) report that almost half of foster families found web-based communication helpful and unproblematic. They also stress the need to upgrade the practitioners' skills to derive full benefit from the Internet.

The need to use ICT tools is becoming more evident with the rise of evidence based practices. In general, to be widely adopted in practice, these technologies should be integrated into existing referral and other resources and embedded in them (Foster & Stiffman, 2009). On the other hand, cooperation between technology and substance experts or user involvement in planning IT systems is a necessary prerequisite for success (Fitch, 2006; Hall et al., 2010; Wessels et al., 2008). The discussion also contains critical voices promoting practitioner participation. If ICT does not support the work practices and fragments the work to atomised entities, such as clients or work processes, it alienates practitioners from both clients and the service system with its descriptive and interpretive demands for the accurate filling in of forms (Ince & Griffiths, 2011;

Jang, 2012; White et al., 2009). For the workers, one way to manage this is to express resistance against the strict standardization of procedures, which in itself does not lead to positive changes. (Wastell et al., 2010).

Teaching ICT skills requires special competences depending on the area and the aspired level of learning. That is why e-teacher competences have to be defined. They include competences, knowledge, skills and attitudes in areas such as facilitating, supervising, collaborating and ICT guidance (Ahmedani et al., 2011; Larsen et al., 2008), and challenges and benefits have to be clearly identified in each particular educational setting (Huntington & Sudbery, 2005). Existing curricula see the role of technology as an adjunct one, not as an independent practice methodology with its own theoretical base. This is one reason why there exists a gap between skills and needs of communication, and why practice methodologies have fallen behind in the fast-changing societal and practice contexts (Rafferty & Waldman, 2006), and there is evidence that cyber communication has dramatically changed the nature of professional relationships and relationships to clients (Mishna et al., 2012). Perron et al. (2010) remind that the social work curriculum focuses almost exclusively on relationships in the absence of IT mediated exchange, and that the field of social work is at risk of not remaining competitive in the provision of services in a situation where health care technologies grow with speed. They also point out that without proper training, social workers are at risk of delivering poor quality services or facing legal or ethical issues. Social workers should therefore have both ICT competence and literacy (ibid.). To remember the most important point, it is not the medium but the interaction and content that counts (Greig & Skehill, 2008).

The smallest sample, with four articles, relates to *the models and structures*, which unites the entities actors and data. Leung (2009), studying knowledge management in social work, classifies ten types of knowledge on the basis of two differing views on the nature of knowledge. Where the evidence-based trend sees knowledge as a rational product and an independent carrier of information, the opposite view emphasizes the know-how knowledge of the social worker, a processual reasoning and judgement. All types of knowledge have to be taken into account in knowledge management settings (ibid.). Pleace (2011) reviews the aggregation of data derived from monitoring unemployed people from the perspective of UK social policy. When data aggregation is carried out, it is important to realize the constraints of interpretation to avoid a distorted worldview – people are many other things than just workless beings. He points out that the person who objects to such action must also be respected.

Another angle on the most theoretical dimension of the paradigm is related to the value chain of knowledge, to how information is transformed into knowledge. According to Jang (2013), knowledge integration takes place when a social worker integrates the information received into his or her previous personal knowledge capital. Knowledge management, in its turn, is an organization´s capability to support this integration. In social work, knowledge is often informal or difficult to categorize under existing categories, and this is why the most essential factor is a practitioner´s ability to combine personal knowledge with that residing in the organization. Here, technology can only play an assisting role. Pithouse et al. (2011) describe the development of knowledge production by means of the internal discourse of a practice community, which is often also based on tacit knowledge; they say that if the process of designing information systems does not recognize this dimension, the system will not work.

In this literature review, the general emphasis in the articles was on the framework of the paradigm, which is where we place the policy issues. They cover the entire field of informatics, and present the administrative, economic and legislative resources, but also the prerequisites for informatics development. From the viewpoint of the paradigm, the emphasis was on the relations between technology and either actors or action. The paradigm entity data received considerably less attention, which might signify the practical orientation of research: there continues to be less interest in the foundation of knowledge formation than in the concrete output generated by the technologies. This we consider a serious threat for the development of the knowledge base of social services ICT and the entire professional understanding of the influence of ICT in service production.

What is also noteworthy here is that such themes as consent, confidentiality, privacy or data security were almost exclusively presented in connection to social work ethics (e.g., Judd et al., 2012). This is not to undermine the value of ethics, but to point out that in these issues there are several possible standpoints, which are not included in the discussion of practice ethics, but they are closely connected to data protection, organizational and technology arrangements and legislative issues. (e.g., Rock, 1999.) We consider it an important factor in the action–technology dimension.

In general, as regards the paradigm themes and angles, this selection of literature seemed to cover their whole spectrum. Inside the different angles there are many sub-themes described in connection with Figure 1, but not included in this small sample. Theoretically, the articles exploit heavily general system theory and its derivatives (e.g., Ferguson, 2008; Fitch, 2006; Monnickendam, 2004), but interestingly, the theoretical main stress lies on a conceptual discussion (e.g., Leung, 2009; Naccarato, 2010; Nguyen, 2007; Parton, 2009; Steyaert & Gould, 2009). In the case studies, the primary methods used are ethnography and focus groups and other interview methods. The spectrum of both theories, methods and methodologies is wide-ranging (e.g. Gillingham, 2011), as is also suggested by our paradigm definition.

## CASE STUDY RESULTS

Finland has traditionally been included among the Nordic welfare states (e.g., Anttonen & Sipilä, 1996). In Finland, the municipalities have a statutory obligation to arrange health and social services. They can fulfil this duty by either producing services through their own service delivery agencies or purchasing them from other municipalities or from private or third-sector (not-for-profit) providers. On the European level, the countries applying the Nordic welfare state model have most often been the last to increase private social services. Nowadays, for instance, it is estimated that about a quarter of the social services in Finland are provided by private enterprises and third-sector organizations, some for-profit and others non-profit (e.g., THL, 2010). In the 1990s, the Finnish municipalities initiated an extensive merger process of primary health care and social services, which has continued up to the present. Altogether, Finland is an exceptionally decentralised (e.g., Kaarakainen. 2008), perhaps the most decentralised country in the world (e.g., Kokko. 2009) with a strong municipal self-government prescribed in the Constitution, including extensive duties and obligations to provide services (e.g., education, health, social and cultural services) and also the right to levy taxes to cover the costs of service provision.

The size of Finnish municipalities, which numbered 320 at the beginning of 2013, varies from 50 inhabitants to more than 610,000 inhabitants (Väestötietojärjestelmä, 2014), but all of them have the same statutory obligations concerning social services. This has evidently some consequences to current service production and the informatics used. Smaller entities have a narrower variety of services and no need for a more fine-tuned ICT systems in the way of large units, with locally designed services and ICT system development of their own. Moreover, the small units have no qualified ICT personnel of their own, but have to rely on expertise from the central municipal administration, whereas there are well functioning and productive units in the big municipalities. However, currently the political debate focuses on the possibilities to integrate municipalities or at least have broader health and social districts than previously.

Considering the above description of the status of the ICT environment in Finnish social services, Table 1 summarizes the most significant milestones in the development of ICTs for social services in Finland, which will be further described below.

- **Decades of Practical Development:** In the 1960s and 1970s, the development relied on the ICT companies working with public authorities on a practical basis, and only after that have there been research and legislative initiatives on both the national and local levels. Even the terms used in the field reflect the state of the art. Such terms as rationalization, automatic data processing and electronic data processing were in public and professional use (e.g., Jensen, 1978). Developers were interested in the work routines of social departments, and it was supposed that the automation of routine documentation would save the work contribution of several persons in big social departments (ibid.).
- **Decade of National Projects:** The use of ICT in social services processes at the local and national levels gave rise to various research and development activities, starting

*Table 1. Milestones of social services ICT development in Finland*

| Decade | Political Steering and Legislation | Development Project Activities | Education | Research |
|---|---|---|---|---|
| **1960** | | ICT companies working with public authorities on a practical basis | | |
| **1970** | | | | |
| **1980** | Personal Data File Act 1987 | National Working Group for ICT in Social Services 1980–1993 | | |
| **1990** | Finland – towards an information society, A National Outline 1995.<br>Quality of Life, Knowledge and Competitiveness 1998.<br>Personal Data Act 1999.<br>The Macro Pilot Project 1999–2001 | | Continuing education on informatics 1997– | |
| **2000** | National Information Society Strategy 2007–2015<br>Act on the Status and Rights of Social Welfare Clients 2000 | National Project for IT in Social Services 2004–2011 | University of Eastern Finland, Health and Human Services Informatics discipline 2000–<br>University of Lapland, Master´s program in Social Work eCompetence, 2008- | Research Programme for Social Care Informatics 2008 |
| **2010** | Unit for the Operational Management of Health and Welfare Information (OPER) 2011- | Sosiaaliportti.fi web page to collect and organize information on social services ICT research 2010 | | First national edited research anthology on social work ICT 2010 |

in the 1980s. The population data required for the setting up of social services client records was discussed (Korpi, 1985). The first traces of research initiatives can be found in 1980, when the National Working Group for ICT in Social Services was established by several federations of municipalities. It produced progress reports about ICT status and development needs in the municipalities. The primary information was gathered at the beginning of the 1980s (Sosiaalitoimen atk-toimikunta, 1981), followed by a report in 1986 (Sosiaalitoimen atk-toimikunta, 1986). The main purpose was to document the status of ICT in the municipalities and to describe the necessary development and research needs. When the Personal Data File Act came into effect in 1987, it did not cause major concern, but was discussed in a very practical manner, from the legislative point of view (Taimiaho, 1987). This practice of concentrating on the legislative aspects of social service production seems to have remained strong in Finnish debate through the years, judging by a review of professional periodicals.

- **Decade of Innovations:** The 1990s can be considered the most innovative and productive decade up to that point in time. In a report written for software suppliers, it was estimated that software had been produced for all major tasks in the social services which had a sound legislative basis, a large production volume and many administrative and financial transactions. The obverse side was that the software did not support co-operation with necessary partners, e.g., health or social security authorities. Software was designed to serve such large service entities as home care and supplementary benefits, and its main objective was to help in calculating benefits and client fees and accounting. It was also estimated that software development was changing towards multi-task programs with several fairly independent program components, instead of rigid one-task programs. (Lunnas & Kuusisto-Niemi, 1991.)

In 1993, the first report evaluating the importance of defining the core data set in social services was published, but the time was not yet quite ripe for such a big turn. (Sosiaalitoimen atk-toimikunta, 1993). The ICT inquiry was replicated in 1999, and it was directed to municipal social service departments, federations of municipalities, third-sector service providers and software suppliers. It was estimated that software was in use in most social service departments, but its quality varied greatly. The same was true of other actors in the field. Mobile phones and personal computers were gaining ground, but the same type of software for large-volume tasks was still dominant, even though the need to develop information systems able to document several independent tasks was also manifest, in contrast to separate one-task systems. (Iso-Markku & Kurhila, 1999.) A demand for expert systems and management information systems also emerged at the time, and it was concluded that due to the considerable differences in the information needs between municipalities, different types of software would be needed in large units as compared to small units with fewer than 20,000 inhabitants. The large units would need specialized systems for social care, health or education, whereas small units could utilize one and the same system across all services. (Anttiroiko & Kallio, 1999.)

Following European development in utilizing information technology in society, the Government of Finland adopted a national strategy for ICT development in 1995 (Valtiovarainministeriö, 1995). On the basis of this, the Ministry of Social Affairs and Health produced a strategy of ICT utilization in the field of social affairs and health in 1996 (Sosiaali- ja terveysministeriö, 1996). The strategy was followed by two memoranda by the Ministry on seamless chains of care and data security. These actions focused on the strategic development of health care information systems. The following large-scale ITC project, which concerned the entire Satakunta hospital district, had only a modest effect on social services ICT practices (Tenhunen et al., 2006). Nevertheless, ICT had become more visible, even if this was a side effect of the debate on health care information systems.

Another issue crucial to the development of ICTs is the lack of activity concerning documentation in the social services. The Act on the Status and Rights of Social Welfare Clients came into force at the beginning of 2001. It gave the Ministry of Social Affairs and Health the right to regulate documentation practices, but so far the only regulation is based on the vast body of acts and decrees on different social services, which leads to a fragmented picture of the coverage and level of regulation.

- **Decades of National Adoption:** To secure the future of the social welfare sector, a national programme was established at 2003. The goals included safeguarding the availability and quality of social services, the renewal of service structure and activities and the development of personnel qualifications and working conditions in the long run, with a view to preventing social problems (Ministry of Social Affairs and Health, 2011). The web page Sosiaaliportti, the Social Gateway, was also established as a consequence of the national development project. It is designed for social sector professionals, to support them in their daily work, and its goal is to bring together different actors and organizations. It includes, among other things, eConsultancy pages, an eHandbook for Child Welfare, the Handbook on Disability Services, discussion groups, daily news, an online expert directory and web pages for development projects. The pages also contain research, mainly doctoral dissertations and master's theses in social work. (Sosiaaliportti, 2014.)

As part of the project, the Ministry of Social Affairs and Health established a national social services ICT project for the years 2003–2007 and a second phase for the years 2007–2011. With this project, a comprehensive development was initiated. The Finnish Government has developed an architecture framework for governmental organisations and municipal public authorities, based on open international and national specifications for enterprise architecture. The framework consists of four viewpoints: Business Architecture, Data Architecture, Software Architecture and Technology Architecture. The enterprise architecture is planned on three levels for all viewpoints: public management on the top level, domain level (such as social care) and unit level. The goal of the National Project for IT in Social Services was to create architecture specifications for the domain level of social care on all viewpoints. This will help municipal authorities in their efforts of specifying their organisational enterprise architecture. Since 2011, this work has been continued by the Unit for the Operational Management of Health and Welfare Information (OPER) (Sosiaalihuollon tiedonhallinta, 2014).

In the framework of the national ICT project, a survey on ICT research was organized in 2006 (Päykkönen & Pohjola, 2007). According to the survey, the research is for a large part practical and mainly in the form of surveys and reports. This is partly due to the fact that the teaching of informatics is at the moment poorly represented in the curricula of all the six universities teaching social work. The report lists several themes which should be included in the curriculum, and the concern familiar from international literature about the lagging behind of social work is mentioned. In addition, the importance of ICT skills for professionals in working life has been highlighted already earlier (Borgman et al., 2005).

At the moment, there are two master's programmes in social services ICT in Finland. A programme that links social work and ICT education is located at the University of Lapland, and master's and doctoral programmes in Health and Human Services Informatics at the University of Eastern Finland. The latter, which has provided the framework for this article, focuses on social and health care informatics in general. The establishment of the programme in 2000 was an important factor in the development of social services informatics. It is also the only permanent master's degree programme of its kind in Finland. The educational framework is based on the International Medical Informatics Association's recommendations (IMIA Education Recommendations, 2010), modified for Finnish conditions (Kuusisto-Niemi & Saranto, 2008). The programme has received International Medical Informatics Association´s (IMIA) accreditation for years 2012-2017. The combination of social services and health care is unique both nationally and internationally. By the end of 2013, over 120 master's theses and seven doctoral dissertations have been completed in the programme.

In 2009, a Research Programme for Social Care Informatics was established in the framework of the national ICT project. The following four main research themes have been identified. Firstly, it has been recognized that developing and evaluating technologies that support the citizens' needs and continued functioning requires research. Technology makes it easier to locate information which supports wellbeing and enables interactive electronic transactions for several population groups, such as elderly or disabled people. On the other hand, it also generates incredible risks, which must also be inventoried. Secondly, the changing operating environment and new technological applications present challenges to social service professionals. Their ability to utilize ICT is the key issue. So far, this has been very little studied. Research is also needed concerning innovative technology-mediated work methods, the promotion of digital documentation practices and the construction of virtual consultation systems. Thirdly, it is the responsibility of service organizations and management to enable new service concepts, creating flexible services, developing working processes and promoting usability. From the viewpoint of organizations the central elements are data models, system architecture, data management and compatibility of local software, but also privacy protection and data security. Fourthly, the theoretical basis of information management and informatics needs a strong input. Attention should be paid to the special intellectual characteristics of social services. These include, among others, the issue concerning the concept of knowledge and ethics in ICT use in social services. (Sosiaalialan tiedonhallinnan tutkimusohjelma, 2009).

The first research anthology in the field, Social work, knowledge and technology, was published in 2010 in the yearbook series of the Finnish Society of Social Work Research (Pohjola et al., 2010). It brings out the view of people as subjects of knowledge, and the 13 articles discuss both the political, conceptual and technological relations of social work to practice. However, reflecting the current debate on tools for practitioners, the main part of the articles discuss web applications and their use in social work practice.

In general, during the over 40 years studied here, the development has shifted from the practice towards a more rational and organized way of doing things. The initiatives of the central government have been very important in the Finnish context. This has also created wider cooperation and communication between local actors, as they have participated in the national project and so realized that similar problems exist in their specific area of ICT.

## DISCUSSION AND IMPLICATIONS FOR FUTURE RESEARCH AND PRACTICE

In this section, we summarize the lessons learned from the literature review and the case study. Even though the material was analysed in different frameworks, the international literature being reviewed through the paradigm framework and the Finnish literature in a more practical manner, several common features can be distinguished. When examined in the framework of the paradigm, all themes related to practice can be included in it.

It has to be borne in mind that the social services systems in each country are different. As described earlier in this chapter, the Finnish municipalities have a strong role in directing resources to services and supporting activities such as ICT development. The role of the state has mainly been to enact laws, which have had a modest influence on knowledge management. Only at the turn of the 2000s has the state taken a more steady hold of the development of social services ICT. Compared to the international experience, this has been a rather late awakening. A strong state input seems necessary, since small municipal units on their own have a modest influence on ICT development. The debate on the drawbacks of ICT has also been more latent, and such critical tones as are present in British debate are not heard. We consider this, too, to manifest a lack of interest in ICT development. The same concern about the social services lagging behind the development as is present in the British debate is also expressed in Finland. This concern should be taken seriously in research as well as in practice.

Judging by research information, the distribution of wellbeing services is increasingly being mediated by technology (Askim et al., 2011; Shah, 2012) and the practitioners´ technology skills must be improved. This is important, firstly, for information systems used in face-to-face client contacts; practitioners must participate more actively than so far in developing their content, the concepts and classifications used, and the information components and their interrelations. This is because these systems also for the basis for the interactive use of web which is increasing (e.g., Mishna et al., 2012). Resources must be allocated to improve the practitioners´ internet skills; at the same time, principles for working over the web must be formulated. The management of social services is responsible for allocating both time and technical resources and for motivating practitioners to work proactively. In fact, tools already exist: for example, the Social Gateway and similarly organized web forums offer a possibility to develop cooperation between actors in the field. Finland´s experiences from the National Project for IT in Social Services, in which dozens of practitioners took part in addition to their regular work, have shown that it is possible to involve practitioners, as long as the impulse for the activity is strong enough and benefits to practical work can be expected.

Another issue that we cover concerns the capacity of social services personnel to utilize the potential of existing ICT. The software has been designed to serve administrative purposes in the first hand, and this goes for both international and Finnish reality. To develop multi-task software with the modern technology would be the next challenge. Also this requires that the personnel participate in system development, which in turn requires educational inputs to ensure that they are able to formulate requirements for software development. Social workers as the leading professionals should take the responsibility of challenging the present situation. This can only happen through a renewal of social work curricula.

West & Heath (2011) note that the greatest problem from the research viewpoint is the lack of research. On the basis of the results of this article, research primarily focuses on the problems of ICT use, while research on information as a phenomenon and on the principles of gathering it is scant. Yet it is precisely the success of defining information that is crucial for the usability of a system. Analysis of the relationship between knowledge and information would also appear to be scant. Therefore, what is needed is theoretical research independent of systems and their usability, with an analysis that starts out from the basis of knowledge formation.

According to some studies (e.g., Gillingham, 2011), practitioners spend a disproportionate number of their working hours using information systems or solving problems caused by them. However, little research information is available on this, nor is there any follow-up research on the effects of technology use on client work or administrative work in the long run. This is also related to the purpose of use of information systems on the local and national levels and to how variation in the focus on care and control (e.g., Keymolen & Broeders, 2013) can be seen in the demand for documentation. Studying failures in the adoption of information systems, Ince & Griffiths (2011) distinguish a political and a technical viewpoint, and this distinction definitely requires additional research. In the future, the use of time will also be affected by the increased importance of public debate (see, e.g. Keymolen & Broeders, 2013) and the industrialization of service provision (West & Heath, 2011), both of which are mostly just briefly referred to in research so far. Thus, there is a great need for research into information management in social services, and no shortage of perspectives to choose from.

The aim of this article was to describe the kind of international research on social services informatics that exists, the development of Finnish social services informatics and research into it, and to examine these in relation to each other and to use that examination to formulate recommendations to support both research and practice. We are conscious of the limitations with fairly limited literature searches and fairly scant national material that primarily focuses on administration and practice. Nevertheless, we consider that we have succeeded in presenting recommendations for concrete measures for both practical information management and research. In our view, the Finnish paradigm of social work informatics research is applicable when studying the topics just mentioned.

The literature covered in this review came mainly from the United States and the United Kingdom, but it would be important to also collect the experiences of others on the development of social services ICT. The themes discussed in both Finnish and international literature were partly the same as regards research and development, but to ensure a common framework for global cooperation and the development of social services ICT, we consider it important to develop common ICT curricula. The most important lesson learned is that at least in smaller countries, it is vital to collect the development activities under a coherent umbrella, instead of launching several separate projects. The former has now been the way to develop social services ICT in Finland, and we believe this to be the only possible way for other countries of similar size.

## ACKNOWLEDGMENT

The authors would like to thank the anonymous reviewers and the editor for their insightful comments and suggestions.

## REFERENCES

Ahmedani, B. K., Harold, R. D., Fitton, V. A., & Shifflet Gibson, E. D. (2011, October). What Adolescents Can Tell Us: Technology and the Future of Social Work Education. *Social Work Education, 30*(7), 830–846. doi:10.1080/02615479.2010.504767

American Nurses Association. (2008). Nursing informatics: Scope and standards of practice. Author.

Anttiroiko, A. & Kallio, O. (1999). *Johdon tietojärjestelmät kunnallishallinnossa. [Management software in municipal administration]*. Tampere: Tampereen yliopisto.

Anttonen, A., & Sipilä, J. (1996). European Social Care Services: Is It Possible To Identify Models? *Journal of European Social Policy*, *6*(2), 87–100. doi:10.1177/095892879600600201

Askeland, G. A., & Payne, M. (1999). Authors and audiences: towards a sociology of case recording. *European Journal of Social Work*, *2*(1), 55–65. doi:10.1080/13691459908413805

Askim, J., Fimreite, A. L., Moseley, A., & Holm Pedersen, L. (2011). One-stop shops for social welfare: the adaptation of an organizational form in three countries. *Public Administration*, *89*(4), 1451–1468. doi:10.1111/j.1467-9299.2011.01933.x

Australian Institute of Health and Welfare 2005. *National Community Services Information Strategic Plan 2005-09*. Retrieved April 12, 2011, from http://www.aihw.gov.au/publication-detail/?id=6442467798

Barcy, W. R., & Barcy, R. T. (2008). The Relationship of Computer Attitudes to Reported Use and Observed Behavioural Proficiency. *Journal of Technology in Human Services*, *26*(1), 19–44. doi:10.1300/J017v26n01_02

Berman, Y., Eaglestein, A. S., & Phillips, D. (1995). Policy Impact on Information Technology Programming in the Social Services. *Knowledge and Policy*, *8*(1), 23–32. doi:10.1007/BF02698554

Blaschke, C. M., Freddolino, P. P., & Mullen, E. E. (2009). Ageing and Technology: A Review of the Research Literature. *British Journal of Social Work*, *39*(4), 641–656. doi:10.1093/bjsw/bcp025

Borgman, M., Kemppainen, T., Mäntysaari, M., Pohjola, A. & Vuorensyrjä, M. (2005). *Sosiaalialan osaamis-, työvoima- ja koulutustarpeiden ennakointihanke. [Foresight of know-how, workforce and educational needs of social care]*. Helsinki: Sosiaali- ja terveysministeriö.

Burgess, H. (2004). Redesigning the Curriculum for Social Work Education: Complexity, Conformity, Chaos, Creativity, Collaboration? *Social Work Education*, *23*(2), 163–183. doi:10.1080/0261547042000209189

Burton, J., & van den Broek, D. (2009). Accountable and Countable: Information Managements Systems and the Bureaucratization of Social Work. *British Journal of Social Work*, *39*(7), 1326–1342. doi:10.1093/bjsw/bcn027

Carrilio, T. E. (2007). Using Client Information Systems in Practice Settings: Factors Affecting Social Workers´ Use of Information Systems. *Journal of Technology in Human Services*, *25*(4), 41–62. doi:10.1300/J017v25n04_03

Congress, E. P. (2012, Fall). Continuing Education: Lifelong Learning for Social Work Practitioners and Educators. *Journal of Social Work Education*, *48*(3), 397–401. doi:10.5175/JSWE.2012.201200085

Cook-Craig, P. G., & Sabah, Y. (2009). The Role of Virtual Communities of Practice in Supporting Collaborative Learning among Social Workers. *British Journal of Social Work*, *39*(4), 725–739. doi:10.1093/bjsw/bcp048

Department of Health and Aging. (2008). *National E-Health Strategy*. Retrieved May 15, 2011, from http://www.health.gov.au/internet/main/publishing.nsf/content/national+Ehealth+strategy

Edwards, H. R., & Hoefer, R. (2011). Are Social Work Advocacy Groups Using Web 2.0 Effectively? *Journal of Policy Practice*, *9*(3), 220–239.

European Union. (1993). *Growth, Competitiveness, Employment, The Challenge and Ways forward into 21st Century*. Retrieved April 12, 2011, from http://aei.pitt.edu/1139/

Ferguson, H. (2008). Liquid Social Work: Welfare Interventions as Mobile Practices. *British Journal of Social Work*, *38*(3), 561–579. doi:10.1093/bjsw/bcl367

Finn, J., & Kerman, B. (2004). The Use of Online Social Support by Foster Families. *Journal of Family Social Work*, *8*(4), 67–85. doi:10.1300/J039v08n04_04

Fitch, D. (2005). The Diffusion of Information Technology in Human Services: Implications for Social Work Education. *Journal of Teaching in Social Work*, *25*(1/2), 191–204. doi:10.1300/J067v25n01_12

Fitch, D. (2006). Examination of the Child Protective Services Decision-Making Context with Implications for Decision Support System Design. *Journal of Social Service Research*, *32*(4), 117–134. doi:10.1300/J079v32n04_07

Foster, K. A., & Stiffman, A. R. (2009). Child Welfare Workers´ Adoption of Decision Support Technology. *Journal of Technology in Human Services*, *27*(2), 106–126. doi:10.1080/15228830902749039 PMID:20198123

Freddolino, P. P., & Han, A. S. (2011). Direct Service Applications of Videoconferencing Technologies: Case Examples from Korea and the United States. *Journal of Technology in Human Services*, *16*(2/3), 19–33.

Garret, P. M. (2005). Social work's 'electronic turn': notes on the deployment of information and communication technologies in social work with children and families. *Critical Social Policy*, *25*(4), 529–553. doi:10.1177/0261018305057044

Gillingham, P. (2011, September). Computer-based Information Systems and Human Service Organisations: Emerging Problems and Future Possibilities. *Australian Social Work*, *64*(3), 299–312. doi:10.1080/0312407X.2010.524705

Graves, J., & Corcoran, S. (1989). The study of nursing informatics. *Image*, *21*(4), 227–231. PMID:2807330

Grebel, H., & Steyaert, J. (1995). Social Informatics: beyond technology. A research project in schools of social work in the European Community. *International Social Work*, *38*(2), 151–164. doi:10.1177/002087289503800205

Greig, M., & Skehill, C. (2008). Increasing Staff and Student Capacity to Use the Communication Facility in Queen's Online in Order to Support Learning and Teaching on a BSW Programme. *Social Work Education*, *27*(6), 634–646. doi:10.1080/02615470802201705

Hall, C., Parton, N., Peckover, S., & White, S. (2010). Child-Centric Information and Communication Technology (ICT) and the Fragmentation of Child Welfare Practice in England. *Journal of Social Policy*, *39*(3), 393–413. doi:10.1017/S0047279410000012

Hämäläinen, P., Reponen, J., & Winblad, I. (2008). eHealth of Finland. In *Checkpoint 2008*. Jyväskylä: Gummerus. Retrieved February 10, 2014, from http://www.julkari.fi/bitstream/handle/10024/79888/f5ca5a36-f2c6-4e94-ae95-a7b439b1169b.pdf?sequence=1

Hardey, M., & Loader, B. (2009). The Information of Welfare: Older People and the Role of Digital Services. *British Journal of Social Work*, *39*(4), 657–669. doi:10.1093/bjsw/bcp024

Hart, C. (2003). *Doing a Literature Review*. London: SAGE Publications Ltd.

Hayes, D., & Devaney, J. (2004). Accessing Social Work Case Files for Research Purposes. *Qualitative Social Work*, *3*(3), 313–333. doi:10.1177/1473325004045667

Henman, P., & Adler, M. (2003). Information technology and the governance of social security. *Critical Social Policy*, *23*(2), 139–164. doi:10.1177/0261018303023002002

Hovmand, P. S., Jonson-Reid, M., & Drake, B. (2007). Mapping Service Networks. *Journal of Technology in Human Services*, *25*(4), 1–21. doi:10.1300/J017v25n04_01

Huntington, A., & Sudbery, J. (2005). Virtual Classrooms: Experiences of European Collaborative Teaching and Learning. *Social Work education*, *24*(3), 363–371. doi:10.1080/02615470500050677

Ince, D., & Griffiths, A. (2011). A Chronicling System for Children's Social Work: Learning from the ICS Failure. *British Journal of Social Work*, *41*, 1497–1513. doi:10.1093/bjsw/bcr016

International Medical Informatics Association. (2010). *IMIA Education Recommendations 2010*. Retrieved February 10, 2014, from http://www.schattauer.de/en/magazine/subject-areas/journals-a-z/methods/contents/archive/issue/1053/manuscript/12538.html

*International Medical Informatics Association (IMIA)*. (2014). Retrieved February 10, 2014, from http://www.imia-medinfo.org/new2/

Iso-Markku, P. & Kurhila, J. (1999). *Sosiaalialan tietotekniikkakartoitus 1999. [Social services ICT review 1999*]. Helsinki: Osaavien keskusten verkosto.

Jang, K. (2013). An Understanding of Optimal Knowledge Management for Social Work Practice: Based on a Process-Oriented Conceptualisation of Knowledge Integration. *British Journal of Social Work*, *43*, 1364–1383. doi:10.1093/bjsw/bcs053

Jensen, C. (2008). Worlds of welfare services and transfers. *Journal of European Social Policy*, *18*(2), 151–162. doi:10.1177/0958928707087591

Jensen, P. (1978). Miten atk palvelee sosiaalitointa? (How does IT serve social services?). *Sosiaaliturva*, *66*(22), 935–938.

Judd, R. G., & Johnston, L. B. (2012, Spring). Ethical Consequences of Using Social Network Sites for Students in Professional Social Work Programs. *Journal of Social Work Values & Ethics*, *9*(1), 5–12.

Kaarakainen, M. (2009). Hajauttaminen valtion ja kuntien välisissä suhteissa 1945 - 2015. Valtiollisesta järjestelmästä kohden kuntaverkostojen perusterveydenhuoltoa. [Decentralization in state and municipal relationships from 1945 to 2015. From national primary health care towards municipality networks]. *Social Sciences*, 153.

Kapp, S. A., & Stipp, K. F. (2010). Trolling the Useful Data in an Automated Information Management System: Experiences of Kansas City Community Mental Health Managers. *Administration in Social Work*, *34*(2), 135–147. doi:10.1080/03643101003608927

Kautto, M. (2002). Investing in services in West European welfare states. *Journal of European Social Policy*, *12*(1), 53–65. doi:10.1177/0952872002012001636

Keegan Eamon, M., Wu, C.-F., Moroney, G., & Gundari, M. (2013). Teaching the Importance and Use of Web-Based Services to Assist Clients in Obtaining Public Benefits. *Journal of Teaching in Social Work*, *2*(33), 143–158. doi:10.1080/08841233.2013.777011

Kerslake, A. (1998). Computerisation of the *Looking After Children* Records: Issues of Implementation. *Children & Society*, *12*(3), 236–237.

Keymolen, E., & Broeders, D. (2013). Innocence Lost: Care and Control in Dutch Digital Youth Care. *British Journal of Social Work*, *43*, 41–63. doi:10.1093/bjsw/bcr169

Kokko, S. (2009). Integrated primary health care: Finnish solutions and experiences. *International Journal of Integrated Care*, (9). Retrieved July 27, 2010, from http://www.ijic.org

Korpi, K. (1985). Yhtenäinen asiakastietokanta sosiaalitoimelle? [Uniform client data base for social services?]. *Sosiaaliturva*, *73*(10), 465–467.

Kuhn, T. A. (1970). *The Structure of Scientific Revolutions*. Chicago: University of Chicago Press.

Kum, H., Duncan, D. F., & Stewart, C. J. (2009). Supporting self-evaluation in local government via Knowledge Discovery and Data Mining. *Government Information Quarterly*, *26*(2), 295–304. doi:10.1016/j.giq.2008.12.009

Kunkel, B., & Yowell, T. (2001). *e*-Tools and Organization Transformation Techniques for Collaborative Case Management. *Journal of Technology in Human Services*, *18*(1/2), 117–134. doi:10.1300/J017v18n01_10

Kuusisto-Niemi, S., & Saranto, K. (2008). Sosiaali- ja terveydenhuollon tietohallinto oppiaineena ja tieteenalana: kehityskulkuja ja näköaloja. [Health and Human Services Informatics as a subject and a discipline: progression and views]. In Sosiaali- ja terveydenhuollon tietotekniikan ja tiedonhallinnan tutkimuspäivät: Tutkimuspaperit 2008 (pp. 60-65). Retrieved May 12, 2011, from http://stty.org/joomla/index.php?option=com_content&view=category&layout=blog&id=44&Itemid=79

Kuusisto-Niemi, S. & Saranto, K. (2009). Sosiaali- ja terveydenhuollon tiedonhallinta - Paradigma tieteenalan perustana. [Health and Human Services Informatics – the Paradigm as the Foundation of the Discipline]. *Finnish Journal of eHealth and eWelfare*, *1*(1), 19-23. Retrieved October 21, 2010, from http://ojs.tsv.fi/index.php/stty/article/view/1734

LaMendola, W. (2010). Social Work and Social Presence in an Online World. *Journal of Technology in Human Services*, *28*(1), 108–119. doi:10.1080/15228831003759562

Larsen, A. K., Sanders, R., Astray, A. A., & Hole, G. O. (2008). E-teacher Challenges and Competencies in International Comparative Social Work Courses. *Social Work Education*, *27*(6), 623–633. doi:10.1080/02615470802201671

Leung, Z. S. (2009). Knowledge Management in Social Work: Types and Processes of Knowledge Sharing in Social Service Organizations. *British Journal of Social Work*, *39*(4), 693–709. doi:10.1093/bjsw/bcp034

Loader, B. D., Hardey, M., & Keeble, L. (2008). Health informatics for older people: a review of ICT facilitated integrated care for older people. *International Journal of Social Welfare, 17*(1), 46–53. doi:10.1111/j.1468-2397.2007.00489.x

Lunnas, H. & Kuusisto-Niemi, S. (1991). *Sosiaalitoimen ohjelmistoselvitys 1991* [*Report on social services software 1991*]. Helsinki: Kunnallishallinnon tietotekniikkaneuvottelukunta.

Luostarinen, H., & Väliverronen, E. (1991). *Tekstinsyöjät. Yhteiskuntatieteellisen kirjallisuuden lukutaidosta. [Text Eaters. About the social science literature literacy.].* Tampere: Vastapaino.

Manthorpe, J., Kharicha, K., Goodman, C., Harari, D., Swift, C., & Iliffe, S. (2010). Smarter Working in Social and Health Care: Professional Perspectives on a New Technology for Risk Appraisal with Older People. *British Journal of Social Work, 40*(6), 1829–1846. doi:10.1093/bjsw/bcp100

McNutt, J. (1996). National Information Infrastructure Policy and the Future of the American Welfare State: Implications for the Social Welfare Policy Curriculum. *Journal of Social Work Education, 32*(3), 375–388.

McNutt, J.G. (2000). Coming Perspectives in the Development of Electronic Advocacy for Social Policy Practice. *Critical Social Work, 1*(1). Retrieved May 12, 2011, from http://www.uwindsor.ca/criticalsocialwork/coming-perspectives-in-the-development-of-electronic-advocacy-for-social-policy-practice-0

Menon, G. M., & Miller-Cribbs, J. (2002). Online Social Work Practice: Issues and Guidelines for the Profession. *Administration in Social Work, 3*(2), 104–116.

Miles, M. B., & Huberman, A. M. (1994). *Qualitative data analysis* (2nd ed.). Sage.

Ministry of Social Affairs and Health. (2011). *Development project for social services underway.* Retrieved May 14, 2011, from http://www.stm.fi/en/pressreleases/pressrelease/view/1287485

Mishna, F., Bogo, M., Root, J., Sawyer, J.-L., & Khoury-Kassabri, M. (2012). "It just crept in": The Digital Age and Implications for Social Work Practice. *Journal of Clinical Social Work, 40*, 277–286. doi:10.1007/s10615-012-0383-4

Monnickendam, M., Savaya, R., & Waysman, M. (2004). Equity Perceptions as a Determinant of Computer User Satisfaction in Human Services. *Journal of Social Service Research, 31*(2), 41–50. doi:10.1300/J079v31n02_03

Moon, S. S., & DeWeaver, K. L. (2005). Electronic Advocacy and Social Welfare Policy Education. *Journal of Teaching in Social Work, 25*(1/2), 57–68. doi:10.1300/J067v25n01_04

Murphy, L., Parnass, P., Mitchell, D. L., Hallett, R., Cayley, P., & Seagram, S. (2009). Client Satisfaction and Outcome Comparisons of Online and Face-to-face Counselling Methods. *British Journal of Social Work, 39*(4), 627–640. doi:10.1093/bjsw/bcp041

Naccarato, T. (2010). Child Welfare Informatics: A proposed subspecialty for social work. *Children and Youth Services Review, 32*(12), 1729–1734. doi:10.1016/j.childyouth.2010.07.016

National Institute for Health and Welfare THL. (2010). *Facts about Social Welfare and Health Care in Finland 2010*. Helsinki: National Institute for Health and Welfare.

Ngyuen, L. H. (2007). Child Welfare Informatics: A New Definition for an Established Practice. *Social Work, 52*(4), 361–363. doi:10.1093/sw/52.4.361 PMID:18232246

Parton, N. (2009). Challenges to practice and knowledge in child welfare social work: From the 'social' to the 'informational'? *Children and Youth Services Review*, *31*(7), 715–721. doi:10.1016/j.childyouth.2009.01.008

Päykkönen, K. & Pohjola, A. (2007). *Selvitys sosiaalialan tiedonhallinnan nykytilasta Suomessa*. [*Account of the present state of social services knowledge management in Finland*]. Retrieved May 13, 2011, from http://www.sosiaaliportti.fi/fi-FI/tikesos/aineistot/selvitykset/

Peckover, S., Hall, C., & White, S. (2009). From Policy to Practice: The Implementation and Negotiation of Technologies in Everyday Child Welfare. *Children & Society*, *23*(2), 136–148. doi:10.1111/j.1099-0860.2008.00143.x

Perron, B. E., Taylor, H. O., Glass, J. E., & Margerum-Leys, J. (2010). Information and Communication Technologies in Social Work. *Administration in Social Work*, *11*(1), 67–81. PMID:21691444

Pithouse, A., Broadhurst, K., Hall, C., Peckover, S., Wastell, D., & White, S. (2012). Trust, risk and the (mis)management of contingency and discretion through new information technologies in children's services. *Journal of Social Work*, *12*(2), 158–178. doi:10.1177/1468017310382151

Pithouse, A., Hall, C., Peckover, S., & White, S. (2009). A Tale of Two CAFs: The Impact of the Electronic Common Assessment Framework. *British Journal of Social Work*, *39*(4), 599–612. doi:10.1093/bjsw/bcp020

Pleace, N. (2011). Workless People and Surveillant Mashups. Social policy and data sharing in the UK. *Information Communication and Society*, *10*(6), 943–960. doi:10.1080/13691180701751171

Pohjola, A., Kääriäinen, A., & Kuusisto-Niemi, S. (Eds.). (2010). Sosiaalityö, tieto ja teknologia. [Social work, information and technology]. Jyväskylä: PS-kustannus.

Rafferty, J., & Waldman, J. (2006). Fit for Virtual Social Work Practice? *Journal of Technology in Human Services*, *24*(2/3), 1–22. doi:10.1300/J017v24n02_01

Rock, B. (1999). The New Confidentiality for the 21st Century in a Managed Care Environment. *Social Work*, *44*(3), 253–262. doi:10.1093/sw/44.3.253 PMID:10348698

Saba, V. K., & McCormick, K. A. (Eds.). (2001). *Essentials of Computers for Nurses: Informatics for the New Millennium*. McCraw-Hill Companies.

Saranto, K., & Kuusisto-Niemi, S. (2012). Tiedonhallinnan koulutusohjelma arvioitavana – kokemuksia kansainvälisestä akkreditoinnista. (Health and Human Services Informatics Master´s Degree Program in Evaluation – Experiences from the international accreditation). *Finnish Journal of eHealth and eWelfare*, *4*(2), 140-144. Retrieved February 12, 2014, from http://ojs.tsv.fi/index.php/stty/article/view/6558/5375

Scottish Government. (2011). *eHealth Programme*. Retrieved May 12, 2011, from http://www.ehealth.scot.nhs.uk/

Shah, N. (2012). Welfare and technology in the network society – Concerns for the future of welfare. *Futures*, *44*, 659–665. doi:10.1016/j.futures.2012.04.004

Shaw, I., Bell, M., Sinclair, I., Sloper, P., Mitchell, W., & Dyson, P. et al. (2009). An Exemplary Scheme? An Evaluation of the Integrated Children's System. *British Journal of Social Work*, *39*(4), 613–626. doi:10.1093/bjsw/bcp040

Sosiaali- ja terveysministeriö. (1996). *Sosiaali- ja terveydenhuollon tietotekniikan hyödyntämisstrategia.* [*Ministry of Social Affairs and Health. The utilization strategy for social affairs and health*]. Helsinki: Sosiaali- ja terveysministeriö.

*Sosiaalialan tiedonhallinnan tutkimusohjelma.* (2009). Retrieved February 14, 2014, from http://www.sosiaaliportti.fi/File/fd89a662-d7e8-4053-b56d-45ea45ecc8db/Tiedonhallinnan+ohjelma.pdf

*Sosiaalihuollon tiedonhallinta*. (2014). Retrieved February 10, 2014, from http://www.thl.fi/fi_FI/web/fi/aiheet/tietopaketit/sosiaalihuollon_tiedonhallinta

Sosiaaliportti. (2014). *Sosiaaliportti - The Social Gateway*. Retrieved February 14, 2014, from http://www.sosiaaliportti.fi/en-GB/

Sosiaalitoimen atk-toimikunta. (1981). *Sosiaalitoimen atk-selvitys* [*National Working Group for ICT in Social Services. Account on social services ICT*]. Helsinki: Suomen Kaupunkiliitto, Suomen Kunnallisliitto.

Sosiaalitoimen atk-toimikunta. (1986). *Sosiaalihuollon tietojenkäsittelyn kehittäminen* [*National Working Group for ICT in Social Services. Development of ICT in social services*]. Helsinki: Suomen Kaupunkiliitto, Suomen Kunnallisliitto.

Sosiaalitoimen atk-toimikunta. (1993). *Sosiaalitoimen järjestelmien peruskäsitteet.* [*National Working Group for ICT in Social Services. The core data set of social services ICT*]. Helsinki: Kunnallishallinnon tietotekniikkaneuvottelukunta.

Steyaert, J., & Gould, N. (2009). Social Work and the Changing Face of the Digital Divide. *British Journal of Social Work*, *39*(4), 740–753. doi:10.1093/bjsw/bcp022

Stillman, L., & McGrath, J. (2008). Is it Web 2.0 or is it Better Information and Knowledge That We Need? *Australian Social Work*, *61*(4), 421–428. doi:10.1080/03124070802441889

Taimiaho, A. (1987). Henkilörekisterilaki voimaan vuoden alusta. (Data security act into operation from the beginning of the year). *Sosiaaliturva*, *75*(22), 1252–1254.

Tenhunen, E., Hämäläinen, P., Kärki, J., & Väinälä, A. (2006). Sosiaaliala ja sosiaali- ja terveydenhuollon tietoteknologiakehitys. [Field of social welfare and the ICT development of social and health care]. In Sosiaali- ja terveydenhuollon tietotekniikan ja tiedonhallinnan tutkimuspäivät: Tutkimuspaperit 2006 (pp. 96-101). Retrieved May 13, 2011, from http://stty.org/joomla/index.php?option=com_content&view=category&layout=blog&id=44&Itemid=79

The Department of Health. (2011). *Defining the electronic social care record* (final version 7.2). Retrieved April 13, 2011, from http://www.dh.gov.uk/en/Managingyourorganisation/Information-policy/Informationforsocialcare/DH_4073714

Tregeagle, S., & Darcy, M. (2008). Child Welfare and Information and Communication Technology: Today's Challenge. *British Journal of Social Work*, *38*(8), 1481–1498. doi:10.1093/bjsw/bcm048

Väestötietojärjestelmä. (2014). *Kuntien asukasluvut aakkosjärjestyksessä 31.8.2013.* [Population Information System. Inhabitants in the municipalities, August 31, 2013.]. Retrieved February 10, 2014, from http://vrk.fi/default.aspx?docid=7675&site=3&id=0

Valtiovarainministeriö. (1995). *Suomi tietoyhteiskunnaksi. [Ministry of Finance. Finland - towards an information society, A National Outline].* Helsinki: Valtiovarainministeriö.

Wastell, D., White, S., Broadhurst, K., Peckover, S., & Pithouse, A. (2010). Children's services in the iron cage of performance management: Street-level bureaucracy and the spectre of Švejkism. *International Journal of Social Welfare*, *19*(3), 310–320. doi:10.1111/j.1468-2397.2009.00716.x

Webster, D., Needell, B., & Wildfire, J. (2002). Data are Your Friends: Child Welfare Agency Self-Evaluation in Los Angeles County with the Family to Family Initiative. *Children and Youth Services Review*, *24*(6/7), 471–484. doi:10.1016/S0190-7409(02)00197-4

Wessels, B., Walsh, S., & Adam, E. (2008). Mediating Voices: Community Participation in the Design of E-Enabled Community Care Services. *The Information Society*, *24*(1), 30–39. doi:10.1080/01972240701774683

West, D., & Heath, D. (2011). Theoretical pathways to the future: Globalization, ICT and social work theory and practice. *Journal of Social Work*, *11*(2), 209–221. doi:10.1177/1468017310386835

White, S., Hall, C., & Peckover, S. (2009). The Descriptive Tyranny of the Common Assessment Framework: Technologies of Categorization and Professional Practice in Child Welfare. *British Journal of Social Work*, *39*(7), 1197–1217. doi:10.1093/bjsw/bcn053

White, S., Wastell, D., Broadhurst, K., & Hall, C. (2010). When policy o'erlaps itself: The 'tragic tale' of the Integrated Children's System. *Critical Social Policy*, *30*(3), 405–429. doi:10.1177/0261018310367675

Whittemore, R., & Knalf, K. (2005). Methodological issues in nursing research: The integrative review: updated methodology. *Journal of Advanced Nursing*, *52*(2), 546–553. doi:10.1111/j.1365-2648.2005.03621.x PMID:16268861

Wong, Y. C., Fung, J. Y. C., Law, C. K., Lam, J. C. Y., & Lee, V. W. P. (2009). Tackling the Digital Divide. *British Journal of Social Work*, *39*(4), 745–767. doi:10.1093/bjsw/bcp026

Youn, E. (2007). The Relationship Between Technology Content in a Masters of Social Work Curriculum and Technology Use in Social Work Practice: A Qualitative Research Study. *Journal of Technology in Human Services*, *25*(1), 45–58. doi:10.1300/J017v25n01_03

## KEY TERMS AND DEFINITIONS

**Human Services:** Services provided for people in need of help in possessing their life, organized in the Finnish context mainly by laws or statutes on the field of social services and social security, employment, health and legal activities. Also the third sector actors and social work of the church are working on the field of human services.

**ICT Education Curriculum:** A plan of conducting for the degree specified ICT studies. They can vary from passing a preliminary exam to taking a degree or a part of it in ICT. In Finland it has been obligatory to pass a basic exam in ICT studies since 1990´s at high school and universities of applied science levels.

**Informatics:** The science and practice of information and its processing. As a science informatics operates on the fields of technologies, philosophy, social and information sciences, studying how to design a system that delivers the right information, to the right person in the right place and time, in the right way.

**Information Management (IM):** Operations, which control and support information acquisition, storage, handling, transfer and delivery in the organization.

**Knowledge Management (KM):** A management process where knowledge, skills, expertise and communication are cared for, administered and steered in a goal-oriented fashion.

**Social Services:** in Finland social services have been defined in Social Welfare Act 710/1982, and they include the following services: 1) social work, 2) child guidance and family counselling, 3) home services, 4) housing services, 5) institutional care, 6) family care, 7) activities supporting the access to employment and specific work for people with disabilities, and 8) measures to establish maintenance for a child. Moreover, a municipality is obliged to arrange also following services, if needed: child and youth welfare, day care for children, special care for the mentally handicapped, services and support for people with disabilities, services related to care for substance abusers, the statutory functions of child welfare officer, other measures related to the investigation and establishment of paternity, adoption counselling, family conciliation and conciliation concerning the enforcement of decisions on child custody and visiting rights, and provision of support for informal care and other social services.

# Chapter 3
# A Social Network Framework to Explore Healthcare Collaboration

**Uma Srinivasan**
*Capital Markets Cooperative Research Centre, Australia*

**Shahadat Uddin**
*The University of Sydney, Australia*

## ABSTRACT

*A patient-centric approach to healthcare leads to an informal social network among medical professionals. This chapter presents a research framework to: (1) identify the collaboration structure among physicians that is effective and efficient for patients; (2) discover effective structural attributes of a collaboration network that evolves during the course of providing care; and (3) explore the impact of socio-demographic characteristics of healthcare professionals, patients, and hospitals on collaboration structures, from the point of view of measurable outcomes such as cost and quality of care. The framework uses illustrative examples drawn from a data set of patients undergoing hip replacement surgery. The practical application of the proposed framework reveals structures of physicians' collaborations that are not favourable to cost and quality of care measures such as readmission rate. The authors believe that such a framework will enable healthcare managers and administrators to evaluate the collaborative work environment within their respective healthcare organisations.*

## INTRODUCTION

Healthcare spending is a major topic of discussion in practically every country in the world. Figure 1 shows the health spending as a percentage of GDP of a few Organisation for Economic Co-operation and Development (OECD) countries based on a report produced by the International Federation of Health Plans[1]. There are growing concerns all around about spiralling healthcare costs, budget constraints and their impact on quality of health outcomes for patients. In this context, a major goal of governments and health providers is to achieve consistency of health outcomes for frequent and

DOI: 10.4018/978-1-4666-6316-9.ch003

*Figure 1. 2010 health spending as a percent of GDP*

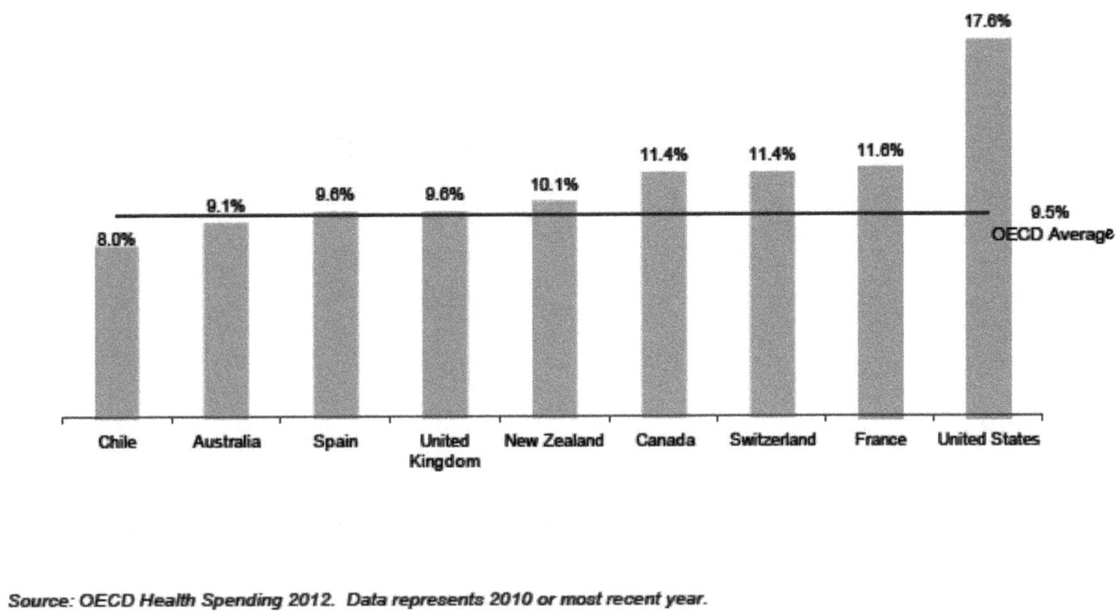


expensive health services and high volume and high cost procedures such as knee and hip replacement surgeries whose numbers have been steadily increasing over the years.

Figure 2 shows the comparative costs of hip replacement procedures from the same report. Comparisons across different countries are complicated by differences in sectors, fee schedules and health plans used for cost comparisons. Nevertheless, it is clear that consistent healthcare strategies are required to deliver high quality of services where health outcomes are consistent and predictable both for the patient and providers involved in caring for the patient.

Although not always formal, there is a protocol among physicians to collaborate while providing care to chronic patients both in a hospital setting as well as in an ambulatory care setting. Given that an informal social network exists or emerges among healthcare professionals to address a specific problem, the question that arises is whether there is a way to measure the network parameters of collaboration networks that consistently perform effectively and efficiently to achieve the desired outcome which could be, in the case of patient care, high quality care with optimal costs. Using principles of social network theories such as Bavelas' Centrality Theory (1950), Freeman's centralization theory (1978), and the social network model of exponential random graph model, we propose a social network-based framework that can serve as a basis to offer insights into the different types of collaboration patterns among healthcare professionals that are conducive to positive health outcomes to patients, as well as provide consistent quality of care measures in healthcare settings.

The rest of the paper is organised as follows: the next section presents a review of network-based collaboration models in a healthcare setting, which is followed by the theoretical background of healthcare collaboration related to network structures and measures of centrality. Then we presents our network-based framework that provides formal measures of physicians' collaboration networks and identifies network measures that indicate positive outcomes in terms of both costs and quality of care. After that, we presents

*Figure 2. Comparative cost for hip replacement procedure in different countries*

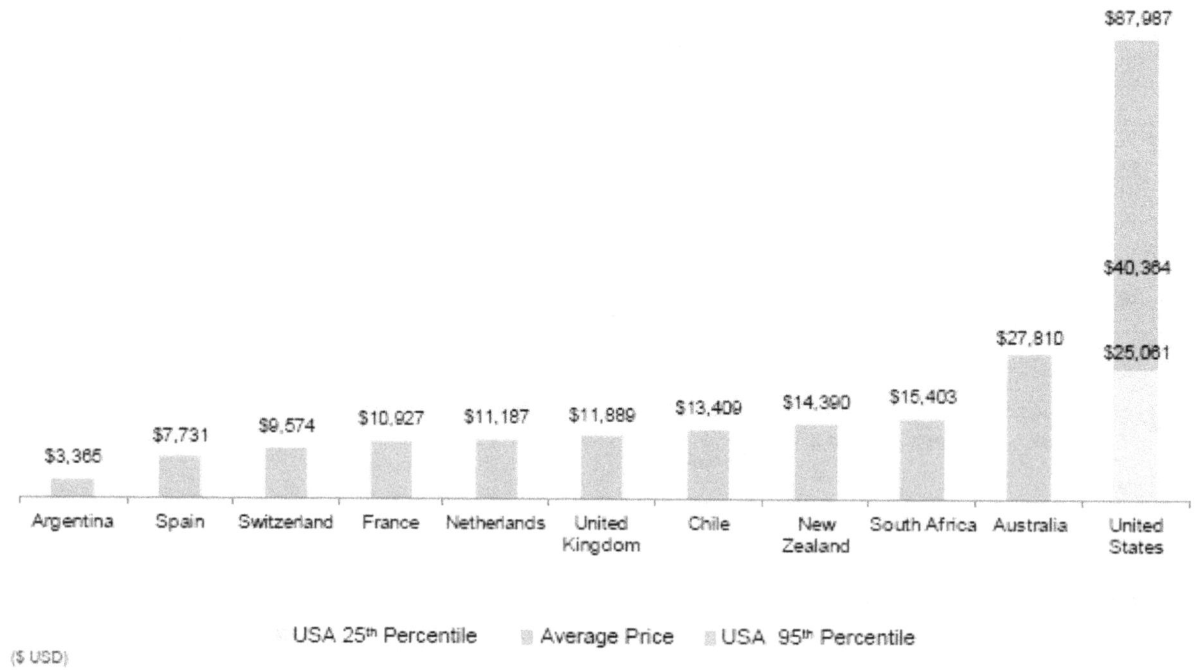


an illustrative application and results of network structure measures on a specific (de-identified and anonymised) health insurance claims data set provided by an Australian not-for-profit health insurance organisation. The last section discusses the contribution of this paper, and presents conclusions and future research directions.

## REVIEW OF HEALTHCARE COLLABORATION

There are numerous studies in current literature exploring collaborations among healthcare professionals. Most of these studies examine hospital performance and patient outcomes by analysing collaboration networks among different healthcare professionals such as nurse-physician collaboration (Knaus et al., 1986), physician-pharmacist collaboration (Hunt et al., 2008), physician-patient collaboration (Arbuthnott & Sharpe, 2009), hospital-physician collaboration (Burns & Muller, 2008), and inter-professional and interdisciplinary collaboration (Gaboury et al., 2009). Cunningham et al. (2012) have conducted an orderly review of 26 studies of professionals' network structures and analysed factors connected with network effectiveness and sustainability specifically in relation to the quality of care and patient safety. They noticed that cohesive and collaborative health professional networks can contribute to improving quality and safety of care.

Another classic study, led by Knaus and his team, identifies a significant relationship between the degree of nurse-physician collaboration and patient mortality in intensive care units (Knaus, et al., 1986). They study treatment and outcome in 5030 intensive care unit patients and find that hospitals where nurse-physician collaboration is present report a lower mortality rate compared to the predicted number of patient deaths. Conversely, hospitals that are noted for poor communication among healthcare professionals exceed their predicted number of patient deaths. In a two group quasi-experiment on 1207 general medicine patients (n = 581 in the experimental group who received care from a specially designed care management plan that facilitated higher collaboration among hospital staff and n = 626 in the control group who received the usual care), Cowan et al. (2006) notice average hospital length of stay, total hospitalization cost and hospital readmission rate are significantly lower for patients in the experimental group than the control group (5 versus 6 days, p< .0001) which contributes a *'backfill profit'* of US$1591 per patient to hospitals. Sommers et al. (2000) examined the impact of an interdisciplinary and collaborative practice intervention involving a primary care physician, a nurse and a social worker for community-dwelling seniors with chronic illnesses. They conducted a controlled cohort study of 543 patients in 18 private office practices of primary care physicians. The intervention group received care from their primary care physician working with a registered nurse and a social worker, while the control group received care as usual from primary care physicians. They noticed that the intervention group produced better results in relation to readmission rates and average office visits to all physicians. Moreover, the patients in the intervention group also reported an increase in social activities compared with the control group.

There are other studies emphasizing collaboration for effective patient outcome across professional boundaries within hospitals. By analysing data collected from 105 interviews (with 40 physician, 32 case managers, 23 physician office staff, 8 administrators and 2 case assistants), Netting and Williams (1996) argue that there is a growing need to collaborate and communicate across professional lines rather than make assumptions about who can do what for better patient outcomes, professional satisfaction and hospital performance. There are other studies that analyse networked collaboration among healthcare specialists to explore different aspects of professional behaviour and quality patient care. For example, Fattore et al. (2009) evaluate the effects of GP network organisation on their prescribing behavior and (Meltzer et al., 2010) develop a selection criteria of group members in order to improve the effectiveness of team-based approach to patient care.

## THEORETICAL MOTIVATION FOR COLLABORATION

Collaboration evolves among healthcare professionals during the course of providing healthcare services to patients. As a result of this collaboration an informal social network emerges among healthcare professionals over time. A social network is viewed as a set of actors and a set of links between those actors. In a social network, an actor is a node which represents an entity such as an individual or an organisation. The formation of a social network is typically associated with the need for an actor to receive some sort of information or resource from others. Each actor is a part of this informal network although they have different positions and locations in the network. Since all actors do not have the same network locations, a reasonable question arises: *"Do actors, who have different network locations, show notable differences in their ability to collaborate?"* A review of classical network theories (i.e. Bavelas Experiment and Freeman's Theory of Centralisation) can provide a better understanding to respond to this performance-related question. These two network theories explain structural influences of collaboration network on group performance.

### Bavelas's Experiment

The *"Bavelas Experiment"* was conducted by Alex Bavelas and his students, particularly Harold

Leavitt, in the Small Group Network Laboratory at *Massachusetts Institute of Technology* (MIT) in the late 1940s (Bavelas, 1950; H. Leavitt, 1949). This experiment, which is also known as the MIT experiment, attempted to seek the impact of different types of human communication patterns on performance. Based on the assumption that (i) success of entire classes of tasks depends upon an effective flow of information, and (ii) communication patterns have effects on task performance and individual outcome, this study focused on the motivating question of "*On what principles may a pattern of communication be determined that will in fact be a fit one for effective and efficient human effort?*" On the basis of the assumption that imposed patterns determine certain aspects of group process, in addition to the first two assumptions, the original driving question further raised three subsequent questions: "*How does a fixed communication pattern affect the performance of a group?*"; "*Do some patterns have structural properties that limit group performance?*"; and "*What effects can pattern have upon the emergence of leadership, the development of organisation, the degree of resistance to group disruption, the ability to adapt successfully to sudden changes in the working environment?*" These research questions sought to answer, through a laboratory-controlled experiment, how social network structures, measured in terms of patterns of communication, affect individual performance, and the work and life of a group (e.g. emergence of leaders and job satisfaction).

The experiment consisted of five people or subjects who had to communicate with each other only through enclosed cubicles in order to solve a puzzle. Each subject was given a card with five different symbols had been printed on it: a circle, a triangle, an asterisk, a plus sign and a diamond (O, Δ, *, +, ◇). Each symbol appeared at most four times in a group of five cards although only one symbol appeared on all five cards. The puzzle was to find the common symbol in the shortest time possible and with minimum communication among subjects. The cubicle of each subject had six switches labelled with one of the six master symbols. The puzzle was considered solved when each subject indicated the common symbol by throwing the appropriate switch. The experiment was trialled 15 times. The same six master symbols were used throughout, however; the common symbol varied from trial to trial. The subjects communicated by writing messages which were passed through slots in the walls of the cubicles. These slots were so arranged that any of the desired patterns of communication structures (i.e. the Y, star, circle and line) shown in Figure 3 could emerge.

The subjects could pass as many messages as they wished and no restriction was placed on the content of these messages. None of the subjects had any idea about the number of people in the study and the configuration of the group communication structure. Total number of individuals and group times, and number of errors (i.e. when a subject threw an incorrect switch) in solving the puzzle were collected and recorded by a laboratory assistant for analysis purpose.

The performance and behaviour of all communication patterns were evaluated on the basis of structure comparison and node-level analysis. Performance of the task-oriented groups was measured in terms of the time taken to solve the puzzle and the number of errors made by each group in the course of completing the puzzle. When completion time (e.g. time needed to complete the puzzle) was considered to compare the performance of groups using various patterns, it turned out that the groups using the *'star'* and *'Y'* structures took less time on average than the groups using other structures (i.e. *'circle'* and *'line'*). Centralisation, as explained by Leavitt (1951), is the chief determinant to this performance difference for various communication structures. It was evident that patterns demonstrating higher centralisation performed better. When there was a central subject present in the structure, all the remaining subjects in the structure channelled

*Figure 3. The Y, star, circle and line structures of communication*

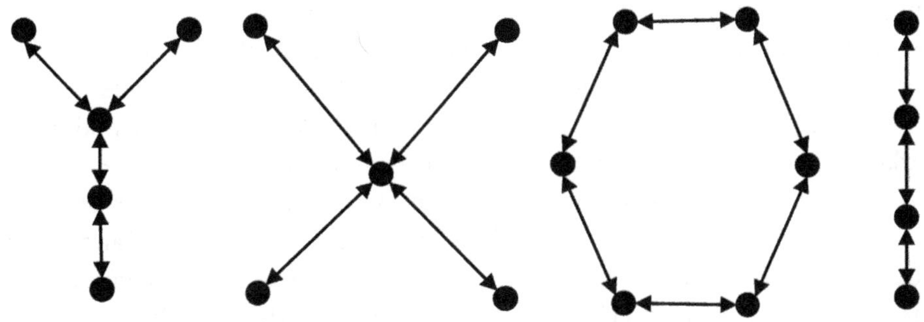

(a) Y-shape (b) Star (c) Circle (d) Line

all required information through that central subject. Therefore, the groups using *'star'* and *'Y'* structures also used fewer numbers of messages compared to groups using other structures and also made the least number of errors.

When node-level analysis was conducted to understand the behavioural differences of communication patterns, they discovered that highly centralised structures had a leader who emerged during the task process. In all structures, leaders emerged at those positions with the highest centrality. As the *'star'* and *'Y'* structures clearly had only one subject with highest degree-centrality, there were more chances of a leader evolving during the experiment, which in turn led to better performance. They also noted that subjects' satisfaction with their roles in the course of completing the puzzle varied among structures as well as among different positions within the same structure (i.e. central position versus peripheral position).

The key finding from this study was that centralised structures such as the *'star'* or *'Y'* were far more conducive to performance (i.e. solving the puzzle faster) than the decentralised or flatter structures such as the *'circle'* structure. The basic logic is that, in decentralised networks the information floats around inefficiently, and is therefore less conducive to efficient performance.

## Freeman's Theory of Centrality and Centralisation

The idea of centrality was applied to human communication by Bavelas (1950) in the late 1950s as described in the previous section. All experiments conducted by Bavelas and his research team concluded that centrality was related to group efficiency in problem-solving, perception of leadership and the personal satisfaction of participants. In the late 1970s, Freeman (1978) wrote a seminal article about the intuitive background for measures of structural centrality which immediately became one of the core concepts in the social network study. His work extended the notion of centrality by proposing three measures: (i) one absolute, (ii) one relative, and (iii) centralisation of the entire network. Each of these has three distinctive concepts for centrality: (a) degree, (b) betweenness, and (c) closeness. He also examined the implications of these nine measures (each of three centrality concepts has three measures) to a study of small groups.

Freeman (1978), motivated by the notion of centrality in Bevalas experiment, reviewed other studies that demonstrated the applicability of the concept of centrality to understand (i) real life problems such as political integration in the context of the diversity of Indian social life (Cohn & Marriott, 1958), (ii) consequences of centrality in communication paths for urban development (Pitts, 1965), and (iii) implications of centrality for the design of organisations (Beauchamp, 1965). Freeman (1978) then reviewed the various measures and overlapping concepts of centrality, while clarifying range, limitations and strength of each measure for application. Centrality had been defined in terms of *'point'*, *'betweenness'* and *'closeness'* as reported by Freeman (1978), while each of them has important implications on social outcomes, process and performance. Point centrality can be measured in terms of degree which is the number of ties to and from an actor in a network. Structurally, centrality is measured in terms of closeness and betweenness. Closeness centrality indicates the extent to which an actor is close to all others in the network, and betweenness centrality reflects the extent to which an actor lies in the shortest path to all others in the network. Each of the centrality concepts has been related to important social occurrences: *'point'* or *'degree'* centrality being viewed as an indicator of the communication activity of an actor; *'betweenness'* centrality being viewed as an indicator of the potential of communication control capacity of an actor; and *'closeness'* centrality is perceived as an index of minimum cost of time and efficiency to communicate with others in the network.

In a subsequent study, Freeman et al. (1979) explored the effects of structural centrality on human communication through the use of a replication of the early MIT experiments by Bavelas (1950). It was shown that although two of the three concepts of centrality measures had a demonstrable effect on individual responses and group processes, the classic measure of centrality based on distance was found unrelated to any experimental variables. Using 100 volunteers from among the student body at Leigh University as subjects, Freeman et al. (1979) analysed the results and demonstrated that centrality is an important structural factor of any network which influences leadership evolvement, and satisfaction and efficiency of actors or subjects. Interestingly, in their research another structural factor, the overall density of communication paths in the structural form, also turned out to be relevant in understanding network performance. Since then, the notion of centrality, density and centralisation were considered as one of the key network measures used for studying network effects on individual and group outcomes such as task efficiency, productivity, and improved performance (Alireza Abbasi et al., 2012; Ahuja et al., 2003; Bonacich, 1991; Brass, 1981, 1985; Cross & Cummings, 2004; Faust, 1997; Hossain et al., 2006; Mullen & Eduardo, 1991; Pfeffer, 1980; Salancik & Pfeffer, 1978; Sparrowe et al., 2001; M. Uddin & L. Hossain, 2009; M. S. Uddin & L. Hossain, 2009; M. S. Uddin & L. Hossain, 2011; Shahadat Uddin, Jafar Hamra, et al., 2013b; S. Uddin & L. Hossain, 2011; Uddin & Hossain, 2012; Uddin & Hossain, 2013; S. Uddin, L. Hossain, & M. Kelaher, 2012). Freeman's work made a substantial contribution to the network structure and task-performance research. Indeed, his contribution was so influential that the notion of centrality is now almost always attributed to him.

In summary, both Bavelas experiment and Freeman's Theory of Centrality and Centralisation open a new area of research to understand and explore individual performance in a collaborative environment. Bavelas (1950) divulged a new research area for investigating how network positions of actors influence their (i) ability to perform, (ii) perception of leadership, and (iii) level of personal satisfaction in the course of working in a collaborative environment towards achieving a common goal. Freeman (1978) proposed three measures for structural centrality: (i) degree centrality – indicating activity of actor and actor popularity, (ii) betweenness centrality – representing actor potential to control, and (iii) closeness centrality – stating the minimum cost to visit all other actors in the network. Since then, these three measures have been utilised extensively by researchers to measure structural positions of actors in a collaborative environment (A. Abbasi et al., 2011; Alireza Abbasi, et al., 2012; Cainelli et al., 2010; Shahian et al., 2010; Shippy et al., 2004; Smith et al., 2003; M. S. Uddin & L. Hossain, 2009; Shahadat Uddin et al., 2012; Uddin, et al., 2013b; S. Uddin, L. Hossain, A. Abbasi, et al., 2012; Shahadat Uddin, Liaquat Hossain, & Kim Rasmussen, 2013; Uddin & Jacobson, 2013; Uddin et al., 2011; S. Uddin et al., 2013; Uddin et al., 2014).

## PROPOSED COLLABORATION FRAMEWORK

The proposed collaboration framework is based on the two network theories of centralisation and centrality, positioned in the context of collaboration that occurs among healthcare professionals while treating a patient with a specific problem. In particular, if the health problem is acute or chronic and requires hospitalisation, the patient goes through a complex journey from one provider to another, while negotiating through the maze of the health system. In the broader sense, most countries around the world have some versions of a '*patient journey*' that come into play when a patient needs hospital treatment. As an illustrative example, we briefly describe the different stages of the patient journey in the Australian healthcare setting.

All Australians are entitled to the government funded public healthcare, which is accessed through the Medicare system. In addition, most people have private health insurance to avoid waiting lists and have access to private hospital cover. Outpatient consultation costs are covered by Medicare and hospital treatment costs are borne by the private health insurance providers. Therefore, the journey involves negotiating both the public and private healthcare settings. Figure 4 shows a patient's journey through the healthcare system.

Each box shows a service provider who provides a specific type of service to the patient.

*Figure 4. Patient journey through the health system. Note: This figure does not include ancillary and allied health services such as dental, optical, physiotherapy, etc. as those services are not funded by the public Medicare system. A privately insured patient, however, can choose additional cover for such ancillary services. Also not shown in the diagram are veterans' affairs and other funding agencies that come into play for motor vehicle accidents, and work related injuries.*

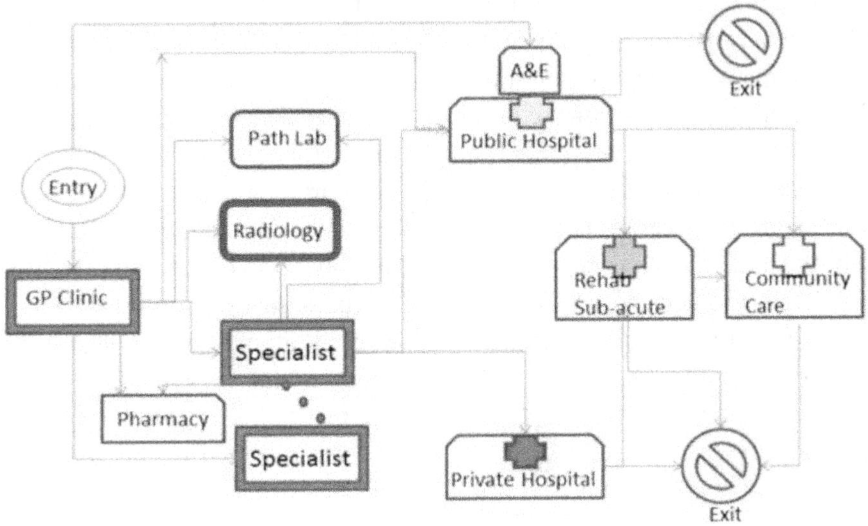

The entry point - the first point of contact - for all Australians is the General Practitioner (GP). Depending on the nature of the presenting problem, the GP could perform any one or all of the following activities: (i) give a script which is dispensed by the pharmacy; (ii) refer the patient for laboratory investigations; (iii) refer the patient for radiology and imaging services; (iv) refer the patient to one or more specialists; (v) send the patient to the public hospital in case of an emergency. All the above services including specialist consultations and emergency public hospital admissions are funded by the public Medicare system. When a patient requires hospitalisation for either investigative or therapeutic procedures, the specialist refers the patient for a hospital admission. At this point the journey changes its direction in different ways for public and private patients. Public patients who do not have private health cover will seek admission in a public hospital which may have long waiting periods for admission. Patients with private health insurance have the option of seeking admission in a private hospital or as a private patient in a public hospital or as public patient in a public hospital. The advantage of seeking admission as a private patient is the shorter waiting time for hospital admissions. For patients with private health insurance all *in-hospital* charges including surgeons' fees, multiple specialist fees, and laboratory and radiology charges are paid for by the private health insurer. Depending on the nature of the illness and treatment, the patient might be discharged and the journey ends; or referred for rehabilitation and sub-acute care and/or community care before their final discharge. A point to note is that although the diagram shows the different stages of the healthcare journey, not all patients will experience all stages of the journey. The level of care required and the coordination among careers could determine the path, as well as the duration of the journey.

As in the Australia, in most countries healthcare delivery requires coordination among several healthcare professionals. The importance of collaboration and coordination is clearly reflected in case of *task-dependency*. For example, when a specialist wishes to explore the presenting problem in greater detail, the patient is sent to a diagnostic centre for further pathology and radiology services. The specialist may also request the patient to come back for a visit a couple of days later. If the diagnostic centre does not provide the results of medical tests within a specified time then the physician may not be able to suggest any additional medication to that patient during the next visit. This kind of *task-dependency* eventually creates an interdependent network among different participating service providers, for example, between the physician and diagnostic centre. Such task dependencies demand efficient collaboration and coordination for better outcomes for the patient. As the different service providers provide different aspects of care (e.g. the diagnostic centre conducts medical tests and the physician recommends the medication to patients), they do not necessarily work together. However, there is a clear need for providers to work together while treating patients with chronic problems or patients who are admitted for acute care. When a patient with a chronic problem such as diabetes or asthma is admitted to a hospital, the treatment may require several visits by multiple specialists. During the course of treatment, they may need to change their medications depending on the patient's health condition and response to other medications. In this case, a proper collaboration among these physicians is mandatory, as they work towards the shared goal of improving the patient's condition.

Gathering appropriate information regarding the collaboration among corresponding healthcare professionals is an arduous task. In Taiwan, for example, the government of Taiwan[2] has made public health services data available to encourage researchers to conduct research in this era. For our research in this paper, we have chosen private health insurance claims data set to study collaboration that occurs among providers while treating patients who are members of a private health insurance provider.

In Australia, for instance, all physicians who treat a patient during a hospital admission send their claims to the patient's private health insurer (PHI). Typically, a claim specifies details about what service is provided to the patient, by whom the service is provided and the cost of those services. There can be several claims from several providers during the course of treating a patient for a specific hospital admission.

The claims data received by PHIs are unique as both business data (e.g. cost of services) and clinical data in the form of specific procedure codes as per Commonwealth Medical Benefits Schedule (CMBS)[3] are available to them via the claim forms (Srinivasan & Arunasalam, 2013). In general, health insurance claim data sets contain a large number of claims that cover a wide variety of medical services, a broad geographic area and a long time period. In addition to utilisation statistics of different medical services and procedures, health insurance claim data set reveals information about interactions among different health service providing units (e.g. physician and hospital) during the course of providing treatment to patients.

This paper presents a social-network based framework that uses the rich claim data set as the source to analyse collaborations that occur while treating admitted patients. Figure 5 shows the framework to explore the collaboration and communication networks among healthcare professionals while treating admitted patients.

*Figure 5. A generic research framework to explore different collaboration networks among healthcare professionals and patients*

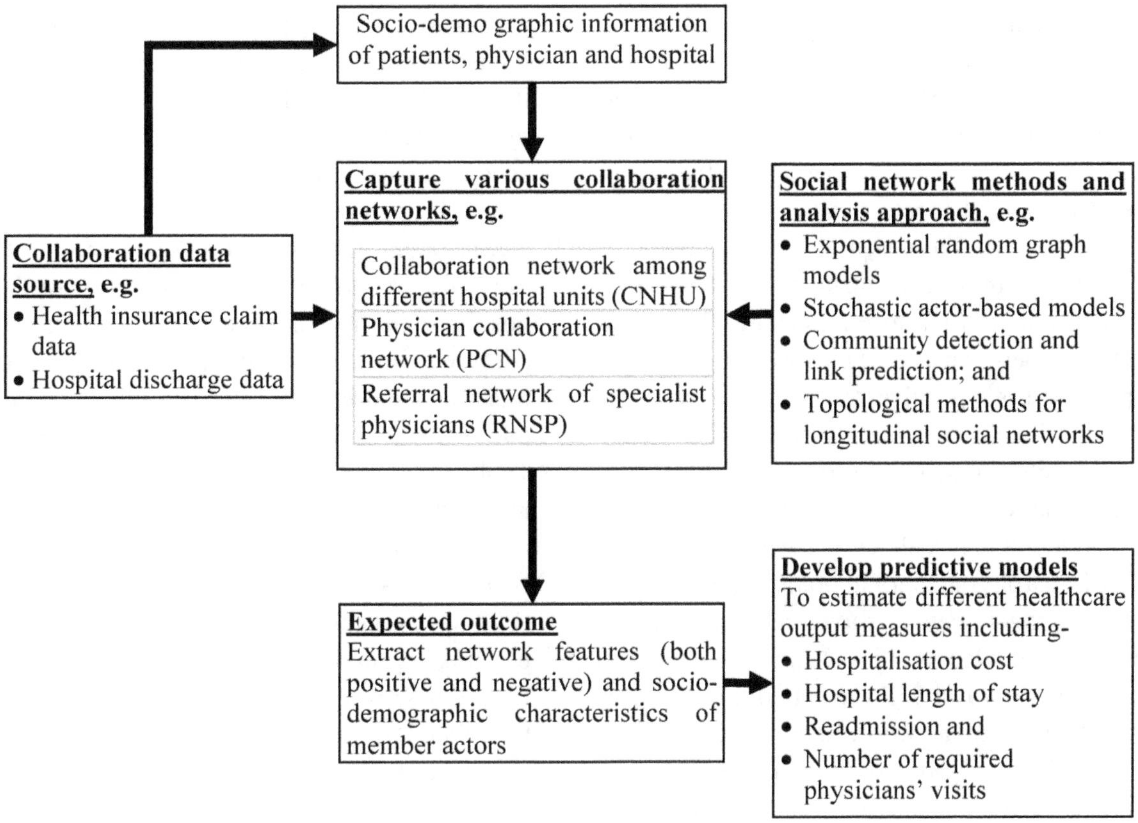

As indicated earlier this framework is based on two network theories (i.e. Bavelas' centralisation theory (Bavelas, 1950) and Freeman's centrality theory (Freeman, 1978)). These theories explain structural changes of actors within a network and their impact on individual and group performances. In order to understand the collaboration that occurs during a treatment episode, we first extract specific data items required to construct different coordination and collaboration networks that evolve during the course of providing healthcare services to patients. For example, the networks that can be constructed from this data could include: (i) coordination network among different hospital units, and (ii) physician collaboration network. These networks can then be analysed using different social network analysis techniques such as social network centrality measures and exponential random graph models.

For research analysis purposes, only social network analysis methods and approaches have been chosen since, according to Bavelas (1950) experiment and Freeman's (1978) Centralisation theory, network positions of actors have impact on their ability to perform. In this analysis, socio-demographic characteristics (e.g. age of patient, location of the hospital and experience of the physician) of the member actors of these networks are also considered. These will ultimately enable us to explore the impact and influence of these characteristics on network formation and subsequent healthcare performance. We expect this analysis to provide both positive and negative network features of the corresponding collaboration networks. Positive network features are the properties of coordination and collaboration networks that are conducive to healthcare performance. For example, if a physician collaboration network with a higher *network density* shows better healthcare performance in terms of less hospitalisation cost then the *density* is a positive network feature for that collaboration network. In contrast, negative network features are not conducive to better healthcare performance. Finally, this framework develops predictive models using the extracted network features for estimating different healthcare outcome measures (e.g. hospitalisation cost and readmission rate) that can be utilised in any predictive health analytics tool.

## METHODOLOGY AND APPLICATION OF THE PROPOSED RESEARCH FRAMEWORK: A CASE STUDY

In this section, we present a specific case study that explores physicians' collaboration which occurred while treating patients undergoing hip replacement surgery, covering a four year period. The data is provided by an Australian not-for-profit health insurance organisation. The data set includes three distinct categories of claims: (i) ancillary claims; (ii) medical claims; and (iii) hospital claims. Ancillary claims are submitted by providers for auxiliary services such as dental, optical, physiotherapy, dietetics, etc. Medical claims are lodged by physicians, surgeons, anaesthetists and other medical providers involved in treating the patient. Hospital claims are submitted by the hospital for all hospital services such as accommodation, theatre, ICU charges, etc. For research analysis purpose, this study considers claims data of hospital admissions only for total hip replacement (THR) patients from 85 different hospitals. In these hospitals, 2352 patients were admitted during the data collection period. In total, these patients lodged 1388 ancillary claims, 69619 medical claims and 24559 hospital claims. Table 1 shows the basic statistical details of the research data set.

Collaborations among physicians, which is termed as *Physician Collaboration Network* (PCN), emerge when they visit common hospital patients (Landon et al., 2012; Uddin, et al., 2012). Figure 6 shows the construction of a PCN and the related network and performance measures.

The left-hand portion of Figure 6 (i.e. Construction of physician collaboration network)

*Table 1. Basic statistics of the research data set*

| Item | Value (Std) |
|---|---|
| Number of patients | 2352 |
| Average LoS of patients | 10.51 (12.11) |
| Average age of patients | 65.02 (16.09) |
| **Gender distribution of patient** | |
| Female | 1302 |
| Male | 1050 |
| **Number of different types of claims** | |
| Hospital claim | 24559 |
| Medical claim | 69619 |
| Ancillary claim | 1388 |

illustrates an example of such a PCN construction. In a hospital (say *H1*), physicians *Ph.A* and *Ph.C*, visit patient *Pa.1*; *Ph.A* and *Ph.B* visit patient *Pa.2*. This is depicted in the *patient-physician* network in the top-left corner of Figure 6. The corresponding physician collaboration network (PCN) for this *patient-physician* network is demonstrated in the bottom-left corner of Figure 6. In this PCN, there are network connections between *Ph.A* and *Ph.B* and between *Ph.A* and *Ph.C* because they visit a common patient. As people have hospital admissions for a wide range of illness and patients need to be seen by several specialists, different types of PCNs evolve. For example knee surgery patients could have a particular type of PCN, and patients with coronary diseases may have a different type of PCN. Since the research data set of this study contains health insurance claim data for THR patients from 85 different hospitals, 85 PCNs evolved during the data collection period. Figure 7 shows the construction of PCN from the research data set.

*Figure 6. Proposed research framework for PCN based on the generic research framework as presented in Figure 5*

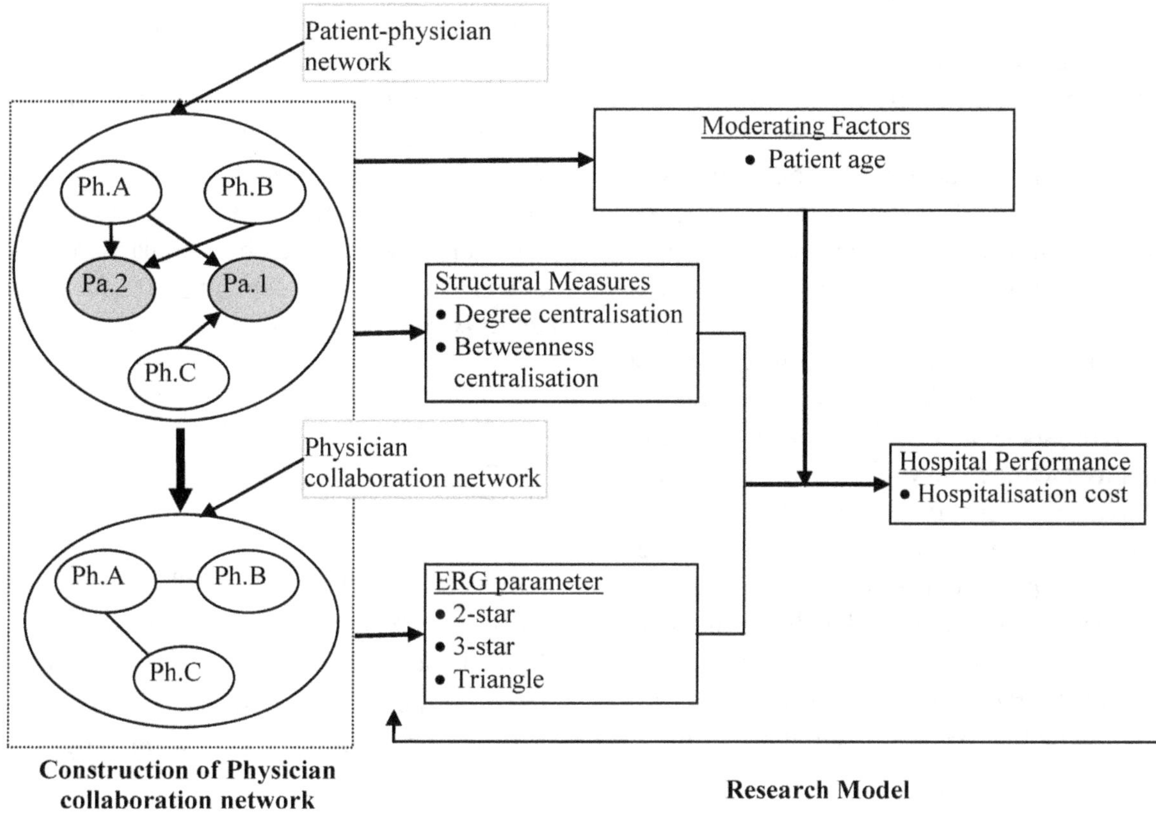

*Figure 7. Illustration of physician-patient network for two hospitals from research dataset: (a) for hospital ID 11450A_H; and (b) for hospital ID 7030Y_H. The red (circle) one indicates physician and the yellow (triangle) one indicates patient actor in these networks. From these two networks and their respective network attributes and performance values (given at the lower right corner), it is evident that structures of physician-patient network have impact on the hospital performance (i.e. total hospitalisation cost).*

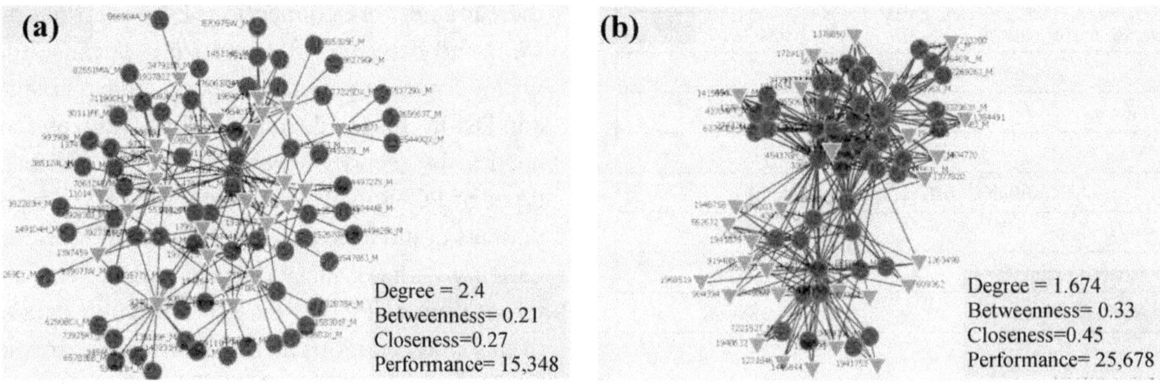


Out of these 85 PCNs, the top-5 PCNs having higher *readmission rate* are compared with the top-5 PCNs having lower *readmission rate* using exponential random graph (ERG) model in order to explore prominence of micro-structures within these two types of PCNs.

## Social Network Analysis of Physician Collaboration

In examining physician collaborations, we consider two social network analysis measures – *degree centralisation* and *betweenness centralisation*. Centralisation is a network-level measure whereas centrality is a node-level measure. Thus, the later one needs to be explained first before describing the former one. Centrality is an important concept in studying social networks. In conceptual term, centrality measures how central an individual is positioned in a network. *Degree centrality* is one of basic measures of network centrality. For an actor, it is the proportion of nodes that are adjacent to that actor in a network. It highlights the node with the most links to other actors in a network (S Wasserman & Faust, 2003). *Betweenness centrality* views an actor as being in a favoured position to the extent that the actor falls on the shortest paths between other pairs of actors in the network. That is, actors that occur on many shortest paths between the other pair of nodes have higher *betweenness centrality* than those they do not (Freeman, 1978). A centralisation measure quantifies the range or variability of individual actor indices that were calculated using one of the centrality measures. *Degree centralisation* is used to determine how centralised the *degree* of the set of actors is in a network. The set of *degree centralities*, which represents the collection of *degree* indices of *N* actors in a network, can be summarised by the following equation to measure network *degree centralisation* (Freeman, et al., 1979):

$$C_D = \frac{\sum_{i=1}^{N}[C_D(n^*) - C_D(n_i)]}{[(N-1)(N-2)]}$$

where, $\{C_D(n_i)\}$ are the *degree* indices of *N* actors and $C_D(n^*)$ is the largest observed value in the *degree* indices. For a network, *degree centralisation* (i.e. the index $C_D$) reaches its maximum value of 1 when one actor chooses all other *(N-1)* actors and the other actors interact only with this one (i.e. the situation in a *star* graph). Similarly, the set of *betweenness centralities*, which represents the collection of *betweenness* indices of $N$ actors in a network, can be summarised by the following equation to measure network *betweenness centralisation* (Freeman, et al., 1979):

$$C_B = \frac{\sum_{i=1}^{N}[C'_B(n^*) - C'_B(n_i)]}{(N-1)}$$

where, $\{C'_B(n_i)\}$ are the *betweenness* indices of $N$ actors and $C'_B(n^*)$ is the largest observed value in the *betweenness* indices.

We develop simple linear regression models to examine the effect of the above two SNA measures: *degree centralisation* and *betweenness centralisation* on the hospital outcome measure. The outcome measure chosen is the *hospitalisation cost*. Table 2 shows the performance of these two models.

The first model which is based on *degree centralisation* does not have any statistically significant effect on the *hospitalisation cost*. This is evident from the low R square value. On the other hand, *betweenness centralisation* has a negative effect on the *hospitalisation cost* as indicated by the second model.

From the perspective of a PCN structure, a high *betweenness centralisation* indicates that the PCN follows a *star-like* or *centralised* structure since *betweenness centralisation* reaches its highest value of 1 for a *star* network. A *star-like* or *centralised* network has few actors with higher *betweenness centrality* values. This indicates that only a small number of actors play a major collaboration role. What is interesting about this finding is that it shows that a star-like network among providers reduces the value of the outcome variable – which in this case is total *hospitalisation cost*. Therefore, this offers some interesting insights to healthcare managers and hospital administrators. Encouraging collaboration, with only one or two key people coordinating the communication (in other words establishing a *star-like* or *centralised* PCN) can help in reducing the total *hospitalisation cost*. However, a PCN with a flat network structure, where members of that PCN have almost equal network participation, appears to have high a *hospitalisation cost*. We do need to understand the influence of age as a moderating variable when it comes to hospital costs. Table 3 shows the effect of *patient age* as control (or moderating) variable.

Next we developed regression models by considering each of the network measures and its product with *patient age*. To show controlling effect, the product of network measure and *patient age* must show significant association with hospital outcome variable (i.e. *hospitalisation cost*) in the egression models (Baron & Kenny, 1986). This product shows a significant association for the second model in Table 3. That means *patient age* moderates only the relation between *betweenness centralisation* and *hospitalisation cost*. Although medical studies (e.g. Landon et al., 2013) suggest that *patient age* has an impact on patient outcomes, we notice some inconsistent outcomes. Out of the two models shown in Table 3, model 2 shows statistically significant effect

*Table 2. Linear regression models between each of network attributes (i.e. degree centralisation and betweenness centralisation) of PCN and hospital performance measure (i.e. hospitalisation cost)*

| Model | Dependent Variable | Independent Variable | $R^2$ value | β | Constant | Significance |
|---|---|---|---|---|---|---|
| 1 | Hospitalisation cost | Degree centralisation | 0.012 | 5906.42 | 19545.39 | 0.309 |
| 2 | Hospitalisation cost | Betweenness centralisation | 0.107 | -12384.79 | 27101.96 | 0.015 |

*Table 3. Linear regression models for checking controlling effect of patient age on the relation between each of network attributes (i.e. degree centralisation and betweenness centralisation) of PCN and hospital performance measure (i.e. hospitalisation cost)*

| Model | Dependent Variable | $R^2$ Value | Constant | Independent Variable | β | Significance |
|---|---|---|---|---|---|---|
| 1 | Hospitalisation cost | 0.102 | 20016.04 | Degrees centralisation | -26621.75 | 0.084 |
| | | | | Degree centralisation*Age | 463.16 | 0.102 |
| 2 | Hospitalisation cost | 0.227 | 27106.44 | Betweenness centralisation | -102698.68 | 0.000 |
| | | | | Betweenness centralisation*Age | 1318.36 | 0.000 |

while model 1 does not. This can be explained by the fact that we consider the average age of all patients in calculating *patient age* for a PCN. On the other hand, studies of present healthcare literature consider *patient age* at the individual level, not at the aggregate level as in this study.

Models of social network analysis have been utilised extensively to understand the structural dynamics of various collaboration networks (Shahadat Uddin, Jafar Hamra, et al., 2013a; S Wasserman & Faust, 2003). One of the widely used social network models is exponential random graph model which can effectively identify structural properties of network formation process (Stanley Wasserman & Pattison, 1996). Next, we will use exponential random graph models to understand the micro structures that influence the development process of the PCN.

## Exponential Random Graph (ERG) Modelling of Physician Collaborations

An ERG model simplifies a complex structure down to a combination of basic parameters. It can effectively identify structural properties in social networks (Snijders et al., 2006). This theory-driven modelling approach also allows us to test the significance of structural parameters in the process of the formation of a given network (Snijders, et al., 2006; S Wasserman & Faust, 2003). For instance, a given cost effective PCN may be explored using ERG model to examine what micro structures play a statistically significant role in the development process of that PCN. A commonly used sub-class of ERG models is the Markov random graph in which a possible tie from *i* to *j* is assumed conditionally dependent only on other possible ties involving *i* and/or *j* (Frank & Strauss, 1986). This sub-class of ERG models is also known as the low-order model which is utilised to explore PCNs having higher and lower readmission rates. The configurations and parameters of low-order model are shown in Figure 8.

These parameters relate to some well-known structural regularity in the network literature and represent structural tendencies in the network (e.g. mutuality and transitivity). They were chosen because they are conceptualised as forces which drive the formation of the network itself. For example, *transitivity* is conceptualised as a force which drives the formation of the network itself (the friends of our friends are more likely to be our friends). An example of a Markov random graph model for non-directed networks, with *edge* (or density), *2-star*, *3-star* and *triangle* parameters, is given below (Robins et al., 2007):

$$\Pr(X = x) = \frac{1}{k} \exp\left\{\theta L(x) + \sigma_2 S_2(x) + \sigma_3 S_3(x) + \tau T(x)\right\}$$

*Figure 8. Configurations of low-order Markov graph (Robins et al., 2007). This study considers only these four configurations for ERG modelling*

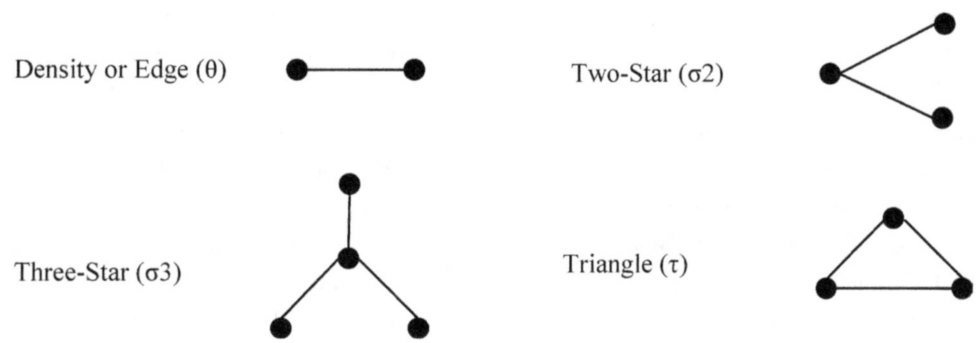


In Eq.(1), $\theta$ is the density or edge parameter and $L(x)$ refers to the number of edges in the graph $x$; $\sigma_k$ and $S_k(x)$ refer to the parameter associated with *k-star* effects and the number of *k-stars* in $x$; while $\tau$ and $T(x)$ refer to the parameter for triangles and the number of triangles, respectively. Goodness-of-fit (GOF) measure is used to test whether a given model fits the network data. A parameter estimate in the model can be assumed to have converged if the GOF index is below 0.10 (Snijders, et al., 2006).

Using Pnet[4], five PCNs with highest *readmission rate* and five PCNs with lowest *readmission rate* were fitted with a low-order model, i.e. *2-star*, *3-star* and *triangle* model. Here, the GOF is less than 0.1, showing a good fit of the parameters of the model. Out of the three parameters, only the *triangle* parameter (subset of 3 nodes in which each node is connected to the rest 2 node) is found to have significant effect for all PCNs. The significance for each parameter is replicated by another variable, called *t-statistics*. A *t-statistics* value of $\geq 2$ is considered to have significance effect for a given parameter. Only *triangle* parameter shows t-statistics value $\geq 2$ for all 10 PCNs. As a part of ERG output, Pnet also produces values of *t-statistics* for each parameter of the model. The positive *triangle* parameter can be interpreted as providing evidence that the ties tend to occur in triangular structures and hence will cluster into clique-like forms. A *t-test* further reveals that there is a significant difference for the *triangle* parameter between PCNs with higher readmission rate and PCNs with lower readmission rate ($t(10) = -3.05$, $p<0.05$). The result shows that, on average, the *triangle* parameter for PCNs with higher *readmission rate* (Mean = 16.49, Standard Error = 1.47) is more positive than the parameter for PCNs with lower *readmission rate* (Mean = 5.90, Standard Error = 1.48). Therefore, the presence of a higher number of *triangle* structures in PCNs with higher *readmission rate* indicates that most actors are likely to have more connections with others. That means all network actors have almost same number of connections with others. On the other hand, PCNs with lower *readmission rate* do not have prevalence of such actors in the network structures, indicating that the possibility of the presence of some actors that have more connections within the network compared to others.

In summary, this case study illustrates the application of the proposed research framework for analysing healthcare collaboration. We have used social network analysis measures and exponential random graph models to explore physician collaborations. Further, we have made some observations on social network attributes of effective and efficient collaborations among physicians, in relation to *hospitalisation cost* and *readmission rate*.

## DISCUSSION AND CONCLUSION

In this chapter, we have presented a framework based on network theories to: (i) explore the nature of collaboration among physicians while providing patient care; (ii) develop a set of network measures that provide insights into both positive and negative impact of collaboration on healthcare performance; and (iii) analyse the network values of centrality and centralisation and provide some intuitive evidence of their impact on healthcare performance as well as health outcomes for the patient.

The work presented in this paper is firmly grounded in both theory and practice as we illustrate the impact network measures in real life data from the private health insurance domain. In order to make the framework practical for health care providers, we have provided illustrative examples of physicians' collaboration while treating patients with a specific problem of hip replacement surgery. While a focussed healthcare domain example has been used, the framework itself is generic and offers a platform to study the impact of collaboration among actors involved in providing services towards achieving a common goal.

Physician collaborations have been analysed by following the proposed research framework of this study. In doing so, we considered measures of social network analysis and exponential random graph models as methodological techniques or tools, patient age as moderating factor and hospitalisation cost as the outcome measure. Based on the assumption that collaboration emerges between two physicians when they visit a common patient, PCNs are constructed in this study from the information of physicians' visits to patients during their hospitalisation periods. It is a standard professional practice that when physicians visit patients they give advice or suggestions to patients based on their health condition and previous medication history deposited in the patient *log book*. All previous advice or suggestions prescribed by any physician to a patient have been taken into consideration during any subsequent physician visit to that patient. It is noticed that the differences in performance measures (e.g. *hospitalisation cost* and *readmission rate*) among PCNs having various network structures can be explained by social network measures (i.e. *betweenness centrality*) and exponential random graph model (i.e. *triangle* parameter of the model).

The findings from the research example of this study could be utilised by hospital administrators to reflect on the nature of collaborations that occur during the course of treating a patient and encourage collaboration models that lead to better outcomes for patients. For example, a low *betweenness centralisation* in a PCN indicates a lower hospitalisation cost for the hospitalised patients, which could indirectly reflect an improved level of healthcare coordination among healthcare professionals in that PCN. Managers could encourage a practice culture where a few physicians have significantly higher number of links with their colleagues.

Although insights gained from this research have interesting applications, there are several limitations. Firstly, this study developed network structures of physician collaborations based on the presence of shared patients using administrative health insurance claim data. Although this technique has been validated (Shahadat Uddin, Liaquat Hossain, Jafar Hamra, et al., 2013), it nevertheless cannot be known what information or behaviour, if any, have an impact on the ties defined by shared patients. Secondly, although the proposed research framework can examine various collaboration networks among healthcare professionals in respect of their perceived level of desired outcomes, it cannot explain the mechanism by which these collaborations evolve over time. Finally, the possibility of unobserved confounders that could help to explain the mechanisms driving the associations that were found in this study cannot be ruled out, although patient age was used as a covariate to adjust these associations.

This research has the potential to open up several new research opportunities for healthcare researchers. Using the proposed framework of this study, researchers could explore other type of collaboration networks (e.g. collaboration networks among different hospital units) in order to find out effective and efficient collaboration structures among healthcare professionals for providing healthcare services. Another area of research is to consider qualitative measures (e.g. patient satisfaction (Reid et al., 2010)), in addition to quantitative measures, to explore the performance of healthcare collaborations. The proposed framework could be used to study physician collaboration networks for chronic patients, as well as for patients in intensive care and others requiring high level of care due to multiple comorbidities. Other social network measures (e.g. closeness centrality) and modelling approach (e.g. stochastic actor-oriented models) could be utilised for analysing and modelling physician collaboration networks for treating more complicated conditions. Finally, node-level attributes of physicians (e.g. level of education and year of experience of healthcare professional) may be considered while exploring collaboration networks.

## ACKNOWLEDGMENT

The authors would like to thank the anonymous reviewers and the editor for their insightful comments and suggestions.

## REFERENCES

Abbasi, A., Hossain, L., Uddin, S., & Rasmussen, K. J. R. (2011). Evolutionary dynamics of scientific collaboration networks: multi-levels and cross-time analysis. *Scientometrics*, *89*(2), 687–710. doi:10.1007/s11192-011-0463-1

Abbasi, A., Uddin, S., & Hossain, L. (2012). Socioeconomic analysis of patient-centric networks: effects of patients and hospitals' characteristics and network structure on hospitalization costs. *The European Journal of Health Economics*, *13*(3), 267–276. doi:10.1007/s10198-011-0303-5 PMID:21347691

Ahuja, M., Galletta, D., & Carley, K. (2003). Individual centrality and performance in virtual R&D groups: An empirical study. *Management Science*, *49*(1), 21–38. doi:10.1287/mnsc.49.1.21.12756

Arbuthnott, A., & Sharpe, D. (2009). The effect of physician-patient collaboration on patient adherence in non-psychiatric medicine. *Patient Education and Counseling*, *77*(1), 60–67. doi:10.1016/j.pec.2009.03.022 PMID:19395222

Baron, R. M., & Kenny, D. A. (1986). The moderator-mediator variable distinction in social psychological research: Conceptual, strategic, and statistical considerations. *Journal of Personality and Social Psychology*, *51*(6), 1173–1182. doi:10.1037/0022-3514.51.6.1173 PMID:3806354

Bavelas, A. (1950). Communication patterns in task-oriented groups. *The Journal of the Acoustical Society of America*, *22*, 725–730. doi:10.1121/1.1906679

Beauchamp, M. (1965). An improved index of centrality. *Behavioral Science*, *10*(2), 161–163. doi:10.1002/bs.3830100205 PMID:14284290

Bonacich, P. (1991). Simultaneous group and individual centralities. *Social Networks*, *13*(2), 155–168. doi:10.1016/0378-8733(91)90018-O

Brass, D. (1981). Structural relationships, job characteristics, and worker satisfaction and performance. *Administrative Science Quarterly*, *26*(3), 331–348. doi:10.2307/2392511

Brass, D. (1985). Technology and the structuring of jobs: Employee satisfaction, performance, and influence. *Organizational Behavior and Human Decision Processes*, *35*(2), 216–240. doi:10.1016/0749-5978(85)90036-6

Burns, L. R., & Muller, R. W. (2008). Hospital-Physician Collaboration: Landscape of Economic Integration and Impact on Clinical Integration. *The Milbank Quarterly*, *86*(3), 375–434. doi:10.1111/j.1468-0009.2008.00527.x PMID:18798884

Cainelli, G., Maggioni, M. A., Uberti, T. E., & De Felice, A. (2010). *The strength of strong ties: Co-authorship and productivity among Italian economists*. University of Padova.

Cohn, B., & Marriott, M. (1958). Networks and centres in the integration of Indian civilization. *Journal of Social Research*, *1*(1), 1–9.

Cowan, M., Shapiro, M., Hays, R., Afifi, A., Vazirani, S., Ward, C., & Ettner, S. (2006). The effect of a multidisciplinary hospitalist/physician and advanced practice nurse collaboration on hospital costs. *The Journal of Nursing Administration*, *36*(2), 79–85. doi:10.1097/00005110-200602000-00006 PMID:16528149

Cross, R., & Cummings, J. (2004). Tie and network correlates of individual performance in knowledge-intensive work. *Academy of Management Journal*, *47*(6), 928–937. doi:10.2307/20159632

Cunningham, F. C., Ranmuthugala, G., Plumb, J., Georgiou, A., Westbrook, J. I., & Braithwaite, J. (2012). Health professional networks as a vector for improving healthcare quality and safety: a systematic review. *BMJ Quality & Safety*, *21*(3), 239–249. doi:10.1136/bmjqs-2011-000187 PMID:22129933

Faust, K. (1997). Centrality in affiliation networks. *Social Networks*, *19*(2), 157–191. doi:10.1016/S0378-8733(96)00300-0

Frank, O., & Strauss, D. (1986). Markov graphs. *Journal of the American Statistical Association*, *81*(395), 832–842. doi:10.1080/01621459.1986.10478342

Freeman, L. (1978). Centrality in social networks: Conceptual clarification. *Social Networks*, *1*(3), 215–239. doi:10.1016/0378-8733(78)90021-7

Freeman, L., Roeder, D., & Mulholland, R. (1979). Centrality in Social Networks: II. Experimental Results. *Social Networks*, *2*(80), 119–141. doi:10.1016/0378-8733(79)90002-9

Gaboury, I., Bujold, M., Boon, H., & Moher, D. (2009). Interprofessional collaboration within Canadian integrative healthcare clinics: Key components. *Social Science & Medicine*, *69*(5), 707–715. doi:10.1016/j.socscimed.2009.05.048 PMID:19608320

Hossain, L., Wu, A., & Chung, K. (2006). *Actor centrality correlates to project based coordination*. Academic Press.

Hunt, J. S., Siemienczuk, J., Pape, G., Rozenfeld, Y., MacKay, J., LeBlanc, B. H., & Touchette, D. (2008). A randomized controlled trial of team-based care: impact of physician-pharmacist collaboration on uncontrolled hypertension. *Journal of General Internal Medicine*, *23*(12), 1966–1972. doi:10.1007/s11606-008-0791-x PMID:18815843

Knaus, W. E., Draper, W. D. P., & Zimmerman, J. E. (1986). An evaluation of outcome from intensive care in major medical centers. *Annals of Internal Medicine*, *104*(3), 410–418. doi:10.7326/0003-4819-104-3-410 PMID:3946981

Landon, B. E., Keating, N. L., Barnett, M. L., Onnela, J.-P., Paul, S., & O'Malley, A. J. et al. (2012). Variation in patient-sharing networks of physicians across the United States. *Journal of the American Medical Association*, *308*(3), 265–273. doi:10.1001/jama.2012.7615 PMID:22797644

Landon, B. E., Onnela, J.-P., Keating, N. L., Barnett, M. L., Paul, S., & O'Malley, A. J. et al. (2013). Using Administrative Data to Identify Naturally Occurring Networks of Physicians. *Medical Care*. doi:10.1097/MLR.0b013e3182977991 PMID:23807593

Leavitt, H. (1949). *Some effects of certain communication patterns on group performance*. Boston: MIT Press.

Leavitt, H. (1951). Some effects of certain communication patterns on group performance. *Journal of Abnormal and Social Psychology*, *46*(1), 38–50. doi:10.1037/h0057189 PMID:14813886

Meltzer, D., Chung, J., Khalili, P., Marlow, E., Arora, V., Schumock, G., & Burt, R. (2010). Exploring the use of social network methods in designing healthcare quality improvement teams. *Social Science & Medicine*, *71*(6), 1119–1130. doi:10.1016/j.socscimed.2010.05.012 PMID:20674116

Mullen, B., & Eduardo, J. (1991). Effects of communication network structure: Components of positional centrality* 1. *Social Networks*, *13*(2), 169–185. doi:10.1016/0378-8733(91)90019-P

Netting, F. E., & Williams, F. G. (1996). Case manager-physician collaboration: Implications for professional identity, roles, and relationships. *Health & Social Work*, *21*(3), 216–224. PMID:8854126

Pfeffer, J. (1980). A partial test of the social information processing model of job attitudes. *Human Relations*, *33*(7), 457. doi:10.1177/001872678003300702

Pitts, F. (1965). A graph theoretic approach to historical geography. *The Professional Geographer*, *17*(5), 15–20. doi:10.1111/j.0033-0124.1965.015_m.x

Reid, R. J., Coleman, K., Johnson, E. A., Fishman, P. A., Hsu, C., & Soman, M. P. et al. (2010). The group health medical home at year two: cost savings, higher patient satisfaction, and less burnout for providers. *Health Affairs*, *29*(5), 835–843. doi:10.1377/hlthaff.2010.0158 PMID:20439869

Robins, G., Pattison, P., Kalish, Y., & Lusher, D. (2007). An introduction to exponential random graph (p*) models for social networks. *Social Networks, 29*(2), 173-191. DOI: 10.1016/j.socnet.2006.08.002

Salancik, G., & Pfeffer, J. (1978). A social information processing approach to job attitudes and task design. *Administrative Science Quarterly*, *23*(2), 224–253. doi:10.2307/2392563 PMID:10307892

Shahian, D. M., Wolf, R. E., Iezzoni, L. I., Kirle, L., & Normand, S. L. T. (2010). Variability in the measurement of hospital-wide mortality rates. *The New England Journal of Medicine*, *363*(26), 2530–2539. doi:10.1056/NEJMsa1006396 PMID:21175315

Shippy, R., Cantor, M., & Brennan, M. (2004). Social networks of aging gay men. *Journal of Men's Studies*, *13*(1), 107–120. doi:10.3149/jms.1301.107

Smith, H., Rogers, Y., & Brady, M. (2003). *Managing one's social network: Does age make a difference*. Academic Press.

Snijders, T. A. B., Pattison, P. E., Robins, G. L., & Handcock, M. S. (2006). New specifications for exponential random graph models. *Sociological Methodology*, *36*(1), 99–153. doi:10.1111/j.1467-9531.2006.00176.x

Sommers, L. S., Marton, K. I., Barbaccia, J. C., & Randolph, J. (2000). Physician, nurse, and social worker collaboration in primary care for chronically ill seniors. *Archives of Internal Medicine*, *160*(12), 1825–1833. doi:10.1001/archinte.160.12.1825 PMID:10871977

Sparrowe, R., Liden, R., Wayne, S., & Kraimer, M. (2001). Social networks and the performance of individuals and groups. *Academy of Management Journal*, *44*(2), 316–325. doi:10.2307/3069458

Srinivasan, U., & Arunasalam, B. (2013). Leveraging Big Data Analytics to reduce Healthcare Costs. *IT Professional*, *15*(6), 21–28. doi:10.1109/MITP.2013.55

Uddin, M., & Hossain, L. (2009). Towards coordination preparedness of soft-target organisation. Electronic Government, 54-64.

Uddin, M. S., & Hossain, L. (2009). *Exploring physical, mental and psychological health for elders through their personal networks*. Paper presented at the e-Health Networking, Applications and Services. Sydney, Australia.

Uddin, M. S., & Hossain, L. (2011). Social Networks Enabled Coordination Model for Cost Management of Patient Hospital Admissions. *Journal for Healthcare Quality*, *33*(5), 37–48. doi:10.1111/j.1945-1474.2010.00118.x PMID:23845132

Uddin, S., Chung, K. S. K., & Piraveenan, M. (2012). *Capturing Actor-level Dynamics of Longitudinal Networks*. Paper presented at the Advances in Social Networks Analysis and Mining (ASONAM). New York, NY.

Uddin, S., Hamra, J., & Hossain, L. (2013a). Exploring communication networks to understand organizational crisis using exponential random graph models. *Computational & Mathematical Organization Theory*, *19*(1), 25–41. doi:10.1007/s10588-011-9104-8

Uddin, S., Hamra, J., & Hossain, L. (2013b). Mapping and modeling of physician collaboration network. *Statistics in Medicine*, *32*(20), 3539–3551. doi:10.1002/sim.5770 PMID:23468249

Uddin, S., & Hossain, L. (2011). Disaster coordination preparedness of soft target organisations. *Disasters*, *35*(3), 623–638. doi:10.1111/j.1467-7717.2011.01229.x PMID:21272059

Uddin, S., & Hossain, L. (2012). Effects of Physician Collaboration Network on Hospital Outcomes. In *Proceedings of Australasian Workshop on Health Informatics and Knowledge Management*. Academic Press.

Uddin, S., & Hossain, L. (2013). Dyad and Triad Census Analysis of Crisis Communication Network. *Social Networking*, *2*(1), 32–41. doi:10.4236/sn.2013.21004

Uddin, S., Hossain, L., Abbasi, A., & Rasmussen, K. (2012). Trend and efficiency analysis of co-authorship network. *Scientometrics*, *90*(2), 687–699. doi:10.1007/s11192-011-0511-x

Uddin, S., Hossain, L., Hamra, J., & Alam, A. (2013). A study of physician collaborations through social network and exponential random graph. *BMC Health Services Research*, *13*(1), 234–247. doi:10.1186/1472-6963-13-234 PMID:23803165

Uddin, S., Hossain, L., & Kelaher, M. (2012). Effect of physician collaboration network on hospitalization cost and readmission rate. *European Journal of Public Health*, *22*(5), 629–633. doi:10.1093/eurpub/ckr153 PMID:22037593

Uddin, S., Hossain, L., & Rasmussen, K. (2013). Network Effects on Scientific Collaborations. *PLoS ONE*, *8*(2), e57546. doi:10.1371/journal.pone.0057546 PMID:23469021

Uddin, S., & Jacobson, M. J. (2013). Dynamics of email communications among university students throughout a semester. *Computers & Education*, *64*, 95–103. doi:10.1016/j.compedu.2013.01.014

Uddin, S., Murshed, S. T. H., & Hossain, L. (2011). Power-law behaviour in complex organizational communication network during crisis. *Physica A: Statistical Mechanics and its Applications*, *390*(15), 2845-2853.

Uddin, S., Piraveenan, M., Chung, K., & Hossain, L. (2013). *Topological Analysis of Longitudinal Networks*. Paper presented at the Hawaii International Conference on System Sciences (HICSS-46). Hawaii, HI.

Uddin, S., Thompson, K., Schwendimann, B., & Piraveenan, M. (2014). The impact of study load on the dynamics of longitudinal email communications among students. *Computers & Education*, *72*, 209–219. doi:10.1016/j.compedu.2013.11.007

Wasserman, S., & Faust, K. (2003). *Social network analysis: Methods and applications*. Cambridge: Cambridge University Press.

Wasserman, S., & Pattison, P. (1996). Logit models and logistic regressions for social networks: I. An introduction to Markov graphs and P. *Psychometrika*, *61*(3), 401–425. doi:10.1007/BF02294547

## KEY TERMS AND DEFINITIONS

**Betweenness Centralisation:** It quantifies the range or variability in the betweenness centrality values of individual actors in a social network.

**Betweenness Centrality:** It views an actor as being in a favoured position to the extent that the actor falls on the shortest paths between other pairs of actors in the network. That is, actors that occur on many shortest paths between the other pair of nodes have higher betweenness centrality than those they do not.

**Degree Centralisation:** It quantifies the range or variability in the degree centrality values of individual actors in a social network.

**Degree Centrality:** It is one of basic measures of the network centrality. For an actor, it is the proportion of other actors that are adjacent to that actor in a network. It highlights the actor with the most links to other actors in a network.

**Exponential Random Graph Model:** An exponential random graph model simplifies a complex structure down to a combination of basic network structure (e.g. edge). It can effectively identify structural properties in social networks.

**Physician Collaboration Network:** Physicians collaborate among themselves in order to provide effective healthcare services to patients. This leads to the development of an informal collaboration network among physicians, which is termed as physician collaboration network in this study.

**Social Network:** A social network is a set of actors (e.g. individuals or organisation) and relations (e.g. friendship, kinship, common interest, sexual relationship and financial exchange) that hold the actors together.

**Social Network Analysis:** Social network analysis is the mapping and measuring of relationships among actors in a social network, which provides both a visual and mathematical analysis of network relations among participating actors.

## ENDNOTES

1 http://hushp.harvard.edu/sites/default/files

2 http://nhird.nhri.org.tw/en/

3 http://www.mbsonline.gov.au/

4 http://www.sna.unimelb.edu.au/pnet/pnet.html

# Chapter 4
# Privacy Perceptions of Older Adults when Using Social Media Technologies

**Dan Dumbrell**
*The University of Sydney, Australia*

**Robert Steele**
*The University of Sydney, Australia*

## ABSTRACT

*Social media technologies represent an emerging means by which older adults can access health and community information, engage in peer-to-peer information sharing, and also potentially decrease social isolation. Privacy concerns, however, have been consistently identified as a barrier for older adults' use of the Web and social media technologies. The authors conduct a preliminary study involving 150 older adult participants, investigating their use and perceptions of social media technologies. The trial involved first providing the participants with brief training in three common social media technologies: Facebook, Twitter, and Skype. The authors carried out a quantitative and qualitative analysis of the participant's use and privacy perceptions of these technologies. Overall, the results are promising as to the potential to address privacy concerns to enable older adults to further utilize these technologies for improved mental, physical, and social health. Implications for future research and usage within the older adult community are also discussed.*

## INTRODUCTION

Social media technologies, such as Facebook and Twitter, have experienced widespread uptake by users worldwide since their relatively recent introduction as platforms for online peer-to-peer communication and information sharing. More recently, the utilization of social media technologies for health information dissemination has been explored (Steele, 2011) and it has been found that social media postings do refer to many types of health-related information (Dumbrell and Steele, 2013). According to recent reports such as Zickuhr and Madden (2012), there has been a large increase in the proportion of older adults (aged 55 and over) that are adopting social media technologies and

DOI: 10.4018/978-1-4666-6316-9.ch004

using them as a means of socially connecting with others. In addition, with the ageing population of the world (and thus Internet users), it can be noted that the use of these media for older adults to access health information can potentially provide benefits in relation to physical and mental health and general well being for individuals.

Whilst there are many potential benefits that could result from the use of social media, there are issues that must be explored that possibly affect older adult's willingness to use these technologies. One of these major issues is concerns about privacy, which has been consistently identified as a barrier for older adult use of the Internet and social media systems. These privacy concerns have also been investigated with online users and the access and sharing of digital health information (Fink and Beck, 2013; Park, 2013). In addition, the recent revelations of Web-based breaches of privacy, as well as the development of laws in relation to online privacy, can potentially affect the perceptions and uptake of use of these technologies by older adults. Therefore further research must be carried out to uncover the specific reasons for the concerns and barriers affecting use.

In this chapter we describe results from a study that was carried out to identify and analyze the effects of introducing social media technologies to an older adult participant sample group (aged 55 and over). The broader goal of this study was to consider whether or not the use of these technologies had any impact on the levels of social isolation and loneliness of older adults. With this as an underlying context, the purpose of this chapter is to explore and analyze the privacy perceptions of these older adults when using Twitter, Facebook and Skype within this study. The study was carried out involving 150 older adult participants, who were free to use these different technologies during a six-month trial period after they were provided with initial training. Quantitative data was gathered from the pre and post questionnaires, and results such as security perceptions and usage rankings of the respective social media technologies were identified. From the qualitative data collected from both questionnaires and the focus groups, recurring themes were identified, and sub-themes within these themes were also identified. These themes and sub-themes are also compared to the existing literature to assist in analyzing our findings as well as to identify current gaps in knowledge on this area.

## BACKGROUND

It is believed that technology usage and adoption amongst older adults will continue to grow, as the majority of baby boomers have already used computers (Harkin and Huber 2004), and are also likely to have more exposure and experience with information technologies. However previous studies indicate that the older the individual, the less likely they are to have interest and experience in using computers (Brosnan, 1998; Billipp, 2001; Czaja and Lee, 2001). Moreover, it has been found that older adults are likely to experience fear and anxiety when interacting with computers (Ellis and Allaire 1999). However it is envisioned that the future older generations may not experience the same level of anxiety and fear that current older generations experience as many baby boomers already have experience with technologies before their retirement. For example, many of them have already used computers and email due to the prevalence of technologies in today's environment, and those below the retirement age and still working are likely to be influenced by the use of new technologies in their workplace (Harkin and Huber, 2004). Recently it has been found that half of adults aged 65 and older are now online, and one in three of these online users are on social networking sites such as Facebook (Zickuhr and Madden, 2012).

A previous qualitative study (Steele, Lo, Secombe and Wong, 2009) was conducted upon a group of senior participants, aged between 65-85 as an exploratory investigation of their perceptions, attitude and concerns towards wireless sensor network technologies in terms of their application to health care. It was found that while older adults perceive sensor networks as a viable solution enabling "ageing-in-place", their acceptance towards a technology was mainly based on its cost and their ability to interact with that piece of technology. Some of our previous findings, in particular those that provide an indication on factors determining an older adult's acceptance of technologies, were considered in designing this study.

The perceptions in relation to online privacy and related issues have been found in previous studies of older adults and Internet use. Gatto and Tak (2008) found that there were varying levels of mistrust experienced by older adults when using sites like Google, Yahoo, and health-related Web sites. These privacy issues caused many older adults to avoid activities on the Internet that required personal information, as well as question the trustworthiness of retrieved information from these sites.

## METHODS

This investigation made use of an analysis of the previous literature, then surveys and focus groups to collect and subsequently analyze data from participants drawn from the older adult population. The research project was advertised in local newspapers, local radio, magazines, local seniors clubs and other community groups, as well as sent to the large Senior's Card (a purchase discounts card issued by State and Territory governments) mailing list. Initially, approximately 230 individuals responded to these advertisements. A further screening telephone interview was carried out on these initial individuals, asking relevant questions about various factors such as: computer literacy, current use of social media technologies, access to the Internet, living arrangements, vision impairment and level of social isolation. From these individuals, 150 participants were selected to be a part of the research project. The selected participants were those: matching the 55 and over age requirement, indicating higher levels of isolation, living in their own home / not a seniors facility, with no or the lowest levels of existing use of social technologies, and those indicating they had access to a computer with Internet either at home or from a public facility.

Participants were recruited mainly from the Sydney metropolitan area but also from two regional locations where training in the technologies could take place. Following this screening-based selection, Sydney-based participants formed the majority with 127 participants, and with other participants coming from the two regional locations, north Lake Macquarie (approximately 150kms from Sydney) having 11 participants and Port Macquarie (approximately 380kms from Sydney) providing 12 participants.

Participants were divided into groups of approximately 10 people for training sessions. Each group would attend two three-hour training sessions, typically the sessions a week apart – the first teaching Twitter and Skype and the second teaching Facebook. At the commencement of the first session, participants were given a questionnaire asking them basic demographic details (e.g. age, gender, living arrangements), current experience with technology and social media sites, as well as questions in relation to loneliness, current social networks and quality of life. Participants were given the opportunity and assistance to sign up, after a brief introduction and demonstration of the potential uses, on each social media application. The instructor then went through basic functions and settings of each application following a written guide that was also provided to participants. The allocation of time required to teach the different applications was set by researchers, as it was considered that Facebook would require more time due to the larger number of settings and functions compared to Twitter and Skype.

Seven groups were comprised of participants who had indicated that they were also willing to participate in an initial focus group. These participants were notified and had consented to be audio recorded when filling out consent forms, and were again reminded of this by the interviewer before the commencement of the focus group recording. Sydney-based training sessions were held at the Australian Seniors Computer Clubs Association (ASCCA) in the Sydney CBD, Cooranbong-based training sessions and focus groups were held at Westlakes Seniors Computer Club in Lake Macquarie, and Port Macquarie-based training sessions and focus groups were held at the Port Macquarie-Hastings Library in Port Macquarie.

After the final training session, there was a six-month period (August 2012 – January 2013) in which participants were given the opportunity to trial the use of these applications. It was reiterated to participants that it was not compulsory to use all (or any) of the applications and it was up to their personal desire to use them. During this period, participants could also request technical assistance from ASCCA in relation to any computer or online issues encountered. At the end of this trial period, participants were contacted via email that follow-up data collection was to occur. Participants in initial focus groups were contacted to organize session times in which they would complete a post-trial questionnaire and partake in a follow-up focus group. Post-trial questionnaires were mailed to the remaining participants. 110 participants completed the final questionnaire, with retrieved data from these questionnaires entered into Excel and analyzed using SPSS.

Free-text and worded responses were entered into Microsoft Excel spreadsheets separately to quantitative data. A researcher manually transcribed the pre and post focus groups. Recurring themes of this collected qualitative data were identified as each participant's qualitative response data was analyzed systematically.

## FINDINGS

Participants were asked about their view of the relative privacy of the three social media platforms. Skype was identified as the overall "most secure" technology in terms of privacy with a majority of respondents (78%) finding it the "most secure". Only 14% and 8% of respondents who ranked Skype's security found it as the "second most secure" and "least secure" application respectively. Although an overwhelming proportion of the sample considered Skype as the most secure application in terms of privacy, it was identified as only the second most used technology. From those who did use Skype, approximately half responded that they used it the most during the six-month trial period. 31% of respondents who used Skype said that it was their second most used application, with the remaining 19% using Skype the least of the three social media technologies. 28 participants chose not to use Skype.

Facebook was considered the "second most secure" in terms of privacy. Only 26% of participants who used Facebook responded that it was the "most secure" in terms of privacy. A slightly larger proportion of respondents (36%) identified this social technology as the "second most secure" with the remaining respondents (38%) ranking it as "least secure" in terms of privacy. Although Facebook was perceived to be significantly less secure than Skype, participants ranked it as the "most used" technology during the six-month trial period with 57% responding with this. Smaller proportions of users ranked Facebook as the "second most used" (29%) and "least used" (14%) social media application. Facebook also had the highest rate of adoption amongst the older adult sample, with only 20 participants choosing not to use this platform.

*Figure 1. Skype privacy perceptions and usage level*

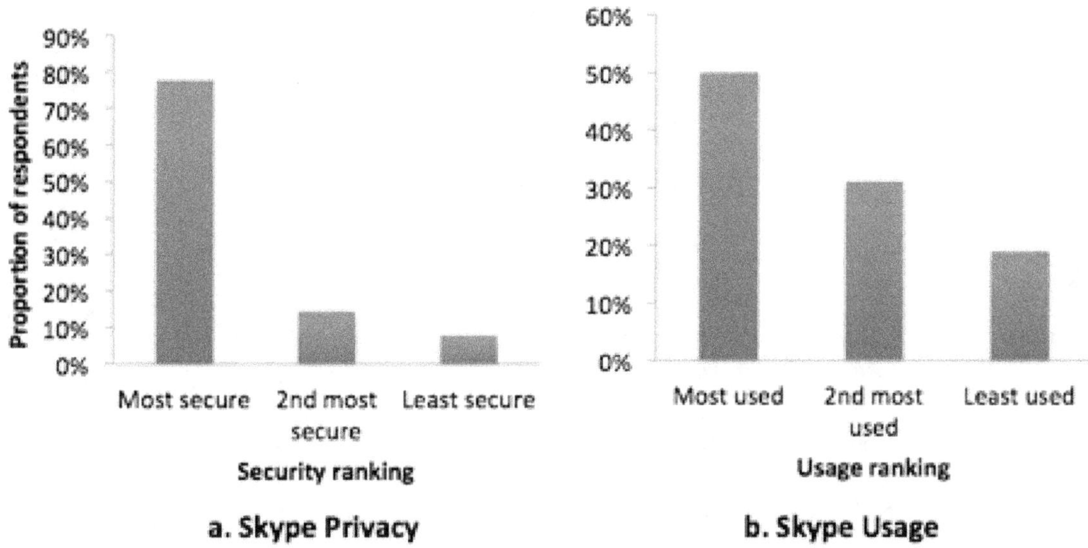


Twitter was both perceived to be the least secure in terms of privacy, and was the least used social media technology. A mere 6% of respondents ranked Twitter as the "most secure" in terms of privacy, and nearly half (49%) identified this social media technology as the "least secure" in terms of privacy. With regards to usage, 41 participants chose not to use this social media technology during the six-month trial period. When looking at those who did use the Web-based platform, only 5% ranked it as the "most used" technology of the three available. 27% identified it as the "second most used", whilst the majority (68%) used this platform the least of the three platforms.

*Figure 2. Facebook privacy perceptions and usage level*

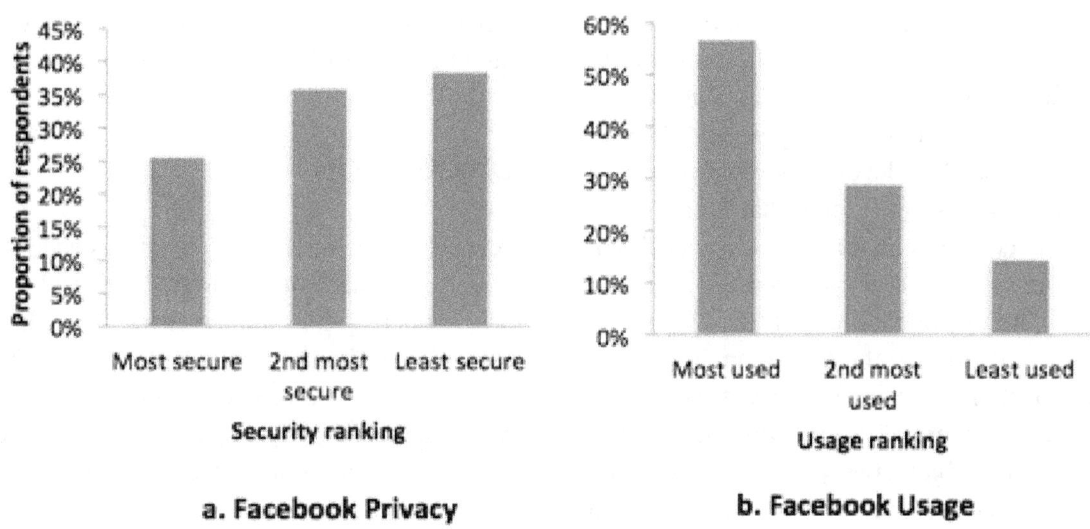

*Figure 3. Twitter privacy perceptions and usage level*

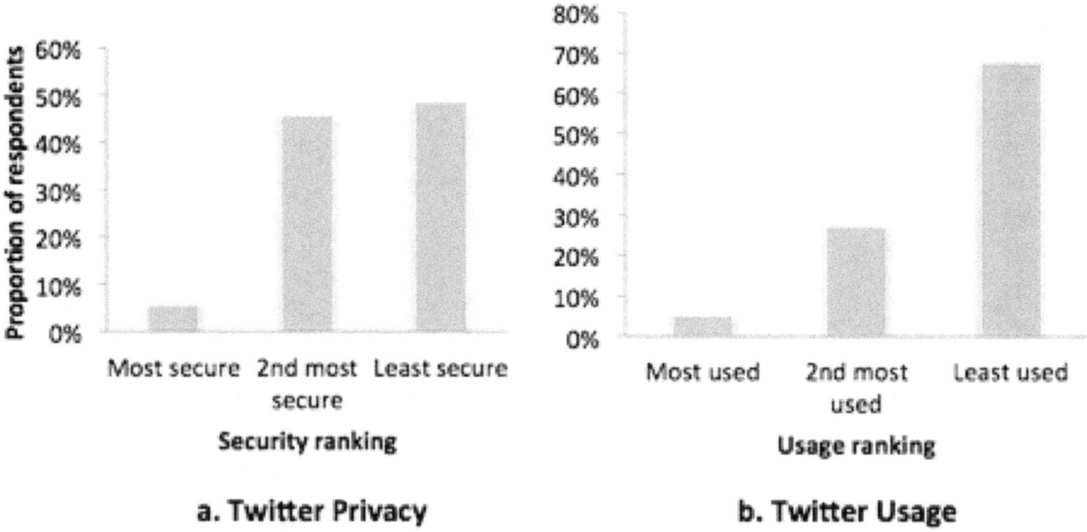


There were differing views in relation to the three platforms when comparing the technologies within each question. When asked to rank the social media technologies participants thought were the most, second most, and least secure, an overwhelming majority considered Skype as the most secure in terms of privacy (Figure 4b). Overall, Facebook was considered the second most secure in terms of privacy whilst Twitter was considered the least secure in terms of privacy. However when asked to rank their use of social media technologies in the six-month trial period from most to least used, Facebook was found to be the most highly used (Figure 4a). The second most used application was Skype, and Twitter was the least used by the older adult trial participants. It is interesting to note that whilst there were some concerns about the use of Facebook in terms of privacy, it was the most used social media technology overall. In addition, the results from these sections of the questionnaires raised further questions such as: why Twitter had very low levels of adoption?, why Twitter ranked the lowest in terms of perceived privacy?, why Skype was seen as the most secure but was the second most used technology?. These questions are further considered based upon the qualitative analysis of the free-text responses of the trial participants described in the Discussion section.

In carrying out a qualitative analysis of the open-ended survey questions we identified five broad themes in relation to the social technology privacy perceptions of the older adult trial participants: (i) user control; (ii) openness of the social media system; (iii) chosen mode of use; (iv) user interface issues; and (v) external factors. These will be further discussed, in conjunction with the quantitative results, in the Discussion section.

## DISCUSSION

As seen in the quantitative findings section, the three social media technologies used had varying privacy perceptions and levels of usage. In addition, various themes were identified from the collected qualitative data from free-text questionnaire responses and focus groups responses. These five themes and a total of twelve sub-themes are now described and discussed.

*Figure 4. Relative privacy perceptions and usage levels*

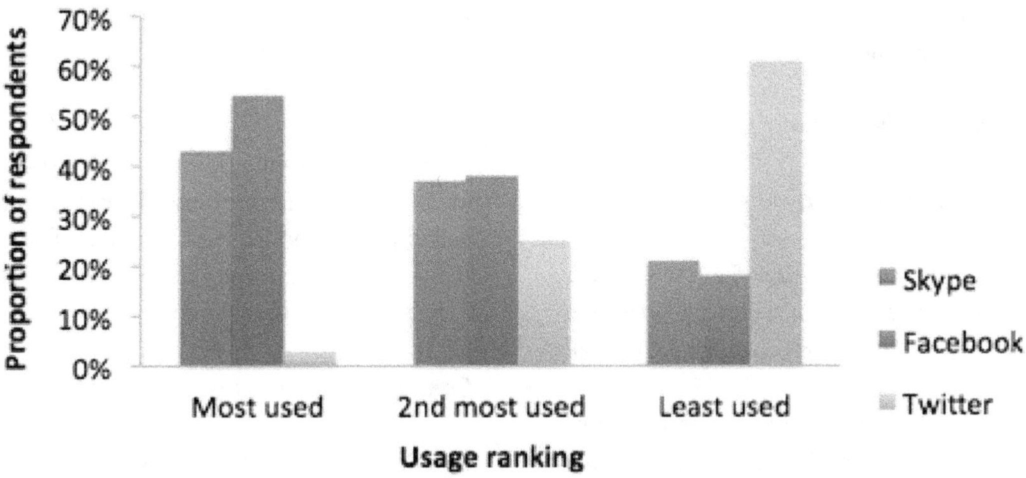


**a. Relative usage**

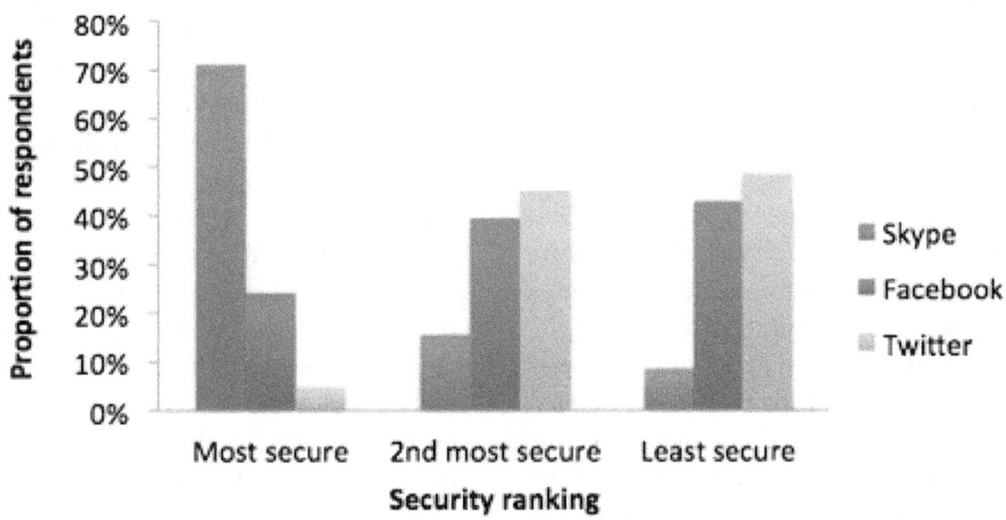


**b. Relative perceived privacy**

## Theme One: User Control

User control featured in various ways in numerous participant responses. This broad theme encompassed two major sub-themes that dealt with different types of control that participants indicated affected their perception of privacy when using the technologies: control of settings and control of online contacts.

### Control of Settings

A common sub-theme was the level of control of the privacy settings of the social media system, and its apparent positive effect upon perceived privacy. Facebook was considered to have the most settings to control privacy, and possibly surprisingly this led to it being perceived as superior in terms of privacy than Twitter, which had minimal such settings. Participants' responses about Facebook-related privacy settings and why this led them to consider it private included comments such as:

*Because you can change your settings*

*Can use settings to make it very secure*

*I feel I have more control and safeguards in place to feel safe using this medium. My age group are still wary of the information available to others*

Whether such settings were understood, used or appreciated also seemed to have led to divergent views as to the privacy of the social media technology. Participants who saw the use of Facebook settings as a key priority for controlling their privacy also found them to be a governing factor in using the social media technology:

*If settings not used considered to be too open "too in your face for me"*

Previous studies (Shapira, Barak and Gal, 2007) have shown that positive feelings may be caused by a sense of control and independence when older adults are using the Internet.

There was also a view that the number of privacy settings on Facebook may have overwhelmed some participants, and hence why some may have ranked the application as the least secure of the three. This raises the issue that having more settings in some cases can instead lead to a negative reaction in terms of privacy, as the complexity of these may act as a deterrent to using them and hence remove the positive impact of improved privacy via use of settings. In addition, Facebook settings that are constantly changing also create an issue of unpredictability and less confidence in relation to user control of privacy:

*[Facebook] least secure as complicated to setup security filters and facebook operators/program unreliable as often changes features (unpredictable)*

However when looking at the social media technology Twitter, it could be suggested from participant responses that the lack of settings was seen as a negative for protecting and controlling user privacy as they:

*Can be passed on - no control*

## Control of Online Contacts

In addition to the control of settings, another recurring sub-theme from participant responses in relation to control was that of control of online contacts. The general theme seen throughout the qualitative data was that the more control of online contacts reflected positively on perceived privacy, as opposed to the previously discussed varying levels of settings control leading to divergent views. When looking at control of online contacts in Skype, it could be seen that the high level of control over whom individuals could accept as a contact, not having to respond to unsolicited contacts, as well as who could find and request a certain individual to be a contact, were possible positive factors in why Skype was seen as the most secure social media technology compared to the others:

*Can limit to just family for example*

Previous research by Brandtzaeg, Luders and Skjetne (2010) found that older adults also identified having too many friends as an issue with Facebook. The inability of individuals to control what information people in their network shared and published about them (without deleting or unfriending them) was also an issue as they felt there was no control over their own personal information. When considering Facebook and Twitter, the participants in our study thought that these social media technologies did not provide as much control when compared to Skype. For example, the number of unwanted or less familiar online contacts that could be linked and pushed to that individual, was recognized by the participants in relation to these applications.

## Theme Two: Openness of the Social Media System

Openness refers to the degree to which the finding and contacting of new contacts is supported or encouraged via the social media system. Two recurring sub-themes that were identified under this broad theme were the auto-suggesting of contacts, and the privacy linked to communicating with already known people.

### Auto-Suggesting of Contacts

Auto-suggesting of contacts was an implicit and non-configurable characteristic and capability of both Facebook and Twitter. This involved suggesting to an individual, contacts to connect with, using entered details (i.e. name, date of birth, email address) or already established online connections (i.e. mutual friends). This was generally seen to have a negative effect on perceptions of privacy, which may have contributed to why participants saw Skype as the most secure technology (as Skype only suggests to users if they would voluntary like to find online contacts via their email address). In relation to Facebook, auto-suggesting of contacts was seen as a greater infringement on privacy, as participants were concerned about the auto-suggestion of acquaintances and unfamiliar online contacts:

*had only just connected and unwelcome faces from the past appeared*

There was also confusion as to how the social media technology knew which people to suggest to them, and this raised the questions as to the type of information that was being used to suggest these contacts:

*I felt personally exposed to potential 'friends'*

When considering the auto-suggesting of contacts on Twitter, there was not as much concern in relation to privacy as seen in relation to Facebook. This may have been due to the characteristics of Twitter to suggest organizations, companies and celebrities to follow based on personal preferences and hobbies (e.g. knitting, scrabble) rather than suggesting potential online contacts that were/might be real-life connections.

### Privacy Linked to Communicating with People Already Known

Skype was perceived as the most secure social media application by a majority of the participants. This is surprising in some regards, as the common means of communication via Skype is more personal (and thus risky) than compared to communication via Facebook and Twitter (i.e. audio and video chat via Skype versus uploading photos and posting for Facebook and Twitter). This however can be possibly attributed to both the lack of openness of Skype (i.e. minimal auto-suggesting of contacts and adding people you already know details of in real life) as well as the one-to-one means of communication that occurs.

As social media technologies often promote a degree of openness, previous researchers have suggested that older adults may feel more comfortable sharing information with recipients that they are able to select from a list of actual names, rather than having previously defined groups (Lehtinen, Nasanen and Sarvas, 2009).

## Theme Three: Chosen Mode of Use

It was found that the chosen mode of use for each social technology often differed between the various participants (i.e. not all participants used the social media technologies in the same way as each other). The way certain participants used these applications actually altered their respective privacy perceptions for each technology. Sub-themes that were identified under this theme were: anonymity capabilities, perceived normative mode of use, and one-to-one versus one-to-many.

### Anonymity Capabilities

Anonymity (or using pseudonyms) has been previously found to facilitate participation in online computer-mediated learning environments (Yu and Liu, 2009) as it creates a more equitable and safe basis for an online user to share and receive opinions and feedback (Guardado and Shi, 2007). Of interest in our study, is the impact of an anonymity capability on privacy perceptions and participation in the use of social media technologies. The word 'anonymous' was repeatedly used in responses of participants when asked about the usability of Twitter. This is because Twitter allows one to use a Twitter 'handle', which is a term that simply means a username (which does not have to reflect in any way the user's real name or identity). This was seen as a positive amongst participant perceptions of privacy, as many felt safer being able to remain anonymous and still using the social media technology:

*Needed a pen name*

*You only use a secret name*

*Using a username made me feel comfortable*

Whilst this was seen as one of the strong positives for privacy in relation to Twitter, in contrast this social media technology was overall perceived as the least private when compared to Skype and Facebook. This is an interesting finding, as both Skype and Facebook provide far less anonymity than Twitter, yet they were still perceived as more secure. This underscores that it was the user's chosen mode of use that was significant in relation to perceived privacy – many of the other trial participants appear not to have conceived that they could remain anonymous and so there was a generally low view of Twitter's privacy.

In addition, it can be said however, that anonymous participation may only occur if users are confident their identity will be protected (Richardson, Zorn and Weaver, 2011, p. 326), and that although Twitter can be anonymous, there may be a lack of confidence by users that the technology will protect this anonymity.

### Perceived Normative Mode of Use

As suggested, there were variations in both the participants' perceptions of privacy as well as how they used each social media technology. Users in some cases felt their privacy to be protected via recognizing and choosing the option to use the media for information gathering and receipt, rather than for the posting of their own information and content. This sub-theme also relates to the anonymity capabilities of Twitter, as rather than providing personal details and sharing of one's own information, some participants chose to use this open platform as an information gathering source:

*I do not have to disclose any details and can still enjoy reading comments*

*Used only to read other comments*

In stark comparison however, those who saw Twitter as mainly a medium for sharing information and self-posting, had perceptions that postings would be open to the public which led to significant privacy concerns:

*Twitter is last, all tweets are in the public domain so you have no choice in who reads your information*

This can be compared to respondents who identified and opted to use the technology solely or largely for the receipt of information – this appears to have hence led to a more favorable conception of Twitter's privacy. Whether this is applicable to Facebook and Skype is not as clear, as both these social media technologies require some sort of two-way interaction (i.e. post and read) when compared to the type of interaction provided by Twitter (i.e. able to read, don't have to post).

### One-to-One vs. One-to-Many

There are various modes of communicating via these social media technologies. Communication can be done on a one-to-one basis (i.e. private/direct messaging on Facebook and Twitter, one-to-one chat and video calls on Skype) or a one-to-many scale (i.e. posting a micro-blog post or 'tweet' on Twitter, updating one's status or uploading a photo on Facebook, participating in conference calls on Skype). Participants did not see the communication through Skype as an issue for privacy, and were even open to the use of video cameras, which may have been why it was ranked as the most secure technology because of its "one to one" or "personal" nature:

*Because its one to one*

*Personal*

Although the one-to-one means of communication on Facebook and Twitter were made known to participants, a majority of responses focused on the one-to-many aspect of these technologies. Some participants found issues with what they posted being able to be shared with friends of friends (if statuses or photos were shared by their friends). Although others seemed to acknowledge that this was a risk of posting on Facebook, and embraced the one-to-many communication that the application provided:

*Its all there for all to see! I admit though I use it the most!*

Whilst direct messaging was understood by some users to add privacy, the public nature of Twitter and the micro-blog post were a concern. More so than Facebook, participant perceptions of Twitter and the one-to-many nature of public posting negatively affected the perception of privacy of those that chose to use Twitter for sharing information. The terms 'follow', 'followers', and 'following' used on this application was also an issue that affected perceptions of privacy amongst the older adult participants:

*Don't much like the concept of followers or following or being in public domain online*

## Theme Four: User Interface Issues

The design and interface of social media technologies is important for functionality, usability, and generalizability. However many older adults found various issues with these interfaces, and thus this affected their perception of the applications' security in terms of privacy. The two sub-themes found within this broader theme were: the effect of perceived familiarity of the technology and issues with the changing of interfaces.

### Perceived Familiarity of the Technology

A sub-theme that was positively associated with privacy perceptions was the perceived familiarity of the social media technologies. Pfeil, Zaphiris and Wilson (2009) investigated the needs and preferences of older adults in relation to online support. One technical issue that was bought up was the unfamiliarity of the Web-based technology for support, with most participants in that study stating that they would rather use a telephone or meet face-to-face. In our study, it can be seen that there was a relatively high uptake of Skype as a communication technology, even though it is a Web-based application. However, when analyzing participant responses about Skype, it was suggested that the application tended to be perceived to have similarities to the telephone, and this appeared to lead to less privacy and security concerns.

*Skype is most secure, as it works like a phone*

This may suggest another possible reason as to why Skype was perceived as the most secure social media technology of the three, as aspects of the application can be perceived to be more familiar to older adults (e.g. calling, answering, speaking directly to the other person by the telephone) whereas the other two communication abilities provided by Facebook and Twitter (i.e. posting) are less similar to traditional communications. However this familiarity with technology may have had a carry-over effect – as participants used video chat on Skype, and because this function was also available on Facebook, this may have made Facebook seem more familiar than Twitter (which might also be a factor as to why Facebook ranked as the second most secure technology).

### Changing Interface

There were issues found with the constant re-designing and re-invention of both the look and the functionality of the social media applications. As with the perceived familiarity issue affecting privacy perception, changing interfaces may be a greater problem potentially for older adults. Not only may this make these social media technologies harder to adapt to and use, but these changing interfaces may also raise privacy concerns for older adult users. Facebook was one of the technologies that provided the greatest issues with changes to interfaces even during the training period, where some participants had signed up with Timeline (a newly introduced Facebook design) and others had signed up with older interfaces. Those who had signed up with older interfaces had to change over to Timeline during the six-month trial period, and this change of interface may have caused a negative impact on privacy perception as well as use:

*I was just getting to understand Facebook when they changed the format. I have rarely used it since.*

However some participants acknowledged that some of the changes made by Facebook (such as in the account and privacy settings) were reflective of the social media technology responding to potential threats by providing options for better and more suited security protections. The changing interfaces of various social media technologies are not the only interface issues that have been identified by previous work. However it can be seen in previous studies that older adults may find support to overcome usability problems if they see benefits of the platform to meet their needs (Fuchsberger, Sullner, Moser and Tscheligi, 2012). Therefore future studies may focus on the effect of technological support on older adult perception of privacy.

## Theme Five: External Factors

There were also external factors that affected the perception of privacy identified by the responding participants. Unlike the first four broad themes, these external factors did not deal with the interactions between the social media technologies and the older adults, but rather the effects upon other outside influences that may have affected both use and privacy perceptions of these applications. The three identified sub-themes within this category were: mass media effect upon perceived possible privacy concerns, the level of training (if any) for older adults as well as the views about the social media companies themselves.

## Mass Media Affect upon Perceived Possible Privacy Concerns

Social media technologies have had various negative media and press releases about various privacy issues and breaches of such applications (Boyd, 2008; Humphreys, Gill and Krishnamurthy, 2010). This was reflected by the responses of the older adult participants, whom had expressed varying levels of suspicion with recent privacy-related events reported on by mainstream media. The recurring concern for using any social media technology that required individuals to provide personal information was that this information would be "leaked" for all to see:

*Seems like the entire world knows about you if not careful*

This sub-theme of our study is similar to various results found by previous literature.

## Level of Training or Experience (If Any)

The level of training and experience of participants within the sample may have also impacted on their perceptions of social technology privacy. Those with less understanding of social media sites and technology in general may have possibly found functions such as privacy settings more difficult to use. This can also be attributed to personal experience with the social media technologies – as those with more (or more rewarding/positive) experiences with these applications may have perceived a higher level of trust and a lower level of resistance in relation to privacy perceptions. One participant identified the following for resistance to using Facebook and the eventual acceptance of the social media technology with further use and experience:

*Many students resisted social media (Facebook) because of privacy, bullying and lack of knowledge on how to operate it... all students are now Facebook devotees*

The Pew Research Center's Internet and American Life Project (Madden and Smith, 2010) released a report about online reputation management. It was found that 20% of older adults aged 65 and older (and 25% of older adults aged between 50 and 64) took steps to limit the amount of personal information available to them online. However when compared to the 44% of younger users aged 18 to 29 (and the 33% of those aged 30 to 49), it can be seen that there is a significant proportion of these older adults that either do not bother enough to, or do not know how to, limit the amount of personal information available about them online. As the privacy concerns of older adults in relation to using the Internet and social media technologies have been consistently raised throughout past literature as well as this study, we can suggest that the reason for not limiting personal information can possibly be attributed to the lack of training or experiences of older adults on these applications, especially when compared with some of the younger user cohorts.

## Views about Social Media Companies

Another sub-theme that affected privacy perceptions of these technologies were the participant's views about the perceived motives of the social media companies themselves. Many raised issues as to where the information they posted was going, as well as why these applications asked them to fill in their real name and details (like date of birth). One of the major concerns was that of sharing photographs of family and friends:

*Something I'm worried about what Facebook will do with my information + photographs*

## IMPLICATIONS

The research carried out provides various implications for health information delivery within older adult communities. With an ageing population comes a greater number of ageing-related health conditions, which can potentially be supported via online health information interventions. As previously identified, the proportion of older adults adopting social media technology is increasing rapidly. By identifying older adult privacy perceptions when using social media technologies, this paper can help to address the various issues that need to be considered when developing and maintaining interventions through such interfaces.

One major implication is that, with regards to health information interventions, there have been no studies observing the impact of social media technologies on specifically older adult communities. Although there have previously been studies about social media technologies and chronic health conditions relevant to the older adult community (e.g. dementia and diabetes), there must be further research specifically considering older adults due to the various, and perhaps differing, privacy perceptions as outlined above. A better understanding of older adult privacy concerns can also have benefits in improving older adult adoption of other health information technologies (Steele, Min and Lo, 2012) that can potentially have particular benefits for this demographic.

## CONCLUSION

From the study, of the three introduced social technologies, it was found that older adults perceived Skype as the most secure in terms of privacy. This was followed by Facebook as the 2nd most secure, and Twitter as the least secure in terms of privacy. The perception of privacy and privacy protection in relation to these applications may have possibly affected the older adult's use, as Twitter was the least used during the six-month trial period by a significant margin. However perceived benefits of use may have been a suggested reason as to why Facebook was the most used (followed by Skype as the second most used). There were various recurring themes seen within the older adults' responses with regards to privacy perceptions and their experiences with social media. After analyzing the qualitative data gathered from questionnaires and focus groups, five broad themes were identified: (i) user control; (ii) openness of social media system; (iii) chosen mode of use; (iv) user interface issues; and (v) external factors. Within these themes, twelve sub-themes were also identified and we have discussed these to consider possible reasons for such privacy perceptions and concerns amongst older adults.

## ACKNOWLEDGMENT

The authors would like to thank the anonymous reviewers and the editor for their insightful comments and suggestions.

## REFERENCES


Billipp, S. H. (2001). The psychosocial impact of interactive computer use within a vulnerable elderly population: A report on a randomized prospective trial in a home health care setting. *Public Health Nursing (Boston, Mass.), 18*(2), 138–145. doi:10.1046/j.1525-1446.2001.00138.x PMID:11285108

Boyd, D. (2008). Facebook's Privacy Trainwreck. *Convergence: The International Journal of Research into New Media Technologies, 14*(1), 13–20. doi:10.1177/1354856507084416

Brandtzæg, P. B., Lüders, M., & Skjetne, J. H. (2010). Too many Facebook "friends"? Content sharing and sociability versus the need for privacy in social network sites. *International Journal of Human-Computer Interaction, 26*(11-12), 1006–1030. doi:10.1080/10447318.2010.516719

Brosnan, M. J. (1998). The impact of computer anxiety and self-efficacy upon performance. *Journal of Computer Assisted Learning, 14*(3), 223–234. doi:10.1046/j.1365-2729.1998.143059.x

Czaja, S. J., & Lee, C. C. (2001). The Internet and older adults: Design challenges and opportunities. In N. Charness, & D. C. Parks (Eds.), *Communication, and aging: Opportunities and challenges for the future* (pp. 60–78). New York: Springer.

Dumbrell, D., & Steele, R. (2013). Twitter and health in the Australian context: What types of information are health-related organizations tweeting? In *Proceedings of System Sciences (HICSS), 2013 46th Hawaii International Conference* (pp. 2666-2675). IEEE.

Ellis, R. D., & Allaire, J. C. (1999). Modeling computer interest in older adults: The role of age, education, computer knowledge, and computer anxiety. *Human Factors: The Journal of the Human Factors and Ergonomics Society, 41*(3), 345–355. doi:10.1518/001872099779610996 PMID:10665203

Fink, A., & Beck, J. C. (2013). Developing and Evaluating a Website to Guide Older Adults in Their Health Information Searches A Mixed-Methods Approach. *Journal of Applied Gerontology, 32*(4). PMID:24652883

Fuchsberger, V., Sellner, W., Moser, C., & Tscheligi, M. (2012). Benefits and hurdles for older adults in intergenerational online interactions. In *Computers Helping People with Special Needs* (pp. 697–704). Springer Berlin Heidelberg. doi:10.1007/978-3-642-31522-0_104

Gatto, S. L., & Tak, S. H. (2008). Computer, internet, and e-mail use among older adults: Benefits and barriers. *Educational Gerontology, 34*(9), 800–811. doi:10.1080/03601270802243697

Guardado, M., & Shi, L. (2007). ESL students' experiences of online peer feedback. *Computers and Composition, 24*(4), 443–461. doi:10.1016/j.compcom.2007.03.002

Harkin, J., & Huber, J. (2004). Eternal youths: How the baby boomers are having their time again. *Demos (Mexico City, Mexico).*

Humphreys, L., Gill, P., & Krishnamurthy, B. (2010). How much is too much? Privacy issues on Twitter. In Proceedings of Conference of International Communication Association. Singapore: Academic Press.

Lehtinen, V., Näsänen, J., & Sarvas, R. (2009). A little silly and empty-headed: Older adults' understandings of social networking sites. In *Proceedings of the 23rd British HCI Group Annual Conference on People and Computers: Celebrating People and Technology* (pp. 45-54). British Computer Society.

Madden, M., & Smith, A. (2010). *Pew Research Center. Reputation Management and Social Media.* Retrieved from http://pewinternet.org/~/media//Files/Reports/2010/PIP_Reputation_Management_with_topline.pdf

Park, Y. J. (2013). Digital literacy and privacy behavior online. *Communication Research*, *40*(2), 215–236. doi:10.1177/0093650211418338

Pfeil, U., Zaphiris, P., & Wilson, S. (2009). Older adults' perceptions and experiences of online social support. *Interacting with Computers*, *21*(3), 159–172. doi:10.1016/j.intcom.2008.12.001

Richardson, M., Zorn, T., & Weaver, C. K. (2011). Older people and new communication technologies: Narratives from the literature. In C. T. Salmon (Ed.), *Communication yearbook 35* (pp. 121–152). Routledge Taylor & Francis Group.

Shapira, N., Barak, A., & Gal, I. (2007). Promoting older adults' well-being through Internet training and use. *Aging & Mental Health*, *11*(5), 477–484. doi:10.1080/13607860601086546 PMID:17882585

Steele, R. (2011). Social media, mobile devices and sensors: categorizing new techniques for health communication. In *Proceedings of the 5th International Conference on Sensing Technology*, (pp. 187-192). Palmerston North, New Zealand: IEEE.

Steele, R., Lo, A., Secombe, C., & Wong, Y. K. (2009). Elderly persons' perception and acceptance of using wireless sensor networks to assist healthcare. *International Journal of Medical Informatics*, *78*(12), 788–801. doi:10.1016/j.ijmedinf.2009.08.001 PMID:19717335

Steele, R., Min, K., & Lo, A. (2012). Personal health record architectures: Technology infrastructure implications and dependencies. *Journal of the American Society for Information Science and Technology*, *63*(6), 1079–1091. doi:10.1002/asi.22635

Yu, F. Y., & Liu, Y. H. (2009). Creating a psychologically safe online space for a student generated questions learning activity via different identity revelation modes. *British Journal of Educational Technology*, *40*(6), 1109–1123. doi:10.1111/j.1467-8535.2008.00905.x

Zickuhr, K., & Madden, M. (2012). Older adults and internet use. *Pew Internet & American Life Project*. Retrieved from http://pewinternet.org/Reports/2012/Older-adults-and-internet-use.aspx

## KEY TERMS AND DEFINITIONS

**Facebook:** A widely used social media application.

**Isolation:** Lack of social contact with other persons.

**Loneliness:** Perceived social isolation, as such subjective.

**Micro-Blog:** A system with a blog-like nature, where incremental updates are provided over time, but for which the text updates are typically shorter.

**Skype:** A widely used voice-over-IP communications application.

**Social Technologies:** includes social media systems, micro-blogging systems and audio and video-based communications technologies.

**Twitter:** A widely used micro-blogging application.

# Section 2
# User Acceptance of Health Information Systems

# Chapter 5
# Perceived Importance of User Expectations from Healthcare Information Systems

**Güney Gürsel**
*Gülhane Military Medical Academy, Turkey*

## ABSTRACT

*Health institutions invest huge amounts in Information Systems (IS). Despite the huge budgets of investments, it is estimated that nearly 60-70% of Information Technology (IT) implementation projects fail in healthcare. In the literature, success factors and the failure reasons have largely been discussed. One of these, both in failure reasons and success factors, is the User Expectations. Expectation Failure, which can be defined as the gap between expectations of the end users from the system and actual performance of it, is introduced as one of the failure reasons of IS. The expectations of users must be well understood and discreetly worked out to design and implement a successful, acceptable, and useful IS. There is no study about the expectations from Healthcare Information System (HCIS) in the literature. The aim of this chapter is to investigate the end user expectations from HIS and their rankings. Seventeen potential end user expectations in four dimensions are examined and ranked according to the importance of expectations to the users.*

## INTRODUCTION

Importance of expectations is clear enough in the success of Information system (IS). The expectations of users must be well understood and discreetly worked out to design and implement a successful, acceptable and useful IS. The expectations, priorities of these expectations, their importance to the users must be well understood. Despite the huge investment amounts, the high failure rate in Healthcare Information Systems (HCIS) is a big problem. To catch the success, user acceptance is an instrument in information systems and can be provided with high expectation meeting ratios. That will lead higher usage ratios, resulting in successful IS implementations.

Despite this fact, there is no dedicated study about the expectations from HCIS, user expectations from IS are great interest to the researchers. The purposes of the study are; to examine the end

DOI: 10.4018/978-1-4666-6316-9.ch005

user expectations from HCIS and their relative importance, to explore the ranking of expectations according to the importance both for all users and for different titled users.

## BACKGROUND

Not only in healthcare institutions, but in all, doing the daily work without an information system (IS) is almost impossible in our era. An IS is not only a way of recording the operations made by the employees, in the recent technology. Today, the users expect more than e-recording, from IS. Taking into account the complexity of the healthcare, we need serious features in HCIS'. That is why healthcare institutions (HI) invest huge amounts in information systems. Literature tells that the amount of investment made in HCIS is not directly proportional with positive effects, many negative effects of IT implementation in HCIS are available (De Keizer & Ammenwerth, 2008). Literature also tells, despite the unquestionable need to IS, and huge budgets of investments, it is estimated that nearly 60-70% of software projects fail in healthcare (Ammenwerth, Iller & Mahler, 2006).

Literature is very well concerned about the success factors and failure reasons of IS. There are many studies about the success factors and failure reasons. In this chapter, we only deal with the factors and reasons, directly related to the subject of the chapter; the User Expectations.

The success factor related to the User Expectations is user satisfaction. It is one of the most studied success factor of IS in the literature. It is presented as an element of system success first by Cyert and March (1963). Collins dictionary defines satisfaction as (Despont-Gros, Mueller & Lovis, 2005)

- The act of satisfying or state of being satisfied.
- The fulfillment of a desire.
- The pleasure obtained from such fulfillment.
- A source of fulfillment.

Seddon (1997) defines user satisfaction as ''a subjective evaluation of the various consequences evaluated on a pleasant –unpleasant continuum''. Gelderman (1998) defines user satisfaction as ''the extent to which information requirements are met''. Similarly, Ives, Olson & Baroudi's (1983) definition of 'user information satisfaction' is ''the extent to which users believe the information system available to them, meets their information requirements''.

Drawing from the definitions, it is clear that satisfaction is directly dependent on expectations, so does the IS satisfaction. As seen in the definitions given above, satisfaction occurs when the expectations are met. User expectations have great influence on user satisfaction with IS. The influence of user expectations on user satisfaction is proved by many studies in the literature (Conrath & Mignen, 1990; Delone & Mclean, 2004; Adam Mahmood, Burn, Gemoets & Jacquez, 2000; Lee 2010; Halilovic & Cicic, 2013). In the literature survey of Petter, Delone & McLean (2013), User Expectations is stated as one of the fifteen success factors that have been found to influence IS success consistently.

IS usage directly depends on the user satisfaction (Bergeron, & Raymond, 1992). End users use the system in a qualified manner, if and only if they are satisfied. The management may force the users, but if they are not eager to use, they do not use the system effectively, then the result would not be satisfactory. User should accept the system for its success. That is why the term "user-acceptance" is so popular. On system usage, users' satisfaction has great impact, meaning that the users do not use the system effectively, if it cannot satisfy its users. When the expectations are not met, dissatisfaction occurs. Unmet expectations create psychological discomfort concluding with the unsatisfied users and unused system (Szajna & Scamell, 1993).

When expectation and satisfaction is under consideration, expectation-(dis)confirmation and dissonance theory, dealing with these two concepts should be examined. Expectation-(dis) confirmation theory has four components (Fan & Suh, 2014)

- Expectations,
- Performance,
- Disconfirmation,
- Satisfaction.

According to the theory, confirmation of user expectations has three possible levels (Staples, Wong, & Seddon, 2002):

- If the product performs as expected, confirmed .
- If the product performs worse than expected, negatively disconfirmed.
- If the product performs better than expected, positively disconfirmed.

Szymanski & Henard (2001) stated that disconfirmation is dominant in satisfaction. Their findings point a negative correlation between user satisfaction and disconfirmed expectations. Disconfirmation theory also states that unrealistically high expectations lead to dissatisfaction. Users are becoming more demanding from their information systems, advances in technology cause these higher expectations and managers try to determine how to establish realistic expectations, they should not oversell the benefits of future systems to get user support for new projects (Staples et al, 2002). Management should take required measures to keep the expectations in realistic level. This issue will be examined in the discussion part.

The cognitive dissonance theory states that unmet IS expectations create dissonant (unharmonious) ideas. In the disconfirmation theory, a user with poor expectations about a product is satisfied if it reaches his expectations (Despont-Gros et al., 2005; Safran, Jones, Rind, Bush, Cytryn & Patel, 1998).

Failure reasons are of great interest to literature as well as success factors. Many reasons are shown for failure. Alshawi (2007), states that failure rarely depends on purely technical reasons. This finding makes us focus on reasons other than technical. "User expectations" is one of the striking reasons in this classification. Lyytinen & Hirschheim (1988) introduced the term "Expectation Failure" to the literature. In their study, the failure reasons of IS are classified into four groups as;

- Correspondence Failure,
- Process Failure,
- Interaction Failure,
- Expectation Failure.

Expectation Failure can be defined as the gap between expectations of the end users from the system and the real performance of it. The work of The Project Management Institute (2008) also supports this claim, by pointing out the user expectation meeting as one of the primary criteria for project success.

Having stressed the importance of the user expectations from IS, we may mention about the background of the study which this work originates from. In the previous study, an expectation based evaluation framework for Hospital Information System (HIS) is presented (Gürsel, Zayim, Gülkesen, Arigoğlu, & Saka, 2014). In this work, first it was tried to model the user expectations from HCIS, because there is no clear explanation or list in the literature about what a user expects from HCIS. In four dimensions, 17 user expectations from HCIS are constituted to evaluate the expectation meeting ratio of the HCIS'. The potential user expectations from HCIS are given Table 1 (Gürsel et al., 2014). Framework is applied to three different types and size of hospitals. In the given study the results belonging to the two of hospitals were given (Gürsel et al., 2014).

For the current study, using data of the biggest hospital of the previous study mentioned above, the expectations (called as expectation variable) given in Table 1 is rank ordered to get the perceived importance. Because everyone has different point of view and approach, perceived importance ratings change from one person to another. Rank ordering is a good technique to eliminate this personal relativity (Li, 1997).

## MATERIALS AND METHODS

### Data

In this study, part of the data gathered in the previous study (Gürsel et al., 2014) is used.

"Expectation Questionnaire" was formed and used for data collection in the previous work (Gürsel et al., 2014). This questionnaire was the data collection tool for the expectation based HCIS evaluation framework. In the "Expectation Questionnaire" for each expectation variable (There are 17 see in Table 1), an importance question was asked to capture the relative importance weight of the variable to the user. Each user is asked to evaluate the importance of the related variable, with the question "What is the importance of this feature of the information system in your opinion?" The choices are 5-point Likert-type scale (very important, important, average important, not so important, not important).

In the background section, it is mentioned that the Expectation Questionnaire was applied to three hospitals of different types and sizes, to evaluate the information systems used. In this study, the data captured from the biggest hospital (having 1700 (900-1000 online) HIS users) is used. Only one hospital data is used to avoid bias in the study, because each hospital was using different information systems. 504 returned questionnaires out of 660 were available; of them 428 completely filled questionnaires, without any missing importance rating for the expectation variables, are used for the study.

The internal consistencies of the answers to the Expectation Questionnaire are measured by Cronbach´s Alpha coefficient using Statistical Package for Social Sciences 19.0 (SPSS, SPSS Inc, Chicago, Illinois, USA). Cronbach´s Alpha greater than 0.70 is considered reliable.

### Ranking the Variables

The Likert scales used are assigned weights ranging from 5 (very important) to 1 (not important) as given in Table 2. These weights are used for rank ordering of the variables, to determine the perceived importance, in the formula given in (1).

Expectations are rank ordered, according to the final rating (RF) of the variables, first in expectation variable base, and then in dimension base.

*Table 1. Potential user expectations from HCIS (Gürsel et al. 2014)*

| Usage Expectations | System and Data Expectations | Improvement Expectations | Managerial Expectations |
|---|---|---|---|
| Ease-of-use | Consistency | Improve service quality | Reporting Facilities |
| Need For Training | Privacy | Decreasing work load | Decision Support |
| Help Manuals | Security | Bringing Positive Change | Function Sufficiency |
| Speed | Availability | Research facilities | |
| User Support | Interoperability | | |

*Table 2. Answers given to the Usage Expectations dimension*

| Variable | VI | I | AI | NSO | NI |
|---|---|---|---|---|---|
| Ease of Use | 307 | 111 | 7 | 2 | 1 |
| Need for Training | 294 | 124 | 8 | 1 | 1 |
| Help Manuals | 193 | 178 | 31 | 21 | 5 |
| User Support | 307 | 108 | 12 | 1 | 0 |
| Speed | 348 | 74 | 2 | 4 | 0 |
| **TOTAL** | **1449** | **595** | **60** | **29** | **7** |

VI = Very Important, I = Important, AI = Average Important, NSO = Not So Important, NO = Not Important

Rank ordering is done both for all users general and for different user title groups. Expectation based ranking gives the idea about the users' priorities of the expectation itself; dimension based ranking gives the idea about the priorities in a more general way.

In expectation based ranking, the final rating (RF) of the expectation variable *j* is computed by

$$RF_j = \sum_{i=1}^{k} W_i R_i / n \tag{1}$$

where *k* is the number of Likert scales used (5 for this study), W is the weight (1 to 5) of the Likert scale *i*, R is the number of answers given as that Likert scale and n is the total number of answers.

In dimension based ranking, the final rating RF of the expectation dimension *j* is computed by weighted average formula

$$RF_j = [\sum_{z=1}^{l}(\sum_{i=1}^{k} R_i)W_i] / \sum_{i=1}^{k} n \tag{2}$$

where *l* is the number of Likert scales used, *k* is the number of variables of the dimension *j* (Table 1), *W* is the weight of the variable *i*, *R* is the number of answers given as that Likert scale *i*, *n* is the number of answers for the variable *i*.

A toy example for calculating the rank of an Expectation Dimension is given below to make it more comprehendible. Table 2 shows the answers for the Usage Expectations variables. Using (2) the final rating of the dimension is;

[(1449 * 5) + (595 * 4) + (60 * 3) + (29 * 2) + (7 * 1)] / (1449 + 595 + 60 + 29 +7) = **4.612**

## RESULTS

Cronbach´s Alpha coefficient, showing the reliabilities (internal consistencies), for the importance weights is 0.871. This value is greater than 0.7, meaning the answers to the questions are internally consistent.

Table 3 gives the distribution of the users participating in the study, according to their business titles. Most of the users are physicians with 34.3%, second come the nurses with 32.7%. Other group comprises the titles, not many in number to be

*Table 3. Distribution of users, participating in the study according to their business titles*

| Business Title | n | % |
|---|---|---|
| Office worker | 39 | 9.1 |
| Laboratory Technician | 29 | 6.8 |
| Nurse | 140 | 32.7 |
| Physician | 147 | 34.3 |
| Other | 37 | 8.6 |
| Missing | 36 | 8.5 |

statistically significant alone such as dieticians, patient consultants, different types of technicians, biologists, physiotherapists etc. 8.5% of the users do not state their titles in the questionnaire.

The frequency distribution of the answers to the Expectation Questionnaire and the ranking results of the expectation variables are given in Table 5. The top five ranked expectations are Availability, Speed, Bringing Positive Change, Ease of Use and User Support. The five least ranked expectations appeared to be Privacy, Help Manuals, Security, Research Facilities and Decision Support, respectively from the least ranked. The results given in Table 4 and 5 are independent of any user feature and represent the general answers given by all the users. In the rest of the study these results will be called as "general ranking".

Results of dimension based ranking and the average frequency rating of dimensions are given in Table 5. The topmost ranked expectation dimension appeared to be the Usage Expectations, whereas the least ranked dimension is Managerial Expectations.

In Table 6, final ratings (RF) of the expectations and their ranks according to the user titles are given. In all titles except Nurses, Availability is the topmost. In Nurses, Speed appears to be the topmost ranked expectation. Speed is the second topmost ranked expectation variable in three of the titles (Physicians, Laboratory Technicians and Office Workers), Nurses have ranked Availability as the second and Others have ranked Decreasing Work Load as the second. Decreasing Work Load (Physicians and Nurses) and User Support

*Table 4. Importance frequency distribution and ranking in expectation base*

| Expectation | r | VI | I | AI | NSO | NO | RF |
|---|---|---|---|---|---|---|---|
| Availability | **1** | 344 | 79 | 5 | 0 | 0 | 4.792 |
| Speed | **2** | 348 | 74 | 2 | 4 | 0 | 4.790 |
| Decreasing work load | **3** | 307 | 117 | 3 | 1 | 0 | 4.706 |
| Ease of Use | **4** | 307 | 111 | 7 | 2 | 1 | 4.685 |
| User Support | **5** | 307 | 108 | 12 | 1 | 0 | 4.685 |
| Need for Training | **6** | 294 | 124 | 8 | 1 | 1 | 4.657 |
| Improve service quality | **7** | 288 | 126 | 11 | 3 | 0 | 4.633 |
| Function Sufficiency | **8** | 282 | 129 | 12 | 4 | 1 | 4.605 |
| Consistency | **9** | 258 | 150 | 13 | 6 | 1 | 4.537 |
| Bringing Positive Change | **10** | 240 | 165 | 13 | 7 | 3 | 4.477 |
| Interoperability | **11** | 248 | 146 | 25 | 6 | 3 | 4.472 |
| Report Facilities | **12** | 227 | 165 | 22 | 13 | 1 | 4.411 |
| Decision Support | **13** | 208 | 183 | 26 | 8 | 3 | 4.367 |
| Research Facilities | **14** | 221 | 147 | 28 | 23 | 8 | 4.288 |
| Security | **15** | 208 | 158 | 38 | 11 | 13 | 4.255 |
| Help Manuals | **16** | 193 | 178 | 31 | 21 | 5 | 4.245 |
| Privacy | **17** | 181 | 156 | 37 | 31 | 23 | 4.030 |

r = rank, VI = Very Important, I = Important, AI = Average Important, NSO = Not So Important, NO = Not Important, RF = Final rating

*Table 5. Dimension based frequency distribution and ranking*

| Dimension | R | VI | I | AI | NSO | NO | RF |
|---|---|---|---|---|---|---|---|
| Usage Expectations | 1 | 289,80 | 119,00 | 12,00 | 5,80 | 1,40 | 4,612 |
| Improvement Expectations | 2 | 264,00 | 138,75 | 13,75 | 8,50 | 2,75 | 4,526 |
| System and Data Expectations | 3 | 247,80 | 137,80 | 23,60 | 10,80 | 8,00 | 4,417 |
| Managerial Expectations | 4 | 239,00 | 159,00 | 20,00 | 8,33 | 1,67 | 4,461 |

r = rank, VI = Very Important, I = Important, AI = Average Important, NSO = Not So Important, NO = Not Important, RF = Final rating

*Table 6. Expectation variables' ranks according to the user titles*

| Expectation | Physician | Nurse | Laboratory Technician | Office Worker | Other |
|---|---|---|---|---|---|
| Availability | 4.830/**1** | 4.779/**2** | 4.759/**1** | 4.821/**1** | 4.891/**1** |
| Speed | 4.779/**2** | 4.814/**1** | 4.690/**2** | 4.795/**2** | 4.730/**3** |
| Decreasing work Load | 4.796/**3** | 4.700/**3** | 4.517/**5** | 4.641/**5** | 4.784/**2** |
| Ease of Use | 4.776/**4** | 4.686/**5** | 4.483/**6** | 4.769/**3** | 4.568/**4** |
| User Support | 4.735/**6** | 4.693/**4** | 4.621/**3** | 4.744/**4** | 4.730/**3** |
| Need for Training | 4.646/**8** | 4.679/**2** | 4.483/**7** | 4.769/**3** | 4.730/**3** |
| Improve service Quality | 4.741/**5** | 4.550/**8** | 4.586/**4** | 4.615/**6** | 4.730/**3** |
| Function Sufficiency | 4.714/**7** | 4.650/**6** | 4.345/**10** | 4.487/**9** | 4.405/**7** |
| Consistency | 4.544/**11** | 4.579/**7** | 4.448/**8** | 4.564/**7** | 4.459/**5** |
| Bringing Positive Change | 4.544/**11** | 4.436/**12** | 4.379/**9** | 4.487/**9** | 4.568/**4** |
| Interoperability | 4.517/**12** | 4.471/**9** | 4.379/**9** | 4.462/**10** | 4.568/**4** |
| Report Facilities | 4.619/**9** | 4.221/**14** | 4.276/**12** | 4.513/**8** | 4.432/**6** |
| Decision Support | 4.483/**13** | 4.286/**13** | 4.310/**11** | 4.385/**11** | 4.378/**8** |
| Research Facilities | 4.571/**10** | 4.108/**15** | 4.345/**10** | 3.923/**14** | 4.270/**10** |
| Security | 4.048/**14** | 4.450/**10** | 4.241/**13** | 4.256/**12** | 4.432/**6** |
| Help Manuals | 4.272/**3** | 4.364/**11** | 4172/**15** | 3.923/**14** | 4.162/**11** |
| Privacy | 3.680/**13** | 4.293/**12** | 4.241/**14** | 4.000/**13** | 4.324/**9** |

Final Rating/Rank

(Laboratory Technicians and Others) comes as the third again in two of the titles. Office Workers have ranked the Ease of Use as the third.

In Table 7, final ratings (RF) of the expectation dimensions and their ranks according to the user titles are given. Nurses, Laboratory Technicians and Office Workers think the Usage Expectations as the most important by ranking them as first. Physicians and Others rank Improvement Expectations as first. Managerial Expectations are the last ranked by Nurses, Laboratory Technicians and Others, for Physicians System and Data Expectations, for Office Workers Improvement Expectations are the last.

*Table 7. Expectation dimensions' ranks according to the user titles*

| Expectation | Physician | Nurse | Laboratory Technician | Office Worker | Other |
|---|---|---|---|---|---|
| Usage Expectations | 4.650/**2** | 4.647/**1** | 4.490/**1** | 4.744/**1** | 4.584/**2** |
| System and Data Expectations | 4.324/**4** | 4.514/**2** | 4.413/**3** | 4.503/**2** | 4.535/**3** |
| Improvement Expectations | 4.663/**1** | 4.449/**3** | 4.456/**2** | 4.141/**4** | 4.588/**1** |
| Managerial Expectations | 4.605/**3** | 4.386/**4** | 4.310/**4** | 4.269/**3** | 4.405/**4** |

Final Rating/Rank

## CONCLUSION

In this study, the perceived importance of the expectations of the medical staff is examined. This study gives important clues to the informations system designers and developers for healthcare. There is no purpose of giving any insight to the medical staff.

In general ranking, Availability is the topmost ranked variable. Four out of the five business titles also ranked the Availability as first. Fifth group, Nurses, ranked Availability as second. We mentioned about the need for qualified computer support in healthcare in the introduction part. The HCIS must be available all the time to meet this qualification and assist in the "indispensible uninterrupted healthcare". This considerable result is a good sign for the reliability of the study.

The general ranking results of expectation variables show that end users of HCIS have the high priority for the Usage Expectations dimension. Four out of the top six rated expectations are the Usage Expectations variables as; Speed is the second, Ease of Use is the fourth, User Support is the fifth and Need for Training is the sixth. Ranking of the expectation dimensions given in Table 8 supports this result. The ranking results according to the titles are also compatible. Speed and User Support is in the top three highest ranked values in titles' ranking. This result shows that in a HCIS, users give the utmost importance to its usage virtues. The lesson to learn from this result should be briefly; a HCIS must be easy to use, easy to learn, fast and well supported to get users' support and appreciation.

The surprising result is the least ranked five expectations in general ranking such as, Privacy, Security, Research Facilities and Decision Support. These expectations are expected to be higher ranked. When looked at the final ratings, there is big difference, 4.792 for the first variable (Availability) whereas 4.030 for the last (Privacy). Had the difference been slight, then this situation could have had an excuse.

In the general expectation dimensions ranking, as stated before, Usage Expectations is the first and then comes the Improvement Expectations. One of the huge expectations from an information system is to make improvements both in the quality of work done and in the business processes (Weerakkody & Currie, 2003; Škrinjar & Trkman, 2013). The users think compatible with the literature and they have ranked the Improvement Expectations as the second.

*Table 8. Weights assigned to Likert Scales*

| Very Important | Important | Average Important | Not So Important | Not Important |
|---|---|---|---|---|
| 5 | 4 | 3 | 2 | 1 |

When ranking results of dimensions according to titles is examined, Nurses, Laboratory Technicians and Office Workers ranked the Usage Expectations as the first, Physicians and Others ranked Improvement Expectations as the first. The physicians are in the core of the health service and they need more qualified help when compared to the other groups. The results are compatible with this need as they expect HCIS to make improvement in the hospital as the first priority.

Managerial Expectations are ranked as the last in general ranking. In titles ranking, this result is also compatible. Managerial Expectations are ranked as the last by the three title groups, the other two groups ranked as the third. Bergersen defines the end-user as "the final or ultimate user for which something is intended (i.e. the normal user of a product). It usually implies an individual with a relatively low level of computer expertise, and they do not generally have administrative responsibilities or privileges" (Bergersen, 2004). This definition explains why Managerial Expectations are ranked as the last. By giving the last rank to the Managerial expectations, end users give the message "I think about the effective usage of the system and the improvement in my work". End users do not care about the managerial virtues of the system, because of the nature of their work descriptions. Managerial tools and facilities are of great importance for sure, but they seem to have no priority for the end users over the other three dimensions. They should be important for the managers and shareholders.

The ratings of the perceived importance are usually different from one person to another, because each has a different measurement standard and personal approach (Li, 1997). Elimination of such individual relativity is possible by means of the rank ordering process (Li, 1997).

Although difficult it is, managing user expectations became essential. Managing or limiting the gap between user expectations is shown as one of the factors that influence successful IS implementation in healthcare, by the literature (Kirkendall, Goldenhar, Simon, Wheeler, & Spooner, 2013; Standing & Cripps, 2013). Staples et al. (2002) state that for implementing a new information system, managing expectations is an important issue. Their study shows the adverse effects of unrealistically high expectations on success of the implementation of a new system. They recommend that managements develop strategies to keep the expectations in a realistic level Unmanaged unrealistically high expectations may result in low levels of success. Vendors, while trying to sell their products, raise expectations unrealistically by focusing the best features of their products and avoid stating issues such as systems conversion, compatibility, or integration with existing systems(Ryker, Nath & Henson, 1997). The management can organize some committees and arrange interviews with users to set realistic expectations (Ryker, Nath & Henson, 1997). IS staff can organize on-site trainings and improve the communication channels with users. User involvement, leadership and building trust with users are the main techniques to set realistic expectations (Petter, 2008). User involvement is clear enough that does need further explanation. Leadership is again a kind of user involvement. Differently in this technique, representatives of user are employed to play an important role in project management and inform (lead) users about the features of the planned system, goal etc. to prevent users from growing unreal expectations. Trust can be defined briefly as sharing every detail with users, even the problems. That helps build a trust between users and project management body. This will also help maintain real expectations.

## FUTURE RESEARCH DIRECTIONS

User expectation is a hard and relative issue. It is not easy to study with user expectations. It can change from user to user, site to site and even title to title. The limitation of this study is being a one site limited study. It does not necessarily reflect the general HCIS user's perspective. For further work, this study can be enlarged to different types and size of hospitals, and it can be deeply investigated if there is a difference in the types of hospitals, in the user titles, user working departments etc. It can also be enlarged to examine the effects of the user virtues such as age, education, etc over the perceived importance.

The least ranked five expectations in general ranking such as, Privacy, Security, Research Facilities and Decision Support, should be further studied in detail to understand the discrepancy. The user groups may be further detailed and a hierarchical grouping can be made such as Physicians working in different units, users having different levels of IS experience etc. One reason may be related to the quality of the HIS used. If it is unable to give the basic virtues such as working without outage (availability) and fast processing (speed), the top perceived importance may appear as being basic usage expectations. Data in different hospitals, using different systems, may also be further analyzed to examine if the reason is the HCIS they used.

## ACKNOWLEDGMENT

Part of this work was presented in the 7th Asia Pacific Association for Medical Informatics Conference (APAMI 2012) on 22-25th October 2012 in Beijing. I would like to thank the anonymous reviewers and the editor for their insightful comments and suggestions.

## REFERENCES

Adam Mahmood, M. O., Burn, J. M., Gemoets, L. A., & Jacquez, C. (2000). Variables affecting information technology end-user satisfaction: a meta-analysis of the empirical literature. *International Journal of Human-Computer Studies*, *52*(4), 751–771. doi:10.1006/ijhc.1999.0353

Alshawi, M. (2007). *Rethinking IT in construction and engineering: Organisational readiness*. Psychology Press.

Ammenwerth, E., Iller, C., & Mahler, C. (2006). IT-adoption and the interaction of task, technology and individuals: a fit framework and a case study. *BMC Medical Informatics and Decision Making*, *6*(1), 3. doi:10.1186/1472-6947-6-3 PMID:16401336

Bergeron, F., & Raymond, L. (1992). Evaluation of EIS from a managerial perspective1. *Information Systems Journal*, *2*(1), 45–60. doi:10.1111/j.1365-2575.1992.tb00066.x

Bergersen, B. (2004). User satisfaction and influencing issues. *Network and System Administration Research Surveys*, *1*, 5–26.

Cardozo, R. N. (1965). An experimental study of customer effort, expectation, and satisfaction. *JMR, Journal of Marketing Research*, 244–249. doi:10.2307/3150182

Conrath, D. W., & Mignen, O. P. (1990). What is being done to measure user satisfaction with EDP/ MIS. *Information & Management*, *19*(1), 7–19. doi:10.1016/0378-7206(90)90010-F

Cyert, R., & March, J. (1963). *A behavioural theory of the 4rm. Englewood Cli8s*. Prentice-Hall.

De Keizer, N. F., & Ammenwerth, E. (2008). The quality of evidence in health informatics: How did the quality of healthcare IT evaluation publications develop from 1982 to 2005? *International Journal of Medical Informatics*, *77*(1), 41–49. doi:10.1016/j.ijmedinf.2006.11.009 PMID:17208040

Delone, W. H., & Mclean, E. R. (2004). Measuring e-commerce success: applying the DeLone & McLean information systems success model. *International Journal of Electronic Commerce*, *9*(1), 31–47.

Despont-Gros, C., Mueller, H., & Lovis, C. (2005). Evaluating user interactions with clinical information systems: a model based on human–computer interaction models. *Journal of Biomedical Informatics*, *38*(3), 244–255. doi:10.1016/j.jbi.2004.12.004 PMID:15896698

Fan, L., & Suh, Y. H. (2014). Why do users switch to an advanced technology? An empirical study based on Expectation-Disconfirmation Theory. *Information & Management*, *51*, 240–248. doi:10.1016/j.im.2013.12.004

Gelderman, M. (1998). The relation between user satisfaction, usage of information systems and performance. *Information & Management*, *34*(1), 11–18. doi:10.1016/S0378-7206(98)00044-5

Gürsel, G., Zayim, N., Gülkesen, K. H., Arifoğlu, A., & Saka, O. (2014). A new approach in the evaluation of hospital information systems. *Turk J Electr Eng Co*, *22*(1), 214–222. doi:10.3906/elk-1110-15

Halilovic, S., & Cicic, M. (2013). Antecedents of information systems user behaviour–extended expectation-confirmation model. *Behaviour & Information Technology*, *32*(4), 359–370. doi:10.1080/0144929X.2011.554575

Ives, B., Olson, M. H., & Baroudi, J. J. (1983). The measurement of user information satisfaction. *Communications of the ACM*, *26*(10), 785–793. doi:10.1145/358413.358430

Khalifa, M., & Liu, V. (2004). The state of research on information system satisfaction. [JITTA]. *Journal of Information Technology Theory and Application*, *5*(4), 4.

Kirkendall, E. S., Goldenhar, L. M., Simon, J. L., Wheeler, D. S., & Andrew Spooner, S. (2013). Transitioning from a computerized provider order entry and paper documentation system to an electronic health record: Expectations and experiences of hospital staff. *International Journal of Medical Informatics*, *82*(11), 1037–1045. doi:10.1016/j.ijmedinf.2013.08.005 PMID:24041453

Lee, M. C. (2010). Explaining and predicting users' continuance intention toward e-learning: An extension of the expectation–confirmation model. *Computers & Education*, *54*(2), 506–516. doi:10.1016/j.compedu.2009.09.002

Li, E. Y. (1997). Perceived importance of information system success factors: a meta analysis of group differences. *Information & Management*, *32*(1), 15–28. doi:10.1016/S0378-7206(97)00005-0

Lyytinen, K., & Hirschheim, R. (1988). Information systems failures—a survey and classification of the empirical literature. In *Oxford surveys in information technology* (pp. 257–309). Oxford University Press, Inc.

Nevo, D., & Wade, M. (2005). *Why Good Technologies Disappoint*. Academic Press.

Petter, S. (2008). Managing user expectations on software projects: Lessons from the trenches. *International Journal of Project Management*, *26*(7), 700–712. doi:10.1016/j.ijproman.2008.05.014

Petter, S., DeLone, W., & McLean, E. R. (2013). Information Systems Success: The Quest for the Independent Variables. *Journal of Management Information Systems*, *29*(4), 7–62. doi:10.2753/MIS0742-1222290401

Project Management Institute. (2008). *A Guide to the Project Management Body of Knowledge: PMBOK® Guide*. Project Management Institute.

Ryker, R., Nath, R., & Henson, J. (1997). Determinants of computer user expectations and their relationships with user satisfaction: an empirical study. *Information Processing & Management*, *33*(4), 529–537. doi:10.1016/S0306-4573(97)00016-2

Safran, C., Jones, P. C., Rind, D., Bush, B., Cytryn, K. N., & Patel, V. L. (1998). Electronic communication and collaboration in a health care practice. *Artificial Intelligence in Medicine*, *12*(2), 137–151. doi:10.1016/S0933-3657(97)00047-X PMID:9520221

Seddon, P. B. (1997). A respecification and extension of the DeLone and McLean model of IS success. *Information Systems Research*, *8*(3), 240–253. doi:10.1287/isre.8.3.240

Škrinjar, R., & Trkman, P. (2013). Increasing process orientation with business process management: Critical practices'. *International Journal of Information Management*, *33*(1), 48–60. doi:10.1016/j.ijinfomgt.2012.05.011

Standing, C., & Cripps, H. (2013). Critical Success Factors in the Implementation of Electronic Health Records: A Two-Case Comparison. *Systems Research and Behavioral Science*. doi:10.1002/sres.2209

Staples, D. S., Wong, I., & Seddon, P. B. (2002). Having expectations of information systems benefits that match received benefits: does it really matter? *Information & Management*, *40*(2), 115–131. doi:10.1016/S0378-7206(01)00138-0

Szajna, B., & Scamell, R. W. (1993). The effects of information system user expectations on their performance and perceptions. *Management Information Systems Quarterly*, 493–516. doi:10.2307/249589

Szymanski, D. M., & Henard, D. H. (2001). Customer satisfaction: a meta-analysis of the empirical evidence. *Journal of the Academy of Marketing Science*, *29*(1), 16–35. doi:10.1177/0092070301291002

Weerakkody, V., & Currie, W. (2003). Integrating business process reengineering with information systems development: issues & implications. In *Business Process Management* (pp. 302–320). Springer Berlin Heidelberg. doi:10.1007/3-540-44895-0_21

Yi, Y. (1990). A critical review of consumer satisfaction. *Revista de Marina (Valparaiso, Chile)*, *4*(1), 68–123.

# Chapter 6
# Don't Leave Me Untouched:
## Considering Emotions in Personal Alarm Use and Development

**Sonja Pedell**
*Swinburne University of Technology, Australia*

**Antonio A. Lopez-Lorca**
*Swinburne University of Technology, Australia*

**Tim Miller**
*The University of Melbourne, Australia*

**Leon Sterling**
*Swinburne University of Technology, Australia*

## ABSTRACT

*Older adults want to live independently in their home for as long as possible, and technologies can support them with this goal. However, solutions to help with living alone are often designed from a technical perspective, ignoring the needs and preferences of older adults. This results in strong attitudes and feelings against, and limited adoption of, these technologies. In this chapter, the authors use ethnographic methods to inform the development of solutions taking into account the emotional needs of end-users. They present a three-staged approach by applying it in the domain of personal emergency alarms. First, the authors identify the shortcomings of current emergency alarm systems as perceived by older adults. Then, they develop a prototype that addresses some of the issues identified, focusing on emotional needs. Finally, the authors conduct a trial with the prototype. The results show that considering emotions during system design can improve user experience.*

## INTRODUCTION

*We've put more effort into helping folks reach old age than into helping them enjoy it – Frank A. Clark*

In recent years there has been growing interest in the design of technologies for older people. Reasons for this are:

- Older adults are a growing segment of both the Australian and world populations;
- Governments are concerned about the escalating cost of healthcare and are looking to technology to help contain costs;
- Older adults are currently more willing to spend money than previous generations of older adults;

DOI: 10.4018/978-1-4666-6316-9.ch006

- Older adults are an interesting group as they are more varied than any other user group; and
- Designing for the ageing provides a space for developing seriously innovative and interesting solutions.

However, all this is still not reflected in the availability of technological solutions suitable for an older generation of users. Technology specifically designed for older users focuses on providing support in the context of failing health and increasing frailty. While these concerns are important for older people we propose that emotions of older people and their specific needs and preferences have been neglected in technological development supposedly designed for older adults.

It is important that older adults are not left behind in the adoption of new technologies. Advantages for older people associated with enhanced use of technology include improving the health and quality of life, increased self-confidence, a sense of well-being and belonging (Heo, 2012; Kim, 2012; Russell, 2011). In order for older people to adopt technology into their lives such technology needs to be easy to use and useful (Hanson, 2010). The key determinants for the success of older adopters of technology are willingness and enthusiasm for acquiring new knowledge (Bolton, Gassert, & Cipriano, 2008). Neither of the two is usually present when adopting assistive technologies that are associated with a stigma. It is proposed that the feelings, interests and independence of older people have been neglected in technology design (Waycott et al., 2012). Their individual needs, interests and feelings need to be understood in order to create technologies that can be integrated in their lives.

## MOTIVATION OF THE PROJECT

In the modern world the cost of healthcare is rapidly increasing. In Australia alone the estimated expenditure on healthcare rose from $77.5 billion in 2000-01 to $130.3 billion in 2010-11 (AIHW, 2012). Aged care constitutes a significant part of the healthcare expenditure, costing $10.1 billion in 2008-09 (AIHW, 2010). Advances in science have led to increased life expectancy. The average life expectancy for Australians has increased from 73.9 to 79 for males and 80.1 to 84 for females in the last 20 years (AIHW, 2013a, 2013b). This is contributing to the ageing Australian population. The Australian Bureau of Statistics records that by June 2012, 14.2% of the population was 65 years and older (ABS, 2013). The median age of Australians was 32.7 in 1992 and 37.3 in 2012 and it is predicted that it will reach 41.9 - 45.2 by 2056 (ABS, 2011). This growth of the elderly population, along with a decreased labour force and tax base, increases the stress on the Australian health and aged care systems. The Australian older population shows increased preference for independent living arrangements supported by community care – as opposed to residential care – and a desire for greater autonomy and choice in aged care services generally (PC, 2008). Existing community care services and systems, such as those involving personal alarms, are expensive and many older people cannot afford them without the support of the government or other organisations. The government-supported systems are typically one-size-fits-all solutions that lack flexibility and restrict the older person's autonomy. Instead of catering for the needs and habits of older adults, older adults are forced to comply with arbitrary constraints. Moreover, the system designs look dated and are often rejected by the older people. Modern technologies have to be married with thought-through designs to support older people sustainably in their own homes in a manner adapted to their particular circumstances and lifestyle.

The goals of domestic and healthcare systems tend to be unaligned with the goals of traditional business systems. The former seek to achieve difficult to define emotional goals that are related to supporting the recovery and well-being of the individual customer, whereas the latter pursue a more material goal aiming to achieve an economic benefit. As their motivation is different their development processes should be different as well (Proynova, Paech, Koch, Wicht, & Wetter, 2011). Wetter and Paech (2010) asked healthcare practitioners about a healthcare system that was developed using classic business development strategies adapted for the healthcare domain. In general they expressed their discontent with the existing system. This is consistent with Baxter and Somerville's observations on socio-technical systems in general (2011): Computer-based systems developed without taking into account both the social and technical factors that influence their usage risk being considered a failure - even when they meet their technical requirements - because they do not deliver the expected support for the real work in the organisation. Baxter and Sommerville (2011) also suggest that human-centred design and the use of ethnographic techniques could contribute to the development of more successful socio-technical systems. Some recent work aims to support people's well-being through participatory design and consideration of emotions, effectively changing the focus for design of technology in the healthcare domain from "well-fare" to "well-being" (De Couvreur et al., 2013; Hassenzahl et al., 2013). Negative emotions not only result in stigma and a lack of use, but also a more general discomfort with technology, preventing some older adults from being motivated to gain new technology skills and adopt new technologies (Demiris et al. 2004; Pullin, 2009). Emotional Goals, often described as the *look and feel* of a product, have always played an important role in design considerations (Desmet & Hekkert, 2009) and have been suggested by Marshall (2014) as an integral part socio-technical system design. In this spirit, we advocate using ethnography to study the emotions that the users want to feel in relation to system use. The emotions identified are then integrated in the requirements models and by doing this we can potentially uncover hidden requirements that contribute to the system being better accepted by users.

## Research Questions

Motivated by the discussion above we asked the following three research questions in the context of the issue of emergency alarm systems for older adults:

1. How can ethnography data inform the requirements of the engineering process?
2. How can ethnography data be used to identify emotional goals?
3. Can we develop a repeatable method that supports the transitioning from ethnographic data to requirements models?

The chapter is structured as follows: In the *Related Work* section we present current research in the areas of older people's attitudes toward technology, personal alarms systems and ethnographic-informed system design. The *General Method* section introduces our method for transitioning from ethnographic data to analysis models. In the *Field Study* section, we describe the first part of our case study of a personal alarm system for older adults. The *Results of Initial Field Study* section presents the findings of the field study presented in the previous section. In the *Prototype* section we introduce a prototype to address some of the issues uncovered by our case study. The *Field Study Follow-up* section describes a second study to evaluate the response of older adults to the prototype, followed by a *Results of Follow-up Field Study* section evaluating the prototype in the light of its emotional requirements. The chapters wraps up with the *Conclusion* section.

## RELATED WORK

Information and communication technologies (ICT) could be useful in improving the quality of life of older adults. It is a common belief that older people are technology adverse in general. However, a survey involving 2500 people (Collins, Bhatti, Dexter, & Rabbitt, 1992) indicates no evidence of a relationship between age and technophobia. In fact, in many instances older people perceive technology as a solution to some of their problems. Meyer et al. (2011) studied the perception of 33 older adults residing in nursing homes that were so far away from their families that they received few visitors. The researchers concluded that half the interviewees were dissatisfied with their level of interactions with families and friends and over 80% of them were interested in trying videoconferencing systems.

The Australian government has also shown concerns about the quality of life of older people and how ICT can contribute to improve it (CoA, 2011; Grealy et al., 2008). In a study of the Comonwealth of Australia (2011) the focus is on personal alarms. The research discusses how some issues associated with age, such as poor eyesight, arthritis, diabetes, depression or dementia, can affect older people's awareness of their surroundings, making them more prone to accidents. They explain how a range of personal alarms work, their associated procedures and how they can help in alleviating the risks that come with ageing. In Grealy et al. (2008) the focus moves away from personal alarm systems. The authors argue that although there are many examples of such assistive technologies they tend to lack effectiveness. Sharing the view given by Collins et al. (1992), they state that devices that improve older people's quality of life are well received, especially when they are provided early and supported by training and ongoing maintenance. Smart technologies, in particular, can improve overall peace of mind for older people and carers, improve quality of life and provide more opportunities to defer moving into residential care. The authors refer to preliminary research that indicates that ICT can improve social connection and communication and the mental and physical health of older people.

We can find in the literature several examples of ICT that were successfully used by older people (Hanson & Magnusson, 2011; Hanson et al., 2007). Hanson et al. (2007) reports a successful application of ICT to support 'people with early dementia' (PWED). The technology consisted of a program that provided memory training and mental stimulation to improve the self-esteem and well-being of PWED. As the program required computer skills the authors developed a 12 week training module. Many participants originally expressed doubts about their capability to learn how to operate the computer. However, they enjoyed their training and at the end many asked for further training to learn new skills, noting that the computer had become part of their everyday lives. The response of participants to the use of the program at home was also positive. Many relatives observed that the program was effective at maintaining the cognitive capabilities of PWED. Some of the older users found the exercises relaxing and others obtained a sense of purpose and satisfaction. Addressing dementia, using ICT, was part of a larger project in which Hanson and Magnusson (2011) aimed at empowering older people with long-standing chronic conditions who live at home, and their families, in their daily lives. The authors present the lessons learned over a 14 year period of implementation of the project. The program is running as a mainstream service in one Swedish municipality and is planned to be implemented in 20 other municipalities. The service has four components: multimedia educational caring programs, the hardware and software system, a call centre run by aged care practitioners and education and supervision. Most of the 400 participants in the project were highly satisfied with the service and believed that it had improved their quality of life. Older people and carers felt less isolated due to the informal support network composed of other participants in similar situations. After a minimum of three months of use family carers felt more confident in their caring skills. The professional carers felt more appreciated and the municipality reduced costs. The authors highlighted that one of the reasons behind the success of the project was that the system was developed together with older people and their carers to meet their needs, preferences and situation. The work of Henkeman et al. (2007) is also aligned with this idea of co-design. The authors argue that eHealth systems are often rejected because they are designed from a technological perspective, without taking into account the final user. They suggest that by placing the older people in a scenario that simulates a living environment the people visualise themselves using the technology, hence increasing its acceptance. We agree with these works that consider the older adults' needs and preferences. Giving them a voice in development is essential in achieving a well-accepted system. Also, our experiences indicate that older adults can use new technologies when provided with minimal instruction. In fact by using touch screens we remove the need for the use of the 'mouse', an entry barrier identified by Hanson et al. (2007).

Although older people are willing to adopt ICT if their quality of life is improved, the design of the solutions may pose threats to their adoption. The first adoption barrier is cost. The cost of technology within the home should match the economic position of the user. However, currently most personal alarm systems are too expensive and cannot be purchased without third-party support (Vergados, Alevizos, Mariolis, & Caragiozidis, 2008). Even if we ignore the economic factor the perceptions of older people have a determinant effect on their adoption of technologies. Demiris et al. (2004) studied how older people perceive aged care technologies in the context of a smart home. The participants in the study acknowledged that areas such as emergency help, prevention and detection of falls or physiological parameters monitoring, would benefit from smart home technologies. However, the older people were also concerned about potential violation of their privacy – an idea also explored by Melander-Wikman et al. (2008) – the replacement of human contacts by computers, the degree of user-friendliness of the systems and the need for specific training for older learners. Regarding the user-friendliness of the devices, the older people were concerned that many of the limitations that come with age, such as vision loss, memory loss or difficulty using small buttons or a computer mouse, would be ignored. In addition, participants raised the issue of stigmatisation provoked by certain devices. Other authors have identified additional factors. For example, some older people do not like personal alarms that have to be worn around the neck visible to everyone (Peeters, 2000). Others find them uncomfortable and do not wear them in bed, which places them at risk when they get up in the middle of the night to go to the bathroom without them (Miguel & Lewin, 2008). It is paramount to identify older people's feelings around the use of technology and design the solutions in such way that negative feelings around such use are avoided or minimised. In this paper we have identified how users of personal alarm systems feel about them and have aimed to address their concerns and sought to fulfil their emotional needs in an attempt to maintain their wellbeing.

The development of the program for ameliorating early dementia, presented in Hanson et al. (2007), used ethnography during the complete development process to engage PWED in a participatory design approach. The authors organised meetings over a nine month period that involved seven PWED and two dementia-specialised nurses. The meetings occurred weekly during the first four months and fortnightly or monthly during the remaining five months. They discussed topics extracted from early stage dementia literature. The discussion sessions were recorded and this data was used to structure the material within a multimedia program. The PWED also produced visual material during these meetings that was included in the multimedia program. The initial version of the program underwent validation and improvement by the PWED during the meetings. The PWED explored existing computer-based exercises, recommended for early dementia subjects, and were encouraged to choose their favourites and adapt them to their tastes. All this led to producing a program that was closely aligned with the interests and needs of PWED. However the authors do not elaborate on how the transition from ethnographic data to the program was done.

Several prototypes have been developed and ideas of adoption explored in a multitude of HCI projects that used ethnographic field studies to facilitate subtle interactions between family members (Hoog, Keller, & Stappers, 2004; Vetere, Davis, Gibbs, & Howard, 2009), in some cases explicitly to support older people to stay longer in their homes (Mynatt, Rowan, Craighill, & Jacobs, 2001). These prototypes, promoting subtle interactions of family members to be in touch, correspond well with the aims of our projects on addressing emotional needs of older users at home using emergency alarms.

Mynatt et al. (2001) created a picture frame that constitutes a surrogate support system that transmits informal daily communication. According to the authors a surrogate support system is a form of mediated awareness intended to re-establish certain aspects of the naturally occurring social support that is disrupted, in this case, by the introduction of geographic distance into an extended family. Their goal is to leverage emotional connections with close family members and friends by augmenting a common household object that is typically associated with the family and the role that portraits already play in decorating the home. This is in strong alignment with the aims of our project making use of existing social structures and routines that are significant and familiar to older adults.

The 'Gustbowl' (Hoog et al., 2004) is an ethnographic research product that enables parents and children who have left their parents' house to bring back the feeling of coming home. The Gustbowl is described as a system allowing for low threshold, uncomplicated communication through using an aesthetically pleasing product. Technology is used to reconnect a parent and grown-up child by anchoring communication in routine daily actions. Importantly the Gustbowl is an example of a product that doesn't require people to change their daily routine but that incorporates everyday rituals to be used casually to be in touch. This connection would be a more subtle and non-intrusive way to communicate with a primary carer than an explicit monitoring system.

In a similar fashion 'Collage' (Vetere et al., 2009) is a shared domestic display using mobile camera-phones as an input device and a touch screen for synchronous interaction between family members with a focus on grandparents and grandchildren. Via the phones, photographs and text messages are sent to the touch screens simultaneously. The photographs and messages provide a constant presence, flowing down continuously on the screen (older pictures are smaller than new pictures and shown less frequently), much like a waterfall. These shared objects can be stopped, moved around, enlarged and arranged. Collage enables a sharing of subtle and often serendipitous interactions without being intrusive. Collage facilitates particular simple forms of playful interaction and communication via the shared touch screen. When communicating via moving pictures or sending photos and texts simultaneously the implicit message sent to family members is "I am ok" without putting a strong emphasis on this aspect of the interaction. The constant presence of the screen with family related content reminder of loved ones and consequently created a feeling of being less alone for some of the older people (Pedell et al., 2014).

These three examples show how domestic prototypes have been developed to cater for meaningful but subtle interactions with family members, including their needs, routines, emotions and interests. Hassenzahl et al. (2012) point out that, from a psychological point of view, the exchange of seemingly trivial "information" about mundane day-to-day events is crucial to the feeling of being involved in the loved one's life. That this can be technologically mediated was shown by Dey and de Guzman (2006). They developed a series of presence display concepts (e.g., PictureFrame, AugmentedMirror).

The idea how such displays can be used for being aware of the wellbeing of older family members was established over a decade ago. Sharing information about past mundane activities will help family members to recognize any change from regular patterns that can be of importance. For instance, for judging the well-being of (grand) parents (Mynatt et al., 2001). These projects are useful in informing a social emergency alarm. In applying ethnographic methods they give insights into the personal perspective of the older user. However, while these prototypes were developed and tested in field trials they were not developed into more widely available solutions in aged care nor was much insight given on how the insights about the user could inform the development of design. We suggest this can be achieved by combining these ideas with our proposed software engineering process.

## GENERAL METHOD: FROM ETHNOGRAPHIC DATA TO MODELS

A key contribution of this paper is a method to bridge the gap between the ethnographic process and the software requirements of engineering activities. By proposing such a method we aim to formalise and make the transition from ethnographic data to requirements models repeatable. Figure 1. provides an overview of the method, which is built around three main activities:

1. The ethnographic data is analysed to identify the key elements in the domain;
2. These elements are used to inform requirements analysis models; and
3. The models are used to drive discussions and engage with project stakeholders for the purpose of feedback and refinement.

In this section, we describe in detail the different activities associated with the method.

### Content Analysis Based on Structured Data

In the first step of the method, we apply content analysis techniques to identify important categories and topics in our ethnographic data that

*Figure 1. The general analysis procedure*

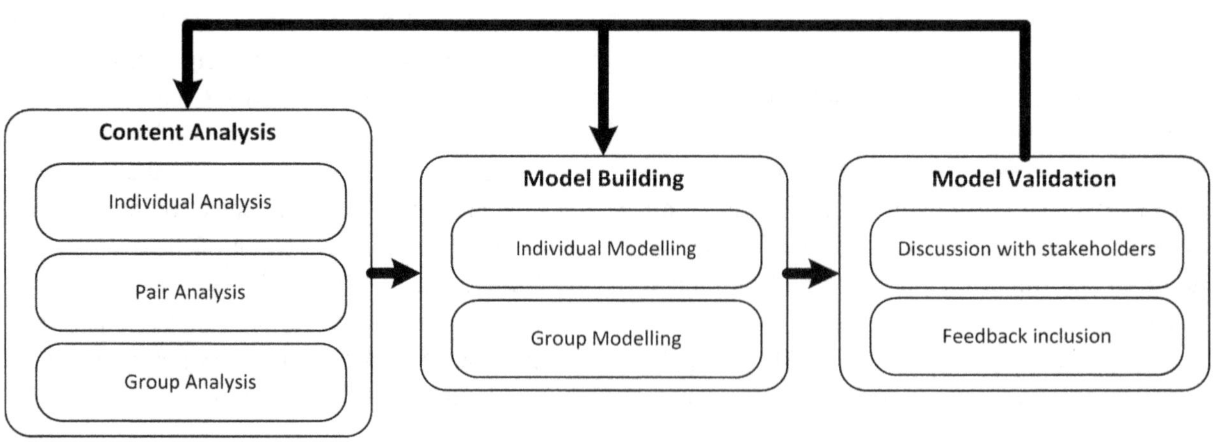

inform the creation of the requirements models in the following step. Our content analysis approach builds on Patton's content analysis (Patton, 2002). Content analysis can be applied to any type of data, possibly a heterogeneous mix of texts, audio material, questionnaires or video recordings, to extract their contents. The data is examined to identify and categorise recurring and important themes and topics. A comprehensive categorisation is typically achieved after several iterations consisting of the complete examination of all data. Each iteration contributes to the understanding of the data contents (Patton, 2002).

We have modified this technique to cater for a three-step process (from individual over pair to group analysis) to increase the validity of the data across multiple people analysing the data. The rest of this section provides guidelines to conduct our modified content analysis process. In our case studies we have focused on analysing the content of interview transcripts, questionnaires, and information about the domestic spaces in which our interview participants live. However this approach can be applied to analyse any data in different domain contexts.

## Domain Dependent and Domain Independent Elements

Our goal is to use the results of the content analysis process to build the requirements models that will result in a new system being developed. This means that we have to identify two distinct types of elements: *domain dependent* elements and *domain independent* elements. Domain dependent elements are those elements of the domain that are important for the analysis, such as wellbeing checks and alarm pendants, while domain independent elements are those relating to our method, such as roles and goals.

Domain dependent analysis is similar to the approach traditionally used in content analysis techniques. On a case-by-case basis content analysts define new categories suiting their purpose. For example, in the initial set of interviews for a given development project, researchers might define categories corresponding to their interests; i.e. stakeholders' backgrounds, their relationship with technology, the obstacles that they face when dealing with certain problems or their expectations of the solution to be developed. A second batch of interviews for the same project could be more geared towards the validation of a prototype and hence developers could focus their content analysis to identify aspects of the prototype that users liked or disliked, paths to be explored or comparison with other systems. Once categories are identified, topics will naturally arise as recurring elements within categories. In the Field Study section we discuss the categories and topics that we identified from our case study.

Domain independent analysis is particular to our research. As we are conducting content analysis to build requirement models, there are certain key elements that should always be identified, regardless of the problem domain. These key elements are the roles in the system, the emotions that drive and permeate the system, the functionalities that are sought and the qualities that the functionalities should have. When we identify these, we can map them directly to the goal model. This is independent of the domain, i.e. there are roles in all domains: Older people, Carer/Relative, Insomniac, Psychosis consumers, Mental health workers, GP, Depressed person

Throughout the content analysis process (of e.g. interview data), researchers also categorise each important domain dependent element. The categories that we try to identify depend on the domain, for example, in one domain we try to find, how older people interact with technology, or what problems do they have with technology. In another domain we look for how people with psychosis deal with the illness, in another, we look at how GP's interact with people with depression.

- **Roles:** These represent capabilities required to solve the problem. They are typically associated with people involved in the problem being studied, but they can also represent automatic capabilities that the system should have. Typically, roles do not capture the capability of an individual but of a set of individuals that can take on that role. For example, the role of a *Working Mother* is not an individual, but a characterisation of the traits and responsibilities; namely that they are female, go to work and also play the role of *Mother*.

- **Emotional Goals:** The stakeholders' *emotions* also have to be identified as they are crucial to the interactions of users with the system. People often express themselves in terms of *negative emotions*. These are emotions that the system has to work around, to completely avoid or to ameliorate. In relation to software development, we define *emotional goals* as the response of the system to these negative emotions, or simply to model the emotional needs of stakeholders. For our purposes, we distinguish between two types of emotional goals (Miller, 2014). *Personal emotional goals* represent emotions that people seek to achieve regardless of the system and that to some extent motivate the existence of the system itself such as the desire to be felt accepted. *System-dependent emotional goals* represent emotions that are related to the use of the system. If the system did not exist these emotional goals would be irrelevant.
- **Functional Goals:** For the problem to be solved it has to be addressed in terms of the functionalities that should be covered. We refer to these functionalities as *functional goals,* which are often driven or affected by the stakeholder's emotional needs.
- **Quality Goals:** Finally, *quality goals* determine constraints on how the functional goals are to be achieved. In later sections we present examples of all these elements.

## Data Distribution

Our version of content analysis is conceived as a team effort (refer to Figure 2). Before the analysis commences the available data, for example interview transcripts, is divided among the team members involved in the process. This division has to be done in such way that at least two team members receive the same data. This will support the second step of the process: the pair analysis. Ideally team members that participated in the data gathering of certain subsets of data should be assigned to other subsets to avoid their own subjective experiences influencing the content analysis. In our case study, for example, we assigned interview transcripts to team members who had not participated in those particular interviews.

- **Individual Analysis:** The first step of the content analysis is done individually. A researcher analyses an assigned set of interview transcripts to identify categories and topics. In our projects we have used context analysis according to Patton (2002), but other thematic analysis techniques could be used.

As well as noting and categorising key concepts an important part of our project has been the highlighting of salient passages in the transcripts to be used as support for conclusions, which is important for the remaining steps.

- **Pair Analysis:** In the second step of the process team members pair up to compare the results of their individual analyses. Researchers can inadvertently introduce personal interpretation or subjective opinions while identifying categories and topics in the individual content analysis process. We deem it important to reach consent via discussion to reduce the risk of distorted results. When the conclusions of both team members coincide we gain con-

*Figure 2. Data allocation for analysis across individual and teams of researchers*

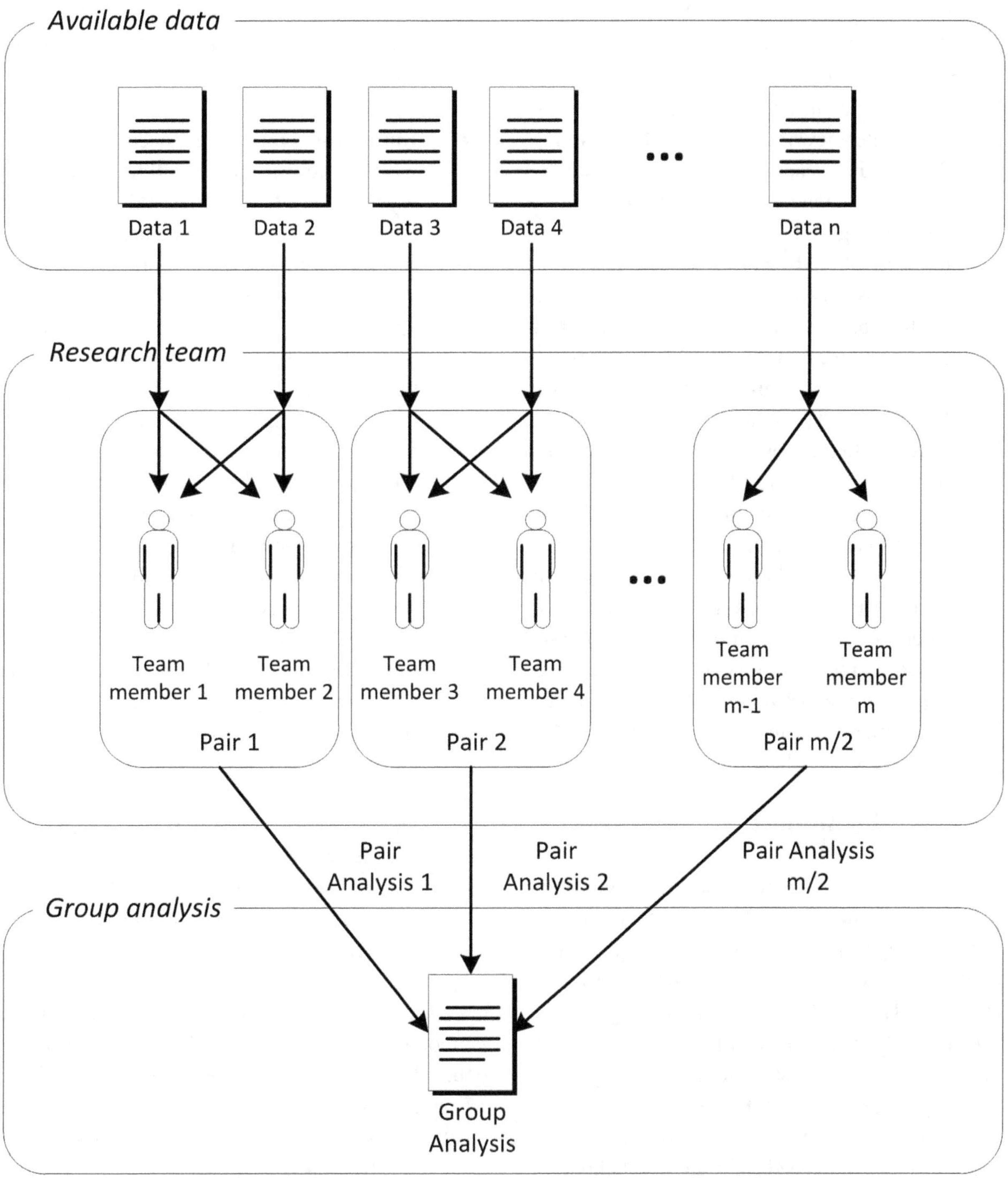

fidence in the results as they are supported by two separate analyses. When the results do not match researchers bring forward the pieces of information that supported their decision, for instance highlighted passages in the interview transcripts. A discussion is then held to reach a consensus that solves all inconsistencies. This step concludes when an agreed summary of both individual content analyses is produced.

- **Group Analysis:** In the final step of the content analysis process all sub-teams meet to share their conclusions. The purpose is to compile the results of the pair analysis for all subsets of data. Results generated by different teams contribute to a more complete understanding of the problem. If inconsistencies in conclusions arise, i.e. elements that contradict others, the teams that identified them should back their position with data excerpts, as in the pair analysis. Then, a discussion among all participants based on the data evidence is conducted to solve the inconsistency. When all generated themes are agreed on the content analysis process concludes.

## Building the Models

The content analysis process described in previous section is intended to facilitate the transition of the ethnographic data to software requirement models. We use the requirement models presented in (Lopez-Lorca, Miller, Pedell, Sterling, & Curumsing, 2014). These models explicitly include the emotional needs of stakeholders (see Figure 3). We propose that in socio-technical systems, and healthcare systems in particular, failing to consider the emotional needs of system stakeholders can lead to missing important requirements and hence, the rejection of the system by its intended users (Miller et al., 2014). We further suggest building the models as a two-step process, in a similar procedure to the content analysis described above, to achieve models that are less influenced by personal bias.

- **Individual Modelling Based on Data:** In the first step of the modelling process every member of the team builds a version of the models based on their interpretation of the final results of the content analysis. Not all levels of models described in (Lopez-Lorca et al., 2014) should be built at this stage. High-level goal models suffice for the purpose of processing ethnographic data to requirements analysis. These models capture the essential elements on which the remainder of the analysis models are based, i.e. roles, emotional goals, functional goals and quality goals. All of these elements should have been identified in the content analysis process. In alignment with Marshall (2014) building on the work on modelling notation of Sterling and Taveter (2009) we suggest classifying the identified elements in four lists: A "Who" list (who are the relevant participants in the system - roles); a "Do" list (what the system should do - functional goals); a "Be" list (how the system should be - quality goals); and a "Feel" list (the feelings relevant for the system - emotional goals and negative emotions).

A detailed explanation on how to build these models is out of the scope of this paper. For further detail on building these models we refer to Lopez-Lorca (2014). What is important to know is that these models are constructed to be understandable by non-technical stakeholders and quick to develop. Using the results derived from the content analysis process, team members should be capable of sketching these models on paper

*Figure 3. High-level goal model*

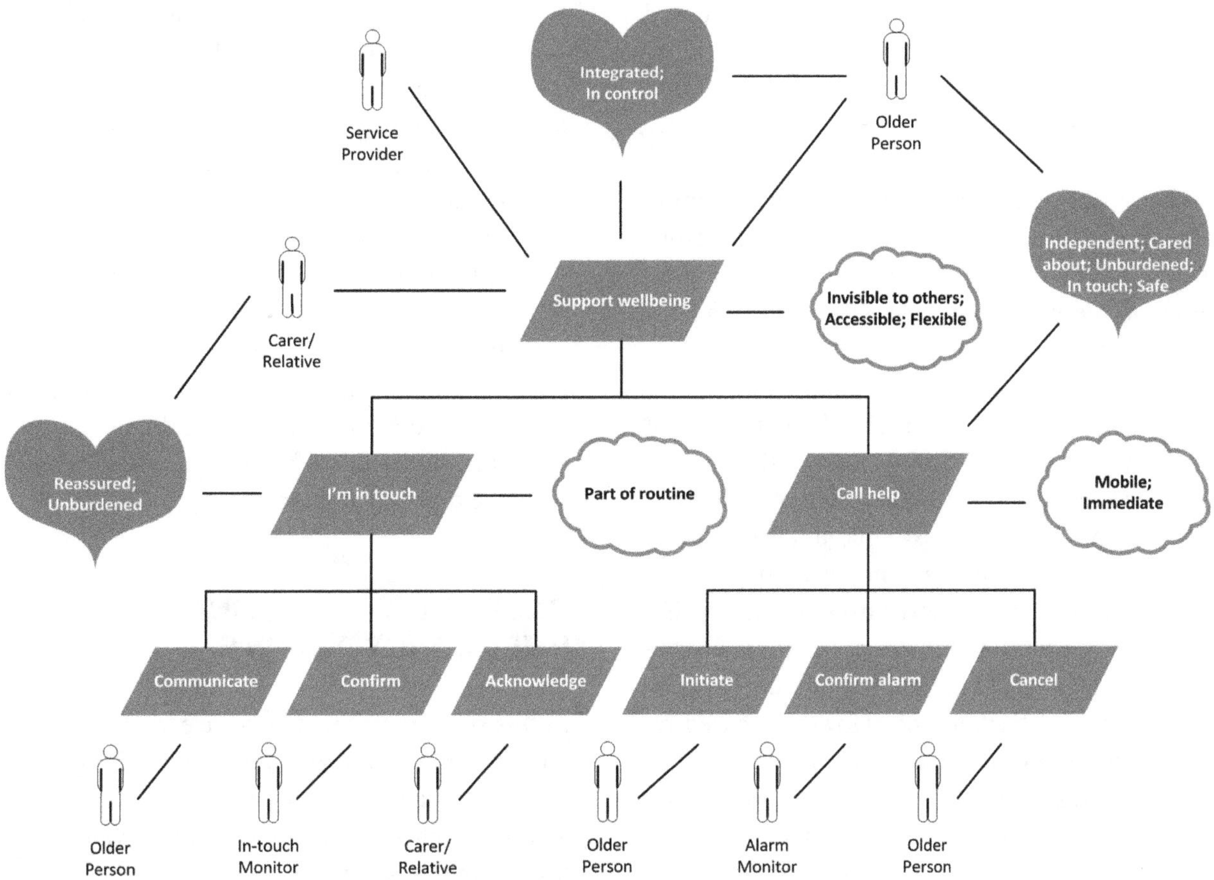


without difficulty. If the content analysis process was applied to the initial phases of a software development project then these models would be developed from scratch. However, if the analysis was intended to assess the reaction of users to a prototype, for example, then team members would have an existing set of models to refine based on the ethnographic data.

- **Round Table Analysis of the Models and Consolidation:** In the second step of the modelling process all team members meet in a collaborative modelling effort. In the previous step participants modelled the elements identified by the content analysis. This forces the team members to rationalise the modelling process. When all individual models are compared and discussed aspects held in common by all participants are directly transferred to the models being collaboratively built. Interpretations that are not homogeneous across all participants will be discussed. Because every team member produced their models following their own rational process they each have to be able to defend their interpretation. This leads to richer discussions and, eventually, to a mature set of models that were built on team consensus considering many different perspectives and whose authorship is shared by all team members. These models constitute the stepping stone on which the other analysis and design models are based on. However, before the project proceeds to that stage, the early models produced in this step are discussed with stakeholders to validate them.

## Validation

The last step of our method focuses on validating the produced models to ensure that the development process has a sound starting point. Any issue in the model can ensue revisiting stages 1 or 2 of the process.

- **Validation with Stakeholders:** In the first step of the validation process the models are discussed with the source of the ethnographic data, for example interviewees. If the original source is not available for discussion representative users of the system are appropriate for this task. Typically the people that are involved in this step have no technical background. However, based on our research and other existing work (Paay, Sterling, Vetere, Howard, & Boettcher, 2009), the models that we use are easily understood by non-technical stakeholders. In the discussion the researcher briefly explains what the model elements mean and how to interpret them. The stakeholders then give feedback about the content of the models.

Our general approach is to allow stakeholders to modify the models during roundtable meetings. By being involved in the modelling itself the stakeholders feel responsible for some of the analysis decisions, which gives them a sense of authorship over the model and a feeling of being listened to (Miller, Pedell, Sterling, & Lu, 2011). We also advocate recording and transcribing the discussion for future reference and analysis.

- **Iteration:** The feedback received in the previous step is used to improve the models. At this point, depending on the nature of the feedback, the process may backtrack to different activities. Researchers discuss the suggestions made by the stakeholders, consider consequences and incorporate them in a consistent way into the final models. If the stakeholders did not modify the models then the recording of the discussion should still be analysed to extract the feedback as it might lead to some small changes in the model such as finding a more accurate term. The process concludes only when all stakeholders are satisfied with the models and make no further suggestions for changes after viewing the updated version.

## CASE STUDY: PERSONAL EMERGENCY ALARMS

In this section, we present a case study focusing on personal emergency alarms for older people, which we have used to evaluate our approach. This research aims to provide data to evaluate the following questions:

1. Does our method for modelling ethnographic data capture the most important themes?
2. Does the consideration of emotions lead us to findings that we would not have discovered otherwise?
3. Do current emergency alarm systems support their users' primary emotional needs?

To answer these questions, we conducted two field studies. One in which we collected data on user needs, primarily via semi-structured interviews, modelled this data using above described procedures, and then qualitatively compared our models with an initial baseline that was constructed prior to the interviews. A second field study explored the how well a prototype built on the results of study one met the needs in particular the emotional needs of older people.

## Overview of Emergency Alarm Systems

Emergency alarm systems aim to support people, generally older people, to live independently in their home who may be prone to falling due to e.g. seizures or frailty or who may be vulnerable to other events requiring help.

Emergency alarm systems typically consist of two broad types of functionality:

1. **An Emergency Alarm:** This is some semi-mobile device, generally in the form of a pendant worn around the older person's neck or wrist, which contains a button that when pressed alerts a service provider that the older person has raised an alarm.
2. **A "Wellbeing" Check:** This is some device, generally of the form of a button on a *base station*, which allows the older person to signal that they are *well*. The older person is required to push the button each day between a fixed period; e.g. between 7am-11am, and if they do not, the service provider's software system sends a report to support staff to check on the older person via a phone call.

In the case that the emergency alarm button is pressed, or the wellbeing check button is not pushed and the older person cannot be contacted, the service provider tries to contact nominated relatives and friends to check on the older person, and ultimately, emergency services if relatives/friends cannot check in. Calls to the older person are used to reduce the number of false alarms, caused by e.g. accidental emergency alarm pushes or simply forgetting to perform the wellbeing check.

Such systems enable older people to live safely in their own home while offering reassurance to worried relatives and friends. This is a valuable service to older people and their relatives and significant others. While these emergency systems offer valuable services to older people and their families, they often suffer from usage problems. The main problems concern not using the device or not having it available when needed and not understanding the implications of use or non-use. Emergency services are usually introduced in a critical period of a traumatic event such after a fall, the bereavement of the partner or when the first time the discussion comes up to move to a nursing home. A lot of older people feel overwhelmed in these situations to adopt a routine around a new technology.

Our field study results confirm that in many cases, emergency alarm systems fail in their objectives of maintaining safety even though the hardware and software form a well-engineered and reliable system. We suggest that on major reason is that their designers did not adequately consider the emotional needs and context conditions of the older people or their relatives and carers. Therefore our research approach focuses on the exploration and understanding of the emotions of users and other stakeholders.

## Details of the Field Study

We conducted semi-structured interviews with four people about emergency alarms and technology in general, modelled the important aspect of the resulting data using our models, and used these models as communication tools within our research group and with external stakeholders. As well as interviewing older people, who have had or currently have an emergency alarm system installed in their home, we interviewed several family members whose relatives have had an emergency alarm installed (4), and some older people (4) who had never had an emergency alarm installed. The interviews provided us with rich, qualitative data about the positives and negatives of current emergency alarm systems and an insight into the types of goals that stakeholders in these systems want supported.

## Study Design

Our first step was to have an initial brainstorming session to define the emotional, functional, and quality goals that we believed older people and the families would want in an emergency system. This provided us with a loose boundary to come up with interview questions as well as providing us with a lens through which we could view the results, although we did not restrict the interview to questions solely inside the boundary.

Next, we interviewed our participants using semi-structured interviews (for more detail on the interviews see the Structure of the Interview section). Interviews were analysed, extracting the key emotional, functional and quality goals of the main stakeholders. This step was modelled on the method defined in the previous section.

The resulting models were used as communication tools throughout the project, both internally and with external teams, such as our project partners and a separate team who developed a prototype emergency alarm based on our findings.

## Interview Participants

We interviewed twelve participants, broken broadly into three groups:

1. Older people who either currently or previously had an emergency alarm installed in their home. Their age ranged from 85 to 91. All participants lived on their own, except for one who lived with her husband.
2. Family members of older people who either currently or previously had an emergency alarm installed into their home. These are important stakeholders as they are often the people who drive the purchase and installation of the system. All of the older relatives of these family members lived on their own.
3. Older people who have never had an emergency alarm installed into their home. Their ages ranged from 66-79.

## Data Collection

The primary data collection method consisted of semi-structured interviews with our participants. However, researchers also recorded additional information such as the physical setup of the alarm in the home. Each participant was interviewed once for a period of 30-60 minutes, focussing on the emotional, functional and quality goals of emergency alarm systems and technology in general. Some of the participants were contacted for short follow-up questions, mainly about their individual emergency alarm service. All interviews were audio recorded and transcribed.

## Structure of the Interview

The interview guideline consisted of several sections. The first section asked for information on the participants' background, their interests and living circumstances. In the second part of the interview the technology use was explored. This encompassed questions such as "Do you remember the reason you got this technology initially?", "What works well with the technology and what doesn't work well?" and "How should the technology be modified that you would like to use it?" The third part covered safety procedures and experiences with emergency alarms, if the participant had used one or was using one currently. All these questions aimed to explore the three key questions - What should technology do? How should it be? and How should it feel?

## RESULTS OF THE INITIAL FIELD STUDY

We present the results from the field study in two sections:

1. What we learnt about stakeholders' emotional goals related to emergency alarm systems and evaluating how well existing emergency alarm systems support these emotions;
2. What we learnt about our method for ethnographic data analysis and modelling.

The results of the field study are a summarised version of the more detailed ethnographic analysis presented in (Pedell, Sterling, Keirnan, & Dobson, 2013).

### Emotions around Current Emergency Alarm Systems

Figure 3 presents an overview of the final goal model for the emergency alarm system. We use this model to summarise and present our results in this section. Our analysis focuses on the two main stakeholders: older people and their relatives, with a particular focus on the emotional goals and how these relate to the functional and quality goals. For each goal that we discuss we provide a short quote from one of the interview participants as an example of why this goal is important.

The major emotional goals for the relatives are 'feeling reassured' and 'feeling unburdened'.

- **Reassurance:** Reassurance was the primary emotional goal of relatives. They want the system installed into the home of their family member to provide them with reassurance about the wellbeing of this family member. Our analysis provides an insight that the emergency systems used by the older persons gave a strong sense of reassurance to the families:

*It was a huge relief, a huge weight of my shoulders, going to sleep at night thinking if something has happened. Or I didn't have to think, "I haven't heard from Mum. Is she ok?" I just knew that there was someone else helping with that caring, if you like. [Christine – daughter of an emergency system user]*

This theme was consistent throughout the interviews with the relatives, with only one exception. One of the relatives felt that the introduction of the emergency system caused stress for his mother, so the service was removed from her house. He felt that visiting his mother regularly was a more suitable and reliable way of keeping in touch than relying on an emergency system.

- **Unburdened:** The secondary result regarding relatives is that they feel that the system *unburdens* them. Before the introduction of the system many of the relatives would take it upon themselves to check in with their family member every day, mostly via short visits or phone calls. They found these visits time consuming and often done in a rush.

*Like where we can actually offload some of that work that's a bit more mundane and a bit more not-so-personal; get other people to do it. [Christine – daughter of an emergency system user]*

Some relatives commented that this reduced the number of visits and phone calls, but in addition, made the visits and calls that they still made feel more personal and made space for more quality time.

The main emotional goals for the *older people* are to feel safe, independent, cared about and in touch. Secondary to these are the emotions that older people want to feel about the emergency alarm systems: that the system is integrated into their lives.

- **Safe:** Feeling safe in their own home is a major emotional goal of older people and emergency alarms have the potential to aid with this:

*But basically because I've got this, I've got confidence when I'm on my own. [Jane – an emergency system user]*

Several participants reported that they, or their family member, felt safer knowing that they could use the system to call for help, or that if they did not "check in", someone would be notified. However, as acknowledged in the quotes about feeling independent and in control, some older persons chose not to wear their emergency pendant, accepting that they would not be able to call for help if something happened. Ultimately, this resulted in some failures of the overall goals of the system, in that the older person required assistance but could not access it, despite the fact that the technology had not failed in a functional way. There was also a feeling on behalf of the relatives that they perceived that the older person feels safer having an alarm than otherwise.

- **Independent:** Independence is a key theme throughout the interviews. Older people want to maintain a level of independence and emergency alarms support this by enabling them to remain in their own home instead of being in institutional care. This is why many of them opted to install an emergency alarm:

*And, you know, she wasn't all anti it. She liked it because it gave her a little bit of independence. [Christine – daughter of emergency system user]*

However, a majority of participants commented that the emergency alarm in fact threatened their independence, rather than enabling it:

*The fact that it wasn't aesthetically pleasing, but it, far more importantly was the psychology of the device and what it meant to her and the fact that she didn't just not wear it in public, but chose not to wear it alone whilst inside the house. I think it's much more an internal thing more than what it looked like or what it said [Joe – nephew of emergency alarm user]*

Our analysis showed two distinct trends with our participants. The older people who initiated the procurement of an alarm felt that it gave them some independence as the system gave to them the opportunity to live alone in their own home for longer. While those who were given an ultimatum by their family - get an alarm system or move to a nursing home - felt overwhelming negative about it. They felt the personal alarm system was taking away their independence in controlling them. They also felt that there was a stigma attached to having an emergency system. However in the end the older people took the alarm option to keep the more relevant independence which was remaining in their familiar environment.

- **Cared About:** The theme of being *cared about* by their family and friends was a major emotional theme. However, more importantly was the idea that our participants wanted to be cared *about,* not cared *for*. That is, they did not want to receive care (as reflected in their desire to be independent), but they did want their families to show that they cared. In discussing his aunt, who had been a nurse, one participant stated:

*This transition was difficult for her, because she went from being a carer to being someone who didn't want to be cared for. [Joe – nephew of emergency system user]*

While the introduction of an emergency system by the family was intended to demonstrate to the older person that their family cared about them the design of the systems did not assist with this. One reason stated for this was that pushing the wellbeing-check button each day offered little feedback that anything was happening. In particular, some emergency systems did not provide feedback as to whether the button had been pushed that day.

*She always would joke about her cowbell, and complain about it. "Look at what my kids are making me do," kind of comment. A slight resentfulness about it. [...]. She'd occasionally make comments about, "Look what I'm resorted to," comments about it. [Lucas – describing feelings of his mother]*

Participants did particularly note that personnel from the service providers showed exceptional care in their interactions, and provided them with a feeling of being cared about, but this only happened in the event that the older person forgot to press the wellbeing check button.

- **In Control:** Related to independence, the feeling of being in control of their lives is important to people. This is particularly the case for older people as they often lose control of some part of their independence due to ill health or lack of mobility. This goes for their life in general:

*But it's just, again, by them shopping and choosing their own food, they've still got some control of their life. [Christine – daughter of emergency system user];*

But also with respect to emergency alarms, some older people felt that the introduction of the alarm itself had other implications:

*With the emergency alarm take up there are, in my opinion, other issues. It is about the end. I am not miserable about it. Life is wonderful, but we are all dying one day. People want to have the right to make a decision when they want to leave. [Marie – non user]*

There was a definite feeling of frustration on behalf of many older persons and their families that there was little control offered to the older person. There are no configurable parameters for any of the emergency systems. For example, each older person was required to press the wellbeing-check button between the hours of 7am and 11am every day. These times could not be changed and if they wanted to leave the house for that period they were required to phone the service provider to let them know. For many of the older persons this inconvenience was exacerbated by the fact that the system was forced upon them in the first place.

- **In Touch:** A major part of an emergency alarm system is the well-being check. This part of the service is a basic way for an older person to get in touch with the service provider, who can then alert the family if the person has not been in touch. However, from our analysis it is clear that the older people did not feel in touch using this system, even though they desired to be in touch. This is partly because the pressing of a button offered no social context and partly because the family did not receive the resulting signal. This lack of contact gave the older person little incentive to push the button, except to satisfy their families. The need to feel in touch is stronger than the need to have an emergency alarm system:

*Like even Christmas, I'm picking Mum and Dad up for Christmas, and Mum said: "What can I get?" I said: "Could you get the plum pudding and some custard?". So she's got that task to do when she goes shopping; makes her feel like she's still contributing. When she's out with this lady shopping: "Yes, I'm going out for Christmas lunch. I'm still part of things." [Christine – daughter of emergency system user]*

However, we believe feeling in touch is ultimately something that emergency alarm systems could support besides feeling safe.

Overall, the feeling of being in touch with friends and family was an important theme, and one, that having an emergency system helped to support, albeit weakly. In fact it was the calls from the personnel from the service providers that provided the strongest support for being in touch for some. However with regard to the technology, most emergency system users felt detached from the system and its greater meaning. Most understood its purpose and why it was there, but for many the daily activity that included pressing the button had no meaning and they could not relate it to a person at the other end:

*It would give greater intimacy, but something of a word like that, to it... If it were a real voice, it would be even more re-assuring than a recorded voice [Jane – emergency system user].*

In our assessment of this, we found that most older persons and their families were not sure what would happen if the emergency button was pressed as they did not know what the human element of the system was. This led to one instance in which Lucas's mother fell but did not press her emergency button because she did not know what would happen.

- **Integrated:** One of the larger problems we identified is that existing emergent alarms were not well integrated into the lives of the older people:

*The biggest problem is it didn't get integrated into my mother's life and part of the routines that she had. If I use jargon, she didn't ever really appropriate the technology. It didn't become part of her life. And she never really viewed it positively. [Lucas – son of emergency system user].*

This lack of integration into people's lives is a major cause of older people's failure to comply with requirements of the system. For example, some older people forgot to push the wellbeing button most days, because it was not part of their routine. This led to embarrassment, as the service provider would then call to ensure the person was well. While the service provider is courteous and friendly while making these check-up calls it caused distress and frustration to some of the older persons, because this happened so frequently:

*And no matter what system I try [claps with hand on his knee in frustration several times] I still managed out of 10 days that I miss out 2 or 3 times by completely forgetting and that is what ANNOYS [emphasis] me [Liam – emergency system user]*

In addition, having to check in during those hours lead to many people feeling that they had to be at home at some point during that time, giving low flexibility and control.

In summary, our data shows that many of the older persons in the field study did not necessarily want to adopt the alarm systems but did so to satisfy their families. Those who did choose to adopt the systems themselves had quite positive experiences while those who were forced to adopt the systems had quite negative experiences and tended not to wear the emergency pendant or did not wear it all the time as required for proper usage. Failure to conform to such requirements was mostly due to the failure of the systems to address the older person's emotional needs.

The system addressed best the primary emotional need of the relatives which is to be reassured about the safety of the older person. Two thirds of the emotions considered relevant for emergency alarm systems were only weakly or not supported at all (refer to Table 1). Older persons felt that the systems were not integrated with their lives and meaningful to them causing many problems

*Table 1. Overview of emotions that are desirable for emergency alarm systems and how well current systems are perceived to support these goals*

| Emotional Goal: User Should Feel.... | Support by Current Personal Alarm Systems |
|---|---|
| Reassured | Strong support |
| Safe | Reasonable support |
| Independent | Conditional support |
| Cared about | Weak support – no support |
| In control | Weak support |
| In touch | Weak support |
| Integrated | Weak support |

such as forgetting to push the wellbeing check, leaving the house and being unable to push it or deliberately not wearing the emergency pendant.

## About Method

### Consistency of Domain Dependent and Domain Independent Elements

Although we did not take a formal measure of consistency we did see strong consistencies for the major themes of our analysis method. In particular, there was a high consistency on high-level domain independent concepts, such as roles and goals. While there was some disparity between the domain dependent elements in many cases, these were resolved by identifying new elements/concepts that captured these disparities. For example, one pair identified the emotional goal that relatives want to feel that the older person "*is safe*", while another identified that the relatives want to feel that the older person "*could get help*". The two themes were merged into the concept of the relatives feeling "*reassured*" during the modelling process.

### Filtering Out Data

There were many minor themes that were brought forward from the pair analysis into the group analysis that did not appear in the final models. While many were merged with others the group analysis played an important role in not only including what was important over several interviews, but filtering out what was either deemed not generalisable, because it was not present over more than one or two interviews. Or it was not relevant because it related to something outside of the scope of emergency alarm systems.

This filtering of data is an important step in the process. While it is important to include elements that are relevant into the models, it is important that the models do not overwhelm stakeholders in the project by being too large and difficult to comprehend. Our aim is that the models should capture only the most important aspects of the socio-technical system being modelled. If more detailed analysis is required, this can be added to the models using annotations or just free text.

### Validation

The validation step proved useful as a step for us to increase our confidence in our models. Despite the fact that the validation conducted as an interview is a qualitative and rather informal step the qualitative data that comes from this clearly supports the models. For example, the following quote demonstrates how the idea of being *cared for* is not what older people want:

*The other thing that strikes me is this distinction that you made about between being cared for and cared about. That really, I immediately kind of went absolutely that was my experience of that. That my aunt very much viewed the device that she was using as something that was procedural and that it took away independence, so it wasn't about caring about it was about caring for, and I think that distinction is a really great one [Joe -- relative of emergency system user].*

In addition, the validation step is an important part of informing the stakeholders that they had been listened to, and importantly, that their views are shared. One respondent summarised it as:

*It was interesting from the things that you were saying, how much my experience of that and my aunt's experience and the information that we talked about during that interview, obviously is a very standard and very common thing [Joe -- relative of emergency system user].*

## PROTOTYPE

In this section we describe the design of the prototype based on the motivational goal model – in particular how the development was informed by the emotional goals (see Figure 3). The prototype built is a photo frame application which is focusing on the functional goal "I am in touch" and its associated qualities and emotions. This system is meant to replace the current base station used for the daily well-being check. The main aim of the photo frame is to balance the complex relation between well-being of the older person and the communication of this state to relatives with a focus on the emotions of both stakeholders.

For the second main functional goal "to initiate an alarm" an alternative modern pendant was created. The development of this pendant is not reported here but described in detail by Keirnan & Pedell (2014).

The prototype technology was developed in an agile development process. One of the researchers of the team was in daily contact with the programmers for the period of two months to give feedback and reflect on how the progress matched with the goals defined in the motivational model. The prototype was developed with the emotional goals as a starting point. Functions and their qualities were discussed between the researcher and the developers in how well they would satisfy the emotional goals. In the following the photo frame prototype is described with a lens on how the system is expected to address the emotions of the older user.

### Overview

The system aims to gauge the well-being of an elderly person, by having them interact with a photo frame - which receives messages and photos from their contacts (family, friends or service provider). The photo frame runs on an iPad (any model from iPad 1 to iPad 4), but can also run on any Web browser. Each photo frame installed in an older persons' home has an individual user email address. For each photo frame (or user) a certain period of time is designated as a check-in period, during which the elderly person is encouraged to use the photo frame. As this period can be defined the system should integrate better into peoples individual life styles and habits and also should "feel more integrated", but also older people should feel more "in control". If the person does not use (scrolls, picks up frame, or sends message) the application during the specified period – and only then - an investigation event is triggered and a message appears inquiring if the user is ok. However if the older person uses the photo frame regularly no investigation is triggered. The emphasis is on the emotional goal "to feel cared about" in receiving personal content by loved ones and significant others. It is expected that the contact person or relative "feels reassured" receiving regular messages. As the system still initiates an investigation, the main responsibility lies with the service provider and relatives should "feel unburdened" and the older person is expected "to feel safe". Additionally, multiple people can send messages and the task of sending new material can be shared.

There are two main areas for the application:

1. Photo frame (touch tablet).
2. Researchers section (administration of alerts and data logging),

## Photo Frame

The photo frame displays images and messages and circulates them in a carousel like manner (see Figure 4). The frame switches between photos based on the 'amount of photo refreshes' setting in the edit installation page giving new photos priority. In addition the image displays a caption which is a truncation of the email subject. The photo frame also displays the contact person who sent the message.

When a new message is received it denotes the start of a conversation and the elderly person can reply to the images and messages received (Figure 5). Then the relative can respond to the elderly person's replies in turn again (this can be repeated continually). When a reply is received by the system the photo frame switches to displaying the first picture that was received in relation to this conversation and it will display the new message as the caption. If a message without picture is received the system will display a default image with the message. The personal messages are intended to make the older person to "feel in touch" with people instead of interacting with an anonymous box and merely press a button without receiving feedback. The meaningfulness of the interaction is expected to add to a "feeling of independence". Older people are not encouraged to press a well-being check button because they are regarded as being frail and need to do so, but some interaction is leveraged for this information.

## Alerts and Administration Section

Based on the events triggered, the system will create alerts for installations (photo frame locations). These alerts are displayed in the administration

*Figure 4. A picture with message sent by a relative in the carousel of the photo frame*

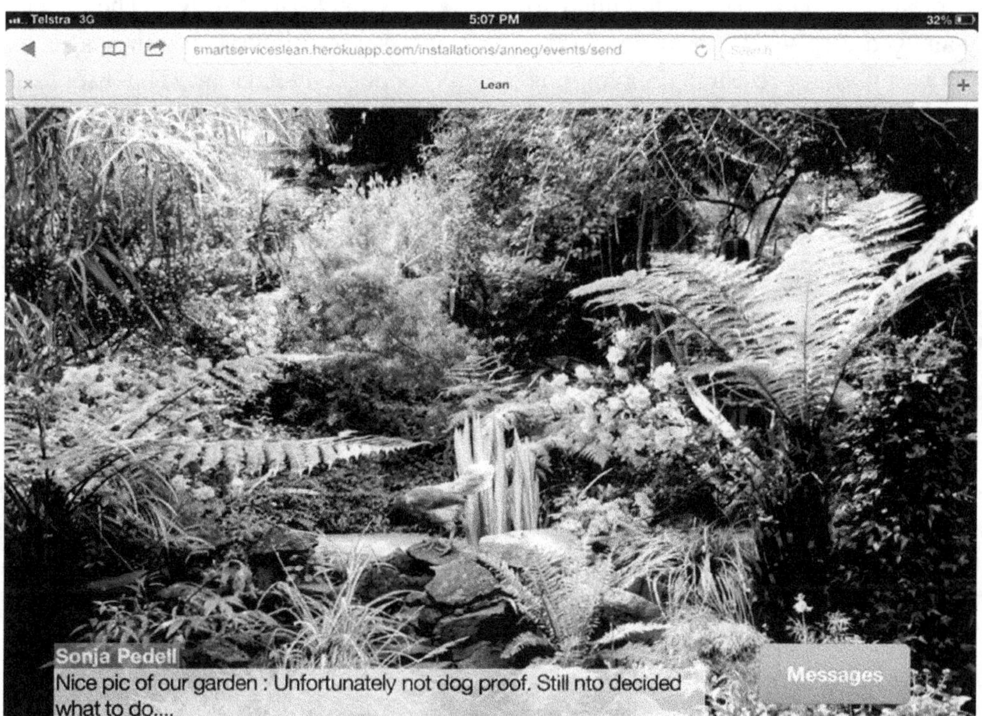

*Figure 5. The conversation screen – writing and sending messages*

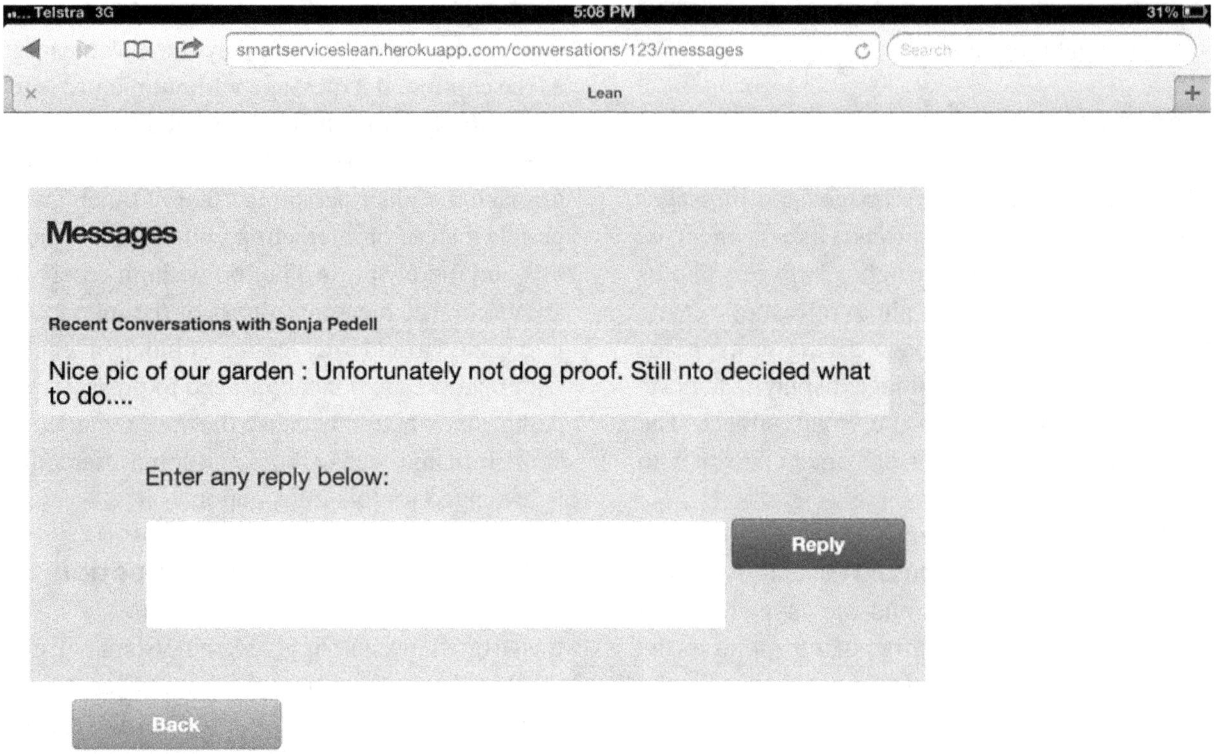


part of the prototype. This part is intended to be used by an aged care service provider. In the field study it was used for research data logging in order to see when and how often users would use the system.

The following alerts exist:

1. **Investigation:** Triggered if the user has not checked in during the required period.
2. **Investigation Cancel:** Triggered if an OK event has been received during an investigation period.

In addition the following data were collected: duration and times the photo frame was used (accelerometer data) and times messages were sent.

- **Check-In Mode:** The check-in mode shows pictures and messages as per a carousel behaviour. The user can click the messages button to display messages related to this picture.

The system will pulse (lightening and darkening the background image) to show that there was no interaction yet and that the check-in period is nearly over. An OK button is displayed that when clicked will trigger an OK event and revert back to a sleeping state.

- **Investigation Mode:** The investigation mode shows pictures and messages as per the carousel behaviour. In addition there is an overlay over half the screen that alerts the user to the fact that an investigation has been started (Figure 6).

The user can click the messages button to display messages related to this picture or click the OK button, both of which will send an OK event and the system will then revert back to the sleeping mode.

## FIELD STUDY FOLLOW-UP

This section describes the follow-up to the first field study to assess to what extent the older persons considered their emotional needs addressed by the prototype.

### Participants and Installation

The photo frame was installed in the homes of older people for two weeks at a location of their choice (see for example Figure 7). We encouraged the set up in a place of their home where they would spend a lot of time and see the picture frame. The study involved nine participants using the system, six women and three men, aged between 69 and 92, with all but one living on their own.. The participants had a range of physical and mental limitations related to age, including visual problems, arthritis, dementia and mobility problems. Three of the participants had used a personal alarm system before, although previous or current personal alarm use was not a pre-requisite for taking part in the study.

*Figure 6. The older person has not interacted with the picture frame in the defined time frame*

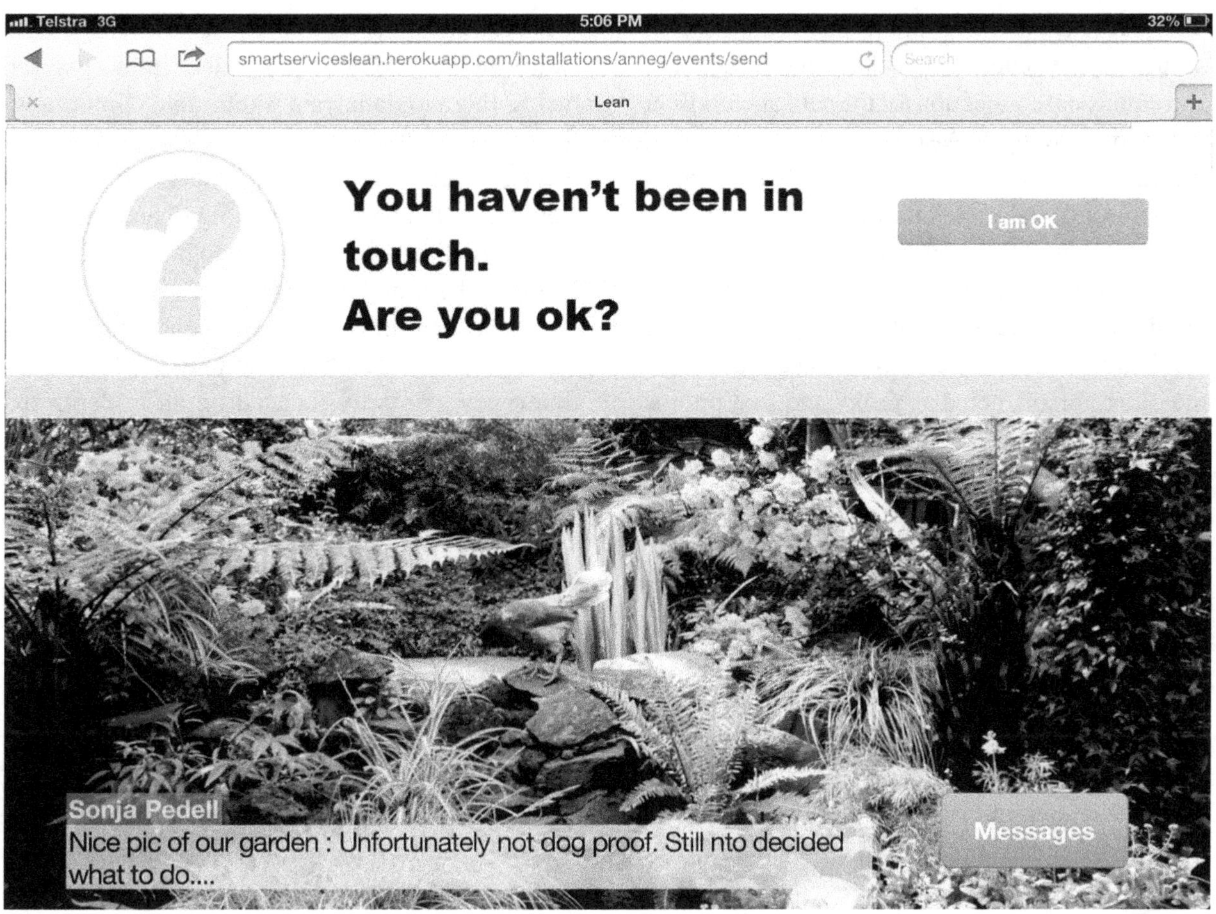

*Figure 7. Ipad with photo frame prototype in a participant's home*

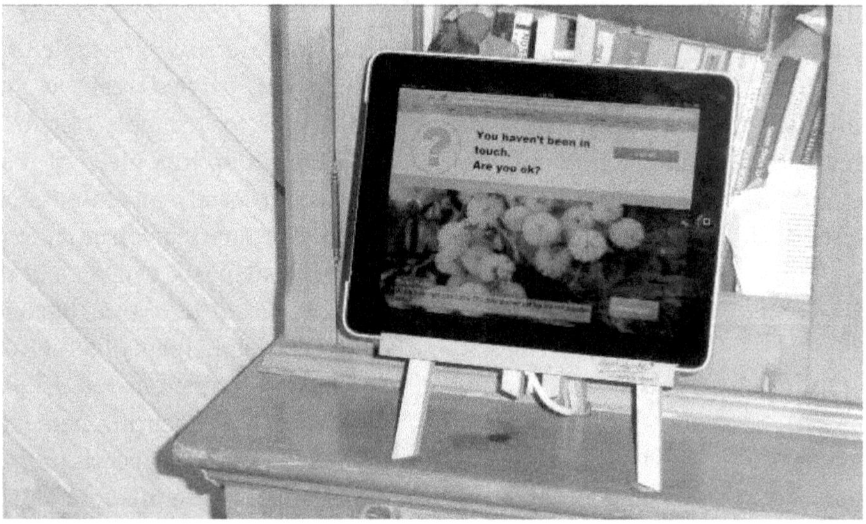


Each of the participants was asked to nominate one or several persons who could co-participate in the study by sending photographs to the iPad. The rationale was that the photographs and messages of significant others would have more meaning and emotional connection for the participants than if sent by a stranger. Also it was anticipated that the older person would be more likely to respond to more personal content and more actively use the system due to the felt connection.

Where participants were unable to engage a relative the researcher installing the prototype and conducting the interviews and hence familiar to the older person, acted as proxy and sent photos and messages instead. As most relatives were not able to send a photo and message every day due to time restrictions most participants additionally were sent photographs to by a researcher, so there was at least one photograph per day received. This continuity was considered to be needed as the investigation period was only two weeks.

## Data Collection

Semi-structured interviews were conducted with all the participants prior to, and immediately following the use of the photo frame. The interviews were done in conjunction with implementation and collection of the prototype. All interviews were between 30 minutes and an hour in length and were audio-recorded, transcribed and analysed using thematic analysis. Preliminary interviews included questions concerning the participants' background (demographic data, interests, daily routines), their current technology use and abilities and a discussion of technologies which might support them in the future.

A second interview was conducted at the conclusion of the photo frame use. The second interview primarily focused on an in-depth exploration of how people managed and felt about using the system. The interview started with open questions such as "How did you expect this technology to work?" and "How did it work for you?". During the interview participants gave a practical demonstration of how they used the photo frame and reflected upon the content of the photographs and messages. In particular the participants were asked to reflect upon any emotions they felt when receiving photographs or messages, sending messages back, and how well the system integrated into their life. Participants who were familiar with personal alarms were also encouraged to compare the use of the personal alarm and the photo frame. Finally we asked participants to imagine a technology which would best suit their needs in the event they were alone and required urgent support or attention.

Semi-structured interviews were also conducted with the relatives. These interviews usually took place at the same time as the participants' interviews. These interviews focussed on relatives' experiences of sending photographs and messages to participants. In particular we were interested in their experiences of choosing which photographs and messages to send, the timing of interactions between both user parties and any feelings or emotions which arose as a consequence of using the system. Additionally we asked for how they thought the photo frame system did or did not work for their older relative. Finally, six semi-structured interviews were conducted with the researchers, who acted as proxy co-participants by sending photographs and messages to participants.

In addition to the 18 participant interviews and the six researcher interviews, data consisted of 580 photographs with captions (i), 200 replies of participants (ii), and extended conversations (up to nine messages) (iii). Additional data that was logged by the photo frame system included dates and times of interactions, photo frame movements (via accelerometer), and pressing the "ok" button and "send messages" button.

A thematic analysis of the transcribed interviews was done by the team in the same way as described for the previous study. The goal model was updated in regards to missing goals and the match of quality goals was assessed.

## RESULTS OF THE FIELD STUDY FOLLOW-UP

In this section, we present a summary of the results of the evaluation of our photo frame system. Overall participants were satisfied with the system. It was easy to use, which is an important pre-condition that needs to be fulfilled in order to investigate the emotions caused by the interaction with the system.

### Participant Use

Generally all users enjoyed receiving and looking at the photographs and messages and appreciated the social aspect of the system. Even the novice users enjoyed learning how to use a new piece of technology. What participants used the photo frame for ranged from a longer conversation to short conversations to using the "ok" button or sending empty replies. Every single user could make use of the application to the best of their abilities.

Overall the prototype was better accepted than current emergency alarm systems that include a daily well-being check. In particular the photos from relatives were more meaningful for participants. Older people felt comfortable using the technology. It was easy to use and all participants replied to messages even with participants who were living with significant impairments (such as severe vision impairments, early Alzheimers) and when relatives were doubtful the picture frame could be of benefit.

### Relatives' Perspective

Sending a picture once a day was a big task and unsustainable for most relatives. It would be useful for them to be able to load a number of photos at once so that they could send them daily over a period of time. They also would have liked to have better integration in their lives and be able to send photos from mobile devices and other email accounts. The prototype was restricted to sending pictures from Gmail and a computer only. Relatives should be able to send from mobile devices and other email accounts for better integration. Additionally, the relatives had to open their Gmail accounts to see if there were messages in reply. It would be useful if there was notification of replies that can be sent to any email provider and mobile devices that they are using anyway.

## Match with Established Emotions and New Emotions

Feelings uncovered in the interview study were confirmed as being important for the participants in the prototype study. These feelings included "feeling safe" and the "feeling of independence". It was difficult to establish if the system was able to increase their feeling of safety and independence. Certainly the use of the prototype did not diminish it. In particular the integration into their everyday life worked well. Most participants reported that the interaction with the photo frame became quickly a part of their daily routine, something they would attend to first thing in the morning, and occasionally throughout the day if a new photograph caught their attention.

Participants appreciated the social interactions, personalised content and the subtle feeling of "feeling in touch" mediated by the picture frame. However, the concept of the prototype to escalate non-social behaviour after a defined period of time as a need to check on the person was not wanted by everyone. One participant was content with the social aspect, but not comfortable with the monitoring aspect of the alarm and still felt that control was taken away from her.

*The way I feel at the moment, I wouldn't like that, because I still want to feel I can independently choose whether to get help or whether not to get help. I might change my mind if something really bad happens. I might think, "Help, I've changed my mind." But on that night when I woke up and I knew I was in a lot of trouble, and my blood pressure was in stroke/heart attack zone when I took it, all I thought was, "Go back to bed, if you're here in the morning, fine, if you're not, you're not." [Anna – prototype user]*

The study reinforced the idea that the prototype catered for important emotional goals and that a system like this addresses the social needs of older people. At the same time there were very strong personal preferences how these needs should be met. There is a tension between the desire of the relatives to feel reassured and unburdened and the older person to have full control over their lives. Any automatic response triggered by the system is felt by some as them not feeling fully in control. There is a very fine line between monitoring people for care and interacting with them in a social manner. While the current system tries to find a balance between the two it is not social enough for some and still too much of a monitoring system for others.

The field study also discovered new emotional goals. The main goal that emerged from the data was 'feeling engaged'. This goal is very multifaceted and encompasses the emotions 'Curious', 'Playful', 'Anticipation', 'Connected' and 'Nostalgia'. These emotions provoked by the use of the system are encouraging as they show the lightweight and positive nature of the interactions. The participants did not feel threatened or scared by the system – in contrary these feelings point to what Gaver et al. (2004) described as 'ludic' interaction.

## LIMITATIONS

There are several limitations to our case study evaluations. First, we currently only have results for one system: the emergency alarm system. While we are currently applying our approach to other health systems, generalising more broadly is currently not possible.

Second, we have not repeated the content analysis and modelling of the emergency alarm case study so cannot determine how repeatable our method is; that is whether another team would come up with the same user goals from our data.

Despite this the content analysis approach that we use is a well-accepted ethnographic technique and informs much of this part of the approach, so we are confident that the method is repeatable.

Finally, at the start of the case study we constructed baseline models to compare with the final models. However these models are subject to bias because we knew that these would be compared, which may have distorted our approach.

## CONCLUSION AND FUTURE WORK

Our research explored, trialed and evaluated the concept of personal alarm systems specifically designed for older adults living by themselves. Our research showed that the emotions of this user group are not taken into consideration when designing, choosing or implementing these devices. Focusing on the feelings of the end-user - the older person - helped us to discover the underlying strong emotions triggered by expectations on family members and personal life style affecting intended personal alarm use. This approach helped us to develop a new system prototype addressing some of these emotions. With a photo frame prototype we were able to leverage the benefits of social communication for transferring information of "well-being" to service providers and carers.

From a development perspective the questions about feelings lead to identifying hidden requirements. A clear implication for practitioners in this area is that simply asking questions about the emotional needs of users and stakeholders in general can improve the overall user experience, which can ultimately improve uptake. While we have conducted in-depth ethnographic studies, we believe that even more lightweight processes, such as talking with some representative users about their emotional needs, can help improve health care systems.

In current work we are applying our approach in other areas of health care, such as support for people with psychosis and applications for assessing depression risk.

In future work we plan to look into even more structured ways to gather data and how to model and how to provide systematic and repeatable support to map emotional goals into system design. In order to get a deeper insight into the emotions of users we plan a long term study of up to twelve months. This will give us the opportunity to further improve our system with several iterations as well as understand better the adoption of technologies by older people to improve their well-being.

Overall, we argue that our method is a systematic, repeatable and useful way of capturing emotional goals of system stakeholders and represent them throughout system design. Furthermore, we propose that the notion of capturing emotions to inform system conceptualisation and design is an important step in improving healthcare systems. The consideration of users feelings cannot be an afterthought, but needs to inform design from the very beginning. Without the gained knowledge about emotional goals from the first field study we would have chosen different functions for our prototype. We can do no better in summarising our intentions than the following quote from a relative of an emergency system user:

*I think that that's the conflict because for me as a relative and a carer, the assuredness was related to the functional aspects of the device, whereas for the user, their assurance isn't related to that at all. Their assurance is much more around the emotional ideas and that idea around the connectivity. And I think that in my situation that was the kind of the clash, is in that what I emotionally needed was very different to what my aunt emotionally needed. What's great to hear in terms of this plan is that this idea that you're addressing both of those things – that the emotional thing isn't just about how you feel about it; it also does relate directly to the functionality of it, because if you have a relative or carer who is really happy and on board with that, that's also obviously going to help emotionally the user and so that link is really important. [Joe – relative of emergency system user].*

## ACKNOWLEDGMENT

We would like to thank the participants for their engagement and lively discussions. This project was funded by the Australian Research Council discovery grant DP130102660 'Software engineering of human-oriented technologies and services' and the Smart Services CRC.

## REFERENCES

ABS. (2011). *Population Projections, Australia, 2006 to 2101*. Canberra: Australian Bureau of Statistics.

ABS. (2013). *Australian Demographics Statistics, Mar 2013*. Canberra: Australian Bureau of Statistics.

AIHW. (2010). *Residential aged care in Australia 2008-09: a statistical overview Aged care statistics series no. 31 (Vol. AGE 62)*. Canberra: Australian Institute of Health and Welfare.

AIHW. (2012). *Health expenditure Australia 2010-11 Health and welfare expenditure series no. 47 (Vol. HWE 56)*. Canberra: Australian Institute of Health and Welfare.

AIHW. (2013a). *Australian trends in life expectancy*. Canberra: Australian Institute of Health and Welfare.

AIHW. (2013b). *Life expectancy*. Canberra: Australian Institute of Health and Welfare.

Baxter, G., & Sommerville, I. (2011). Socio-technical systems: From design methods to systems engineering. *Interacting with Computers*, *23*(1), 4–17. doi:10.1016/j.intcom.2010.07.003

Bolton, L. B., Gassert, C. A., & Cipriano, P. F. (2008). Technology solutions can make nursing care safer and more efficient. *Journal of Healthcare Information Management*, *22*(4), 24–30. PMID:19267016

CoA. (2011). *Don't fall for it. Falls can be prevented!* Canberra: Commonwealth of Australia.

Collins, S. C., Bhatti, J. Z., Dexter, S. L., & Rabbitt, P. M. (1992). Elderly people in a new world: attitudes to advanced communications technologies. In H. Boumqa, & J. A. M. Graafmans (Eds.), *Gerontechnology* (p. 35). Amsterdam: IOS Press.

De Couvreur, L., Dejonghe, W., Detand, J., & Goossens, R. H. M. (2013). The role of subjective well-being in co-designing open-design assistive devices. *International Journal of Design*, *7*(3), 57–70.

Demiris, G., Rantz, M., Aud, M., Marek, K., Tyrer, H., Skubic, M., & Hussam, A. (2004). Older adults' attitudes towards and perceptions of "smart home" technologies: a pilot study. *Medical Informatics and the Internet in Medicine*, *29*(2), 87–94. doi:10.1080/14639230410001684387 PMID:15370989

Desmet, P. M. A., & Hekkert, P. (2009). Special issue editorial: Design & emotion. *International Journal of Design*, *3*(2), 1–6.

Dey, A. K., & Guzman, E. d. (2006). *From awareness to connectedness: the design and deployment of presence displays*. Paper presented at the SIGCHI Conference on Human Factors in Computing Systems. Montreal, Canada.

Gaver, W., Bowers, J., Boucher, A., Gellerson, H., Pennington, S., Schmidt, A., et al. (2004). The Drift Table: Designing for ludic engagement. In *Proc. CHI'04 Design Expo*. New York: ACM Press.

Grealy, C., Olver, K., Connell, J., Power, J., Bramich, M., & Yeomans, J. (2008). *Comprehensive scoping study on the use of assistive technology by frail older people living in the community*. Canberra: Commonwealth Department of Health and Ageing.

Hanson, E., & Magnusson, L. (2011). The role of ICT support services to promote ageing in place: The ACTION service. *Eurohealth*, *17*(2-3), 24–26.

Hanson, E., Magnusson, L., Arvidsson, H., Claesson, A., Keady, J., & Nolan, M. (2007). Working together with persons with early stage dementia and their family members to design a user-friendly technology based support service. *Dementia (London)*, *6*(3), 411–434. doi:10.1177/1471301207081572

Hanson, V. L. (2010). Influencing technology adoption by older adults. *Interacting with Computers*, *22*(6), 502–509. doi:10.1016/j.intcom.2010.09.001

Hassenzahl, M., Eckoldt, K., Diefenbach, S., Laschke, M., Lenz, E., & Kim, J. (2013). Designing moments of meaning and pleasure. Experience design and happiness. *International Journal of Design*, *7*(3), 21–31.

Hassenzahl, M., Heidecker, S., Eckoldt, K., Diefenbach, S., & Hillmann, U. (2012). All You Need is Love: Current Strategies of Mediating Intimate Relationships through Technology. *ACM Transactions on Computer-Human Interaction*, *19*(4), 30. doi:10.1145/2395131.2395137

Henkemans, O. A. B., Caine, K. E., Rogers, W. A., Fisk, A. D., & Ruyter, B. d. (2007). *Medical Monitoring for Independent Living: User-Centered Design of Smart Home Technologies for Older Adults.* Paper presented at the Med-e-Tel conference for eHealth, telemedicine and health information and communication technologies. Luxembourg.

Heo, J. a. K., J. and Won, Y. (2012). Exploring the Relationship Between Internet Use and Leisure Satisfaction Among Older Adults. *Activities, Adaptation and Aging*, *35*(1), 43–54. doi:10.1080/01924788.2010.545975

Hoog, W. d., Keller, I., & Stappers, P. J. (2004). *Gustbowl: technology supporting affective communication through routine ritual interactions.* Paper presented at the CHI '04 Extended Abstracts on Human Factors in Computing Systems. Vienna, Austria.

Keirnan, A., & Pedell, S. (2014). *Developing a Personal Alarm Pendadant for Older Adults at Home* (White Paper). Swinburne University of Technology.

Kim, K. O. (2012). *The Emotional Responses of Older Adults to New Technology.* (PhD Thesis). University of Illinois at Urbana-Champaign, Urbana-Champaign, IL.

Lopez-Lorca, A. A., Miller, T., Pedell, S., Sterling, L., & Curumsing, M. K. (2014). (Manuscript submitted for publication). *Modelling People's Emotions for Socio-technical Systems.*

Marshall, J. (2014). Agent-Based Modelling of Emotional Goals in Digital Media Design Projects. *IJPOP special issue on Emotions and People-Oriented Programming, 3*(1), 44-59.

Melander-Wikman, A., Faltholm, Y., & Gard, G. (2008). Safety vs. privacy: elderly persons' experiences of a mobile safety alarm. *Health & Social Care in the Community*, *16*(4), 337–346. doi:10.1111/j.1365-2524.2007.00743.x PMID:18613909

Meyer, D., Marx, T., & Ball-Seiter, V. (2011). Social isolation and telecommunication in the nursing home: A pilot study. *Gerontechnology (Valkenswaard)*, *10*(1), 51–58. doi:10.4017/gt.2011.10.01.004.00

Miguel, K. D. S., & Lewin, G. (2008). Personal emergency alarms: what impact do they have on older people's lives? *Australasian Journal on Ageing*, *27*(2), 103–105. doi:10.1111/j.1741-6612.2008.00286.x PMID:18713202

Miller, T., Pedell, S., Mendoza, A., Keirnan, A., Sterling, L., & Lopez-Lorca, A. A. (2014). *Emotionally-driven models for people-oriented requirements engineering: the case study of emergency alarm systems.* (Under review).

Miller, T., Pedell, S., Sterling, L., & Lu, B. (2011). Engaging Stakeholders with Agent-Oriented Requirements Modelling. In D. Weyns, & M.-P. Gleizes (Eds.), *Agent-Oriented Software Engineering XI* (Vol. 6788, pp. 62–78). Springer. doi:10.1007/978-3-642-22636-6_4

Mynatt, E. D., Rowan, J., Craighill, S., & Jacobs, A. (2001). *Digital family portraits: supporting peace of mind for extended family members.* Paper presented at the SIGCHI Conference on Human Factors in Computing Systems. Seattle, WA.

Paay, J., Sterling, L., Vetere, F., Howard, S., & Boettcher, A. (2009). Engineering the social:The role of shared artifacts. *International Journal of Human-Computer Studies, 67*(5), 437–454. doi:10.1016/j.ijhcs.2008.12.002

Patton, M. Q. (2002). *Qualitative research and evaluation methods.* Thousand Oaks, CA: Sage Publications, Inc..

PC. (2008). *Trends in Aged Care Services: some implications* (Commission Research Paper). Canberra: Productivity Commission.

Pedell, S., Miller, T., Sterling, L., Vetere, F., & Howard, S. (2014). (forthcoming). Tools for participation: Intergenerational technology design for the home. *International Journal of Design.*

Pedell, S., Sterling, L., Keirnan, A., & Dobson, G. (2013). *Emotions around emergency alarm use: A field study with older adults (Report for Smart Services CRC).* Swinburne University of Technology.

Peeters, P. H. (2000). Design criteria for an automatic safety-alarm system for elderly. *Technology and health Care, 8*(2), 81-91.

Proynova, R., Paech, B., Koch, S. H., Wicht, A., & Wetter, T. (2011). *Investigating the influence of personal values on requirements for health care information systems.* Paper presented at the Proceedings of the 3rd Workshop on Software Engineering in Health Care. Waikiki, HI.

Pullin, G. (2009). *Design meets disability.* MIT Press.

Russell, H. (2011). Later Life ICT Learners Ageing Well. *International Journal of Ageing and Later Life, 6*(2), 103–127. doi:10.3384/ijal.1652-8670.1162103

Sterling, L. S., & Taveter, K. (2009). *The art of agent-oriented modeling.* Massachusetts Institute of Technology.

Vergados, D., Alevizos, A., Mariolis, A., & Caragiozidis, M. (2008). *Intelligent services for assisting independent living of elderly people at home.* Paper presented at the 1st international conference on Pervasive Technologies Related to Assistive Environments. Athens, Greece.

Vetere, F., Davis, H., Gibbs, M., & Howard, S. (2009). The Magic Box and Collage: Responding to the challenge of distributed intergenerational play. *International Journal of Human-Computer Studies, 67*(2), 165–178. doi:10.1016/j.ijhcs.2008.09.004

Waycott, J., Pedell, S., Vetere, F., Ozanne, E., Kulik, L., Gruner, A., & Downs, J. (2012). *Actively Engaging Older Adults in the Development and Evaluation of Tablet Technology.* Paper presented at the 24th Australian Computer-Human Interaction Conference (OzCHI' 12). Melbourne, Australia.

Wetter, T., & Paech, B. (2010). *What if "business process" is the wrong metaphor? Exploring the potential of Value Based Requirements Engineering for clinical software*. Paper presented at the 13th International Congress on Medical Informatics. Cape Town, South Africa.

## KEY TERMS AND DEFINITIONS

**eHealth:** eHealth is a recent term for healthcare practice supported by electronic processes and communication.

**Emotion-Informed Software Development:** The process of incorporating the emotions and well-being of the end-users in software development.

**Ethnography:** Ethnography is the systematic study of peoples and cultures and representing the culture of a group graphically and in writing.

# Chapter 7
# User Behavioral Intention toward Using Mobile Healthcare System

**Pantea Keikhosrokiani**
*School of Computer Sciences, Universiti Sains Malaysia, Malaysia*

**Norlia Mustaffa**
*School of Computer Sciences, Universiti Sains Malaysia, Malaysia*

**Nasriah Zakaria**
*Medical Education Department, College of Medicine, King Saud University, Saudi Arabia & School of Computer Sciences, Universiti Sains Malaysia*

**Ahmad Suhaimi Baharudin**
*School of Computer Sciences, Universiti Sains Malaysia, Malaysia*

## ABSTRACT

*This chapter introduces Mobile Healthcare Systems (MHS) and employs some theories to explore the behavioral intention of Smartphone users in Penang, Malaysia to use MHS. A survey was conducted in the form of questionnaire to Smartphone users in Penang, Malaysia for the duration of three weeks starting in September 2013. A total number of 123 valid surveys out of 150 were returned, which is equivalent to a response rate of 82%. The authors use Partial Least Squares (PLS) for analyzing the proposed measurement model. The factors that are tested are self-efficacy, anxiety, effort expectancy, performance expectancy, attitude, and behavioral intention to use. The results indicate which factors have a significant effect on Smartphone users' behavioral intention and which factors are not significant. The results assist in assessing whether MHS is highly demanded by users or not, and will assist in development of the system in the future.*

## INTRODUCTION

Patient monitoring and intelligent health care system can prevent chronic diseases on time. With the advancement of wireless technology and mobile-based systems, the process of monitoring patients becomes ubiquitous. Mobile Health System (MHS) provides the facility of constant monitoring of patients in case of emergency. Medical professionals are concerned about risk and uncertainty of new technologies in healthcare. Thus, they usually tend to adapt new technologies

DOI: 10.4018/978-1-4666-6316-9.ch007

first until those technologies become mature. Introduction of information technology (IT) in healthcare has a deep effect on the performance of the healthcare systems. Many researchers have studied IT adoption and diffusion recently. Adoption is defined as the decision to accept, or invest in a new technology (Masrom & Hussein, 2008). Accessing to the value of the IT to the projects or organization is one of the main objectives for those IT researchers. IT resources can improve overall effectiveness of the organizations. IT adoption and usage by individual users is another key objective considered by researchers.

The main goal of this article is to conduct a survey in order to evaluate user behavioral intention toward using MHS. In consideration of user's behavior toward using MHS, we will conduct a survey among Smartphone users in Penang, Malaysia. The main construct of this study will be user behavioral intention to use the MHS. Behavioral intention to use is a measure of the strength of individual intention to perform a specified behavior which is use of a new technology or system (Davis, Bagozzi, & Warshaw, 1989). For this study, we proposed to use a research model based on three models i.e. Unified Theory of Acceptance and Use of Technology (UTAUT), Theory of Planned Behavior (TPB) and Theory of Acceptance Model (TAM). We will use Partial Least Squares (PLS) for analyzing the proposed measurement model. Firstly, construct validity that comprises convergent and discriminant validities will be used for this purpose. In addition, the structural equation modeling technique will be performed to evaluate the causal model. The factors that will be tested are self-efficacy, anxiety, effort expectancy, performance expectancy, attitude, and behavioral intention to use. The results will indicate which factors have significant effect on Smartphone user's behavioral intention and which factors are not significant. The results will assist in assessing whether MHS is highly demanded by users or not, as well as assist us in development of the system in the future.

## LITERATURE REVIEW

This section discusses briefly the literature review approach and background of the study. In the background section, theoretical bases along with development of appropriate hypothesis will be mentioned. Based on the previous researches, research framework for this study is designed which includes formulating conceptual model, research hypotheses, and methodology.

Several literature reviews cover the usage of mobile technologies in healthcare. Moreover, many researchers have studied acceptance of mobile technology in healthcare or user behavioral intention to use of new technologies in healthcare. However, those studies have been conducted with different aims, and it is not easy to compare their results. In order to find important factors of user acceptance or user behavioral intention to use of mobile technology in healthcare, we have done a systematic literature search in several databases such as MEDLINE, PubMed, ScienceDirect, SpringerLINK, IEEE Xplore and so on. We searched using the terms "mobile healthcare system", "acceptance of mobile technology in healthcare", "behavioral intention to use of mobile device in healthcare." In the next step, we have combined the search results and shortlisted the most recent and relevant papers with the aim to evaluate user behavioral intention to use of mobile device in healthcare.

## MOBILE HEALTHCARE SYSTEM (MHS)

With growth of mobile device penetration as well as worldwide enhancement of wireless networks, the wireless infrastructure can support many healthcare systems. This can provide ubiquitous healthcare, which means healthcare services available at anytime at anywhere. The wireless technologies offer various services such as reliable access along with transmission of medical data, tracking patient's current location, support of patient mobility, providing quick services in emergency and so on (Varshney, 2007). Location management can add value to healthcare by offering a location-based healthcare services using location tracking technologies such as global positioning systems (GPS), cellular networks, wireless local area networks (LANs), and radio frequency identification (RFID) (Tu, Zhou, & Piramuthu, 2009; Varshney, 2003). Various remote devices are utilized in wireless healthcare systems such as wireless sensors for blood oxygen saturation monitoring (Asada, Shaltis, Reisner, Sokwoo, & Hutchinson, 2003; Sokwoo, Boo-Ho, Kuowei, & Asada, 1998), infrared and radio-based locator badges (Stanford, 2002), using wearable devices for long-term health monitoring (Jovanov, O'Donnel, Morgan, Priddy, & Hormigo, 2002), remote heart monitoring systems (Ernest, et al., 2011; Ross, 2004), healthcare monitoring for patients with hypertension and arrhythmia (Keikhosrokiani, Mustaffa, Zakaria, & Sarwar, 2012), providing emergency services based on patient's current location (El-Masri & Saddik, 2012; Keikhosrokiani, et al., 2012), wireless telemetry systems for EEG epilepsy monitoring (Liszka, et al., 2004), real-time monitoring of patients in the home environment (Korhonen, Parkka, & Van Gils, 2003), and lastly, using GlucoBeep device for checking and transmitting the patient's diabetic information (Jansà, et al., 2006). In addition, there are other studies have been conducted in order to improve emergency healthcare systems (Bergrath, et al., 2011; Li, Cheng, Lu, & Lin, 2011).

The use of wireless technologies in healthcare can provide useful treatment for patients in hospitals, thus the outcome of the healthcare will increase effectively (Gravelle & Siciliani, 2008). Moreover, using mobile device and wireless technologies in healthcare can reduce the long-term cost and increase productivity in healthcare systems. In order to support patient's healthcare need, wireless patient monitoring systems must be designed for the homes, nursing homes and hospitals (Kevin & Yuan-Ting, 2003; Pollard, Rohman, & Fry, 2001; Varady, Benyo, & Benyo, 2002). Utilizing mobile device and wireless technologies in healthcare can improve the quality of healthcare. Hence, exploring the use of mobile devices is a major issue for medical personnel, nursing staff, and patients in hospitals.

## THEORIES ON TECHNOLOGY ACCEPTANCE MODELS (TPB, TAM, AND UTAUT)

Theory of Planned Behavior (TPB) was introduced in 1985 by Ice Ajzen and it was also known as social cognition model (SCM) (Ajzen, 1985). TPB and Technology Acceptance Model (TAM) are originally based on Theory of Reasoned Action (TRA) that is a model for predicting and explaining human behavior in different domains (Fishbein & Ajzen, 1975). TPB adds perceived behavioral control to the TRA model where perceived behavioral control is determined by availability of skills, resources, and opportunities to achieve outcomes. It is closely linked to self-efficacy belief concept (Ajzen, 1991). The concept of self-efficacy is concerned with people's belief in their ability to produce effects. TPB illustrates attitude (AT), subjective norm (SN), and perceived behavioral control (PBC) as direct determinants of intentions that will influence behavior. The focus of this study is on the attitude (AT) as well as behavioral intention (BI) in TPB model. AT refers to "the degree to which the person has a favorable or unfavorable evaluation of the behavior in question" (Ajzen, 1989). Whereas BI refers to "the subjective probability of one's engagement in any behavior." The stronger the behavior, the more likely is the execution of the behavior (Fishbein & Ajzen, 1975)

TAM is an information system theory that depicts how user accepts and uses a computer-based technology. It was developed by Davis Jr, in order to explain computer-based behavior

(Davis Jr, 1986). As mentioned before, TAM is the extension of TRA (Fishbein & Ajzen, 1975). The main purpose of TAM is to provide a basis for tracing the impact of external variables on internal beliefs, attitudes, and intentions. In TAM model attitude towards behavior in using the system is a central feature. Two most effective factors on attitude are perceived usefulness (PU) as well as perceived ease of use (PEOU). PU refers to "the degree to which a person believes that using a particular system would enhance his or her job performance." PEOU refers to "the degree to which a person believes that using particular system would be free from effort." Behavioral intention to use (BI) the system is directly determined by the person's attitude toward using the system as depicted in TAM model. BI is defined as "a measure of the strength of one's intention to perform a specific behavior, that is, use an information system" (Davis Jr, 1986).

Unified theory of acceptance and use of technology (UTAUT) was developed by Venkatesh, Morris and Davis, (2003) in order to merge previous TAM related studies. UTAUT is combination of TAM, TRA, TPB, TAM-TPB, motivational model, innovation diffusion theory, and social cognitive theory. It is developed for use in information and communication technology research. It seeks to clarify user intention to use an information system (IS) and consequent usage behavior. The theory consists of four main constructs including performance expectancy, effort expectancy, social influence, and facilitating condition. These constructs are direct determinants of usage behavior (Venkatesh, Morris, Davis, & Davis, 2003).

The focus of this study is on performance expectancy (PE) as well as effort expectancy (EE) in UTAUT model. PE refers to "the degree to which an individual believes that using the system will help him/her to attain gains in job performance"; whereas, EE is defined as "the degree of ease associated with the use of the systems."

In line with this, a study has been conducted in order to understand student perceptions in using course management software. The studied course management software is Blackboard which is a web-based tool that becomes popular and important application in higher education (Marchewka, Liu, & Kostiwa, 2007). This study utilized UTAUT model as well as adding self-efficacy and anxiety constructs to the model. Self-efficacy (SE) and anxiety (Ax) are another two more important constructs that can be added to UTAUT (A Iahad, Rahim, Zairah, & Oye, 2012). SE is defined as "perceptions of user's ability to use new technology in the accomplishment of the task." Ax can be defined as "the degree to which a user's fear, concern and hesitation of damaging the device, being embarrassed to use the new system" (A Iahad, et al., 2012).

## CONCEPTUAL MODEL AND RESEARCH HYPOTHESIS

### Definitions and Research Model

Based on the foregoing discussion, this study integrates TPB, TAM, and UTAUT with two additional variables including self-efficacy and anxiety affecting behavioral intention to use MHS among Smartphone users. Table 1 summarized the definition of each construct and the conceptual research model is illustrated in Figure 1.

The conceptual model depicts four independent variables (self-efficacy, effort expectancy, performance expectancy, and anxiety) which affect dependent variable that is behavioral intention to use MHS. There is a mediating effect of the attitude towards using MHS between three independent variables (self-efficacy, effort expectancy, and performance expectancy) and dependent variable (behavioral intention to use MHS).

The following section discusses the development of relevant hypothesis for this study. Majority of information system model do not specifically regard differences between stationary computing and mobile devices in technology acceptance mod-

*Table 1. Definition of the constructs*

| Construct | Definition |
|---|---|
| **Self-Efficacy (SE)** | The Smartphone user's perceptions of his or her ability to use MHS in the accomplishment of healthcare task. |
| **Effort Expectancy (EE)** | The degree to which a Smartphone user believes that the use of MHS would be free of physical and mental effort. |
| **Performance Expectancy (PE)** | The degree to which a Smartphone user believes that the use of MHS would enhance his or her performance. |
| **Attitude towards Using MHS (AT)** | A Smartphone user's positive or negative feeing about using MHS. |
| **Anxiety (Ax)** | The degree to which a Smartphone user's fear, concern and hesitation of damaging the device, being embarrassed to use MHS. |
| **Behavioral Intention to Use (BI)** | The degree to which a Smartphone user's motivation intend to use the MHS. |

*Figure 1. Conceptual model for behavioral intention to use MHS*

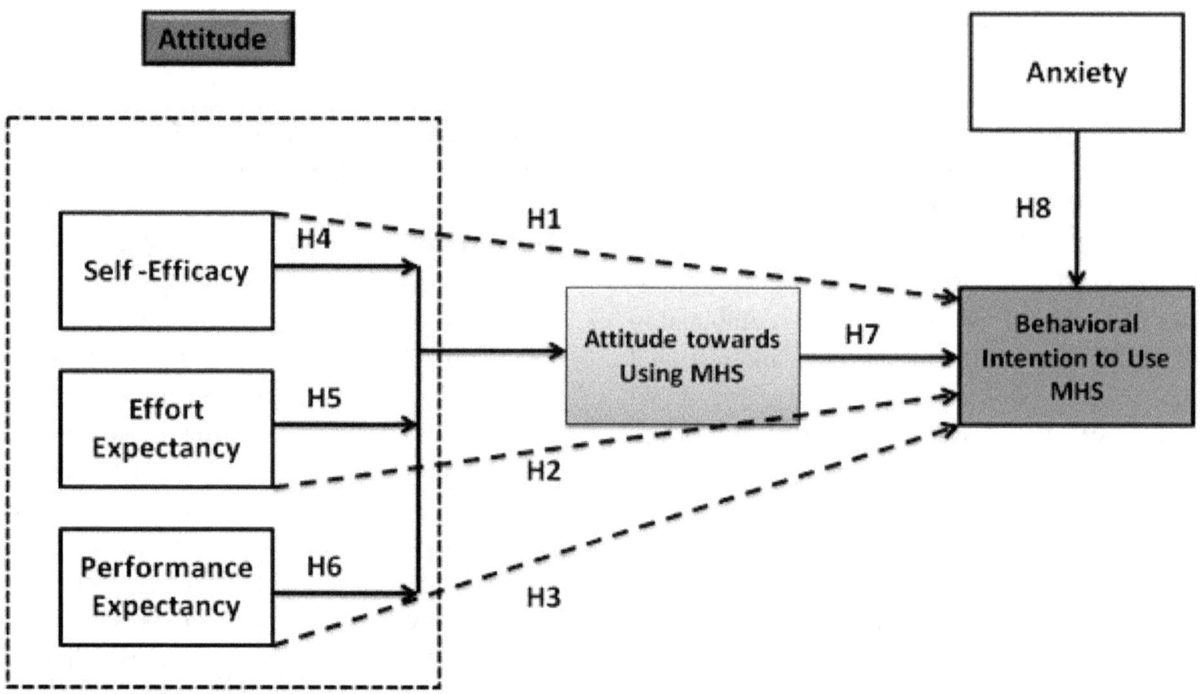


els. Thus, in order to draw the mobile context and study on technology acceptance models, Biljon, et al., (2007) designed a Mobile Phone Technology Acceptance Model (MOPTAM) (Biljon & Kotz, 2007). The need for considering control-based beliefs to understand personal behavior related to the adoption of mobile healthcare was indicated in many studies (Hung & Jen, 2012), (Wan Ismail, Chan, Buhari, & Muzaini, 2012), (I.-L. Wu, Li, & Fu, 2011), (Holden & Karsh, 2010), (Ozok, et al., 2009), and (J.-H. Wu, Wang, & Lin, 2007). User's belief in using mobile technologies can be related to individual categories such as perceived self-efficacy in using mobile technology, or organizational category such as technology and management support as well as training.

Based on the above discussion as well as literature review that have been conducted, there are three direct variables i.e. self-efficacy (SE), effort expectancy (EE), and performance expectancy (PE) for determining behavioral intention to use of MHS (Marchewka, et al., 2007). For the purpose of this study, there are three linkages between these three variables and behavioral intention to use the MHS. Therefore, three hypotheses are proposed as follow:

**H1:** Self-efficacy has a positive effect on Smartphone user's behavioral intention to use the MHS.

**H2:** Effort expectancy has a positive effect on Smartphone user's behavioral intention to use the MHS.

**H3:** Performance expectancy has a positive effect on Smartphone user's behavioral intention to use the MHS.

Moreover, based on TAM and TPB, as mentioned previously, attitude has a direct impact on behavioral intention to use MHS. Based on the literature review, self-efficacy, effort expectancy, and performance expectancy can be considered as direct variables for determining attitude (Yu, Ha, Choi, & Rho, 2005). For this study, we established that there are three linkages between these three variables and attitude towards using MHS. Therefore, three hypotheses are proposed as follows:

**H4:** Self-efficacy has a positive effect on Smartphone user's attitude towards using MHS.

**H5:** Effort expectancy has a positive effect on Smartphone user's attitude towards using MHS.

**H6:** Performance expectancy has a positive effect on Smartphone user's attitude towards using MHS.

Based on the theories such as TRA, TPB, and TAM, it is ascertained that attitude has a positive effect on the behavioral intention to use of the new technology. Thus, the hypothesis is set as follows:

**H7:** Smartphone user's attitude towards using MHS has a positive effect on the behavioral intention to use of MHS.

Mobile healthcare anxiety here refers to "the main reason for prevention of computer technology adoption is defined as trepidation, fear, concern and hesitation of damaging the device, being embarrassed" (Heinssen, Glass, & Knight, 1987). Jen and Chao (2008) defined mobile healthcare anxiety as "a high anxious response towards interaction with the mobile patient safety information system" which has a negative effect on the quality of care that physician provides for the patient. Therefore, it has a negative effect on user' s attitude towards using that healthcare system (Jen & Chao, 2008). Based on the previous studies, mobile patient safety information systems play a role in improving patient services and reducing patient risk, as well as showing that use of these communication systems may unintentionally be a factor in physician anxiety (Jen & Chao, 2008). Marchewka, et al. (2007) used anxiety as one of the effective factor on behavioral intention to use in UTAUT model for his research (Marchewka, et al., 2007). We can conclude that less anxiety means user has a positive intention towards using MHS and finally would like to use it. Thus, the following hypothesis is set:

**H8:** The level of mobile healthcare anxiety has a negative effect on the behavioral intention to use MHS.

## RESEARCH METHODOLOGY AND DESIGN

### Instrumentation

A survey is used as an instrument to collect data for this study. It was conducted for the duration of three weeks starting in September 2013. The survey was conducted by distributing the questionnaire to the respondents who are Smartphone users in Penang, Malaysia. The questionnaire was designed in the form of four categories of questions addressing demographic, Smartphone users' experience using Smartphone, chronic disease experience, and assessment part. The type of questions in the first three parts is selective while in the assessment part the response is collected using a five point Likert-type scale from one, being "strongly disagree" to five, being "strongly agree".

## DATA ANALYSIS AND RESULTS

### Demographics

This section presents descriptive analyses of demographic data providing a profile of respondents including frequency values. All the tables in this section present a profile of the surveyed respondents with regard of age, gender, and education, Smartphone users' experience using Smartphone and their experience about chronic disease. In this study, we are using basic descriptive analysis with frequency table to provide a demographic profile of respondents. The second part of data analysis is to understand Smartphone users and their opinion about usefulness of Smartphone for healthcare. Third part is analyzing about experience of chronic disease; whether the respondents experience it themselves or someone in their family face the chronic disease. All questions required to be answered, so there is no missed question. Respondents were Smartphone users from Penang, Malaysia, with the total number of 150. A total number of 123 valid surveys out of 150 were returned which is equivalent to a response rate of 82%.

Table 2 illustrates demographic data of the respondents. As Malaysia is a multicultural country, the respondents comprise of different ethnicity namely Malay, Chinese, and Indian with the percentage of 34.1%, 39.0% and 26.8%, respectively. Based on Table 2, majority of the respondents were female with 56.1% while the rest is 43.9% male participants in the survey. Most of the respondents were between 26 to 33 years old and no participant whose age is less than 18 years old. For the academic qualification part, the respondents mostly graduated at least at undergraduate level (60.2%). The respondents' income mainly is in between 1,000 to 3,000 (Ringgit Malaysia) and 3,001 to 5,000 (Ringgit Malaysia) with the percentage of 38.2 and 37.4 respectively.

### Measurement Model

Partial Least Squares (PLS) is a powerful structural equation modeling technique that uses a nonparametric and component-based approach for estimation (W. Chin, Marcolin, & Newsted, 1996; W. W. Chin, 1998a, 1998b). PLS reduce demands on sample size and residual distributions. The sample size needed for PLS is 10 times of the number of indicators for the most complex construct. When there are three variables and each includes 2-4 measuring items, the sample size of 123 respondents might not be enough to use Analysis of Moment Structures (AMOS; another type of analytical tool) for a goodness of mode-fit. PLS is a good analytical tool for fitting the requirement of a small sample size. Thus, PLS is suitable in this study for analyzing the measurement model. Firstly, construct validity test that comprises of convergent and discriminant validities is used and this is followed by hypotheses testing.

- **Convergent Validity:** Convergent validity of a construct is assessed by few cri-

*Table 2. Demographic data*

| Item | Option | Frequency | Percent (%) |
|---|---|---|---|
| **Race** | Malay | 42 | 34.1 |
| | Chinese | 48 | 39.0 |
| | Indian | 33 | 26.8 |
| **Age** | Under 18 | - | - |
| | 18-25 | 34 | 27.6% |
| | 26-33 | 64 | 52.0% |
| | 34-41 | 19 | 15.4% |
| | 42 and above | 69 | 4.9% |
| **Gender** | Male | 54 | 43.9% |
| | Female | | 56.1% |
| **Education** | High School | 2 | 1.6% |
| | Diploma | - | - |
| | Undergraduate | 74 | 60.2% |
| | Postgraduate | 39 | 31.7% |
| | Professional Degree | 8 | 6.5% |
| **Income** | Less than RM 1,000 | 16 | 13.0% |
| | Between RM 1,000 to RM 3,000 | 47 | 38.2% |
| | Between RM 3,001 to RM 5,000 | 46 | 37.4% |
| | Between RM 5,001 to RM 10,000 | 14 | 11.4% |

teria including: (1) All of the item loading in a construct must be more than 0.5 (Janz & Prasarnphanich, 2003; Saadé, 2007) that suggest item reliability while the Cronbach's alpha values must exceed 0.6 for the construct reliability (Nunnally, 2010). The reliability of individual item was assessed by examining the loading of items on their respective constructs that are illustrated in Table 3. The loading must be greater than 0.5 to indicate significant variance was shared between each item and the construct. The only loading that is below 0.5 is Ax2 (0.491) that is recommended to be removed from the model. As shown in Table 3, reliability was evaluated using the Cronbach's alpha. Most of the constructs appear to have a good degree of reliability since each computed statistic is above 0.60. The only questionable construct is Effort Expectancy (EE) as the respective test statistic falls below 0.60. (2) Composite reliability (CR) for a construct should exceed 0.6 and can be interpreted like Cronbach's alpha coefficient (Bagozzi & Yi, 1988). Based on Table 3, CR for all of the constructs is more than 0.6. (3) Next important factor is average variance extracted (AVE) for a construct that should be greater than 0.5 (Bagozzi & Yi, 1988). After removing Ax2 from the model, calculation was done again and AVE for anxiety changed from 0.599 to 0.776. AVE for all of the constructs is more than 0.5 except the AVE of effort expectancy (EE) and anxiety (Ax) that are 0.562 and 0.599 respectively. These AVEs are not strong enough but still acceptable (depicted in Table 3).

*Table 3. Assessment of convergent validity*

| Construct | Items | Item Loading | Composite Reliability | AVE | Cronbach'α |
|---|---|---|---|---|---|
| **AT** | AT1 | 0.933 | 0.936 | 0.880 | 0.863 |
| | AT2 | 0.943 | | | |
| **Ax** | Ax1 | 0.976 | 0.807 | 0.599 | 0.802 |
| | Ax2 | 0.491 | | | |
| | Ax3 | 0.776 | | | |
| **BI** | BI1 | 0.912 | 0.922 | 0.797 | 0.873 |
| | BI2 | 0.919 | | | |
| | BI3 | 0.846 | | | |
| **SE** | SE1 | 0.902 | 0.875 | 0.778 | 0.717 |
| | SE2 | 0.862 | | | |
| **EE** | EE1 | 0.856 | 0.715 | 0.562 | 0.232 |
| | EE2 | 0.626 | | | |
| **PE** | PE1 | 0.903 | 0.914 | 0.730 | 0.717 |
| | PE2 | 0.958 | | | |
| | PE3 | 0.688 | | | |
| | PE4 | 0.844 | | | |

- **Discriminant Validity:** "Discriminant validity is a measure of the extent to which the construct is not a reflection of some other variable." Table 4 depicts discriminant validity of the construct using squared root of the AVE for each construct. This value should be more than the correlations between it and all other constructs. The results illustrate a high degree of discriminant validity as shown in Table 4.

## Statistical Analysis and Hypothesis Testing

In order to examine the causal relationships among the constructs, a structural model was built. For evaluating the structural model, two steps are needed here. The first step is estimation of standardized path coefficients and their statistical significance for testing the hypotheses. Unfortunately, a significance test or confidence interval estimation is not provided by PLS. In this step, we used Bootstrapping analysis to estimate path coefficients, statistical significance, and relevant parameters, such as means, standard errors, item loadings, and item weights. The second step is calculation of the coefficient of determination (R2) for endogenous variables in order to assess the predictive power of the structural model. The R-square values (0.222) for attitude towards using MHS and 0.717 for behavioral intention to use MHS suggest a good model fit as shown in Figure 2.

Table 5 illustrates the results of hypotheses testing. Although, the significance of the proposed relationship between self-efficacy and performance efficacy with Smartphone user's attitude toward using MHS is not supported, effort expectancy ($\beta$ =0.340, $p < 0.05$) poses significant influence on attitude. This supports H5 and confirms the

*Table 4. Assessment of discriminant validity*

| | AT | Ax | BI | EE | PE | SE |
|---|---|---|---|---|---|---|
| AT | ***0.938*** | | | | | |
| Ax | 0.031 | ***0.881*** | | | | |
| BI | 0.768 | -0.154 | ***0.893*** | | | |
| EE | 0.444 | 0.133 | 0.588 | ***0.750*** | | |
| PE | 0.392 | -0.041 | 0.476 | 0.665 | ***0.854*** | |
| SE | -0.064 | -0.524 | 0.046 | 0.073 | 0.014 | ***0.882*** |

Note: The bold-italic numbers in the diagonal row are square roots of AVE

*Figure 2. Results of structural model. Value on path: standardized coefficients (β), R2: Coefficient of determination, **p<0.01, *p<0.05.*

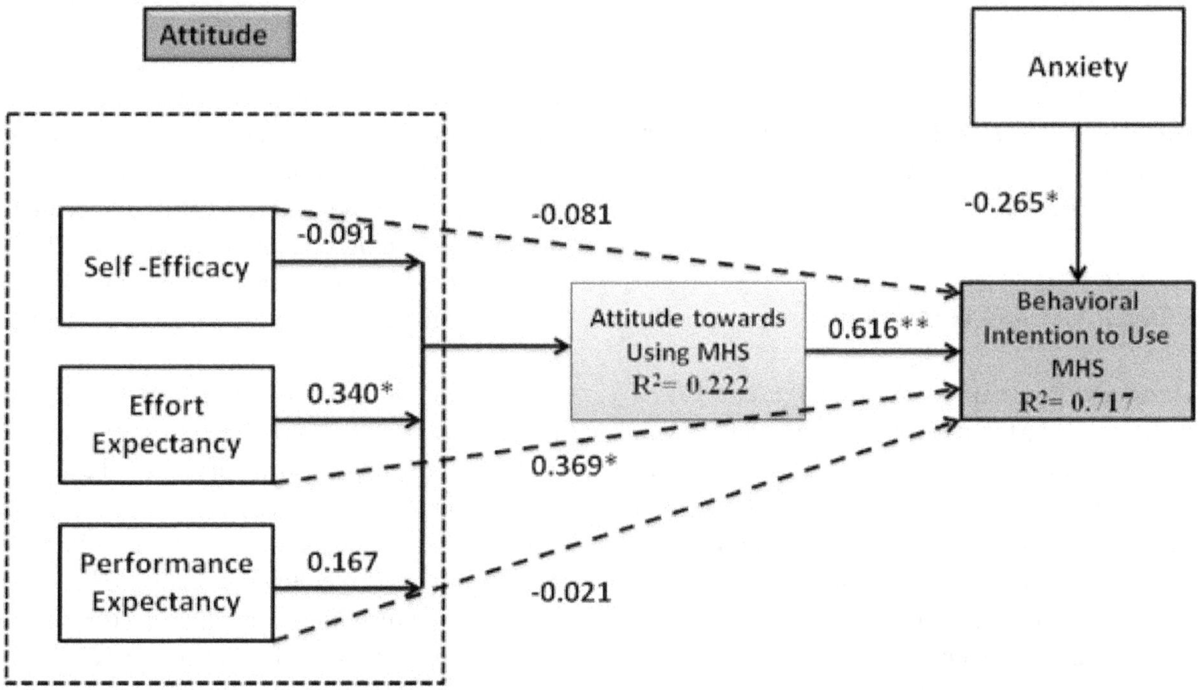


importance of effort expectancy in the attitude towards using MHS.

As shown in Table 5, the results support the prediction that attitude (β=0.616, p<0.01) and anxiety (β=-0.265, p<0.05) have statistically significant relationships with behavioral intention to use of MHS. Thus, hypothesis H7 and H8 are supported. However, effort expectancy (β =0.369, p < 0.01) is reported to be important antecedents of behavioral intention to use and H2 is supported. In contrast, the constructs of self-efficacy (β=-0.081) as well as performance expectancy (β=-0.021) indicates no significant influence on behavioral intention to use MHS.

Moreover, we evaluate the mediating effect of the attitude between three independent variables (self-efficacy, effort expectancy, and performance expectancy) and dependent variable (behavioral

*Table 5. Results of hypotheses testing*

| Path | Beta | Standard Error (SE) | T-Value | P-Value |
|---|---|---|---|---|
| AT → BI | 0.616 | 0.063 | 9.722 | p<0.01 |
| Ax → BI | -0.265 | 0.126 | 2.100 | p<0.05 |
| EE → AT | 0.340 | 0.132 | 2.571 | p<0.05 |
| EE → BI | 0.369 | 0.093 | 3.982 | p<0.01 |
| PE → AT | 0.167 | 0.136 | 1.226 | Not significant |
| PE → BI | -0.021 | 0.096 | 0.215 | Not significant |
| SE → AT | -0.091 | 0.099 | 0.915 | Not significant |
| SE → BI | -0.081 | 0.078 | 1.028 | Not significant |
| SE→AT→BI | -0.056 | 0.060 | -0.936 | Not Significant |
| EE→AT→BI | 0.209 | 0.089 | 2.349 | P<0.01 |
| PE→AT→BI | 0.103 | 0.086 | 1.194 | Not Significant |

intention to use). Based on our evaluation, attitude mediate the relationship between effort expectancy and behavioral intention to use MHS where β=0.209 and $p<0.01$.

## CONCLUDING REMARKS

This study proposed a revised model based on TPB, TAM, and UTAUT models in order to investigate what determined Smartphone's user behavioral intention toward using MHS. The results indicated that effort expectancy, anxiety, and attitude are important determinants to Smartphone user's behavioral intention to use MHS. This current model indicates high explanatory power for behavioral intention to use MHS with $R^2$=0.717 while similar study by Yi et al. (2006) indicates lower level of predictive power (Yi, Jackson, Park, & Probst, 2006) with $R^2$=0.57 and another similar study by Chau and Hu (2002) yields $R^2$=0.43 (Chau & Hu, 2002). This high explanatory power is due to effort expectancy, attitude, and anxiety that are significant in their influence; however, some factors such as self-efficacy and performance expectancy were not supported. The test results showed that Smartphone user's intention to use MHS can be predicted by effort expectancy, attitude and anxiety (Marchewka, et al., 2007). Moreover, we found that attitude can mediate the effect of effort expectancy on behavioral intention to use MHS.

Although, users would like to use MHS, the intention to use this kind of systems was not very high as users' demand was not analyzed carefully (Reuss, Menozzi, Büchi, Koller, & Krueger, 2004). Prior instruction and practice is needed to improve the users' confidence toward using MHS. Thus, they will be more likely to use this kind of systems. In addition, MHS designers must be careful more about user requirement analysis in order to meet their expectation.

Even though, this study provides insight into the factors affecting on intention to use MHS, there are some limitations in the findings. The introduction and implementation of the new MHS is time consuming and it cannot be possible to employ a new MHS and measure the effects immediately. Nevertheless, our study provides useful information for understanding the determinants of implementing new MHS. However, this research finding is only based on our study; therefore, the readers must generalize the findings and inferences from other studies related to MHS as well.

Studies related to the evaluation and the use of new technologies in healthcare can assist healthcare providers to design better systems while considering users' expectations. Many other important factors can be considered in the use of MHS and the factors can be studied further. Promoting the use of MHS among healthcare professionals as well as Smartphone users will result in the improvement of general healthcare and allocation of healthcare resources.

## ACKNOWLEDGMENT

The authors would like to thank the anonymous reviewers and the editor for their insightful comments and suggestions.

## REFERENCES

Ajzen, I. (1985). From Intentions to Actions: A Theory of Planned Behavior. In J. Kuhl, & J. Beckmann (Eds.), *Action Control* (pp. 11–39). Springer. doi:10.1007/978-3-642-69746-3_2

Ajzen, I. (1989). Attitude, structure, influence and role expectations on shopping center patronage intentions. *Journal of the Academy of Marketing Science*, *24*(3), 208–218.

Ajzen, I. (1991). The theory of planned behavior. *Organizational Behavior and Human Decision Processes*, *50*(2), 179–211. doi:10.1016/0749-5978(91)90020-T

Asada, H. H., Shaltis, P., Reisner, A., Sokwoo, R., & Hutchinson, R. C. (2003). Mobile monitoring with wearable photoplethysmographic biosensors. *Engineering in Medicine and Biology Magazine, IEEE*, *22*(3), 28–40. doi:10.1109/MEMB.2003.1213624 PMID:12845817

Bagozzi, R., & Yi, Y. (1988). On the evaluation of structural equation models. *Journal of the Academy of Marketing Science*, *16*(1), 74–94. doi:10.1007/BF02723327

Bergrath, S., Ro¨rtgen, D., Rossaint, R., Beckers, S. K., Fischermann, H., & Brokmann, J. C. et al. (2011). Technical and organisational feasibility of a multifunctional telemedicine system in an emergency medical service - an observational study. *Journal of Telemedicine and Telecare*, *17*(7), 371–377. doi:10.1258/jtt.2011.110203 PMID:21933897

Biljon, J. v., & Kotz, P. (2007). *Modelling the factors that influence mobile phone adoption*. Paper presented at the 2007 annual research conference of the South African institute of computer scientists and information technologists on IT research in developing countries. New York, NY.

Chau, P. Y., & Hu, P. J.-H. (2002). Investigating healthcare professionals' decisions to accept telemedicine technology: an empirical test of competing theories. *Information & Management*, *39*(4), 297–311. doi:10.1016/S0378-7206(01)00098-2

Chin, W., Marcolin, B., & Newsted, P. (1996). *A partial least squares latent variable modeling approach for measuring interaction effects: results from a Monte Carlo simulation study and voice mail emotion/adoption study*. Academic Press.

Chin, W. W. (1998a). Commentary: Issues and opinion on structural equation modeling. *Management Information Systems Quarterly*, vii–xvi.

Chin, W. W. (1998b). *The partial least squares approach for structural equation modeling*. Academic Press.

Davis, F. D. Jr. (1986). *A technology acceptance model for empirically testing new end-user information systems: Theory and results*. Massachusetts Institute of Technology.

Davis, F. D., Bagozzi, R. P., & Warshaw, P. R. (1989). User acceptance of computer technology: a comparison of two theoretical models. *Management Science, 35*(8), 982–1003. doi:10.1287/mnsc.35.8.982

El-Masri, S., & Saddik, B. (2012). An Emergency System to Improve Ambulance Dispatching, Ambulance Diversion and Clinical Handover Communicationâ-A Proposed Model. *Journal of Medical Systems, 36*(6), 3917–3923. doi:10.1007/s10916-012-9863-x PMID:22673893

Ernest, K., Lamei, C., Mohamed, S., Shakshuk, M., Badreldin, I., & ElBabli, I. (2011, 21-24 Feb. 2011). *A ZigBee-based telecardiology system for remote healthcare service delivery*. Paper presented at the Biomedical Engineering (MECBME). New York, NY.

Fishbein, M., & Ajzen, I. (1975). *Belief, Attitude, Intention, and Behavior: An Introduction to Theory and Research*. Boston: Addison-Wesley.

Gravelle, H., & Siciliani, L. (2008). Optimal quality, waits and charges in health insurance. *Journal of Health Economics, 27*(3), 663–674. doi:10.1016/j.jhealeco.2007.08.004 PMID:18191254

Heinssen, R. K., Glass, C. R., & Knight, L. A. (1987). Assessing computer anxiety: Development and validation of the Computer Anxiety Rating Scale. *Computers in Human Behavior, 3*(1), 49-59. doi: 10.1016/0747-5632(87)90010-0

Holden, R. J., & Karsh, B.-T. (2010). The technology acceptance model: its past and its future in health care. *Journal of Biomedical Informatics, 43*(1), 159–172. doi:10.1016/j.jbi.2009.07.002 PMID:19615467

Hung, M.-C., & Jen, W.-Y. (2012). The Adoption of Mobile Health Management Services: An Empirical Study. *Journal of Medical Systems, 36*(3), 1381–1388. doi:10.1007/s10916-010-9600-2 PMID:20878452

Iahad, A, N., Rahim, A., Zairah, N., & Oye, N. (2012). Acceptance and usage of ICT by university academicians using UTAUT model: A case study of University of Port Harcourt, Nigeria. *Journal of Emerging Trends in Computing and Information Sciences, 3*(1), 81–89.

Jansà, M., Vidal, M., Viaplana, J., Levy, I., Conget, I., Gomis, R., et al. (2006). Telecare in a structured therapeutic education programme addressed to patients with type 1 diabetes and poor metabolic control. *Diabetes Research and Clinical Practice, 74*(1), 26-32. doi: 10.1016/j.diabres.2006.03.005

Janz, B. D., & Prasarnphanich, P. (2003). Understanding the antecedents of effectiveness knowledge management: The importance of a knowledge-center culture. *Decision Sciences, 34*(2), 351–384. doi:10.1111/1540-5915.02328

Jen, W.-Y., & Chao, C.-C. (2008). Measuring mobile patient safety information system success: An empirical study. *International Journal of Medical Informatics, 77*(10), 689-697. doi: 10.1016/j.ijmedinf.2008.03.003

Jovanov, E., O'Donnel, A., Morgan, A., Priddy, B., & Hormigo, R. (2002). *Prolonged telemetric monitoring of heart rate variability using wireless intelligent sensors and a mobile gateway.* Paper presented at the Engineering in Medicine and Biology, 2002. 24th Annual Conference and the Annual Fall Meeting of the Biomedical Engineering Society EMBS/BMES Conference. New York, NY.

Keikhosrokiani, P., Mustaffa, N., Zakaria, N., & Sarwar, M. I. (2012). A Proposal to Design a Location-Based Mobile Cardiac Emergency System (LMCES). *Studies in Health Technology and Informatics*, *182*, 83–92. PMID:23138083

Kevin, H., & Yuan-Ting, Z. (2003). Implementation of a WAP-based telemedicine system for patient monitoring. *IEEE Transactions on* Information Technology in Biomedicine, *7*(2), 101–107.

Korhonen, I., Parkka, J., & Van Gils, M. (2003). Health monitoring in the home of the future. *IEEE Engineering in Medicine and Biology Magazine, 22*(3), 66–73. doi:10.1109/MEMB.2003.1213628 PMID:12845821

Li, S.-H., Cheng, K.-A., Lu, W.-H., & Lin, T.-C. (2011). Developing an Active Emergency Medical Service System Based on WiMAX Technology. *Journal of Medical Systems*, *36*(5), 3177–3193. doi:10.1007/s10916-011-9809-8 PMID:22109672

Liszka, K. J., Mackin, M. A., Lichter, M. J., York, D. W., Dilip, P., & Rosenbaum, D. S. (2004). Keeping a beat on the heart. *IEEE Pervasive Computing*, *3*(4), 42–49. doi:10.1109/MPRV.2004.10

Marchewka, J. T., Liu, C., & Kostiwa, K. (2007). An application of the UTAUT model for understanding student perceptions using course management software. *Communications of the IIMA*, *7*(2), 93–104.

Masrom, M., & Hussein, R. (2008). *User Acceptance of Information Technology: Understanding Theories and Models: Venton Publishing (M).* Sdn. Bhd.

Nunnally, J. C. (2010). *Psychometric theory*. India: McGraw-Hill Education.

Ozok, A. A., Gurses, A., Wu, H., Nelson, M., Moen, D., & Wei, J. (2009). Usability and User Acceptance for Personal Health Records: A Perspective from Healthcare Citizens. In A. A. Ozok, & P. Zaphiris (Eds.), *Online Communities and Social Computing* (Vol. 5621, pp. 690–699). Springer. doi:10.1007/978-3-642-02774-1_74

Pollard, J. K., Rohman, S., & Fry, M. E. (2001). *A Web-based mobile medical monitoring system.* Paper presented at the Intelligent Data Acquisition and Advanced Computing Systems: Technology and Applications. New York, NY.

Reuss, E., Menozzi, M., Büchi, M., Koller, J., & Krueger, H. (2004). Information access at the point of care: what can we learn for designing a mobile CPR system? *International Journal of Medical Informatics*, *73*(4), 363–369. doi:10.1016/j.ijmedinf.2004.02.003 PMID:15135755

Ross, P. E. (2004). Managing care through the air [remote health monitoring]. *IEEE Spectrum, 41*(12), 26-31.

Saadé, R. G. (2007). Dimensions of perceived usefulness: Toward enhanced assessment. *Decision Sciences Journal of Innovative Education*, *5*(2), 289–310. doi:10.1111/j.1540-4609.2007.00142.x

Sokwoo, R., Boo-Ho, Y., Kuowei, C., & Asada, H. H. (1998). *The ring sensor: A new ambulatory wearable sensor for twenty-four hour patient monitoring*. Paper presented at the Engineering in Medicine and Biology Society. New York, NY.

Stanford, V. (2002). Using pervasive computing to deliver elder care. *Pervasive Computing, IEEE*, *1*(1), 10–13. doi:10.1109/MPRV.2002.993139

Tu, Y.-J., Zhou, W., & Piramuthu, S. (2009). Identifying RFID-embedded objects in pervasive healthcare applications. *Decision Support Systems*, *46*(2), 586–593. doi:10.1016/j.dss.2008.10.001

Varady, P., Benyo, Z., & Benyo, B. (2002). An open architecture patient monitoring system using standard technologies. *IEEE Transactions on* Information Technology in Biomedicine, *6*(1), 95–98.

Varshney, U. (2003). Location management for mobile commerce applications in wireless Internet environment. *ACM Transactions on Internet Technology*, *3*(3), 236–255. doi:10.1145/857166.857169

Varshney, U. (2007). Pervasive Healthcare and Wireless Health Monitoring. *Mobile Networks and Applications*, *12*(2-3), 113–127. doi:10.1007/s11036-007-0017-1

Venkatesh, V., Morris, M. G., Davis, G. B., & Davis, F. D. (2003). User Acceptance of Information Technology: Toward a Unified View. *Management Information Systems Quarterly*, *27*(3).

Wan Ismail, W. K., Chan, P. H. K., Buhari, N., & Muzaini, A. (2012). *Acceptance of Smartphone in Enhancing Patient-Caregivers Relationship* (Vol. 7). Academic Press.

Wu, I.-L., Li, J.-Y., & Fu, C.-Y. (2011). The adoption of mobile healthcare by hospital's professionals: An integrative perspective. *Decision Support Systems*, *51*(3), 587–596. doi:10.1016/j.dss.2011.03.003

Wu, J.-H., Wang, S.-C., & Lin, L.-M. (2007). Mobile computing acceptance factors in the healthcare industry: A structural equation model. *International Journal of Medical Informatics*, *76*(1), 66–77. doi:10.1016/j.ijmedinf.2006.06.006 PMID:16901749

Yi, M. Y., Jackson, J. D., Park, J. S., & Probst, J. C. (2006). Understanding information technology acceptance by individual professionals: Toward an integrative view. *Information & Management*, *43*(3), 350–363. doi:10.1016/j.im.2005.08.006

Yu, J., Ha, I., Choi, M., & Rho, J. (2005). Extending the TAM for a t-commerce. *Information & Management*, *42*(7), 965–976. doi:10.1016/j.im.2004.11.001

## KEY TERMS AND DEFINITIONS

**Anxiety:** The degree to which the person has a favorable or unfavorable evaluation of the behavior in question.

**Attitude:** The degree to which the person has a favorable or unfavorable evaluation of the behavior in question.

**Effort Expectancy:** The degree of ease associated with the use of the systems.

**Mobile Healthcare System:** The system that is able to Transfer biomedical signals (blood pressure, cardiac performance, insulin level etc.) over a long distance using wired or wireless communication technologies.

**Performance Expectancy:** The degree to which an individual believes that using the system will help him/her to attain gains in job performance.

**Self-Efficacy:** The concept of self-efficacy is concerned with people's belief in their ability to produce effects.

**Theory of Acceptance Model:** Is a model for predicting and explaining human behavior for accepting new technologies in different domains.

**Theory of Planned Behavior:** Is a model for predicting and explaining human behavior in different domains.

**Unified Theory of Acceptance and Use of Technology:** This theory is the combination of few theories and it seeks to clarify user intention to use an information system (IS) and consequent usage behavior.

**User Behavioral Intention to Use:** Is a measure of the strength of individual intention to perform a specified behavior, which is use of a new technology or system.

# Section 3
# Emerging Technologies for Healthcare

# Chapter 8
# Sleep Disorder Diagnosis:
## An Analytical Approach

**Jacqueline Blake**
*University of the Sunshine Coast, Australia*

**Don Kerr**
*University of the Sunshine Coast, Australia*

## ABSTRACT

*Sleep disorders are a significant and growing problem, both for the economy of the nation and for the physical and psychological well-being of individual sufferers. Physicians are under pressure to find ways of dealing with the backlog of patients. The purpose of this chapter is to investigate the operational, administrative, and medical environment within which sleep physicians diagnose patients with sleep disorders and develop an online support system that would efficiently gather patient history data and improve the effectiveness of patient-physician consultations, the diagnoses, and patients' self-management of any subsequent treatment plans. Investigations confirm that the physicians spend a large portion of the available consultation time on routine questions. In the new system, the patient information is captured by the patient completing an online questionnaire. Due to the reduction in time given for data collection, the physician can spend time with the patients discussing patient-specific symptoms and life-styles.*

## INTRODUCTION

Sleep disorders are a significant and growing problem, both for the economy of the nation and for the physical and psychological well-being of individual sufferers. Physicians, who deal with sleep disorders, and their administrative support staff and facilities, are under constant pressure to find more efficient ways of dealing with the backlog of patients, many of whom face significant wait times before being able to attend a consultation.

The main symptom of a sleep disorder is excessive daytime sleepiness there are a number of lifestyle consequences associated with this. Deloitte Access Economics (2011) state that 8.9% of the Australian population are affected. the direct and indirect costs of sleep disorders to the Australian society in 2010 was 36.4 billion dollars

DOI: 10.4018/978-1-4666-6316-9.ch008

(Deloitte Access Economics 2011). The indirect costs include co-morbidities[1] such as hypertension, lost production, transport and workplace accidents and social costs, such as learning difficulties. Physically, sleep deprivation may be associated with an increased risk of myocardial infraction (heart attack), type two diabetes, depressed immune response (Akerstedt & Nilsson 2003) and may present as depression. However treatment for sleep disorders reduces the direct and indirect costs restoring productivity and well-being to the individual and any organisation they are involved with. Sleep disorders are a chronic condition, so that for most conditions a treatment plan must be enduring requiring a considerable on-going commitment from the sufferer and partnership with their physician.

The estimate of 8.9% of the Australian population who have a sleep disorder is in all probability an underestimate with sleep disorders underdiagnosed in Australia (Deloitte Access Economics 2011), other countries report similar statistics (Young, Peppard & Gottlieb 2002) with the people who are referred for treatment being strongly symptomatic (Kramer et al. 1999). This means that there remains a sector of the population who are yet to seek treatment demonstrated by the direct costs of sleep disorders comprising only two per cent of the total cost. Sleep disorders commonly affect people around middle-age so as the population ages there are an increased number of people with sleep disorders with risk factors in adults being obesity, alcohol, smoking, nasal congestion and menopause (Young et al. 2002). The wait times for a consultation in a publically funded facility may be significant (Flemons et al. 2004). The wait times demonstrate a gap between demand for sleep disorder assistance and the ability of the most health services to provide for the current level of people referred to sleep clinics. Australia in common with other developed countries is also facing an aging population in which sleep disorders will become more prevalent (Alzougool, Chang & Gray 2008).

## INCREASING DEMAND FOR SERVICES

This increasing service demand and a shortage of sleep disorder specialists (Australian Medical Workforce Advisory Committee 2000; Patlak 2005) have driven the sleep community interest in changing the traditional model of care for sleep disorders to one that leverages information systems to provide efficiencies and timely communication flows (Colten & Alterogt 2006). Abidi (2001) refers to the strategic use of knowledge derived from healthcare data as being "... *pertinent towards the improvement of the operational efficiency of the said healthcare enterprise*" (Abidi 2001, p. 6) while Hirakis & Karakounos *(2006)* and Haux (2010) state that knowledge management in healthcare allows the development of best practice models, making guidelines explicit and encourages innovation through development of the resultant knowledge base.

The term health informatics was developed by the International Medical Informatics Association (IMIA). They defined the term as "a combination of computer science, information science and health science designed to assist in the management and processing of data, information and knowledge to support healthcare and healthcare delivery (Conrick 2006, p. 4). Health informatics now forms part of the infrastructure for the delivery of healthcare with one of the major fields of research being decision support (Haux 2010). Health informatics allows the timely retrieval and filtering of patient and disorder information so that care givers have appropriate information in a quickly assimilated format within their work flow. Health informatics is the overarching domain within which this project lies as this project aims to use information systems to assist in providing knowledge to support both the patient and physician in the diagnosis of sleep disorders.

One important avenue to leverage the capabilities of this project and its collection of sleep disorder data is that of business analytics. Chen,

Chiang and Storey (2012,p. 1166) defined business analytics as "techniques, technologies, systems, practices, methodologies and applications that analyse critical business data to help the enterprise better understand its business and market and make timely business decision." In this instance we can consider a sleep clinic's business of being the most efficient means of diagnosing and helping a patient deal with the lifestyle implications of a chronic disorder diagnosis.

The purpose of this research was to investigate the operational, administrative and medical environment within which sleep physicians currently diagnose patients with sleep disorders and develop an online support system that would more efficiently gather patient history data, and so improve the effectiveness of patient–physician consultations, the diagnoses, and patients' self-management of any subsequent treatment plans. The research used observations and a participatory research process based on inputs from two sleep physicians and a sleep psychologist to guide the development for the information technology artefact. This process ensured that the resultant online tools fitted into the physician's work flow with the patient information in the required format.

## RESEARCH OBJECTIVES

A design science approach was taken to building the online tools. The resultant online tools incorporates four sub-applications,

1. An online sleep diary, with an output of a physician report showing a graph of the patients sleep patterns and sleep statistics and the online presentation to the patient of the sleep pattern graph.
2. An online patient history questionnaire, asking lifestyle, medical history and sleep disorder specific questions.
3. A decision support system using as an input data from the patient history questionnaire.
4. A report generator summarising and presenting the output from the decision support system.

These tools aim to remove responsibility for form filling from the physician to the patient, Give the patient access to sleep disorder specific questions earlier in their interaction with the sleep investigation unit to aid self-discovery of sleep disorder information. Another outcome is presenting the patient information to the physician within the natural workflow of a consultation in a format which the physicians find useful.

One of the critical factors for physicians to accept a clinical decision support system is openness and transparency of how the decision was derived therefore an explanation of how a decision is reached by the system must be provided. The provision of an explanation module and the diagnostic environment of heterogeneous sleep disorder sufferers drove the adoption of small rule based decision support systems at every decision point in the argument toward diagnosis as described by Stranieri et al. (1999). Graber and Mathew (2008) found that to increase acceptance of clinical decision support systems, reducing physician time to input data and fitting the system into physician work flow were key factors.

## THE IT ARTEFACT

The IT artefact will aid physicians by presenting them with relevant patient information within the natural workflow of a consultation, and in a format that the physicians finds useful, while the individual who has a sleep disorder is able to fill in the questionnaire at their leisure and in their own home.

The development of an online application gives the form designer control over the sequence in which the form must be filled in, which means that the user can be constrained to provide information according to a required pattern. An online application also provides an opportunity to validate the entered data at the point of entry. Using validation in the sleep tool application means that the physician does not need to question the patient about the data contained in the application, but instead has time to talk about what the information means to the patient, for instance the impact of smoking on sleep disorders.

A well-developed sleep tool web application can be cost effective. The data sets from large numbers of respondents represent many repeated iterations of the form; consequently, as the data is captured, it can be automatically stored, manipulated and analysed. Thus data analysis is low cost and happens in real time for each form (Haynes et al. 2006). The automatic storage of collected information also provides an opportunity for good quality, validated data to be used for future research. This is important as at the moment no aggregated analysis is carried out on the present pen-and-paper patient history forms. Anecdotal evidence suggests that manually computing the data from a paper-based patient history, and the data entry of the information into a database, requires a large time commitment from clinic staff. This means that the routine collection of sleep diary information to build an evidence base is unlikely to be given a priority outside of a specific research project.

During 2009, there was strong growth in internet access in Queensland homes, reaching 87.6 per cent, which was an increase of 2½ per cent above the 2008 figure (Queensland Government Chief Information Office 2010). Minimal difference was shown in internet use between genders. The survey showed growth in computer access by people aged over 65; their internet use had grown strongly during the year to 61.1 per cent – a 6 per cent increase (Queensland Government Chief Information Office 2010). These percentages show that online forms are a viable alternative to paper-based forms for a large proportion of the population.

## THE DEVELOPMENT

One of the difficulties in constructing an online information system is the need to design the application for unknown users. Users of an online system will have a range of technical skill levels, and will access the system through a variety of connection mechanisms, using an assortment of hardware. This diversity contrasts sharply with the development of an organisational system, which requires standardised connections and hardware, and whose operators have known, minimum technical standards (Taylor, Wade & England 2003). Useability must be a primary objective of an online tool, Guenther (2004) stating that having a clear set of objectives for the user helps to make the online system a high value one. This project had two sets of users: physicians and patients. Consequently, the online tool had to meet two different sets of objectives and expectations. Calongne (2001) argues that what the user wants to achieve from the site must also be considered. In this project the online systems were tools, so that to achieve user satisfaction the online tools had to look and feel like a solid health orientated implement. In the patients' case, the tool needed to feel like a device that would provide good information to them and to their physician, while in the physicians' case, the tool needed to provide a set of quality information in an easy to assimilate format.

To display information online, equity of access had to be considered, so that online tools had utility for the sight, hearing and physically impaired; users with little technical expertise had also to be catered for. Wagner, Hassanein, and Head (2010) suggest a number of guidelines for older users of web sites, including making sure visual elements are large enough to be seen and deciphered. They suggest using elements that contrast highly with the background, such as black elements on a white background. An uncluttered web page without too many elements claiming attention helps the user to make sense of the page. Also, graphics should be used only when necessary to illustrate or add to the site's function (Yen, Hu & Wang 2007). For the online sleep tool application, the expected age range of the users was expected to be fairly broad and computer literacy to be variable. Most of the potential patients would be older than 45 and reasonably computer literate, but to improve equity of access the sleep diary had to be as accessible as possible across the whole spectrum of potential patients.

In the sleep tool application, the user interface was given the maximum contrast of black sans serif text on a plain white uncluttered background. The uncluttered background means that the sleep tool application can be personalised – with, for example, an organisation's logo – without disturbing the readability of the questions. The plain background also helps to minimise the file size of the web application, so that patients whose computers have slow download speeds are not penalised by having to wait for a graphic to appear.

A user tries to make logical sense of a displayed web page at first glance, so the design of the page must make logical sense; for instance, headings should be in a larger font. Design elements that are related need to be gathered together graphically; for example a question is contained within a frame. The graphical treatment of these elements needs to be consistent and predictable throughout the web site to aid usability (Willems 2000). A linear web site plan, where the user moves through the web application page by page, helps to orientate the user so that they are aware of where in the web site they are (Guenther 2004; Yen et al. 2007). These requirements were carried out in the application.

The heuristic evaluation rules for websites detailed by Sharp, Rogers and Preece (2007) were employed. The website has internal consistency, with terms carrying the same meaning throughout the web site, using simple language. To aid internal consistency, formatting of pages, fonts, font sizes and font colours were made consistent. Shortcuts were not used, as the sleep tool application has a simple linear format which must be followed to gather complete information. The user's memory load is minimised with no information being required to be remembered from one part of the web-page or web-site to the other. Entries into the web form are validated; for example in the sleep diary, a wake time before a sleep time cannot be chosen, and throughout, each page is checked for completeness. The user is given feedback in two forms: for the sleep diary, the user is presented with a sleep pattern graphic that represents the entered sleep patterns; for the patient history questionnaire, the user receives a message that their information has been sent to their sleep clinic.

One of the complications with implementing this application is the need to build the application in accordance with guidelines set by the government for patient privacy; for instance, a patient number cannot be used as an identifier. A different number is required to satisfy the National Privacy Principles stated in the Queensland Government's information architecture for the Department of Health (Queensland Government 2001). This was last reviewed in April 2008 (Queensland Government Chief Information Office 2008), and states that an identifier that has been assigned by an agency cannot be adopted by an outside application. Consequently, for this project, a user number that was unique, and different from the patient number, was required to be system assigned.

## Purpose of the Web Application

One of the most important factors in the design of the sleep tool web application was the role the patient history played during a consultation. Physicians have clear expectations about what they consider to be best practice at this time, so patient history was included as an input to the system. In order to facilitate the knowledge acquisition process, the researcher formed a team with two sleep physicians and a psychologist. All three were considered to be experts in the field of sleep disorder diagnosis, and a collaborative approach was taken to help gain insights into their shared knowledge and experience in the sleep disorder domain and in order to develop the knowledge base for the DSS. All stakeholders (physicians and patients) provided approval for the process (as required by ethics). Gaining the physician stakeholders' approval of the output from the sleep tool application and its utility as a data gathering instrument for the patient history was essential. This approval meant the project gained access to the sleep physicians' patient knowledge and gave the medical team a vested interest in the success of the project (Cornwall & Jewkes 1995). The two sleep specialists provided expertise on the diagnostic criteria and process, while the psychologist specialised in psychological sleep disorders such as insomnia, the psychology impacts of sleep disorders and compliance with sleep disorder treatment by patients. The researcher acted as team leader to keep the team focused on the required outcome, researched questions from the team, set agendas, produced questionnaire drafts, scheduled meetings and kept records of the meetings.

## Structure of the Web Application

The sleep tools application has three main areas of functionality (see Table 1).

There are four main categories of user in the sleep tools application (see Table 2).

The entry page of the online sleep application is a log-on page providing the facility to differentiate between different types of users and the means to authenticate users through the use of an identification number and user name. Differentiating between users is important to customise their interaction with the web site. To facilitate the physician's use of the tool the physician goes directly from log-on to the sleep statistic page for the entered patient number, which allows for the entry of a user name and password. The next page has a different menu, depending on the class of user.

The patient menu page shown in Figure 1 allows the user to choose between either the sleep diary or the patient history areas of functionality or, alternatively, to return to the log-on page.

*Table 1. Sleep tools application main areas of functionality*

| Functionality | Output |
|---|---|
| An online sleep diary, which records 14 days of a person's sleep habits and mood. | *Patient:* A graphical representation of their sleep habits.<br>*Physician:* A graphical representation of a patient's sleep habits and a report containing sleep statistics showing the averages of sleep data. |
| An online patient history questionnaire | Data stored in database. |
| A knowledge-based decision support system | Data retrieved from database, manipulated according to logic embedded in decision support system and presented as a report to the physician detailing if the person's patient history meets the criteria for the main sleep disorders. |

*Table 2. Types of user in the web based sleep tools application*

| Type of user | Function |
|---|---|
| A super-user or administrator | Limited to one user – has overall administration responsibility. |
| Hospital administration staff | Add or edit patients and doctors. They may also access patient results for their clinic, to print out results for patient files. |
| Physicians | Review and print their patients' results. |
| Patients | Complete sleep diary and patient history questionnaire. |

*Figure 1. Patient menu from the sleep tools application*

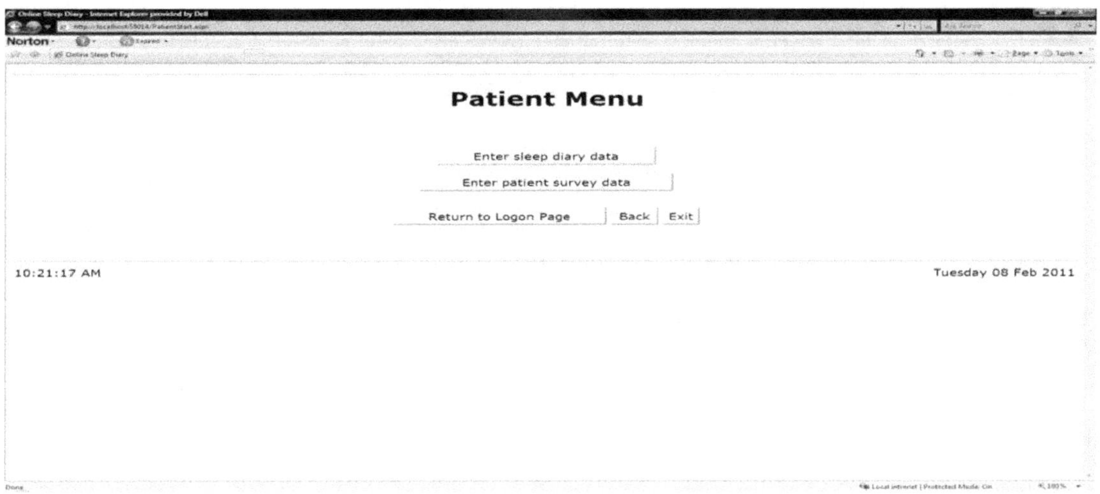


The main administrator or super-user menu screen is shown in Figure 2. This shows that the main administrator can access all areas and has overall responsibility for administering the system.

The physician administration menu screen is shown in Figure 3. A physician must be linked to a clinic in order for this screen to be created. This function can be completed by an administration officer (clinic administrator) or the super-user.

The clinic administrator's menu screen is shown in Figure 4. The clinic administrator must also be associated with a clinic. Their role is to create patient records and support the physicians by printing patient reports. They may also create other administrator screens. These figures showing the management screens demonstrate the overlay of administration and security which controls the views that users have of the main areas of functionality.

*Figure 2. Super-user menu screen*

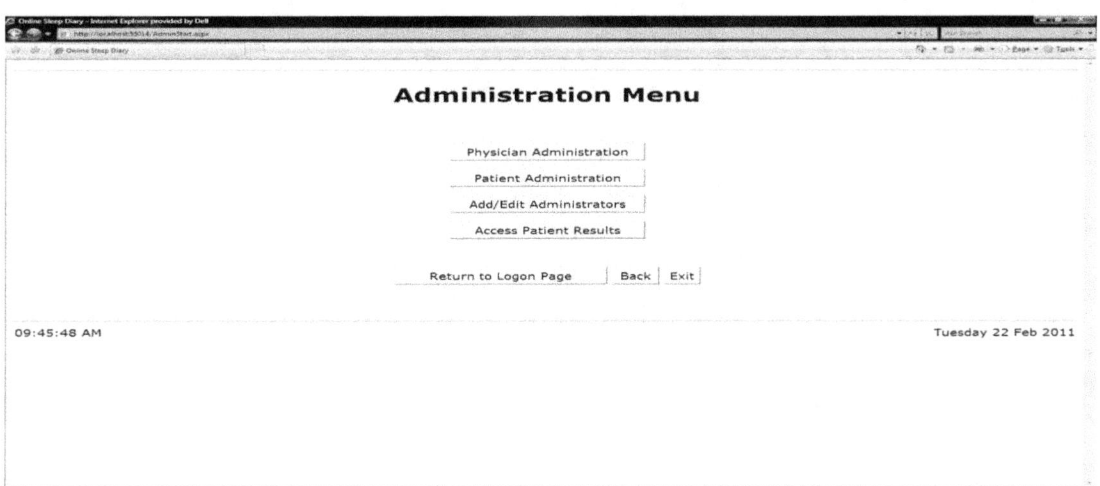

*Figure 3. Physician administration screen*

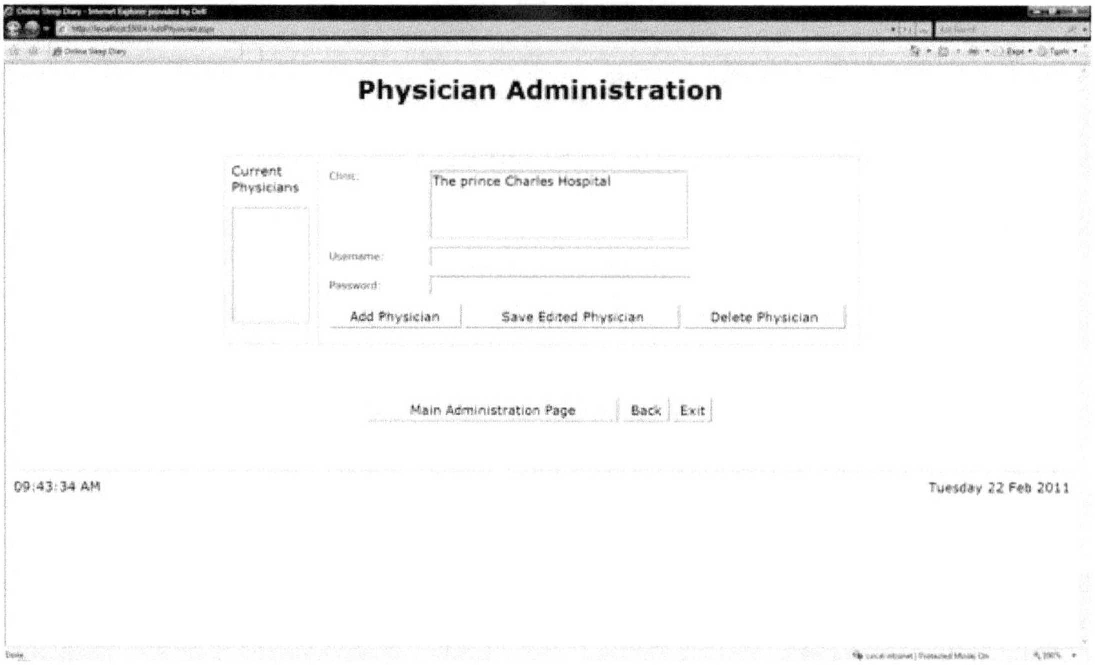


*Figure 4. Administration officer screen*

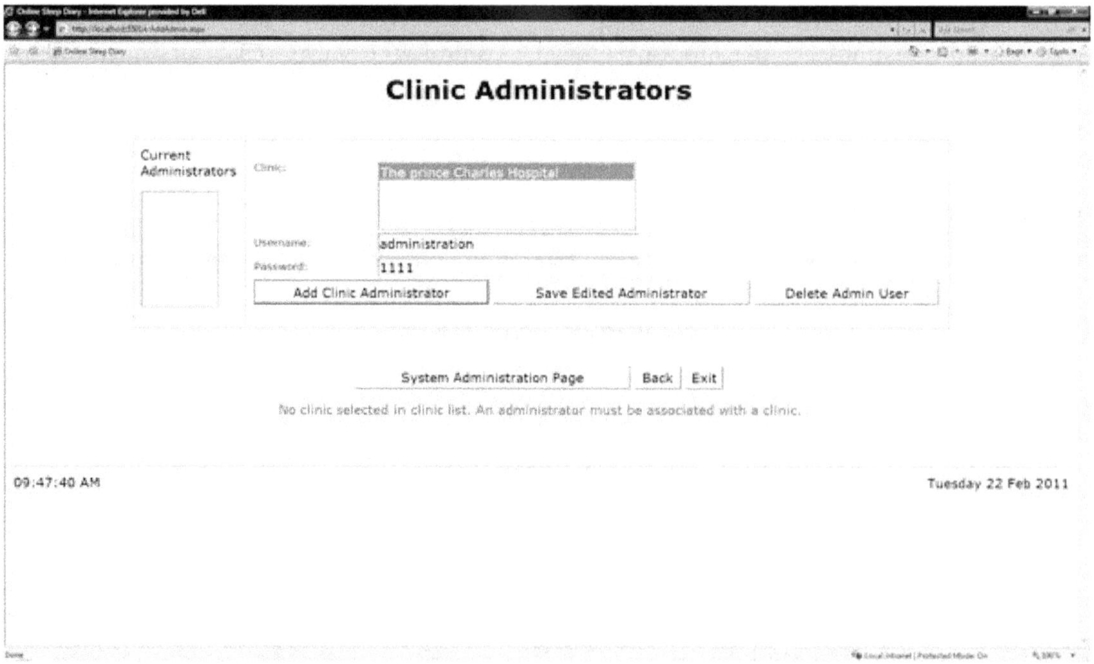

## Online Sleep Diary

A sleep diary is used to record sleep patterns, usually for fourteen nights. The person notes the details of their night's sleep day-by-day, building up a picture of sleep habits (known as *sleep hygiene*). Poor sleep hygiene, or insufficient time made available for sleep, may be a cause of excessive daytime sleepiness, the main symptom of a sleep disorder. Therefore, a sleep diary can be used to identify a cause for daytime sleepiness, lifestyle reasons or a sleep disorder. Sleep diaries are used by a number of health professionals, including psychologists, physicians and sleep specialists and is the primary diagnostic tool for identifying insomnia. It is a very useful aid in the diagnosis of other sleep disorders, as relatively short periods of time taken to fall asleep or frequent awakenings are indicators of poor quality sleep, and of sleep disorders.

During an exploratory interview early in a project to review sleep diagnosis, the remark was made by a director of a large public health clinic that "… sleep diaries were a good tool which were not being used efficiently due to the timing and the short length of time available in the consultation to extract information from the data" (pers. Comm. 23 Sept.). The current format of the sleep diary used in the sleep investigation unit study was a pen-and-paper questionnaire in which the patient coloured in a square between two printed times – for example, nine and ten o'clock – to indicate bed time and waking up time.

This created a situation that requires the sleep physician to clarify which time the patient actually meant to mark. The data contained in the completed sleep diary required manual calculation to extract daily entries, aggregate the data and calculate the required sleep statistics and was in a format that was difficult to quickly assimilate within a time limited consultation. Due to the low utility of this model of use, the physician had difficulty in using a sleep diary effectively. The information in the sleep diary was also in a format from which a patient cannot extract information without physician assistance. An online literature search was carried out for Internet or web and online sleep diaries for evidence of previous peer reviewed papers. This search was periodically carried out throughout this project, the last being undertaken on 30 March 2012. No peer reviewed papers focusing on online sleep diaries were found.

Patient access to the information contained in an online sleep diary means the patient gains increased self-knowledge of their sleep hygiene, which has been shown to improve health outcomes (Smith et al. 2004). Patients should be able to self-monitor their sleep patterns. Wilde and Garvin (2007, p. 343) define self-monitoring as "awareness of symptoms or bodily sensations that is enhanced by periodic measurements recordings and observations to provide information for improved self-management". Self-monitoring of sleep patterns means that the patients have an opportunity for shared decision making with their physician on the management of their sleep disorder. Shared decision making is a significant factor in compliance with treatment plans (Sheppard et al. 2009). This is important in a chronic condition such as a sleep disorder, which has an ongoing treatment burden

With this on-line system, the physician gains earlier access to patient sleep hygiene information and can therefore prioritise those patients who need to be seen first, ensuring that those in most need of the service will have the shortest wait times. It is also forecasted that patient satisfaction with the service will increase as during the wait time for an appointment they are able to self-monitor their condition. Therefore, the online sleep diary has a number of benefits, namely:

1. The data contained within the diary is presented in a summarised, readily accessible format for both physicians and patients.
2. The diary contents are available at any internet access point and in real time (subject to security precautions).

*Figure 5. Flowchart of how sleep tool web application is accessed*

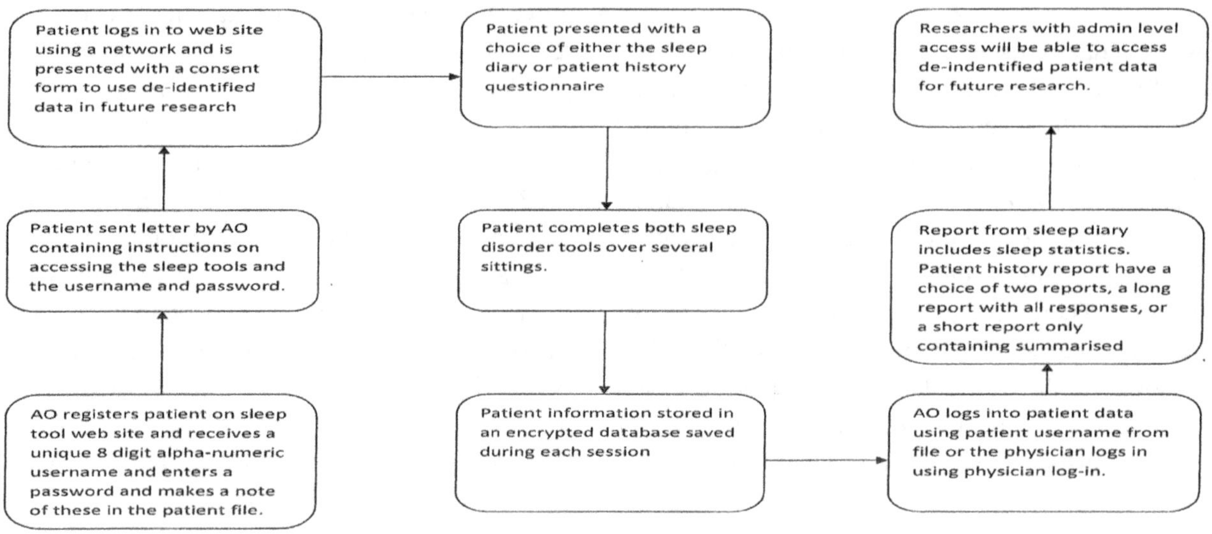


3. The diary facilitates the easy development of a database of sleep patterns and this can be used for historical data analysis.
4. The online diary has all the advantages of digital data such as reuse, multiple storage locations, easier transferability of data to other medical professionals and availability for statistical analysis.

Better quality sleep information is obtained when a sleep diary is filled out every day. This ensures that the person has the best recall of sleep quality and timing of sleep, Libman, Fichten, Bailes, and Amsel (2000) stated that questionnaires that look at respective sleep patterns are susceptible to memory distortion, whereas a sleep diary filled in every day has the ability to capture day-to-day variations, highlighting variations that may indicate problems such as sleep deficits in sleep patterns. This means that the recording of a person's sleep habits over a two-week period in a sleep diary gives a baseline of a person's sleep patterns with greater precision than retrospective sleep quality questionnaires.

One disadvantage of a sleep diary is that subjects may change their sleep patterns in reaction to the self-monitoring and the imposition of filling in the diary day-to-day (Libman et al. 2000). However, Lacks and Morin (1992) comment that a sleep diary is the most widely used, practical and economical method of gauging sleep patterns.

An online sleep diary has a number of benefits: the data contained within the diary are presented in a summarised, readily accessible format for both physicians and patients, and are available in real time, while the database of sleep patterns is being built.

## ONLINE SLEEP DIARY OUTPUTS

The online sleep diary will produce a summary report which may be printed both for the person filling in the diary and for a physician. This summary report gives access to sleep statistics (see Table 3).

Also reported is a count of the number of times that reasons for waking were checked, and the reasons given for the patient being kept awake. An average of the morning's mood and feeling are also given. The report is presented in a quickly assimilated format that has direct utility

*Table 3. Sleep statistics in report for physician*

| Name | Description |
|---|---|
| Mean sleep duration | Average time spent asleep. |
| Range of sleep duration | The minimum and maximum time spent asleep over the sleep diary time period. |
| Number of nights with fewer than seven hours sleep. | A count of the number of nights where fewer than seven hours of sleep were achieved. |
| Mean for sleep onset. | Average length of time taken between settling in bed ready for sleep; for example, light off, television off, and time that sleep was achieved. |
| Range of sleep onset | The minimum and maximum times spent getting to sleep over the sleep diary period. |
| Mean wake up time | Average time that the person wakes for the last time. |
| Mean sleep efficiency | Sleep efficiency is the proportion of time spent asleep in the time available for sleep; for example, of the nine hours spent in bed, eight hours were spent asleep. The sleep efficiency is 8/9 = 0.89. |

for assisting in a diagnosis of a sleep disorder. The summary report may also be filed in a patient record to provide a baseline for future sleep diary reports for the physician and patient.

A summary report of sleep hygiene practices may also be useful for the user to take to their primary care physician if the user is concerned about excessive daytime sleepiness. Potentially, this means that primary care physicians may refer patients with moderate symptoms of a sleep disorder to a sleep specialist, as sleep disorders are under-diagnosed in all but the most symptomatic patients (Kramer et al. 1999). The online sleep diary may also be used by primary physicians to consider diagnosing a sleep disorder in patients who describe symptoms such as fatigue or lack of energy (Chervin 2000) which traditionally lead to a diagnosis of depression. Shepertycky, Banno and Kryger (2005) state that approximately 90% of women with moderate to severe obstructive sleep apnoea are undiagnosed or misdiagnosed as having depression – leading to significant health impacts and costs to the health system.

The facility to export the data contained in the online sleep diary in an eXtensible Markup Language (XML) format was also provided. This means that organisations other than that hosting the sleep diary can receive patient data in an electronic format, facilitating use of electronic record keeping.

## CURRENT SLEEP DIARY MODEL

The current paper-based sleep diary, as stated above, does not present information in a format that the lay person can understand. The online sleep diary in this project presents sleep patterns as an easy to understand multi-coloured horizontal bar graph, with time along the $x$-axis. Midnight is the centre of the $x$-axis to allow the comparison of the regularity of bed and waking up times important in sleep hygiene. This graph builds day by day as the patient completes each day's diary entry. The different colours within the bars represent different states, such as awake during sleep time, sleep latency and sleep time. Therefore, the physician can gain a view of the patient's sleep patterns quickly, while the patient gains access to the information on their sleep patterns presented in a simple graphical format.

The current model of a pen-and-paper sleep diary denies the patient an opportunity to self-monitor their sleep patterns and adopt functional analysis of lifestyle changes such as reducing caffeine intake. With the online sleep diary, patients gain a tool to use in self-monitoring their sleep patterns. Wilde and Garvin (2007, p.343) define self-monitoring as awareness of symptoms that is facilitated by periodic measurements or recordings to provide information for improved self-management. The use of the online sleep diary to self-monitor gives patients the opportunity for shared decision making with their physician on the management of their sleep disorder. Vermeire and Hearnshaw (2001) found that shared decision making is an important factor in compliance to treatment; it is important because compliance to CPAP requires commitment from the user.

The online sleep diary is a sub-application of the sleep tool web application, with the printed graph and sleep statistics providing a hard copy report for the physician.

## Patient History Questionnaire

There are a number of questionnaires that are designed to diagnose specific sleep disorders, such as the Sleep Decisions Questionnaire (SDQ) and the Pittsburgh questionnaire. However, these questionnaires are not designed to act as a complete information gathering point for a physician consultation about sleep or designed for future automated data collection. The increasing burden of these disorders on the medical community – caused by a higher profile and aging population – has led to interest by the sleep community in changing the traditional model of care for sleep disorders to one that leverages information systems to provide efficiencies and timely communication flows (Colten & Alterogt 2006,p. 26). Within the Queensland Health system researched in this project, anecdotal evidence suggests that sleep laboratory time is available to perform more polysomnography tests. However, there is an insufficient number of appointment slots for a patient to see a sleep physician before undertaking a polysomnography sleep study. Consequently, the efficient use of a physician's time during a consultation is critical to maintaining the sleep unit's work flow and an appropriate wait time for patients before seeing a physician.

### Development of the Questionnaire

The questionnaire is required to act as an information gathering point for input into the intelligent decision support system standard and a validated tool for patient appraisal in sleep disorder consultations. This will provide the sleep physician with good quality data before the first consultation with the patient. The responsibility for filling out the forms is transferred to the patient. This shift from the current practice will potentially free up physician time during the consultation and remove the need for the physician to ask information gathering closed-ended questions during the consultation; for example, "How many caffeine containing drinks did you consume during the day?" Instead, the physician will already have access to the patient's background information, so can use the limited consultation time to focus on the patient's sleep problem and to suggest lifestyle changes. This also has the potential to increase the patient's satisfaction with the provided service.

The outline of the proposed data gathering system for the decision support system for the diagnostic process was driven by a series of three one-hour interviews with the director of a Sleep Investigation Unit, Brisbane, Australia to discuss the sleep disorder diagnostic process. convergent interviewing method as described in the methodology chapter was used to discover initial requirements. This informal interviewing technique is useful when the researchers are in some doubt about the information which is to be collected. Notes and impressions from the interviews were written in a journal and emailed to the interviewee for confirmation that these were aligned with the information they intended to convey. These meetings established the outline of the patient–physician interaction and discovered that there were two main types of consultations. The first was an exploratory consultation where the physician was investigating the current symptoms and patient history; the second was a shorter, confirmatory consultation where the physician discussed the diagnosis with the patient.

## Domain Specialist Knowledge Acquisition

The researcher formed a team with two sleep physicians and a psychologist. A collaborative approach was taken with the medical staff to gain their shared knowledge and experience in the sleep disorder domain as knowledge acquisition for the knowledge base of the decision support system. Gaining these stakeholders' approval of the instrument was essential to gain access to sleep investigation clinic patients so as to test the instrument, and to give these team members a vested interest in the success of the project (Cornwall & Jewkes 1995). The team members were two sleep specialists, a sleep psychologist; and the researcher. The two medical doctors provided expertise on the diagnostic criteria and process; the psychologist specialised in psychological sleep disorders such as insomnia, the psychological impacts of sleep disorders, and compliance with sleep disorder treatments by patients. The researcher led the team and in addition had domain experience in constructing questionnaires and providing information systems in knowledge management. The researcher was also responsible for keeping the team focused on producing a data gathering tool for the decision support system, for undertaking research activities outside the meeting, for checking the literature for parameters, and for confirming decisions. The researcher was also responsible for producing the hospital ethics application, producing questionnaire drafts, scheduling meetings and keeping records of the meetings.

A participatory approach was taken to the development of the questionnaire as this can form "knowledge used in action" (Cornwall & Jewkes 1995, p. 1667), while Macaulay (2007) promotes its use by physicians to produce relevant research. White, Suchowierska & Campbell (2004) agree that participatory research can produce relevant research, resulting in the development of user friendly instruments. University of British Columbia Institute of Health Promotion Research (1996) describes participatory research as "systematic inquiry, with the collaboration of those affected by the issue being studied, for purposes of education and taking action or effecting change". In this instance the community being studied comprised sleep specialists who worked within the Queensland Health public system, and who showed concern about the problem by approaching the university with the research concept. The participatory research approach ensured that there was a collegial power sharing approach with a mutual respect of each participant's expertise in their field. The interaction of the team using this approach meant that once a clear definition of the problem under study was made, a solution that was technically possible and immediately useful to the physicians could be designed (White et al. 2004). The technical aspect of the solution was made accessible to the team members by using pen-and-paper and PowerPoint prototypes to make explicit the outcome of the system (Pilemalm & Timpka 2008).

# RESULTS

## Physician Evaluation of Sleep Tools Instrument

Investigations confirmed that the physicians spend a large portion of the available consultation time on routine questions such as capturing details on smoking habits and caffeine consumption. One of the physician's initial comments on seeing a patient history report was that at least they could read it demonstrating how important how important information which is easy to assimilate is within the confines of a consultation.

The sleep tool web application is intended to be used first, by patients with potentially limited computer literacy, and then by physicians who will use the application for diagnostic purposes. It was therefore essential to ensure that the application was usable. The International Standards Organisation (ISO) defines usability in standard 9241–11 as "extent to which a product can be used by specified users to achieve specified goals effectively, efficiently and with satisfaction in a specified context of use" (Zikmund 2003). The online sleep tools was evaluated by sleep physicians, in terms of their perception of how the use of the tools would benefit their practice, the consultation and patient information. A sample of 267 people from a general population used the sleep tools and then completed a usability questionnaire, finally a technical expect evaluated the sleep tools in terms of their usability.

The physicians were sent ten outputs from the sleep tools from randomly selected sleep disorder patients who completed the sleep tools. This is equivalent to the patient information which the physician's will receive before a consultation when the proposed sleep tool consultation interaction is implemented. The physicians were then asked a set of questions focusing on any impact that receiving the information in this format and before a patient consultation would have of their practice. The operational impacts of using the sleep tools were also investigated.

The physicians stated that the application was usable and useful, that it could improve their communication with their patients, and that it provided efficiencies during the patient–physician diagnostic interaction. Importantly use of the sleep tools did not impose a change of the physician's workflow except that they had access to good quality patient information before the patient consultation. There was still an opportunity for physician's to clarify patient information with the sleep tool report acting as an objective second opinion according to established international disorder criteria.

For the validity of the sleep tools instrument, the ten outputs from sleep disorder people were considered by the sleep physicians. The physicians concurred that the patient outputs fell within the expected range of patient responses.

## Patient Evaluation of Sleep Tools Instrument

A total of 267 users entered their information in the sleep tools web application and then completed a questionnaire developed by the researcher based upon the Technology Acceptance Model (TAM). The questions from this questionnaire were pre-tested on colleagues who had previously used TAM for evaluating applications (Soroush, Hafeez-Baig & Gururajan 2010) The questionnaire focused upon the two different areas of functionality: the online sleep diary and the online patient history questionnaire. The usability questionnaire was completed when the person's interaction with the application was finished. The questionnaire was a short pen-and-paper document that was easy to fill in.

The 269 users who evaluated the sleep tools web application indicated that it is easy to use, easy to understand and easy to read. The results demonstrated that the interface of the sleep tools web application is suited to users with low computer literacy and can be considered relatively easy to read and understand. The users' responses indicated that filling in the application resulted in them thinking about and understanding the pattern of their sleeping habits indicating that this tool is usable for users over a range of ages, education and computer literacy. This agrees with Calongne (2001) who postulated in an opinion paper that usability should be a primary objective in web site design, suggesting that knowing the audience and their objective in using a web site should be considered to achieve usability. Guenther (2004) also agreed that for successful web site usability, one should focus on end user objectives in using the application This study also agrees with Williams (2000) that a simple clean design with high contrast between elements that stand out clearly against their background are important. This also agrees with the findings from the technical evaluation that the layout of the web application was in a simple linear layout. The layout of the application in a linear design also agreed with another of Guenther (2004) principles. Yen et al. (2007) in a review of literature and the proposal of a model for web design also agreed that a linear layout assisted user's navigation.

The user evaluation that the sleep tool web application was usable agrees with previous studies that the Internet administration of questionnaires offers a valid mode of delivery (Buchanan 2003; Carlbring et al. 2007; Johnson 2005). Buchanan (2003) reviewed the administration of three online medical questionnaires and found that with the exception of using norms gathered from online questionnaires to compare against those gathered in pen and paper questionnaires, online delivery of questionnaires was a valid delivery mode. Johnson (2005) found that for protocol validity, respondents to an online questionnaire were as consistent as those respondents using a pen and paper questionnaire. Carlbring et al. (2007) investigated the psychometric properties of online questionnaires in a test retest study using online and pen and paper questionnaires. The finding was that online administration of questionnaires was reliable and valid. The outcome from this study is that an online questionnaire offers a mode of delivery which respondents find comfortable and usable.

## Technical Evaluation of Sleep Tools Instrument

The technical evaluation revealed the sleep tools web application to be easy to use with a simple linear design. However, a number of usability issues were noted that were not identified by the patient usability research. Some of these issues, such as the minimalist observation, reflected the following of access considerations and a desire for regional patients with slower Internet access not to be penalised. This evaluation shows that this desire for equity of access may impact on the feel of the instrument, and the input of a graphical user interface expert should requested for the next iteration of the application.

# IMPLICATIONS

In this system the collection of routine patient information is done by the patient completing an online questionnaire. Due to the removal of data collection in a consultation, the physician can spend time with the patient discussing patient-specific symptoms and life-style. This will enable the physician to see more patients or they can perform a more in-depth consultation with each patient. The implication is that a shorter consultation will allow the sleep physician to see more patients and thereby lessening the consultation wait time. In this case a shorter consultation times maximises the use of physician time and represents a saving to the service provider while the patient still receives a good quality service.

The output from the sleep tools web application will allow an efficient, consistent triage process before seeing a patient for the first time. The operational implication of this is that a patient with a high risk of sleep apnoea can be sent to have a polysomnography before a consultation with a sleep physician. This acts to shorten the diagnostic interaction by at least one consultation freeing the physician to see more new patients and reducing the cost of treating each of these patients. As the sleep disorder clinic is government funded this offers a direct saving to the government health budget and will help to alleviate wait times to be seen for patients. The patient is also saved the burden of having to travel to one consultation.

Dement (2008) suggests that an aging population will exacerbate that shortage finding time gains and efficiencies within the sleep disorder consultation interaction is important for patient wait times and the cost of treating the disorder.

The sleep tools web application automatically saves the patient history and sleep diary data in a database. This database will then form a valuable resource for researchers in aggregated patient history data, with the facility to export unidentified data in a eXtensible Markup Language (XML) format. This aggregated information is not currently available within this health service as hard copy patient records are used. One of the most important characteristics of the sleep disorder population is that it is heterogeneous, future data mining of the aggregated patient history data may lead to a discovery of a combination of factors which may be used to screen for individual sleep disorders in the wider population. This analytic approach has implications for screening of populations in whom an undetected sleep disorder poses a risk not only to themselves but also to other members of the community such as commercial drivers.

One of the problems with the management of chronic conditions such as sleep disorders is to gain collaboration between health providers, such as sleep specialist and primary care physicians. The collection of electronic patient data allows an ease of patient information transfer. This means that the primary care physician is able to reinforce the need for life style changes suggested by the specialist to improve patient treatment.

## CONCLUSION

The sleep tool objectives – that of devolving the responsibility for form filling from the physician to the patient, and giving the patient access to sleep disorder specific questions earlier in their interaction with the sleep investigation unit – have been met. This will aid patients in their self-discovery of their own sleep disorder information, as the literature shows that a more knowledgeable patient receives a more personalised consultation and is better able to comply with treatment plans. However the primary objective which was met was to improve the communication flows between the patient and physician. This objective meant the consultation could change from one where the patient was required to answer a series of questions to a consultation where there was time for a discussion on how a patient's condition might be best managed and fitted into their lifestyle. This type of discussion is important for treatment compliance for patients with a chronic condition such a sleep disorder.

## ACKNOWLEDGMENT

The authors would like to thank the anonymous reviewers and the editor for their insightful comments and suggestions.

## REFERENCES

Abidi, S. S. R. (2001). Knowledge management in healthcare: towards `knowledge-driven' decision-support services. *International Journal of Medical Informatics*, *63*(1-2), 5–18. doi:10.1016/S1386-5056(01)00167-8 PMID:11518661

Akerstedt, T., & Nilsson, P. M. (2003). Sleep as restitution: an introduction. *Journal of Internal Medicine*, *254*(1), 6–12. doi:10.1046/j.1365-2796.2003.01195.x PMID:12823638

Alzougool, B., Chang, S., & Gray, K. (2008). Towards a comprehensive understanding of health information needs. *Electronic Journal of Health Informatics*, *3*(2), e15.

Australian Medical Workforce Advisory Committee. (2000). *The Specialist Thoracic Medicine Workforce In Australia*. Retrieved 31 March 2008, from http://www5.health.nsw.gov.au/amwac/amwac/pdf/thoracic_medicine_2000.1.pdf

Buchanan, T. (2003). Internet-based questionnaire assessment: Appropriate use in clinical contexts. *Cognitive Behaviour Therapy*, *32*(3), 100–109. doi:10.1080/16506070310000957 PMID:16291542

Calongne, C. M. (2001). Designing for web site usability. *Journal of Computing Sciences in Colleges*, *16*(3).

Carlbring, P., Brunt, S., Bohman, S., Austin, D., Richards, J., Öst, L.-G., & Andersson, G. (2007). Internet vs. paper and pencil administration of questionnaires commonly used in panic/agoraphobia research. *Computers in Human Behavior*, *23*(3), 1421–1434. doi:10.1016/j.chb.2005.05.002

Chen, Hsinchun, Chiang, Roger H L, & Storey, Veda C. (2012). Business intelligence and analytics: From big data to big impact. *Management Information Systems Quarterly*, *36*(4), 1165–1188.

Chervin, R. D. (2000). The multiple sleep latency test and Epworth sleepiness scale in the assessment of daytime sleepiness. *Journal of Sleep Research*, *9*(4), 399–400. doi:10.1046/j.1365-2869.2000.0227a.x PMID:11123526

Colten, Harvey R, & Alterogt, MBruce M. (2006). *Sleep disorders and sleep deprivation: An unmet public health problem.* Retrieved from http://books.nap.edu/catalog.php?record_id=11617#toc

Conrick, Moya. (2006). *Health informatics: transforming healthcare with technology*. Melbourne: Thomson Social Science Press.

Cornwall, A., & Jewkes, R. (1995). What is participatory research? *Social Science & Medicine*, *41*(12), 1667–1676. doi:10.1016/0277-9536(95)00127-S PMID:8746866

Dement, W. C. (2008). History of sleep medicine. *Sleep Medicine Clinics*, *3*, 147–156. doi:10.1016/j.jsmc.2008.01.003

Economics, D. A. (2011). *Re-awakening Australia: The economic cost of sleep disorders in Australia, 2010*. Australia: Sleep Health Foundation.

Flemons, W., Douglas, N. J., Kuna, S. T., Rodenstein, D. O., & Wheatley, J. (2004). Access to diagnosis and treatment of patients with suspected sleep apnea. *American Journal of Respiratory and Critical Care Medicine*, *169*, 668–672. doi:10.1164/rccm.200308-1124PP PMID:15003950

Graber, M. L., & Mathew, A. (2008). Performance of a Web-Based Clinical Diagnosis Support System for Internists. *Journal of General Internal Medicine*, *23*(Supplement 1), 37–40. doi:10.1007/s11606-007-0271-8 PMID:18095042

Guenther, K. (2004). Know the fundamentals and good design will follow. *Online*, *28*(1), 54–56.

Haux, R. (2010). Medical informatics: Past, present, future. *International Journal of Medical Informatics*, *79*(9). doi:10.1016/j.ijmedinf.2010.06.003 PMID:20615752

Haynes, R. B., Sackett, D. L., Guyatt, G. H., & Tugwell, P. (2006). Clinical epidemiology: How to do clinical practice research (3rd ed.). Philadelphia: Lippincott Williams & Wilkins

Hirakis, O., & Karakounos, S. (2006). Goals and benefits of knowledge management in healthcare. In A. A. Lazakidou (Ed.), *Handbook of Research on Informatics in Healthcare and Biomedicine* (pp. 193–200). Idea Group Reference. doi:10.4018/978-1-59140-982-3.ch025

Johnson, J. A. (2005). Ascertaining the validity of individual protocols from Web-based personality inventories. *Journal of Research in Personality*, *39*(1), 103–129. doi:10.1016/j.jrp.2004.09.009

Kramer, N. R., Cook, T. E., & Carlisle, C. C., Corwin, R. W., & Millman, R. P. (1999). The role of the primary care physician in recognizing obstructive sleep apnea. *Archives of Internal Medicine*, *159*(9), 965–968. doi:10.1001/archinte.159.9.965 PMID:10326938

Lacks, P., & Morin, C. M. (1992). Recent advances in the assessment and treatment of insomnia. *Journal of Consulting and Clinical Psychology*, *60*(4), 586–594. doi:10.1037/0022-006X.60.4.586 PMID:1506506

Libman, E., Fichten, C. S., Bailes, S., & Amsel, R. (2000). Sleep Questionnaire Versus Sleep Diary: Which Measure Is Better? *International Journal of Rehabilitation and Health*, *5*(3), 205–209. doi:10.1023/A:1012955423123

Macaulay, A. C. (2007). Promoting Participatory Research by Family Physicians. *Annals of Family Medicine*, *5*(6), 557–560. doi:10.1370/afm.755 PMID:18025494

Patlak, M. (2005). *Tips to help you detect common sleep disorders*. Retrieved 31 March 2008, from http://www.acpinternist.org/archives/2005/03/sleep.htm#pool

Pilemalm, S., & Timpka, T. (2008). Third generation participatory design in health informatics—Making user participation applicable to large-scale information system projects. *Journal of Biomedical Informatics*, *41*(2), 327–339. doi:10.1016/j.jbi.2007.09.004 PMID:17981514

Queensland Government. (2001). *Information Standard No 42A: Information privacy for the Queensland Department of Health*. http://www.qgcio.qld.gov.au/02_infostand/standards/is42a.pdf

Queensland Government Chief Information Office. (2008). *Current information standards, guidelines and reviews*. Retrieved from http://www.qgcio.qld.gov.au/02_infostand/standards.htm

Queensland Government Chief Information Office. (2010). *2009 Queensland Household Survey - Computer and Internet Use*. Retrieved 7 February 2011, from http://www.qgcio.qld.gov.au/SiteCollectionDocuments/Resources/householdsurvey2009.pdf

Sharp, H., Rogers, Y., & Preece, J. (2007). *Interaction design: Beyond human-computer interaction* (2nd ed.). Chichester, UK: John Wiley and Sons Limited.

Shepertycky, M. R., Banno, K., & Kryger, M. H. (2005). Differences between men and women in the clinical presentation of patients diagnosed with Obstructive Sleep Apnea Syndrome. *Sleep*, *28*(3), 309–314. PMID:16173651

Sheppard, V. B., Williams, K. P., Harrison, T. M., Jennings, Y., Lucas, W., Stephen, J., . . . Taylor, K. L. (2009). Development of decision-support intervention for Black women with breast cancer. *Psycho-Oncology*.

Smith, S., Lang, C., Sullivan, K., & Warren, J. (2004). Two new tools for assessing patients' knowledge and beliefs about Obstructive Sleep Apnea and Continuous Positive Airway Pressure therapy. *Sleep Medicine*, *5*(4), 359–367. doi:10.1016/j.sleep.2003.12.007 PMID:15222992

Soroush, L., Hafeez-Baig, A., & Gururajan, R. (2010). *Clinicians' perception of using digital stethoscopes in telehealth platform: Queensland telehealth preliminary study*. Paper presented at the 21st Australasian Conference on Information Systems. Brisbane, Australia. Retrieved from http://aisel.aisnet.org/acis2010/43/

Stranieri, A., Zeleznikow, J., Gawler, M., & Lewis, B. (1999). A hybrid rule – neural approach for the automation of legal reasoning in the discretionary domain of family law in Australia. *Artificial Intelligence and Law*, *7*(2-3).

Taylor, M. J., Wade, S., & England, D. (2003). Informing IT system web site design through normalisation. *Internet Research: Electronic Networking Applications and Policy*, *13*(5), 342–355. doi:10.1108/10662240310501621

University of British Columbia Institute of Health Promotion Research. (1996). *Guidelines and categories for classifying participatory research projects in health*. Retrieved from http://www.lgreen.net/guidelines.html

Wagner, N., Hassanein, K., & Head, M. (2010). Computer use by older adults: A multi-disciplinary review. *Computers in Human Behavior*, *26*(5), 870–882. doi:10.1016/j.chb.2010.03.029

White, G. W., Suchowierska, M., & Campbell, M. (2004). Developing and systematically implementing participatory action research. *Archives of Physical Medicine and Rehabilitation*, *85*(Supplement 2), 3–12. doi:10.1016/j.apmr.2003.08.109 PMID:15083417

Wilde, M. H., & Garvin, S. (2007). A concept analysis of self-management. *Journal of Advanced Nursing*, *57*(3), 339–350. doi:10.1111/j.1365-2648.2006.04089.x PMID:17233653

Willems, D. (2000). Managing one's body using self-management techniques: practicing autonomy. *Theoretical Medicine and Bioethics*, *21*(1), 23–38. doi:10.1023/A:1009995018677 PMID:10927967

Williams, T. R. (2000). Guidelines for designing and evaluating the display of information on the web. *Technical Communication*, *47*(3), 383–397.

Yen, B., Hu, P. J.-H., & Wang, M. (2007). Toward an analytical approach for effective Web site design: A framework for modeling, evaluation and enhancement. *Electronic Commerce Research and Applications*, *6*(2), 159–170. doi:10.1016/j.elerap.2006.11.004

Young, T., Peppard, P. E., & Gottlieb, D. J. (2002). Epidemiology of Obstructive Sleep Apnea: A population health perspective. *American Journal of Respiratory and Critical Care Medicine*, *165*(9), 1217–1239. doi:10.1164/rccm.2109080 PMID:11991871

Zikmund, W. G. (2003). Business research methods (7th ed.). Mason, OH: Thomson South-Western.

## KEY TERMS AND DEFINITIONS

**Online Tool:** A web-based application capable of accepting, storing and manipulating data so that the output can easily understand and add value to a task.

**Polysomonography:** Is a gold standard test for some sleep disorders and consists of sensors monitoring a person's vital information such as brain waves, breathing, blood oxygen levels during an overnight sleep text.

**Sleep Disorder:** A collection of physical and mental disorders which impact upon a person's sleep quality. The main symptom of a sleep disorder is excessive daytime sleepiness.

**Sleep Hygiene:** The following of habits to promote continuous sleep – such as increasing exercise, avoiding caffeine in the evening and adopting regular times to go to sleep and wake up. Controlling the sleep environment so that it is dark, cool and quiet is also considered part of sleep hygiene.

**Sleep on-Set Latency:** The length of time between the person settling for sleep – for example, turning off the light – and the time when sleep occurred. Sleep latency is used as an indicator of a sleep disorder. A short sleep latency time indicates a sleep deficit, while a long sleep latency time may indicate insomnia.

**Sleep Study:** An overnight test performed in a sleep laboratory where a person undergoes a polysomnography.

**Sleep Tool Web Application:** A web application which presents a patient with a patient history questionnaire to be completed and receives 14 days of sleep hygiene information. This information is then processed and the physician can receive a patient report detailing patient history, sleep hygiene information and if a person has met the criteria for a sleep disorder.

## ENDNOTES

1 Co-existing or additional diseases with reference to an initial diagnosis.

# Chapter 9
# Supporting Physicians in the Detection of the Interactions between Treatments of Co-Morbid Patients

**Luca Piovesan**
*Università degli Studi di Torino, Italy*

**Gianpaolo Molino**
*Azienda Ospedaliera San Giovanni Battista, Italy*

**Paolo Terenziani**
*Università del Piemonte Orientale "Amedeo Avogadro", Italy*

## ABSTRACT

*The treatment of patients affected by multiple diseases (comorbid patients) is one of the main challenges for modern healthcare. Clinical practice guidelines are widely used to support physicians, providing them evidence-based information of interventions, but only on individual pathologies. This sets up the urgent need of developing methodologies to support physicians in the detection of interactions between guidelines, to help them in the treatment of comorbid patients. In this chapter, the authors identify different levels of abstractions in the analysis of interactions, based on both the hierarchical organization of clinical guidelines (in which composite actions are refined into their components) and the hierarchy of drug categories. They then propose a general methodology (data/knowledge structures and reasoning algorithms operating on them) supporting user-driven and flexible interaction detection over multiple levels of abstraction.*

DOI: 10.4018/978-1-4666-6316-9.ch009

# INTRODUCTION

## Background

Nowadays, the rationalization of the healthcare systems is a task of fundamental importance in order to grant both the quality and the standardization of healthcare services, and the minimization of costs. Clinical Practice Guidelines (CPGs) are one of the major tools that have been introduced to achieve such a challenging task. CPGs are, in the definition of the USA Institute of Medicine, "systematically developed statements to assist practitioner and patient decisions about appropriate health care in specific clinical circumstances" (Institute of Medicine, Committee on Quality Health Care in America, 2001). Thousands of CPGs have been devised in the last years. For instance, the Guideline International Network (http://www.g-i-n.net) groups 77 organizations of 4 continents, and provides a library of more than 5000 CPGs. CPGs are commonly recognized as a tool to encode and support the practical adoption of evidence-based medicine (EBM).

The adoption of computerized approaches to acquire, represent, execute and reason with CPGs can further increase the advantages of CPGs, providing crucial advantages to:

1. Patients, granting them that they will receive the best quality medical treatments (since CPGs are actually a way of putting EBM into practice);
2. Physicians, providing them with a standard reference which they may consult, with a way of certifying the quality of their activity (e.g., for insurance or legal purposes), as well as with advanced support to their decision-making activity;
3. Hospitals and health-care centers, providing them with tools to grant the quality and the standardization of their services, as well as with a means to evaluate quality, and to optimize costs and resources.

In recent years, the research about computerized guidelines has reached a relevant role within the Medical Informatics community, and many different approaches and projects have been developed to create domain-independent computer-assisted tools for managing, acquiring, representing and executing computer-interpretable clinical guidelines (henceforth CIGs). See e.g. the systems Asbru (Shahar, Miksch, & Johnson, 1998), EON (Shahar, Musen, & Tu, 1996), GEM (Shiffman, et al., 2000) GLARE (Terenziani, Molino, & Torchio, 2001) (Terenziani, et al., 2003), GLIF (Peleg, Boxwala, & Ogunyemi, 2000), GUIDE (Quaglini, Stefanelli, Lanzola, Caporusso, & Panzarasa, 2001), PROforma (Fox, Johns, & Rahmanzadeh, 1998), and the collections (Gordon & Christensen, 1995) (Fridsma, 2001) (Lucas & Ten Teije, 2008). One of such approaches is GLARE (Guideline Acquisition, Representation and Execution), which has been built starting from 1997 in a long-term cooperation between the Department of Computer Science of the University of Piemonte Orientale, Alessandria, Italy, and the Azienda Ospedaliera San Giovanni Battista in Turin (one of the largest hospitals in Italy). Besides supporting CIG acquisition, representation, storage and execution, GLARE is characterized by the adoption of advanced Artificial Intelligence and Temporal Databases formal techniques to provide advanced supports for different tasks, including reasoning about temporal constraints (Anselma, Terenziani, Montani, & Bottrighi, 2006), the treatment of periodic data (Stantic, Terenziani, Governatori G., Bottrighi, & Sattar, 2012), guideline versioning (Anselma, Bottrighi, Montani, & Terenziani, 2013), model-checking verification (Bottrighi, et al., 2010), decision support (based on Decision Theory) (Montani & Terenziani, 2006) (Anselma, et al., 2011), contextualization (Terenziani, et al., 2004).

By definition, clinical guidelines address specific clinical circumstances (i.e., specific diseases). However, unfortunately, specific patients may be affected by more than one disease. The treatment of patient affected by multiple diseases (*comorbid* patients) is one of the main challenges for the modern health care, also due to the aging of population, and the increase of chronic diseases. Just as an example, the prevalence of chronic diseases such as hypertension, diabetes mellitus or heart failure in society has grown during the last decades as the number of elderly people increased (Robert Wood Johnson Foundation and Partnership for Solutions, 2004). Moreover, most of the patients suffering from such chronic diseases, are affected by two or more of them (Gijsen, Hoeymans, & Schellevis, 2001)

Thus, "health care systems must deal with an increasing number of patients with several simultaneous pathologies (i.e., comorbid patients). … Clinical practice guidelines provide evidence-based information of interventions, but only on individual pathologies. This sets up the urgent need of developing ways of merging multiple single-disease interventions to provide professionals' assistance to comorbid patients." (Riaño & Collado, 2013).

However, though some CPGs covering frequently occurring comorbidities might be devised, the approach of considering all the possible combinations of pathologies does not scale up:

"Developing Clinical Practice Guidelines that explicitly address all potential comorbid diseases is not only difficult, but also impractical, and there is a need for formal methods that would allow combining several disease-specific clinical practice guidelines in order to customize them to a patient". (Michalowski, et al., 2013).

Several studies show that the lack of such methods is one of the obstacles in the adoption of CPGs in the clinical practice, and the development of these methods has been identified as one of the "grand challenges" for clinical decision support (Sittig, et al., 2008).

In the very last years, some computer-based approaches have started to face this problem, aiming at providing physicians with different forms of support for managing multiple CIGs. Notably, in the last Artificial Intelligence in Medicine Europe (AIME '13) Conference, held in Murcia, Spain, from 29/5/2013 to 1/6/2013, a whole session (4 papers) has been devoted to such an issue (Sánchez-Garzón, et al., 2013) (Jafarpour & Abidi, 2013) (Riaño & Collado, 2013) (Michalowski, et al., 2013). The state of the art in the computer-based treatment of comorbidities is presented in section "Related Works". Despite the high quality of the recent research approaches in the literature, the treatment of comorbidities is an extremely difficult and challenging problem, so that substantial forward steps need to be achieved. In the rest of the paper, we address our contribution.

## Goals of Our Overall Approach

In this chapter, we show how we are extending the GLARE approach to cope with comorbidities. The long-term goal of our overall approach is that of providing physicians with a domain-independent and guideline-independent set of tools and methodologies to facilitate the integration of two or more CIGs. Such supports may be adopted at different stages, i.e.

- To detect the interactions between two or more guidelines,
- To solve the interactions,
- To merge multiple guidelines in the treatment of the specific patient at hand.

The philosophy underlying our approach derives from our long-term interdisciplinary cooperation between computer scientists and physicians. We neither aim to provide any fully-automatic tool to synthesize the merging of two (or more) CIGs, nor we want to provide any tool intended to wholly take the place of physicians in any of her/his high-level activities. Indeed, our goal is that of providing a suite of tools and methodologies to support physicians, providing her/him, as much as possible, information and hints that may be helpful in her/his activity when facing multiple guidelines. As a consequence, there are several desiderata that our approach will need to meet:

- **Interactivity:** We think that the system should help the physician in the merging process, but it shouldn't replace her/him, so the system must involve the user in decisions and must be easy to use;
- **Flexibility:** We do not think there can be a unique "golden" standard methodology to merge two guidelines. Indeed, we aim at supporting physicians by providing them physician-driven explorations of the different possible ways of facing the problem;
- **Multiple Abstractions:** given the complexity of the overall task, physicians usually face it in a "top-down" fashion, operating at multiple levels of abstractions; supporting user-driven interactive and flexible merging of CIGs operating at different detail levels (along different dimensions) is one of the core goals of our approach.

## Goals and Content of the Chapter

In this Chapter, we will focus on the first, essential, step in the development of the above approach, namely the development of a methodology addressing the detection of the interactions between different CIGs. It is worth stressing that there are already two kinds of tools that physicians use in order to supervise treatments and detect drug interactions: information tools like PDAs on online access to pharmacological databases (Robert Wood Johnson Foundation and Partnership for Solutions, 2004), and alerting systems such as CPOE (Koppel, Metlay, & Cohen, 2005), that detect and inform about interactions (Medscape (http://reference.medscape.com/drug-interactionchecker/), Drugs.com (http://www.drugs.com/druginteractions.html), etc.). However, such tools mostly focus on drug-drug interactions only. Unfortunately, this is only a very limited support, when a physician has to detect and analyze the interactions between two or more guidelines. Indeed, though a large variety of representation formalisms exists (Ten Teije, Miksch, & Lucas, 2008), most CIG formalism support a hierarchical decomposition of guidelines at multiple levels of detail, in which composite actions may be represented, and then refined (possibly at different levels of abstraction) into their components. At the finest level of detail therapeutic actions in the guideline may recommend, depending on the accuracy, the use of drugs or drugs categories, or active principles(thus, also the interactions between drug categories must be considered). However, at higher levels, composite actions may be better characterized on the basis of their intentions (i.e., of the high-level goals they aim to achieve; consider, e.g., ASBRU (Shahar, Miksch, & Johnson, 1998)). We aim at devising a more suitable and complete support to the detection of interactions between guidelines, in which also high-level action intentions are taken into account, and the interaction analysis is supported at any possible level of abstraction considered in the guideline specification. As previously discussed, besides multiple abstractions, interactivity and flexibility are essential desiderata of our approach. Given the relevance of such desiderata, we illustrate the need for them through an example. The example is deliberately abstract, to stress the generality of our methodology (real medical examples will be widely provided throughout all the rest of the Chapter). In the example, as well as in the approach described in this Chapter, we focus our attention on the actions in the therapeutic parts of CIGs (composite actions and pharmacological actions, recommending drug administrations).

*Example:* Suppose, for instance, that the user physician UP needs to detect the interaction between two composite actions A1 (belonging to the guideline G1) and A2 (belonging to the CIG G2). (S)he selects A1 from G1, and A2 from G2, and then looks for the interactions. At this level of abstraction, i.e., the interaction between the intentions of A1 (*int1* in the upper part of Figure 1) and A2 (*int2* in Figure 1) is taken into account.

The possible continuation of the interaction detection process may strictly depend on the output of such an analysis. For instance:

Case 1 (shown in Figure 1). Suppose that, at this level of abstraction, no interaction is found between *int1* and *int2*. UP wants to further refine his/her search. (S)he expands A1 and A2 into the actions composing them in the CIGs, focuses on some of them (see the lower part of Figure 1), e.g., $A1_1$ and $A1_2$ (one of the possible decompositions of A1 in G1, or part of it) and $A2_1$ and $A2_2$ (one of the possible decompositions of A2 in G2, or part of it), which all are pharmacological actions. Then, UP looks for the interactions between them. In particular, pharmacological actions prescribe the administration of drug categories (for example, in Figure 1, we represent the fact that $A1_1$ prescribes the administration of $cat1_1$, and so on), and the interactions between them is further analyzed.

Case 1.1 (shown in Figure 2). Suppose that no interaction between the drug categories ($cat1_1$ and $cat1_2$ from G1, $cat2_1$ and $cat2_2$ from G2) is found. UP further wants to refine his search by expanding the pharmacological actions to the level of drugs, selecting few drugs (e.g., $Drug_b$ for $Cat1_1$, etc., in the graphical example in Figure 2), and, finally, analyzing their interactions. This process can *iteratively go on* until non-interacting drugs are found for the four actions.

*Figure 1. States of guideline explorations for Case 1*

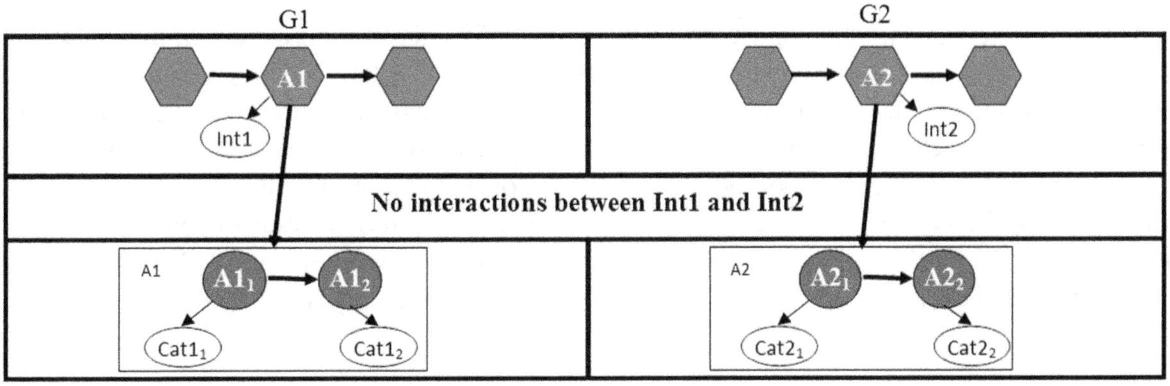


*Figure 2. States of guideline explorations for Case 1.1*

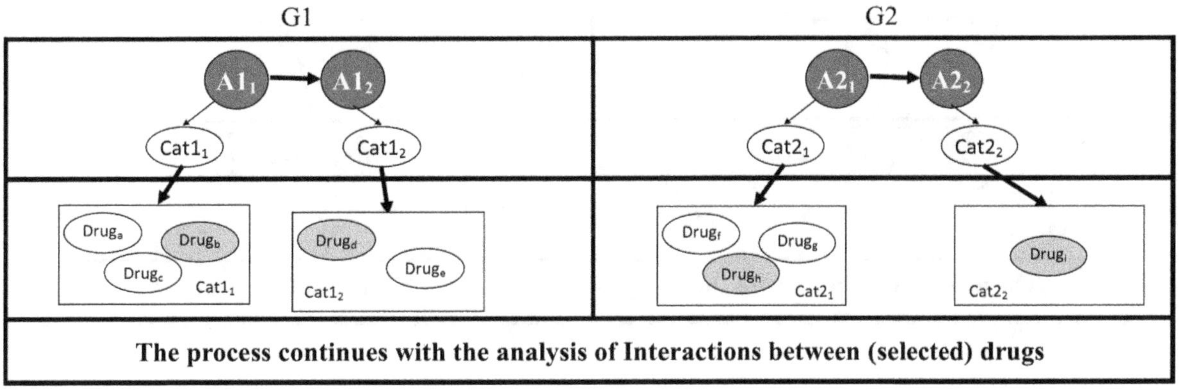

Case 1.2 (shown in Figure 3). On the other hand, suppose that some interaction between the drug categories ($cat1_1$ and $cat1_2$ from G1, $cat2_1$ and $cat2_2$ from G2) is found. UP may use the focusing tool to "go up" to A1 and A2, and focus on an alternative decomposition of them (e.g., in Figure 3, $A1_3$, $A1_4$ and $A1_5$ for A1, $A2_3$ and $A2_4$ for A2). The process continues with the analysis of the interactions between $A1_3$, $A1_4$ and $A1_5$ (from G1) and $A2_3$ and $A2_4$ (from G2).

*Consideration:* Notice that, although the above example seems to indicate that interactions are always "bad" (so that they are a reason for looking for alternatives), this is not necessarily true. As we will analyze in Section "Interactions Ontology", the spectrum of possible interactions types is wide, and only few types can be easily categorized as "bad" (e.g., two intentions are "opposite"), or "good" (e.g., two intentions are "equal", or are "independent"). In all the other cases, interactions are "workable" (e.g., a "reinforcing" interaction between two drugs can be managed by operating on the posology of such drugs), and the user-physician may choose to: (i) manage and "solve" them, e.g., through the modification of drug posology, (ii) try to avoid them, looking for alternatives, or (iii) further investigate them (e.g., at a lower level of detail).

The above example clearly shows that the detection of interaction is intrinsically an *interactive* process, in which each step is "unpredictable", since it depends on the output of the previous step. Additionally, the above consideration shows, that, given the output of one step, there are (in most cases) alternative ways of going on, and it is almost impossible to automatically choose between them (indeed, user-physicians might accept knowledge-based suggestions on the way to go on, but certainly not a system-made decision on that).

Thus, and *interactive* and *user-driven* interaction detection process is required. The goal of the work we present in this paper is to identify a general methodology (data/knowledge structures and reasoning algorithms operating on them) supporting it.

## Summary

The Chapter will be organized as follows. The section "The GLARE formalism" presents the GLARE approach, with specific emphasis on the physician-friendly formalism we have devised in order to represent CIGs. The first step of our approach is the definition of appropriate formalisms to cope with the knowledge that is needed to support the analysis of interactions (Section

*Figure 3. States of guideline explorations for Case 1.2*

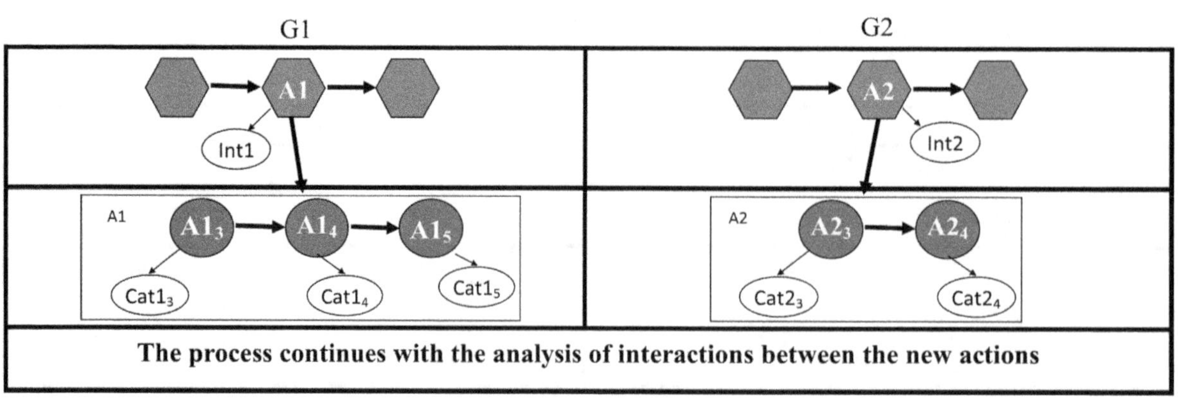

"Interactions: ontological notions"). In Section "Interactions detection algorithm", we describe a new methodology to explore the above-mentioned knowledge sources, and multiple guidelines, in an interactive and flexible way. In Section "Related works", we will describe the state-of-the-art, and, finally, we draw the conclusions.

## MAIN FEATURES OF THE GLARE SYSTEM

GLARE is a long-term project started in 1997 to provide a user-friendly and domain-independent tool to support CIG acquisition, representation and execution, and to provide physician with a wide range of facilities, helping her/him in decision support or CIG analysis tasks. The main goals of the GLARE systems are:

- **To Be Domain-Independent:** In particular, GLARE has been already applied to deal with a wide range of CIG, ranging, e.g., from asthma to ischemic stroke.
- **To Be User-Friendly:** GLARE is intended to be a tool to support physicians (in particular, as regards decision making), not at all to replace them. Such a goal has several implications, including the facts that (i) CIGs representation language must be as close as possible to the physicians' way of looking at it, and (ii) the "technological" complexity of the system must be hidden to the user-physicians, through a user-friendly and easy-to-use interface.
- **To Be Easily Extendable:** Indeed, a plenty of facilities concerning CIG treatment should be provided to physicians. Thus, the system architecture must be modular and easily extendable.

Of course, each one of the above tasks has deeply influenced the design of GLARE, and its main features.

### GLARE Representation Language

In the medical literature, clinical guidelines are often described using different levels of detail (and top-down refinement), and oriented graphs of actions, similar to flow-charts are often used to describe the ordering of actions at the different levels. As a consequence, in GLARE, a CIG can be represented as a hierarchical graph, where nodes are the actions to be executed, and arcs are the control relations linking them.

In GLARE, we distinguish between *atomic* and *composite actions* (plans), where atomic actions represent simple steps in a CIG, and plans represent actions that can be defined in terms of their components via the has-part relation.

In order to be as physician-friendly as possible, a limited and "physician oriented" number of types of atomic actions have been identified:

- **Work Actions:** In other words, actions that describe a procedure which must be executed at a given point of the GL.
- **Pharmaceutical Actions:** Specifying a drug (or drug category, of active principle) to be administered to the patient, and the posology.
- **Decision Actions:** Used to model the selection among different alternatives. We have introduced a distinction between:
    - **Diagnostic Decisions:** Used to make explicit the identification of the disease the patient is suffering from, among a set of possible diseases, compatible with her findings. A diagnostic decision is represented as an open

set of triples <diagnosis, parameter, score> (where, in turn, a parameter is a triple <data, attribute, value>), plus a threshold to be compared with the different diagnoses' scores;
    - **Therapeutic Decisions:** Used to represent the choice between paths in a GL, where each path represents a particular therapeutic process. The choice can be made by evaluating a fixed set of parameters (effectiveness, cost, side-effects, compliance and duration).
- **Query Actions:** In other words, requests of information (typically patient's parameters), that can be obtained from the outside world (physicians, databases, patient's visits or interviews). The GL execution cannot go on until this information has been obtained.
- **Conclusions:** Which explicitly identify the output of a decision action.

In particular, the distinction between diagnostic and therapeutic decisions is very fundamental to physicians, and constitutes one of the features that distinguish GLARE from most CIG approaches in the literature. Each kind of action is described by a set of properties. For instance, a pharmaceutical action is described by:

- **Action Type:** Which for each action of this category takes the value "Administration of Medicament",
- **Substance:** Which describes the administered drug,
- **Posology:** Which describes the dosage and the modality of assumption. This property structure is complex, since it might involve the description of periodicity (Anselma, Terenziani, Montani, & Bottrighi, 2006).

Actions in a GL are connected through control relations. Control relations establish which actions can be executed next, and in what order. In particular, the *sequence* relation explicitly establishes what is the following action to be executed; the *alternative* relation describes which alternative paths stem from a decision action, and the *repetition* relation, states that an action has to be repeated several times. In detail, given a repeated action, the number of its repetitions can be fixed a priori, or, alternatively, it can be asserted that the action must be repeated until a certain *exit condition* becomes true (in this case, the number of repetitions is only known at runtime, during execution). In particular, advanced AI techniques are required to deal with temporal reasoning in repeated actions (Anselma, Terenziani, Montani, & Bottrighi, 2006).

## Architecture of the Kernel of GLARE

The core of GLARE (see box on the left of Figure 4) is based on a modular architecture. CG_KRM (Clinical Guidelines Knowledge Representation Manager) is the main module of the system: it manages the internal representation of CPG, and operates as a domain-independent and task-independent knowledge server for the other modules; moreover, it permanently stores the acquired CPG in a dedicated Clinical Guidelines Database (CG-DB). The Clinical Guidelines Acquisition Manager (CG_AM) provides expert-physicians with a user-friendly graphical interface to introduce the CPG into the CG_KRM and describe them. It may interact with four databases: the Pharmacological DB, storing a structured list of drugs and their costs; the Resources DB, listing the resources that are available in a given hospital (it is therefore used to represent the context-dependent version of a CPG); the ICD DB, containing an international coding system of diseases; the Clinical DB, providing a "standard" terminology to be used when building a new CPG, and storing the descriptions and the set of possible values of clinical findings.

The execution module (CG-EM) executes a CPG for a specific patient, considering the pa-

*Figure 4. Architecture of GLARE. Rectangles represent computation modules, and ovals represents data/knowledge bases. The left box contains the "core" of GLARE, while additional modules in the right of the figure depict advanced AI support for several tasks.*

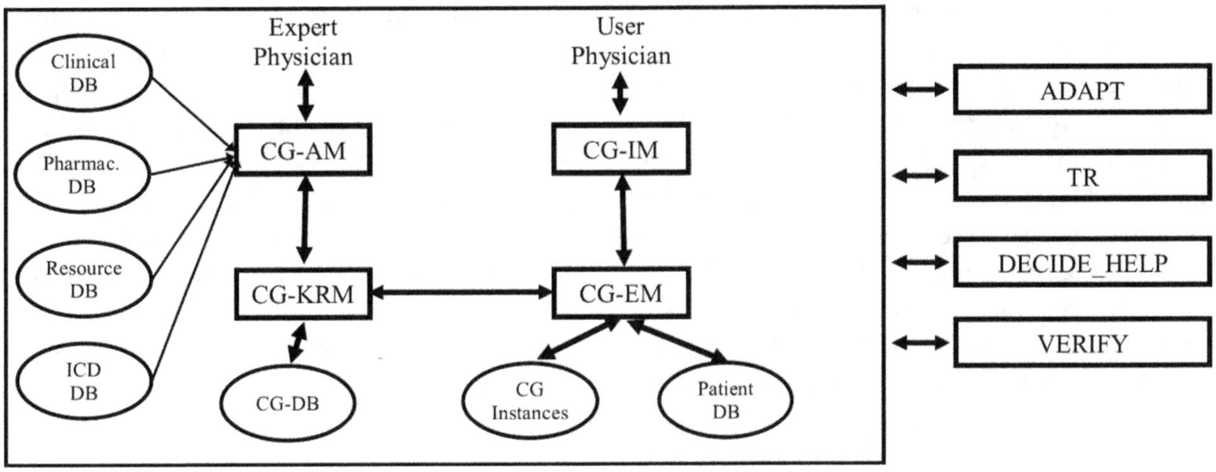


tient's data (retrieved from the Patient DB). The schema of the Patient DB mirrors the schema of the Clinical DB. Therefore, the interaction with the Clinical DB during the acquisition phase makes it possible to automatically retrieve data from the Patient DB at execution time. CG-EM stores the execution status in another DB (CG Instances) and interacts with the user-physician via a graphical interface (CG-IM).

It is worth noticing that, through the CG-AM and CG-IM modules, GLARE provides user-friendly interfaces to user, achieving the goal of "hiding" them the internal complexity of the system.

## Extended Architecture

To enhance extendibility, GLARE's architecture is open: new modules and functionalities can be easily added to the system if/when necessary. In the latest years, we have added new modules and/or methodologies in order to cope with automatic resource-based contextualization (ADAPT module, (Terenziani, et al., 2004)), temporal reasoning (TR, (Anselma, Terenziani, Montani, & Bottrighi, 2006) and (Stantic, Terenziani, Governatori G., Bottrighi, & Sattar, 2012)), decision-making support (DECIDE_HELP, (Montani & Terenziani, 2006) and (Anselma, et al., 2011)), and model-based verification (VERIFY, (Bottrighi, et al., 2010)). While all the methodologies to cope with the above issues have been widely addressed, not all the prototypical software modules have been implemented yet. However, we envision a modular architecture, in which all such modules will be loosely coupled with the core of GLARE, as shown in the right part of Figure 4.

## INTERACTIONS: ONTOLOGICAL NOTIONS

The first step of our approach is the definition of an ontology, clarifying the semantics of interactions, and modeling the different knowledge sources involved in their detection and analysis. In philosophy, *Ontology* is "the study of the nature of being, becoming, existence, or reality, as well as the basic categories of being and their relations". In computer and information science, ontology is a technical term denoting an artifact that is designed for a purpose, which is to enable the modeling of knowledge about some domain, real or imagined (Gruber, 2009). Ontologies have been initially introduced in AI in 1980's, and then they have spread over many fields such as databases, systems and software engineering, semantic web and biomedical informatics. In health informatics, they are defined as "collections of formal, machine-processable and human interpretable representation of the entities, and the relations among those entities, within a definition of the application domain" (Rubin, et al., 2006).

Since 2001, there has been an increasing use of ontological approaches to health (Liaw, et al., 2013). As a matter of facts, the adoption of formal ontologies is almost becoming a standard in medical informatics, since it provides many advantages, including terminological standardization and the definition of a common semantics. For instance, SNOMED (http://www.ihtsdo.org/snomed-ct/) is a widely used clinical terminology, and stresses that "the use of a standard clinical terminology makes a significant contribution towards improving the quality and safety of healthcare by enabling consistent representation of meaning in an electronic health record". In particular, the definition of an ontology for interactions allows us to achieve several different goals:

- **Define a Shared Semantics for Guidelines and Interactions:** We need to define a semantics for interactions and guidelines actions. This semantics must be shared and "understood" both by information systems and by human users (Gruber, 2009; Rubin, et al., 2006).
- **Define a Standard for Terminology and Representation:** GLARE is a standard for guidelines representation. The use of ontologies for the action model supports the standardization between different guidelines. In addition, ontologies are often used to disambiguate terms. The use of existing and consensus ontologies for data representation avoid ambiguities and allows the reuse of the knowledge.
- **Unify Different Sources:** In the medical field, data can derive from different sources. Unify them using ontologies helps to improve data quality (Liaw, et al., 2013).
- **Reason on the Data:** The use of standard ontology representation as RDF or OWL allows processing the content of information through existing reasoners (McGuinness & van Harmelen, 2004): *"by incorporating defined rules, ontologies may also generate logical inferences"* (Pérez-Rey, et al., 2006).

Our ontology of interactions is based on the consideration that physicians usually analyze the interactions between guidelines at different levels of detail. At the highest level, they take into account the intentions (or goals) of actions (e.g., "Decrease the blood volume"). Then, moving towards more specific information, they may also consider the interactions between specific drugs categories (e.g., Diuretics), and, finally, between specific drugs (e.g., Furosemide).

Our goal is to devise a general ontology underlying the detection of guideline interactions. Our methodology is completely general, and we are not committed to any specific pre-existent ontology. However, given its relevance and generality, we use the SNOMED ontology (http://www.ihtsdo.org/snomed-ct/) as a reference one. Sometimes we also consider the Anatomical Therapeutic Chemical (ATC) ontology (http://www.whocc.no/atc) as concerns the drug classification. We extend them in order to model both the different sources of interactions (intentions, drugs categories, drugs) and the different types of interactions between them.

For the sake of interaction detection, the description of guideline actions must include the intention of composite and work actions, or the drug (class of drugs, active principle) of pharmacological actions. We first describe our ontology of intentions (subsection "Intentions Ontology") and of drug classes (subsection "Drug Classes Ontology"). Then, in subsection "Interactions Ontology", we describe our ontology for the interactions (between intentions, and between drug classes and drugs).

## Intentions Ontology

At an high level of abstraction, an action can be represented by its objectives or (desired) effects. In this section, we focus on the objectives of composite actions (plans), work actions and pharmacological ones, and we call them *Intentions* (i.e., the goals that the physician expects to obtain realizing that action)[1].

Intentions can be organized along a hierarchy of ISA and PART-OF relations: high-level intentions can be decomposed into lower-level intentions, and alternative decompositions are possible.

For instance, Figure 5 shows (not exhaustively) the hierarchy of the intention "Decrease Blood Pressure". That intention is typically obtained through the realization of several lower-level intentions and many alternative decompositions (and combinations between them) are possible. Then, lower level intentions can be decomposed by many part-of relations (as can be seen for the "Improve Lifestyle" intention), or not (for example "Block of Calcium Channels"). A particular case is represented by the combination of more intentions in order to reinforce the higher-level one: the intention "Inhibition of Angiotensin Converting Enzyme (ACE)" is both a sub-intention of "Decrease Blood Pressure" and a part of the combined intention "Decrease Blood Volume + ACE Inhibition".

Ultimately, at the lower level, the intentions can be described as (desired) modifications of specific parameters of the patient status. In the following, we call such intentions *atomic intentions*. In our ontology, atomic intentions can be represented by a couple <BodyPartAttribute, Modality> in which BodyPartAttribute is the attribute that is expected to change, and Modality is an element belonging to the set {Increasing, Decreasing, Stability} and describes how the attribute is expected to change. Of course, if needed, the hierarchy of modalities might be further refined. For instance, we can distinguishe between different degrees of increase/ decrease. Figure 6 shows that BodyPartAttribute is in its turn connected with the respective body part. Both concepts have a counterpart in SNOMED Ontology: BodyPart is equivalent to the SNOMED concept "Body Structure" and BodyPartAttribute to the SNOMED concept "Observable Entity", whilst concepts of Intention and Modality are not included in SNOMED.

*Figure 5. Representation of the intention "Decrease blood pressure". The image is not exhaustive due to space limitations, but represents a typical intention hierarchy.*

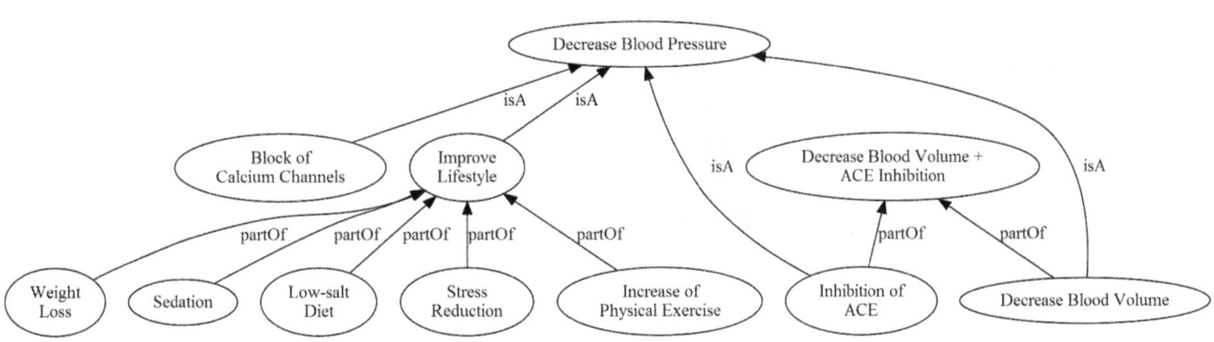

*Figure 6. Ontology of atomic intentions*

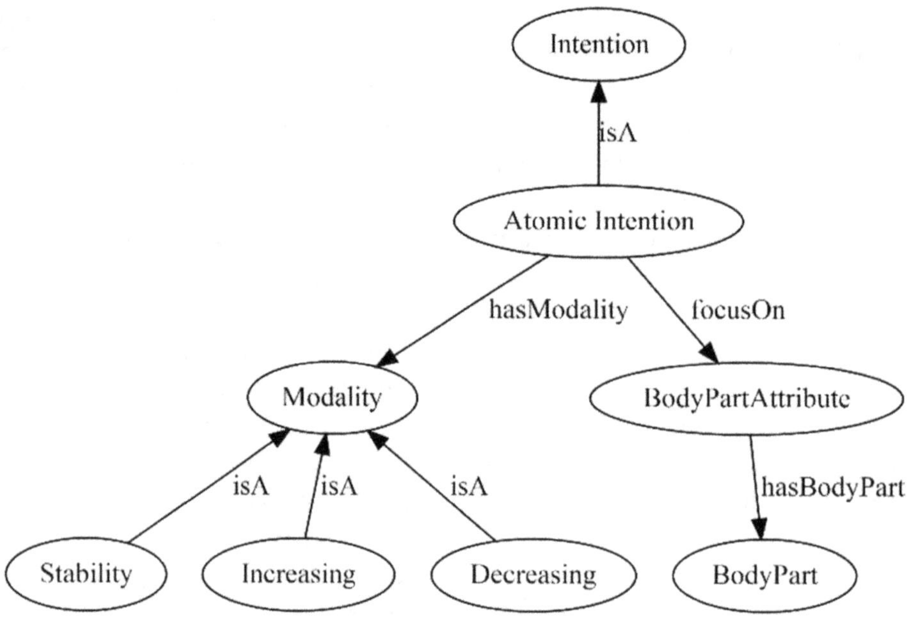


We illustrate the concepts previously described by an example (see Figure 7): the intention of improve the cardiac activity can be to increase (Modality) the cardiac activity (BodyPartAttribute), which is in its turn linked to the BodyPart cardiovascular system. Both Cardiac Activity and Cardiovascular System are individuals of the SNOMED Ontology.

## Drug Classes Ontology

As discussed in Section "GLARE representation language", in GLARE the representation of a pharmacological action includes, among the other, an attribute (*substance*) that specify the drug category (or the specific drug, depending on the level of detail of the CIG itself) prescribed in

*Figure 7. "Improve cardiac activity" intention*

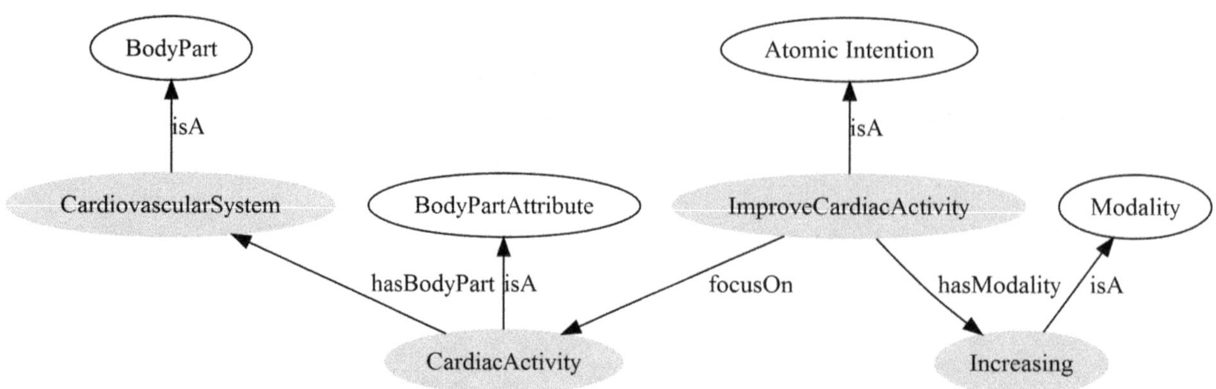

order to achieve the action's atomic intention. The value of such an attribute is a link to a subconcept of the ontological concept DrugCategory (see the higher part of Figure 8).

DrugCategory (and its refinements in the hierarchy) are used in order to achieve (atomic) intentions (see the "aimsTo" arc in Figure 8).

The DrugCategory concept is not flat: it is the root of a hierarchy of categories and its expansion depends on the classification used. In fact, there are in literature several ways to classify the drugs (e.g. those based on the chemical type of the active ingredient, those based on the way they are used to treat a particular condition, etc.). We will use the SNOMED classification for our examples: its concept "Drugs or Medicaments" (that is hierarchically organized) contains our concepts DrugCategory and Drug. However, our approach is independent of the chosen classification, so it is possible to use also other ones (e.g., ATC).

A hierarchical classification of drugs is crucial: several CIGs identify accurate pharmacological prescriptions, pointing out specific drugs, whilst other ones can identify the only drug categories of the pharmacological actions, leaving the physician the task of choosing the drug case by case.

In general, our methodology (see Section "Interaction Detection Algorithm") is independent of the specific ontology, since it supports the navigation of the drug category ontology along the ISA relationships.

## Interactions Ontology

As discussed above, our approach supports the description of CIGs at different levels of abstractions. First of all, GLARE supports *top-down action refinement* in the action description, through the decomposition of nested composite actions (plans) into their parts (components). Plans are "high-level" actions, aiming at achieving "high-level" goals, i.e., *intentions* (see Figure 5). At a finer level of details, GLARE pharmacological and work actions (which are part of plans) have *atomic intentions*, which can be achieved through the administration of drugs (see Figure 8). In turn, drugs can be organized through a multiple-level hierarchy of abstraction, going from drug categories to specific drugs (see Figure 9).

Consequently, it is important to notice that interaction can be identified (with different levels of detail) at each one of the different levels of

*Figure 8. Drug categories and drugs ontology*

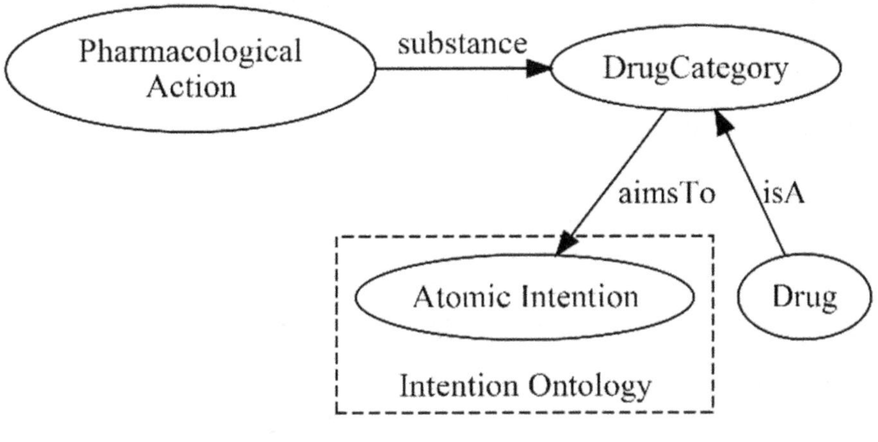

*Figure 9. Complete Warfarin classification (following the SNOMED hierarchy)*

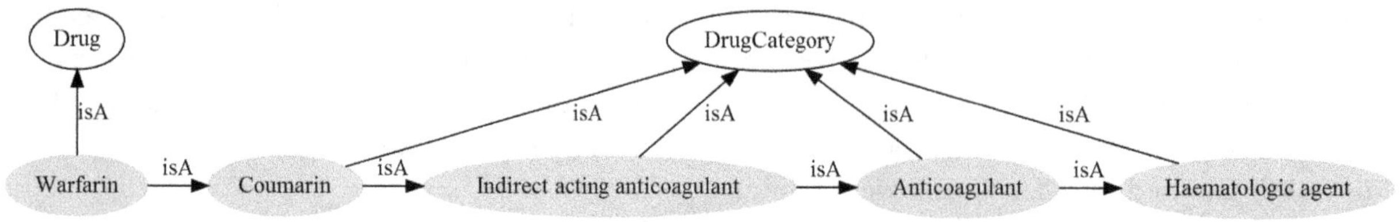


abstraction. As a consequence, in our ontology, we distinguish between IntentionInteractions, AtomicIntentionInteractions, and DrugCategoryInteractions[2]. In Figure 10, we show the higher level of our ontology of interactions.

IntentionInteraction is an interaction between two intentions, and has an InteractionType. In Figure 11, we distinguish between three basic types of interactions between intensions. The "Independence" type covers cases in which the intentions do not interact. The "Concordance" type covers cases in which the two intentions are not independent, but reinforce each other (see example 5 below). The "Discordance" type covers cases in which the two intentions negatively interact with each other (see, for instance, example 1).

Notice that we have deliberately chosen to support a "fuzzy" representation of interactions. Indeed, in many cases, medical intentions are not 100% in agreement or disagreement. However, more "sharp" types of interactions can also be added to the ontology. For instance, the "Op-

*Figure 10. Interactions ontology*

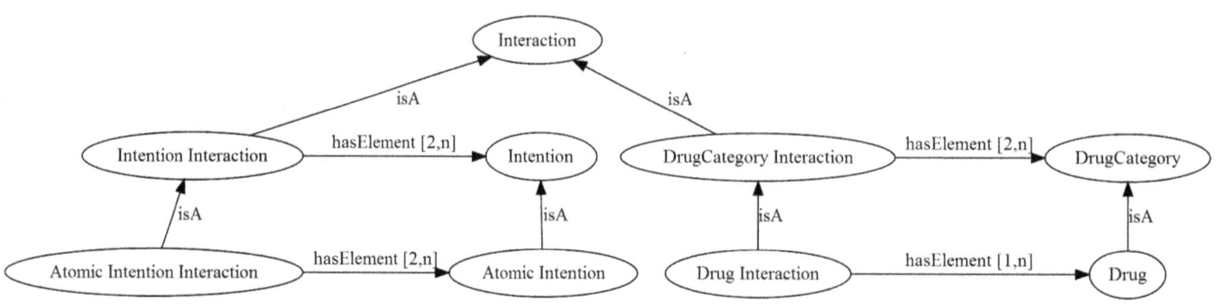


*Figure 11. Intentions interactions*

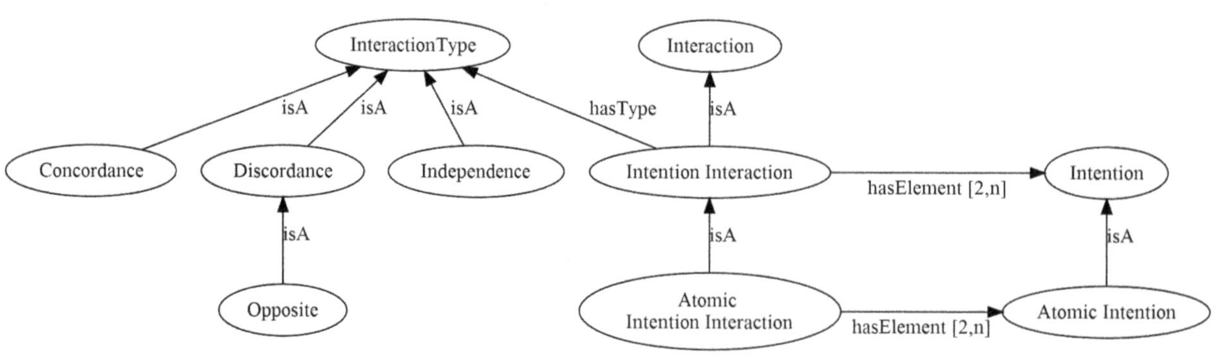

posite" type could be added as a refinement of the "Discordance" type, to cope with opposite intentions (see example 6).

As shown in Figure 11, AtomicIntentionInteraction is a subconcept (ISA arc) of Intention-Interaction, being an Interaction between two AtomicIntentions (which, in turn, are Intentions).

Drug category interactions occur between two DrugCategories (or subconcepts), and cause a variation of their (atomic) intentions. In our formalism, an interaction between two or more drug categories is modeled as the variation of one or more atomic intentions of the actions involved in the interaction itself, so it is completely described by the intentions it changes and the variation it causes. Since an atomic intention is itself described by a modality, an interaction is a variation of that modality (MV) and its domain is the same set {Increasing, Decreasing, Stability} seen for the concept Modality (see below examples 3 and 7).

The representation of drug-drug interactions (i.e., interactions between two Drugs) is similar, and is not reported for the sake of brevity (see examples 4 and 8).

In our ontology, specific interactions may occur at any one of the multiple abstraction levels we support. For instance:

**Example 1:** *Intentions Interaction.* In the treatment of edema due to heart failure, the main intention is to decrease the accumulation of fluids. In the case in which that particular patient also manifests a syncope crisis, it is likewise necessary to increase the blood pressure. However, this later intention forces the heart to a higher activity, which in turn may increase the heart failure, worsening the edema.

**Example 2:** *Atomic Intentions Interaction.* In patients affected by thrombosis, anticoagulant drugs are usually administered, in order to decrease the formation of thrombi. If the patient affected by thrombosis has also a risk of bleeding (e.g. due to a minor surgery) the anticoagulant therapy must be discontinued because of the need to increase the blood coagulation.

**Example 3:** *Drug Categories Interaction.* The administration of antacids (category) at the same time of other drugs orally administered can change the intestinal absorption of the later decreasing their effects (e.g. levofloxacin).

**Example 4:** *Drugs Interaction.* In many cases, interactions involve individual drugs. For example, between trimethoprim and sulfamethoxazole there is a strengthening synergism: the antibiotic effect of their concomitant administration is stronger than the sum of the two single effects.

*Figure 12. Drugs interactions*

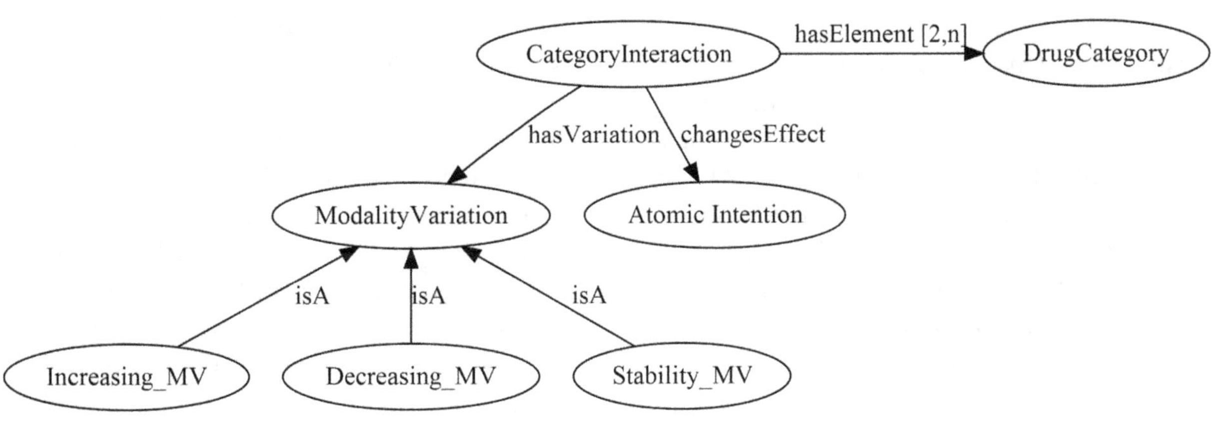

It is worth stressing again that interaction detection should be performed at different levels of abstraction, since, in several cases, top-down refinement along the different hierarchies is needed to detect specific interactions. Of course, results strictly depend on the level of abstraction chosen by the user physician. For instance, some interactions can be discovered considering the higher abstraction level of Intentions.

**Example 5:** Diuretics are a category of drugs frequently used for the treatment of edema (intention). In the case that a patient affected by edema should be treated for hypertension (intention: "decrease blood pressure"), the physician may administer ACE inhibitors or calcium channel blockers. Most of the drugs belonging to these categories do not present explicit interactions with diuretics; however, as shown in Figure 5, the intention of diuretics (i.e., "decrease blood volume" in the Figure 5), of ACE inhibitors (i.e., "inhibition of ACE") and of calcium channel blockers (i.e., "block of calcium channels") are all sub intentions (ISA arcs in the figure) of the same high-level intention "decrease blood pressure". Therefore, the physician can decide to change the posology of the administered drugs.

Other interactions come out only at the lowest abstraction level of Atomic Intentions (e.g., of the pharmacological prescription actions).

**Example 6:** One of the sub-intentions of the high-level intention "decrease the urinary retention" is to stimulate contraction of the bladder. That, in turn, can be obtained through the stimulation of the muscarinic receptors (atomic intention), administering, for example, bethanechol[3] *(*drug). If the patient is affected by peptic ulcer a parallel intention should be to decrease the gastric acid secretion, that can be obtained by the inhibition of the muscarinic receptors (atomic intention), administering pirenzepine[4] (*d*rug). The two atomic intentions are obviously conflicting.

In other cases, interactions may show up only at the drug category level: pharmacological actions may have independent intentions, but the drug categories they imply may interact with each other.

**Example 7:** Vasoconstrictors (drug category), for instance adrenaline (drug), reduce the absorption of the lidocaine (drug), which is a local anesthetic (drug category), enhancing its effect. However, anesthetic intention (for lidocaine) and treatment of anaphylaxis (one of the intentions of adrenaline) do not interact.

Last, some interactions can be detected only at the lowest level, considering specific drugs.

**Example 8:** Warfarin (drug) is an anticoagulant (drug category) used to prevent the formation of thrombi (intention), whilst erythromycin (drug) is an antibiotic (drug category) commonly used, for instance, in the treatment of respiratory tract infections (intention). There is not interaction between the two categories they belongs to; however, the anticoagulant effect of warfarin is enhanced by the simultaneous use of erythromycin.

## INTERACTIONS DETECTION ALGORITHM

Our focusing tool is quite innovative, since it allows physician to navigate both knowledge sources (the CIGs and the ontology) together, thus complementing the general knowledge in the CIGs with the additional knowledge in the ontology.

In this section, we will describe a new methodology to explore the above-mentioned knowledge sources in an interactive and flexible way. In Section "The GLARE formalism", we have shown that GLARE (as well as most CIG formalisms) supports different abstraction levels (through the part-of hierarchy of actions) in the description of CPGs. In Section "Interactions: ontological notions", we have described how our ontology supports the description of different types of interactions at the different abstraction levels, describing not only interactions between general intentions, but also more specific interactions between drug categories, and drugs.

Two main issues must considered for the definition of an approach for detection of interaction considering the above knowledge sources

1. Integration between CIGs and ontology.
2. Interactions with user-physicians.

## Integration between CIGs and Ontology

The integration between CIGs and ontology is important, since, in many cases, CIG actions are described at a quite high level of detail, while specific interactions may arise at lower levels. For instance, frequently, CIG pharmacological actions only indicate drug categories. However, at the very end, a specific drug of that category must be prescribed to the specific patient, and we have previously shown examples in which, while two drug categories do not interact, specific drugs of the two categories do interact. Such interactions can only be detected in case the CIG knowledge is *expanded* with the knowledge (about drug interactions) in the ontology, and achieving such an *integration* is one of the main results of our tool.

Abstractly speaking, in our approach, the integration of the knowledge in the CIG and the one in the ontology provide three main levels of detail (henceforth called "dimensions") at which interactions can be studied:

1. **Action Dimension:** This dimension is specified directly by the CIG, in which each composite action can be refined into its components (which, in turn, may be composite).
2. **Drug Category Dimension:** Such a dimension is specified by the ontology.
3. **Drug Dimension:** Such a dimension is specified by the ontology, as the bottom level of the drug category hierarchy.

In our approach, the two knowledge sources (i.e., CIGs and ontology) are strictly connected: as mentioned above, the types of CIG actions and the values of many properties of actions are links to ontological notions (see, e.g., the description of pharmacological actions in Section "GLARE representation language"). In particular, in our approach the representation of pharmacological actions in the CIGs provide the *crucial link for the expansion*: through the *substance* attribute, each pharmacological action specify a drug category (or, in some cases, a specific drug) to be used, pointing out to the concept representing it in the ontology.

## Interactions with User-Physicians

In our opinion, a black-box tool that, given two (or more) CIGs and the ontology, provides in output all the possible interactions actions in the CIGs (possibly considering also the possible "expansions" provided by the ontology), is not really useful for user-physicians. CIGs often consist of hundreds of actions, and the pharmacological prescriptions they contain may often be achieved through the adoption of several different drugs. Thus, a tool detecting interactions between any pair of actions and drugs belonging to two (or more) CIGs, and blindly operating at all levels of abstraction, would simply output too many interactions to be useful to physician. For such a reason, we aim at devising a flexible and interactive detection tool allowing physicians to navigate through the different abstraction levels, thus supporting the natural methodology they adopt to cope with comorbidities. For instance, at the highest level, a physician may want to start to consider only the interactions between the intentions of the "macro-actions" of the guidelines. Then, focusing on a specific part of the guideline, (s)he may want to move down to a more detailed analysis, considering the decomposition of the "macro action" into its parts, and/or the specific drugs category considered in order to reach the high-level intentions. In general, our approach will provide physicians with the possibility of moving in both directions, i.e., going down from a general to a more specific analysis, or moving up, from a specific analysis to a higher level of abstraction.

## Interaction Detection Process

Wrapping up, as a result of the above consideration, our approach consists of two main tools:

1. A *focusing* tool, allowing physicians to *navigate* into the CIGs to be merged, *selecting* subparts of them and/or expanding/ abstracting them at the chosen level of detail (considering all the three dimensions).
2. An *interaction analysis* tool that, given the output of the focusing on two or more CIGs, analyses the interactions, *at the level of abstraction chosen through the focusing tool*.

When analyzing the interaction between two or more CIGs, the user-physician can iteratively use such tools to create her/his "personalized" interaction detection process, as required by the specific circumstances and goals. In other words, instead of providing a pre-defined (and unique) way of detecting interactions, and super-impose it to user-physicians, we provide her/him the proper tools, allowing her/him to *interactively* work out the detection process (s)he needs (please remember the comments to Example in the "Introduction" Section).

Given the general picture, we now refine it by providing the focusing and the interaction analysis tools.

## The Focusing Tool

The focusing tool is recursive and highly interactive: at each time the physician user chooses a part of one of the guidelines or a specific action and the dimension along which (s)he wants to explore it. Then the system provides the new visualization of the guideline considering that expansion. The exploration status of each guideline is maintained in a *guideline_navigator*: this data structure keeps track of each expansion done. A guideline navigator can be represented as an ordered list of views (*guideline_view*) of the same CIG: initially, it is initialized to the view that represents the higher level of abstraction of the guideline, then, each time the user performs an exploration action (described in the following), a new level representing the new view is added to the guideline navigator. During the navigation, when the user decides to return to a higher level of abstraction, the last level of the navigator is deleted. Figure 13 shows in detail the structure of a guideline navigator.

Given two or more CIGs to be merged, a guideline navigator is used for each one of them, and the user-physician can operate independently on each one of them. Three basic operations are provided for focusing: ZOOM_IN, ZOOM_OUT, and SELECT.

The SELECT operation allows the user to create a new level of the navigator, which contains only the selected action(s).

The ZOOM-OUT operation recover the penultimate expansion in a guideline navigator, deleting the last view.

The ZOOM-IN operation creates a new abstraction level in the guideline navigator, allowing for user-driven refinements. The definition of such an operation is quite complex, since it may consider

*Figure 13. Growth of a Guideline Navigator depending of some actions. View 1 is the view of the entire guideline, view 2 is built due to a ZOOM-IN action (referred to the highlighted action), whilst view 3 after a SELECT one.*

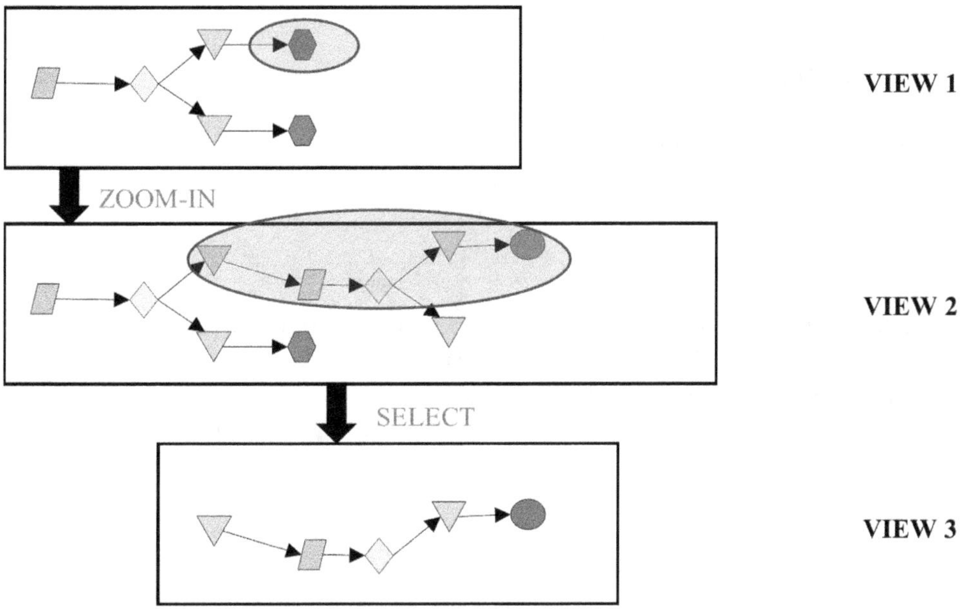


refinements along different and heterogeneous levels of abstraction, and the user can operate recursively (i.e., decide to refine newly determined refinements).

The ZOOM-IN operation is applied on a guideline_navigator (*gn1* in the algorithm in Figure 14), and modifies it, by appending a new guideline_view (*New_View*), which represents the new refinement. At the initialization step, the user has to specify which actions of the last guideline view of *gn1* (s)he wants to modify (*To_Refine_Set* is initialized by such a set of actions). If *To_Refine_Set* is not empty, then *New_View* is created as a copy of the last view of *gn1*. Then, each action *a* in *To_Refine_Set* is independently refined, through the REFINE operation (see later). The REPLACE operation simply substitutes *a* with the newly identified refinements into *New_View*. Whenever a new refinement is added, we allow users to update *To_Refine_Set*, adding actions of the new refinement to it. In such a way, we provide users with the possibility of going on with this process until the desired level of detail is reached,

The REFINE operation takes in input a guideline_view (*gv*) and *a* action in it, and performs one step of refinement. The way in which such a refinement is obtained depend on the type of *a*. If *a* is a composite action in the guideline_view *gv*, its expansion is simply the sub-guideline constituted by the actions composing it. Thus, the refinement can be easily determined on the basis of the description of the guideline *gv* itself. On the other hand, if *a* is a pharmacological action, the representation of *a* contains the attribute *substance*, whose value is a link to the ontological entity representing drug category to be administered (*drug_cat*). Thus, through the *Down* operator, the algorithm determines the set of descendants of *drug_cat* in the ISA hierarchy in the ontology (the case in which *a* is a specific drug is a degenerate one, in which the result of *Down* is empty). Of course, each one of the descendants $c_1, \ldots, c_n$ is a

*Figure 14. The ZOOM_IN algorithm*

```
ZOOM_IN (gn1) returns guideline_navigator
        Input: gl1, a guideline navigator

To_Refine_Set ← user selection of actions from gn1
if To_Refine_Set ≠ {} then
begin
        New_View ← generate_view()
        New_View ← copy(Last(gn1))
        Append(New_View, gn1)
        while To_Refine_Set ≠ {} do
        begin
                a ← take an action from To_Refine_Set and remove it from To_Refine_Set
                refinement ← REFINE(New_View, a)
                REPLACE(a,refinement, New_View)
                To_Refine_Set ← To_Refine_Set ∪ user selection of actions from refinement
        end
end
return gn1
```

possible alternative refinement of *drug_cat*. To convert this notion into a guideline-like format, the function *BUILD_ALTERNATIVES* constructs a new piece of guideline, consisting of a decision node connected to *n* pharmacological action nodes (each one prescribing one of the drug categories $c_1, \ldots, c_n$).

## Interaction Analysis Algorithm

Once the level of abstraction of the analysis has been specified by the user-physician, through the focusing tool, (s)he may look for the interactions at the *chosen level*. Though the Interaction analysis easily applies also to cases in which more than

*Figure 15. The REFINE algorithm*

```
REFINE (gv, a) returns guideline_view
        Input: gv, a guideline view
               a an action in gv

case a of
        a is a composite action in gv:
                refinement ← expansion of a into its components, considering the guideline
        a is a pharmacological action in gv:
                drug_cat ← get(a, substance)
                {c1, ...,cn} ← Down(drug_cat, Ontology)
                refinement ← BUILD_ALTERNATIVES({c1, ...,cn})
end case of
return refinement
```

two CIGs are considered, for the sake of brevity here we consider only the case of two CIGs. After the focusing analysis, the user-physician has determined exactly which parts of the CIGs (s)he is interested in, possibly expanding CIGs with the ontology (e.g., expanding a pharmacological action prescribing a drug category into a therapeutic decision followed by the actions of administering its sub-categories), to reach the desired level of abstraction/detail. At this point, the interaction analysis tool operates as described in the ANALYSE_INTERACTIONS operation below.

Given two guideline views *gv1* and *gv2*, all composite, work and pharmacological actions are considered. The set of pairs of actions *<a1,a2>* such that *a1* belongs to *gv1*, and *a2* belongs to *gv2* is constructed (*intPairSet*), and the result (*intTripleSet*) is initialized to the empty set. Notice that *intTripleSet* is a set of triples *<a1,a2,i_Set>*, where *<a1,a2>* is a pair in *intPairSet*, and *i_Set* is a set of interactions (the possible interactions between *a1* and *a2*). Then, for each pair *<a1,a2>* in *intPairSet*, *Search_interactions* is applied, returning the set *intSet* of possible interactions (see the algorithm below), and the triple *<a1,a2, intSet>* is added to the set *intTripleSet*.

For each pair *<a1, a2>* of actions, *SEARCH_INTERACTIONS* reports the possible interactions (as stored in the ontology), which are added to the output (*interactions*). It operates only on pairs of "homogeneous" actions. Indeed, this is not restrictive, since we provide user with operators (ZOOM-IN, ZOOM-OUT) to choose the desired level of abstraction. If *a1* and *a2* are both composite or work actions, the interactions between their intentions have to be analyzed in the ontology. In our ontology, pharmacological actions have intentions (indeed, atomic intentions), and prescribe the administration of drug categories (or drugs). Thus, both the interactions between intentions and those between drug categories (or drugs) are considered. However, in the case of pharmacological actions added to the CIG by the expansion step (see *BUILD_ALTERNATIVES* in the REFINE operator), no intention is specified (the system cannot automatically determine action intentions), so that only the interactions between the prescribed drug categories (drugs) are considered.

Given two actions *a1* and *a2*, *FIND_INTENTION_INTERACTIONS* finds the interactions between their intentions stored in the ontology. Since actions in CIGs may have multiple intentions, all of them are retrieved (considering the *aimsTo* arcs exiting *a1* and *a2* in the ontology). For each pair <i1,i2> of intensions (such that

*Figure 16. The ANALYSE_INTERACTIONS algorithm*

```
ANALYSE_INTERACTIONS (gv1, gv2) returns set of action interactions
      Input: gv1, gv2: guideline views

actSet1 ← set of all the composite, work and pharmacological actions in gv1
actSet2 ← set of all the composite, work and pharmacological actions in gv2
intPairSet ← actSet1 × actSet2
intTripleSet ← {}
for each <a1, a2> in intPairSet do
begin
      intSet← SEARCH_INTERACTIONS (a1, a2)
      intTripleSet ← intTripleSet ∪ {<a1, a2, intSet>}
end
return intTripleSet
```

*Figure 17. The SEARCH_INTERACTIONS algorithm*

```
SEARCH_INTERACTIONS (a1, a2) returns set of interactions
        Input: a1, a2: actions

interactions ← {}
case a1, a2 of
        a1, a2 are both composite or work actions
        interactions ← FIND_INTENTION_INTERACTIONS (a1, a2)
        a1, a2 are both pharmacological actions in the original CIGs
        interactions ← FIND_INTENTION_INTERACTIONS (a1, a2, Interactions) ∪
                        FIND_DRUG_INTERACTIONS (a1, a2, Interactions)
        a1, a2 are pharmacological actions, but one of them (or both) are the result of an
        expansion
        interactions ← FIND_DRUG_INTERACTIONS (a1, a2)
end case of
return interactions
```

*i1* is an intention of *a1* and *i2* of *a2*), the ontology is explored (by following backward the arc hasElement of the concept IntentionInteraction, and considering inheritance) in order to determine the type (*intType*) of interaction holding between them. Then, the triple <i1,i2,intType> is added to the *interactions*. Of course, if no such information is stored in the ontology, nothing is added to the output. Notice, that, on the other hand, some interactions between atomic actions can be automatically inferred even they are not directly specified in the ontology. Specifically, if two intentions concerns the same BodyPartAttribute, but involve different variations for it, the respective interaction can be automatically inferred. In particular, if they share the same value of Modality, their interaction is classified as "Concordance", whilst, in other cases, its classification is "Discordance", with a specific case in which the modalities are opposite ("Decreasing" and "Increasing") and the interaction type is "Opposite".

Finally, *FIND_DRUG_INTERACTIONS* is defined in a similar way but, obviously, involves searching the ontology for different paths of arcs.

## RELATED WORKS

Excluding few common features, the existing methods are very different from each other. (Sánchez-Garzón, et al., 2013), for example, attempts to capture the collaborative aspect of the merging: each guideline is considered as a physician expert in the treatment of a single disease, and represented by an agent with hierarchical planning capabilities. The result is obtained through the coordination of all the agents, and respects the recommendations of each guideline. Another interesting approach, presented in (Michalowski, et al., 2013) and (Wilk, et al., 2013), uses constraint logic programming to identify and address adverse interactions. In this solution, a constraint logic programming (CLP) model is derived from the combination of logical models that represent each CIG, then a mitigation algorithm is applied to detect and mitigate interactions. Among rule-based systems, (López-Vallverdú, Riaño, & Collado, 2012) represents guidelines as sets of clinical actions that are modeled into an ontology. To combine two treatments, first they are unified

*Figure 18. The FIND_INTENTION_INTERACTIONS and the FIND_DRUG_INTERACTIONS algorithms*

```
FIND_INTENTION_INTERACTIONS (a1,a2) returns set of interactions
        Input: a1, a2: actions
               interactions: set of interactions

begin
        i1_Set ← get(a1, aims_To)
        i2_Set ← get(a2, aims_To)
        for each <i1, i2> such that i1∈i1_Set and i2∈i2_Set do
        begin
                intType ← navigate the ontology to find the type of interaction between i1 and
                  i2 (following backward the arcs hasElement and hasType and using
                  inheritance along ISA hierarchies)
                if intType ≠ empty then
                        interactions ← interactions ∪ {<i1,i2,intType>}
        end
end

FIND_DRUG_INTERACTIONS (a1,a2) returns set of interactions
Input: a1, a2: actions
        interactions: set of interactions

begin
        d1_Set ← get(a1, substance)
        d2_Set ← get(a2, substance)
        for each <d1, d2> such that d1∈d1_Set and d2∈d2_Set do
        begin
                intType ← navigate the ontology to find the type of interaction between d1
and               d2 (following backward arcs hasElement and using inheritance along ISA
                  hierarchies)
                if intType ≠ empty then
                        interactions ← interactions ∪ {<d1,d2,intType>}
        end
end
```

in a unique treatment, then a set of "combination rules" is applied to detect and avoid possible interactions. Jafarpour (Jafarpour & Abidi, 2013) uses semantic-web rules and an ontology for the merging criteria. Given these, an Execution Engine dynamically merges several CIGs according to merge criteria. GLINDA proposes a wide ontology of cross-guideline interactions (Musen, et al., 2011). Despite the methods used are very different from each other, one can classify them according to two (orthogonal) criteria. First, CIG can be merged before or during the execution (Abidi, 2008). In the second case the methodology "*take account also of execution of and patient data*", while in the first the result of merging is a general treatment that needs to be customized for each patient and situation. Another important distinction arises between autonomous methods and other that require (or allow) physician intervention. In the first, given two or more CIGs, the system returns a merged guideline without user intervention. In the second, during the process, (s)he can be consulted to take decisions about merging options. This last category (to which, for example, belongs (López-Vallverdú, Riaño, & Collado, 2012)) is very interesting, because it allows to use a basic medical knowledge that only the physician owns, and that is very difficult to a priori extract and model into an autonomous system.

## CONCLUSION

The treatment of patients affected by multiple diseases (*comorbid* patients) is one of the main challenges for the modern health care, also due to the aging of population, and to the increase of chronic diseases. In many cases, guidelines coping with each one of the diseases (independently of the others) may be available. However, combining guidelines is a challenging task and a hot topic in the most recent research in Medical Informatics. Though several valuable proposal have been pointed out in the specialized literature (see the "Related Works" section), the complexity of the overall problem demands for additional steps forward of the state-of-the-art.

In this Chapter, we address a significant part of the problem, namely the detection of interactions between CIGs. Relevant studies demonstrates that various types of interactions must be taken into account when merging two (or more) CIGs, and propose and ontology of interactions (Musen, et al., 2011). However, to the best of our knowledge, our approach is the first one that identifies different levels of abstractions in the analysis of interactions, based on both the hierarchical organization of CIGs (in which composite actions are refined into their components) and the hierarchy of drug categories (specific drugs often constitute the bottom of such a hierarchy). We show that interactions can occur at each abstraction level, so that the medical interaction detection process must navigate all levels. In addition, the medical experience shows that the detection of interaction must be an *interactive* process, in which, at each step, user-physicians decide how to proceed on the basis of the previous steps.

In this Chapter, we propose a general methodology (data/knowledge structures and reasoning algorithms operating on them) supporting user-driven and interactive interaction detection over multiple levels of abstraction. To the best of our knowledge, no other approach in the literature has explicitly addressed such a challenging goal. In this sense, we believe that our approach, besides being innovative, is somehow *complementary* with respect to several other approaches in the literature, so that an integration with them can be possible as a future work (e.g., with Riaño's methodology to merge CIGs (Riaño & Collado, 2013)).

The main contributions of our work are:

1. We identified three different abstraction levels at which interactions can occur: between actions in CIGs, between drug categories, and, finally, between specific drugs.
2. We worked out an ontology of interactions, considering the three levels above.
3. We clarified that the study of CIG interactions can be performed only by considering the expansion of CIGs with (part of) the ontological knowledge.
4. Last, but most important, we proposed a set of tools and operations supporting *user-physician-driven interactive* interaction detection along the three different *levels of abstraction*.

From the viewpoint of user-physicians, our approach is original, by supporting interaction detection at multiple levels of abstraction. Such a new feature can provide significant advantages in different application contexts. For instance, it may support expert physicians to analyze "abstractly" (i.e., just considering the guidelines, with no reference to a specific patient) the interactions between two or more guidelines that are commonly used together (e.g., with the final goal of providing some "partial merge" between them). In such a case, the possibility of reasoning about "high-level" actions is certainly crucial. On the other hand, thanks to its flexibility, our approach can also support a physician treating a specific comorbid patient. In such a context, though the abstraction facilities are certainly helpful, the possibility of moving from the "general" actions in the guidelines to study of the interactions of specific drug categories (and drugs) can play a crucial role.

On the other hand, from the viewpoint of research, the above results can be regarded as the starting point of a new computer-based methodology to (support user-physicians to) cope with comorbidities, based on the notion of multiple abstractions. Carrying on such a new line of research will involve interesting new scientific challenges, especially concerning the development of suitable *flexible* and *interactive* approaches to support physicians in the *solution of interactions at different levels of abstractions.*

We are currently developing a prototypical implementation to demonstrate our approach, based on GLARE. In our short-term future work, we aim at extending our approach to cope also with "patient – CIG action" interactions and "patient – drug" interactions, and to cope with the temporal issues (e.g., not all interactions between CIGs are possible, due to the temporal constraints between CIG actions).

In our long-term future work, we will attempt to achieve the goals specified in the section "Goals of our overall approach": supporting physicians also in the interaction solving, and, finally, in merging multiple guidelines in the treatment of the specific patient at hand.

## ACKNOWLEDGMENT

The authors are very grateful to Yuval Shahar for his invaluable advice and for many inspiring suggestions.

The work described in this chapter was partially supported by Compagnia di San Paolo, in the Ginseng project.

## REFERENCES

Abidi, S. R. (2008). A Conceptual Framework for Ontology Based Automating and Merging of Clinical Pathways of Comorbidities. *K4HelP, 5626*, 55-66.

Anselma, L., Bottrighi, A., Molino, G., Montani, S., Terenziani, P., & Torchio, M. (2011). Supporting knowledge-based decision making in the medical context: The glare approach. *International Journal of Knowledge-Based Organizations*, *1*(1), 42–60. doi:10.4018/ijkbo.2011010103

Anselma, L., Bottrighi, A., Montani, S., & Terenziani, P. (2013). Extending bcdm to cope with proposals and evaluations of updates. *IEEE Transactions on Knowledge and Data Engineering*, *25*(3), 556–570. doi:10.1109/TKDE.2011.170

Anselma, L., Terenziani, P., Montani, S., & Bottrighi, A. (2006). Towards a comprehensive treatment of repetitions, periodicity and temporal constraints in clinical guidelines. *Artificial Intelligence in Medicine*, *38*(2), 171–195. doi:10.1016/j.artmed.2006.03.007 PMID:16766167

Bottrighi, A., Giordano, L., Molino, G., Montani, S., Terenziani, P., & Torchio, M. (2010). Adopting model checking techniques for clinical guidelines verification. *Artificial Intelligence in Medicine*, *48*(1), 1–19. doi:10.1016/j.artmed.2009.09.003 PMID:19864118

Fox, J., Johns, N., & Rahmanzadeh, A. (1998). Disseminating medical knowledge: the proforma approach. *Artificial Intelligence in Medicine, 14*(1-2), 157–182. doi:10.1016/S0933-3657(98)00021-9 PMID:9779888

Fridsma, D. B. (2001). Special Issue on Workflow Management and Clinical Guidelines. *Journal of the American Medical Informatics Association, 22*(1).

Gijsen, R., Hoeymans, N., & Schellevis, F. G. (2001). Causes and consequences of comorbidity: a review. *Journal of Clinical Epidemiology, 54*(7), 661–674. doi:10.1016/S0895-4356(00)00363-2 PMID:11438406

Gordon, C., & Christensen, J. P. (1995). *Health telematics for clinical guidelines and protocols*. IOS Press.

Gruber, T. (2009). Ontology. In L. Liu, & M. Tamer Özsu (Eds.), Encyclopedia of Database Systems (pp. 1963-1965). Springer US.

Institute of Medicine, Committee on Quality Health Care in America. (2001). Crossing the quality chasm: A new health system for the 21st century. National Academy Press.

International Health Terminology Standards Development Organisation. (n.d.). *Snomed Clinical Terms*. Retrieved October 2013, from IHTSDO website: http://www.ihtsdo.org/snomed-ct/

Jafarpour, B., & Abidi, S. S. (2013). Merging Disease-Specific Clinical Guidelines to Handle Comorbidities in a Clinical Decision Support Setting. In *Proceedings of 14th Conference on Artificial Intelligence in Medicine* (vol. 7885, pp. 28-32). Murcia, Spain: Springer.

Koppel, R., Metlay, J. P., & Cohen, A. (2005). Role of Computerized Physician Order Entry Systems in Facilitating Medication Errors. *Journal of the American Medical Association, 293*(10), 1197–1203. doi:10.1001/jama.293.10.1197 PMID:15755942

Liaw, S. T., Rahimi, A., Ray, P., Taggart, J., Dennis, S., & de Lusignan, S. et al. (2013). Towards an ontology for data quality in integrated chronic disease management: A realist review of the literature. *International Journal of Medical Informatics, 82*(1), 10–24. doi:10.1016/j.ijmedinf.2012.10.001 PMID:23122633

López-Vallverdú, J. A., Riaño, D., & Collado, A. (2012). Rule-Based Combination of Comorbid Treatments for Chronic Diseases Applied to Hypertension, Diabetes Mellitus and Heart Failure. *ProHealth/KR4HC, 7738*, 30-41.

Lucas, P., & Ten Teije, S. M. (2008). *Computer-based Medical Guidelines and Protocols: A Primer and Current Trends*. IOS Press.

McGuinness, D. L., & van Harmelen, F. (2004). *OWL Web Ontology Language*. Retrieved from W3C Recommendation: http://www.w3.org/TR/owl-features/

Michalowski, M., Wilk, S., Michalowski, W., Farion, K., Lin, D., & Mohapatra, S. (2013). Using Constraint Logic Programming to Implement Iterative Actions and Numerical Measures during Mitigation of Concurrently Applied Clinical Practice Guidelines. In *Proceedings of 14th Conference on Artificial Intelligence in Medicine* (vol. 7885, pp. 17-22). Murcia, Spain: Springer.

Montani, S., & Terenziani, P. (2006). Exploiting decision theory concepts within clinical guideline systems: Toward a general approach. *International Journal of Intelligent Systems*, *21*(6), 585–599. doi:10.1002/int.20149

Musen, M., Goldstein, M. K., Tu, S., Martins, S., Nyulas, C., Jung, H., & Kum, P. (2011). *GLINDA Interaction Ontology*. Retrieved from GLINDA: GuideLine INteraction Detection Arch.: http://glinda-project.stanford.edu/guidelineinteractio-nontology.html

Peleg, M., Boxwala, A. A., & Ogunyemi, O. (2000). Glif3: the evolution of a guideline representation format. *Proc AMIA Symp*, 645–649. PMID:11079963

Pérez-Rey, D., Maojo, V., García-Remesal, M., Alonso-Calvo, R., Billhardt, H., Martín-Sánchez, F., & Sousa, A. (2006). ONTOFUSION: Ontology-based integration of genomic and clinical databases. *Computers in Biology and Medicine*, *36*(7-8), 712–730. doi:10.1016/j.compbiomed.2005.02.004 PMID:16144697

Quaglini, S., Stefanelli, M., Lanzola, G., Caporusso, V., & Panzarasa, S. (2001). Flexible guideline-based patient care. *Artificial Intelligence in Medicine*, *22*(1), 65–80. doi:10.1016/S0933-3657(00)00100-7 PMID:11259884

Riaño, D., & Collado, A. (2013). Model-Based Combination of Treatments for the Management of Chronic Comorbid Patients. In *Proceedings of 14th Conference on Artificial Intelligence in Medicine* (vol. 7885, pp. 11-16). Murcia, Spain: Springer.

Robert Wood Johnson Foundation and Partnership for Solutions. (2004, September). *Chronic Conditions: Making the Case for Ongoing Care.* Johns Hopkins University.

Rubin, D. L., Lewis, S. E., Mungall, C. J., Misra, S., Westerfield, M., & Ashburner, M. et al. (2006). National Center for Biomedical Ontology: advancing biomedicine through structured organization of scientific knowledge. *OMICS: A Journal of Integrative Biology*, *10*(2), 185–198. doi:10.1089/omi.2006.10.185 PMID:16901225

Sánchez-Garzón, I., Fernández-Olivares, J., Onaindia, E., Milla, G., Jordán, J., & Castejón, P. (2013). A Multi-agent Planning Approach for the Generation of Personalized Treatment Plans of Comorbid Patients. *14th Conference on Artificial Intelligence in Medicine, 7885*, 23-27.

Shahar, Y., Miksch, S., & Johnson, P. D. (1998). The Asgaard project: a task-specific framework for the application. *Artificial Intelligence in Medicine*, 29–51. doi:10.1016/S0933-3657(98)00015-3 PMID:9779882

Shahar, Y., Musen, M., & Tu, S. W. (1996). Eon: A component-based approach to. *Journal of the American Medical*, 367-388.

Shiffman, R. N., Karras, B. T., Agrawal, A., Chen, R., Marenco, L. N., & Nath, S. (2000). Model formulation: Gem: A proposal for a more comprehensive guideline document model using xml. *Journal of the American Medical Informatics Association*, *7*(5), 488–498. doi:10.1136/jamia.2000.0070488 PMID:10984468

Sittig, D. F., Wright, A., Osheroff, J. A., Middleton, B., Teich, J. M., & Ash, J. S., Campbell, Emily M., Bates, D. W. (2008). Grand challenges in clinical decision support. *Journal of Biomedical Informatics*, *41*(2), 387–392. doi:10.1016/j.jbi.2007.09.003 PMID:18029232

Stantic, B., Terenziani, P., Governatori, G., Bottrighi, A., & Sattar, A. (2012). An implicit approach to deal with periodically repeated medical data. *Artificial Intelligence in Medicine*, *55*(3), 149–162. doi:10.1016/j.artmed.2012.03.002 PMID:22503730

Ten Teije, A., Miksch, S., & Lucas, P. (2008). *Computer-based Medical Guidelines and Protocols: A Primer and Current Trends*. IOS Press.

Terenziani, P., Bottrighi, A., Torchio, M., Molino, G., Anselma, L., & Correndo, G. (2003). Applying artificial intelligence to clinical guidelines: the glare approach. AI*IA, 2829, 536-547.

Terenziani, P., Molino, G., & Torchio, M. (2001). A modular approach for representing and executing clinical guidelines. *Artificial Intelligence in Medicine*, *23*(3), 249–276. doi:10.1016/S0933-3657(01)00087-2 PMID:11704440

Terenziani, P., Montani, S., Bottrighi, A., Molino, G., Torchio, M., & Correndo, G. (2004). A context-adaptable approach to clinical guidelines. *Studies in Health Technology and Informatics*, 169–173. PMID:15360797

WHO Collaborating Centre for Drug Statistics Methodology. (n.d.). *Anatomical Therapeutic Chemical classification system*. Retrieved October 2013, from WHOCC website: http://www.whocc.no/atc

Wilk, S., Michalowski, M., Michalowski, W., Farion, K., Hing, M. M., & Mohapatra, S. (2013). Mitigation of adverse interactions in pairs of clinical practice guidelines using constraint logic programming. *Journal of Biomedical Informatics*, *46*(2), 341–353. doi:10.1016/j.jbi.2013.01.002 PMID:23376273

## KEY TERMS AND DEFINITIONS

**Clinical Practice Guidelines:** Systematically developed statements to assist practitioner and patient decisions about appropriate health care in specific clinical circumstances.

**Comorbid Patient:** A patient affected by multiple diseases.

**Computer-Interpretable Clinical Guidelines:** Computer-assisted tools for managing, acquiring, representing and/or executing clinical guidelines.

**Drug Interaction:** Drug interactions occur when the effect of a particular drug is altered when it is taken with another drug.

**GLARE:** A prototypical system for the acquisition, representation and execution of computer interpretable clinical guidelines (acronym of GuideLine Acquisition, Representation and Execution). GLARE has been built starting from 1997 in a long-term cooperation between the Department of Computer Science of the University of Piemonte Orientale, Alessandria, Italy, and the Azienda Ospedaliera San Giovanni Battista in Turin (one of the largest hospitals in Italy).

**Intentions of a Therapeutic Action:** The goals that physicians expect to obtain realizing an action; usually such intentions can be expressed as (desired) modifications of specific parameters characterizing the patient status.

**Navigation and Focusing on Computer Interpretable Clinical Guidelines:** The exploration of a computer interpretable guideline, in order to identify specific (relevant) parts of it. This process can involve the exploration of the different levels of detail that are usually adopted to represent a guideline.

**Ontology:** Ontology is the study of the nature of being, becoming, existence, or reality, as well as the basic categories of being and their relations. In computer and information science, ontology is a technical term denoting an artifact that is designed for a purpose, which is to enable the modeling of knowledge about some domain, real or imagined.

## ENDNOTES

1 Please notice that, in this chapter, we deliberately use the term "intention" in a broad sense, to cover not only the desired effects of medical actions, but also the effects of pharmacological prescriptions, and of drugs

2 Indeed, in our ontology we also take into account other types of interactions, involving the status of the patient. In particular, the patient status may interact with the Intentions of composite actions, with the atomic intentions of pharmacological prescriptions, and with DrugCategories. Such issues are not taken into account in this paper, where we focus only on "patient-independent" detection of CIGs interactions.

3 Bethanechol is an agonist of muscarinic receptors, belonging to the acetylcholine drug category.

4 Pirenzepine is an antagonist of muscarinic receptors, belonging to the atropine drug category.

# Chapter 10
# Radio Frequency Identification Technology as an Analytical Lens and Solution in Hospitals:
## A Novel Approach in BPR/BPM

**Chandana Unnithan**
*Deakin University, Australia*

**Bardo Fraunholz**
*Deakin University, Australia*

## ABSTRACT

*Radio Frequency Identification—an object recognition technology—has been explored by hospitals worldwide in the past decade for inventory management. As this technology became accepted with successful pilots, integrating the technology with other applications within hospitals gained momentum. For this purpose, however, it is necessary to revise existing processes that are impacted by RFID. The standard approach in business process management is to redesign the existing processes to plug-in the technology and implement the new process with the technology. In this chapter, the authors provide a novel perspective in Business Process Redesign and Management that RFID may not only be a technology solution, but also an analytical lens to review the existing processes within hospitals such that existing inconsistencies may be revealed and an opportunity presented to address them.*

## INTRODUCTION

Radio Frequency Identification (RFID) is commonly defined as wireless technology for automatic identification of objects or people, in which a reader emits a series of commands to extract data/information from tags (Maillart et al. 2010). It is an object recognition technology that uses radio waves (Greene, 2005) automatically. This avant-garde concept was initially trialled by the British in World War II to identify friendly airplanes returning from their missions (Landt, 2001). The ability of this technology to track signals and store data helped in its commercialisation through RFID tags or small silicon microchips, as small as half a millimetre square attached to antennae and could

DOI: 10.4018/978-1-4666-6316-9.ch010

be placed anywhere (Taghaboni-Dutta, Velthouse, 2006). These tags are able to store unique serial numbers and other information, which can be read by readers a few or hundreds of meters away.

It was in the last decade that hospitals realised the benefits of integrating RFID into their operations, to enhance efficiency and provide better quality of care (Cavoukian, 2008; Cangialosi, Monaly, Yang, 2007). In particular, hospitals became interested in tracking high value and frequently used equipment to optimize their utilization in emergency settings such as surgeries (Nagy et al. 2006). Conversely, resource constraints in hospitals are increasingly rendering it difficult to provide care to an adequate standard (Hoskins 2006). Frequently, surgical procedures are delayed due to missing high-end critical equipment or regularly used assets such as IV stands or defibrillators. Majority of the large hospitals globally seem to have spent significantly on stocking inventories of such equipment. Nevertheless, medical staff spends hours searching for wheelchairs, stretchers, gurneys etc, sacrificing the time with patients, particularly in surgeries (Hoskins 2006). High value assets are often underutilized, due to slow device cycle times while hospitals continue to overspend on rental assets (Nagy et al. 2006). In such an environment, relatively inexpensive RFID technology is perceived as a solution for resource optimization and to support appropriate allocation of scarce material resources.

Specifically, poor exploitation of resources and slow device cycle times cause many high-value assets to go underutilised while hospitals continue to overspend on new and rental assets (Hoskins, 2006). Meanwhile, nurses sacrifice time with patients (especially in surgeries) to seek equipment they need and maintenance staff lose productive hours searching for specific items that need maintenance. As a result, the efficiency of processes in the hospitals reduce, costs and complexities continue to rise (Hoskins, 2006, Nagy et al., 2006). Managing the processes efficiently, enhancing quality of care and controlling costs are seen as the rationale for adopting RFID systems.

Pivotal research into drivers for RFID in hospitals have consistently indicated that RFID tags may lead to reduction in clinical errors, reduced costs and increased efficiencies (Nagy et al. 2006; Chen et al. 2008). Fisher and Monahan (2008) concur that due to its many dimensional uses, RFID is rapidly becoming the standard for hospitals to track inventory, identify patients, and manage personnel. Many hospitals have initiated the use of RFID tags on wristbands (or bracelets) which store data and can be scanned with a reader to identify a patient, and what surgical procedure is required (Hancox, 2006; Cangialosi et al., 2007). For example, RFID tags embedded in patient bracelets can help medical staff identify patients before surgery and before administering medications or blood transfusions – reducing possible clinical errors. RFID systems have been implemented such that patient movements can be traced through hospital services. Medical staff is often given RFID tags on their badges in order to collect data on workflow to find inefficiencies in current operations of the hospital. These systems are particularly useful in emergency settings where there is high patient volume, and heightened risk of medical error. Conversely, tracking equipment takes less time, leaving practitioners to spend more time with the patients (McCarthy, 2004).

Hospitals can lower expenses on rental equipment and over supply inventories, with the implementation of RFID systems often known as *indoor positioning systems* (Fisher, 2006). Current research (Fisher and Monahan, 2008) is in concurrence that due to its many dimensional uses, RFID is rapidly becoming the standard for hospitals to track inventory, identify patients, and manage personnel. The potential of RFID has been explored for asset tracking and process enhancements in hospitals, worldwide. The technology has been accepted in such environments, as it is relatively inexpensive and, in principle, uncomplicated to integrate with other clinical support systems. It is perceived to offer many benefits to currently resource critical/strained hospitals.

Despite the perceived benefits, these systems are not easily adapted to hospitals due to infrastructure in terms of space, equipment, personnel and patients, making it much more complicated than a factory or warehouse setting. Fisher and Monahan (2008) opinion that privacy concerns of patients/staff and the possible work intensification for nursing and other hospital staff, as a result of efficiencies experienced by this technology, should be taken into account from the onset, particularly during design and implementation stages. RFID systems may have a valence toward surveillance, such that nurses may feel overtly scrutinised by the tracking technologies.

The Spyglass Consulting Group (eWeek 2005) argued that uncoordinated efforts between hospitals, vendors, shippers and suppliers are restricting RFID adoption in hospitals. In many hospitals, the implementation of RFID is vendor driven and implemented, often not in consultation with all the staff concerned. An RFID pilot may begin with a vendor providing the equipment, handling installation and testing, which may be quite sudden and not known to all the staff concerned. In a resource-constrained hospital, it is also difficult to inform everyone, as many staff work part time. Effectively, this lack of coordination or minimal coordination, results in under-utilisation of the system as such. Specifically, if every employee who works part time is not aware of RFID tracking being available, they may not be using it during their shift hours. Conversely, when a pilot implementation begins, all the equipment to be tagged may not be available at one time to be tagged. And all tags may not have arrived at one time in stock, to enable the tagging from the vendor. This results in less accuracy of tracking, poor adaptation of the systems and also encourages a certain level of resistance from the users.

Nonetheless, RFID integration is no longer a new portent for hospitals. More and more hospitals are implementing or at least initiating installation of this technology for improving efficiencies as the potential of the technology is now accepted in this context. Our research into RFID enabled process redesign and enhancements in hospitals revealed a new perspective. As a technology, RFID has the potential to enhance processes as a tool, but it can also become an analytical lens for process review in hospitals. The research perspectives reported in this chapter are based on action research in a group of hospitals.

The rest of the chapter is organised as follows. In the next section, we provide nomenclature, to take a closer look at the technology itself, as it has evolved. In the following section, we brief on RFID in hospitals to synthesise some contemporary developments and issues. The section thereafter offers the business process redesign context and subsequently emergent findings that has resulted from the first phase of a real action research project in a large hospitals group, that resulted in the our proposition of the novel approach. The final section provides pathways into future research as well as the relevance of this research to practice. The objective of this chapter is to present the potential of RFID technology to act as an analytical lens for process review in hospitals as well as a technology solution.

## BACKGROUND

### Radio Frequency Identification: Nomenclature

As Radio Frequency Identification develops as a useful technology for hospitals, it also keeps evolving. RFID is a generic term of technologies, which uses radio waves to identify people and objects. The most common method is use is to store a serial number on a microchip attached to an antenna (Greene, 2005:30). When the bar coding technology, where RFID evolved from, requires line of sight i.e. require a scanner to "see' the code to read it, an RFID reader does not need this (Greene, 2005). Conversely, according to Accenture, if there is an existing bar coding project, the financial justifications for RFID is already met and bar coding technology was serving as a platform to move to RFID (H&HN, 2004).

The technology consists of two components: a tag that acts as a data transponder; and an RFID reader. While the number of tags can range a few thousands in small RFID systems, the number of readers can increase in large scale systems, to create a more accurate three dimensional positioning system for the tags. In healthcare, the RFID tags take many forms including badges, pendants, labels, cards and even implants (Wicks, Visich & Li, 2006). There are 4 types of RFID tags available; passive, active semi passive and semi active (Mehrjerdi, 2008). Passive tags react when the signal is received they are powered by an electronic reader and store small amount of data. They receive energy from a remote RFID reader. They have a 3 feet range of 3 feet approximately (Roark DC & Miguel, 2006).

Semi passive tags are similar to passive tags except they have an internal power source that increases the storage capacity and the range. They use a small onboard battery to power the chip and are priced at about USD6 to USD50 depending on the capabilities. The read range for a passive tag depends on various factors such as the power of the reader, interference from metal objects or other RF devices. In general, low-frequency tags are read from a foot or less, while high frequency tags are read from about three feet and Ultra High Frequency (UHF) tags are read from 10 to 20 feet. Where longer ranges are needed, active tags are used to boost read ranges to 300 feet or more. Active tags have an internal lithium battery power source that continuously receives and transmits signals on various different frequencies. It uses a battery for both the chip and the transmission of data on the antenna. It has an internal data storage capability (Roark DC & Miguel, 2006). Active tags have a limited life, are heavier and more expensive when compared to passive tags. Semi-active tags use the battery for powering the antenna but the chip relies on the RF energy from the reader (Mehrjerdi, 2008).

The RFID system is based on miniaturized transponders and readers for connection to information systems (Mehrjerdi, 2008). Each RFID tag has a unique identification number stored in it, which identifies the object to which the tag is attached. The communication between the tag and reader begins when the tag enter the electromagnetic field of the reader. The reader interrogates the tag using a modulated carrier and the tags reply by modulated backscattering. The reader that acts as a transceiver can read and write information on the tag. Greene (2005: 30) summarises as follows: "Active tags have a transmitter and their own power source (typically a battery). The power source is used to run the microchip's circuitry and to broadcast a signal to a reader (the way a cell phone transmits to a base station). Passive tags have no batteries, instead they draw power from the reader, which sends out electromagnetic waves that induce a current in the tag's antenna".

Seminal research (Nagy et al., 2006) points out the lack of common global standard for RFID. There exist and proposed RFID standards that deal with the way tags and readers communicate, the way data is organised or formatted, ways to test that product meets the standard and how standards are used on applications (such as labels, for example). The International Standards Organisation has created different standards that apply to each of these. The situation became complex because the Auto-ID Centre at MIT Labs, in USA, which developed the Electronic Product Code (EPC) technologies, chose to also create its own air interface protocols for tracking good through the international supply chain (RFID Journal, 2005:1). Expressly, the Auto-ID Center was set up in 1999 at MIT, in USA, to develop the Electronic Product Code (EPC) and related technologies that could be used to identify products and track them through the global supply chain. Its aim was to develop a low-cost RFID system, based on global and open standards. It developed its own protocol and licensed it to EPCglobal. A set of classes of tags, with different memory and capabilities were proposed and eventually, two were retained: a Class 0 tag, which was a read only tag that was programmed at the time the microchip was made and Class 1 tag, which used a different protocol and was also a simple, passive only, backscatter tag, with one time field programmable, non volatile memory. Since the Class 0 tag used a different protocol from the Class 1 tag, end users had to buy multiprotocol readers to read both. The reason to retain these non-interoperable tags was because of the prohibition of one type of tags in Europe as compared to North America. For example, Class 0 sent out a signal at one frequency, and received a signal back at different frequency within the UHF band; which was prohibited in Europe(RFID Journal, 2005:2).

The Auto-ID Center transitioned into two separate organizations in 2003. While Auto-ID Labs and other universities continued primary research on EPC technologies, the technology itself was licensed to the Uniform Code Council, which set up EPCglobal as a joint venture with EAN International, to commercialise EPC technology. Finally, in September 2003, the Auto-ID Center handed off the Class 0 and Class 1 protocols to EPCglobal. Subsequently, the board of EPCglobal approved Class 0 and Class 1 as EPC standards. However, the issue remained that it is still not a global standard and therefore, could not be submitted to ISO.

Subsequently, in 2004, EPCglobal began developing the second-generation protocol (Gen-2), in an effort to create a single, global standard that aligns with ISO standards and it was approved in December, the same year (RFID Journal, 2005:3). In the process of this transition up until the year 2005, many organisations had already adapted the previous standards. The new generation RFID tags were not backward compatible and therefore, those organisations had to either mover forward and upgrade their RFID systems, replace them or continue with the existing standards issues. To a large extent, this had restricted RFID adoption in various sectors, particularly in healthcare and hospitals.

## Radio Frequency Identification in Hospitals

RFID implementation globally seem to be driven by vendors. A survey based report from Frost and Sullivan, in 2005 (O'Conner, 2005), revealed that the vast majority of RFID education – for users – are vendor driven and lacking in technological detail. The same report also suggested that it is process efficiencies that is driving the mandate for RFID. The views of vendors and systems integrators on the need for end-user training were divergent. Most vendors felt that informing the users was a key component for success, while some integrators felt that end-users could be trained throughout the implementation. However, even the vendors did not find it necessary to involve the end-users in the whole implementation process.

Tracking is an activity in hospitals that is pivotal to its operations. There are varied items that would need to be tracked including people: doctors, nurses, patients, visitors etc; equipment that needs to be prevented from being stolen; medicines that need to be administered in time, in the correct proportions, from the correct packages and so forth (Pappu et al., 2004). According to H&HN (2006:28), hospital staff has always reported trouble in tracking down ventilators, intravenous pumps and similar medical devices. With the increased reliance on shared handheld devices and laptop computers – the scenario is further complex. Therefore, a growing number of hospitals are beginning to combine their existing wireless communication networks, with RFID, to create real-time location systems.

In hospitals, RFID tags can be attached to equipments and people, such as newborns whose security can be better ensured with an RFID wristband. Clinicians in a hospital also can be traced and reached quickly in an emergency, while emergency departments can use RFID tags to follow patient charts and improve efficiencies. According to the managing Director of a large health care practice in California, hospitals should adopt RFID in such manner that the technology is compatible in different parts of the hospital (Greene, 2005). For example: "RFID tags could be used by materials management to track portableX-ray machines and also by the pharmacy to track a unit dose of an expensive drug" (Greene, 2005: 32).

A survey in 2005 (Baker, 2005) revealed that 10 percent of health care organisations in the USA use RFID tags to track expensive equipment and 45 percent are expected to have systems in place. As reported in H&HN (2005:23), in 1993, St Elizabeth Medical Centre in Edgewood, Ky, deployed an early form of RFID to prevent baby thefts in the maternity ward. Since then, it upgraded the technology and extended its use to some patients – mainly those with psychological or substance abuse problems- who are likely to hurt themselves or someone else if they are left untreated. The same report also pointed out the early use of patient tracking in Boston based Beth Israel Deaconess Medical Centre which outfitted its 48,000 square foot emergency department with RFID tags to track clinicians, patients and equipment (H&HN, 2005:24).

RFID has a major advantage that might justify any additional cost - it is automatic and so does not require manual intervention to work, which removes the potential for human error. In a hectic operating room environment, inventory control cannot get in the way of taking care of the patient (Nagy et al., 2006). A Frost and Sullivan report (Simpson, 2007) indicated that RFID tracking could save hospitals time and money which could be expended in tracking lost equipment. Page (2007) reported that pilot testing of RFID tracking had already given way to implementation, with hospitals moving ahead with dependable uses of RFID such as asset tracking. For example, O'Connor (2006) reported on the results of an RFID pilot implementation of RFID in a Toronto area hospital, Hamilton Health Sciences Acute Care Center, Canada. The pilot implementation tagged 200 pumps, as well as diagnostic equipment and other high value mobile assets in the nursing ward. Although the upfront costs were substantial, the full implementation is expected to bring high ROI, as it extends to infant tracking, adult patients or geriatric patient monitoring. The pilot was successful in identifying the shortfalls and leading to broader implementation.

The Shelby County Regional Medical Center in Memphis, implemented RFID patient tracking systems to reduce overcrowding in the emergency department (HFM, 2005). Until that time, the centre could only account for 25 percent of the typical patient stay in the trauma unit. After implementation of RFID, it now accounts for 80 percent of the patient time. The Heart Hospital Baylor Pano, Texas, has implemented an RFID network, which automates tracking and cataloguing of the hospital's high end equipment (Godinez, 2007). Staff in the hospital had embraced this technology well and very satisfied with its performance. Subsequently, the President of the Dallas Fort Worth Hospital Council declared that all hospitals in the region plan to deploy RFID systems. Baldwin and Larkin (2008) find that asset tracking systems can help hospitals keep tabs on their mobile inventories. They comment that RFID monitoring can fit into a hospital's strategic priority. However, which tracking solution and infrastructure is needed can vary widely depending on the context and one RFID solution do not fit all hospitals, nor countries.

The Rockhampton Base Hospital In Queensland, Australia, is using RFID to improve safety of nurses, during a renovation that has left holes in mental health ward building (Bacheldor, 2006). Nurses in the hospital's mental-health ward are using Alarm Cards, which combines a long-range wireless duress transmitter, a photo ID and proximity access control in one device, which is credit-card-sized.. The duress transmitter features a battery-powered RFID tag, operating at 433 MHz. Any nurses in danger or in need of assistance can push a button built into the back of the card, causing the transmitter to send a signal to an RFID reader to alert coworkers. To make the process convenient, nurses receive the cards when they sign in at the beginning of their shifts, and the tags' unique ID numbers are correlated in a database with the nurses' names and photos.

RFID may have much more potential in developing nations where healthcare systems even in advanced hospitals are strained by inefficient utilisation and the shortage of expensive equipment. The need is therefore higher in finding solutions that enable optimum utilisation of assets, resources and increasing the quality of care. For example, in India, where there is a multitude of small, medium and large hospitals that are struggling to assimilate and use expensive, higher technology equipment that is increasingly being demanded by both physicians and their patients. This creates significant shortages in hospitals, leading potentially to denial of the highest standard of care, even when, in theory, the device or equipment in question is part of the hospital inventory.

The Bhagwan Mahaveer Jain (BMJ) Heart Center – a cardiac hospital in Southern India, is using passive UHF RFID tags to assist with maintaining patient records, monitoring patient flows and tracking assets throughout the outpatient department (Bacheldor, 2007). An average of 100 patients is tracked in a day, which includes returning patients as they check into the outpatient department. Patients checking into the outpatient department receive RFID tagged cards. The unique ID number on each tag is associated with that of the patient electronic records in the Clinical Information Processing Platform (CLIP) – a system that includes software and RFID interrogators and tags. The RFID interrogators or readers are positioned in the waiting room, consultation rooms and labs and they document whenever a patient enters, leave and how long they stay in the area. The CLIP system is also integrated with hospital billing system, enabling the staff to use patient care and workflow information for accurate billing. The manual effort of paper registration and use of paper forms has been eliminated.

Conversely, the hospital is attaching EPC Gen 2 RFID tags to stents, pacemakers, wheelchairs, gurney and other high value items, as well as certain mobile devices used in diagnostic labs. The CLIP AssetLIVE application, which uses a mapping technology, is used to track the location of these assets. The system, instead of tracking tagged objects in real time, documents their location by analysing RFID data reads and render their last known position in a graphic (Bacheldor, 2007). The hospital has benefitted from the technology in that it has increased patient throughput, reduced paper work and added visibility to supplies. However, the hospital is still in the process of finding if RFID is providing cost savings and improving workflow processes in the hospital, especially in the asset tracking area.

Early applications of RFID such as infant tracking is now giving away to staff tracking, combined with time and motion studies to optimise workflows in areas such as radiology and surgeries (Cox, 2008). Harrisburg Hospital in Pennsylvania deployed a range of RFID applications from a patient tracking system for surgical patients to a 433MHx wireless infrastructure able to track wheelchairs and a range of portable medical gear. In Christiana Hospital, Newark, Delaware, the emergency department has 76 treatment rooms that handle 100,000 patients annually. Nurses were losing track where patients were in the treatment process, as they were moved among diagnostics and treatment facilities. This resulted in patient stay spiking above normal levels and resulted in 4-5% leaving without treatment. The hospital combined a tracking system with infrared sensor network for locating hardware assets. A web-based application showed tagged patients, staff and medical assets and created a visual workflow for patient progress. The data is filtered through various subset views so departments can expect and manage the number of patients and streamline their progress. According to the report, the length of patient stay has been reduced (Cox, 2008).

Chen et al., (2008:286) imply that while an increased number of vendors, hospital administrators and caregivers are advocating the relative advantages of RFID, the adoption seems to have slowed, which can be attributed to technology resistance, expensive system costs and disparate standards. Their research that addressed RFID adoption in hospitals from the expectation-confirmation perspective revealed that Healthcare providers who have a high perception of the usefulness in front-end interoperability and of performance expectancy affirm a positive confirmation experience with the use of RFID technology. However, for its continues use and progress,“ hospital administrators and equipment vendors need to address those factors that have been revealed as significant such as increasing the perceived frontend interoperability by using experienced consultants and integrators to implement systems that are proven to be interoperable at the front-end. They may also intervene via training and education to increase caregivers' performance expectancy of RFID" (Chen et al., 2008:286).

The first author of this chapter explored an RFID integration pilot in Australia, which revealed that the technology being vendor driven was not accepted completely by end users. When the pilot was deployed, there was no user involvement with the implementation team, as it mainly consisted of vendor recruits. The implementation was product/technology driven. Therefore, the processes which were affected, after RFID implementation, were redesigned based on the product information of the vendor and some inputs from the technology department of the hospital. There was no consistent process redesign in consultation with the users or managers of the relevant areas. In hospitals, where processes are time critical, and if these were to be made more efficient, by RFID integration, the end user involvement is imperative from the onset, as the post implementation conducted by the first author of this chapter revealed.

## Business Process Redesign in the Milieu

Seminal research (Indulska, Recker, Rosemann, Greene, 2009) purports that business process modeling and redesign has undoubtedly emerged as one of the relevant practices in Information Systems. Systematic approaches to generate radical improvement of business processes can be traced back to the early nineties (Davenport and Short 1990; Hammer 1990). BPR is a process for assessing performance issues of a particular process and conducting radical redesign to the process, by redesigning the process itself and systems, policies or organisational structures. The result is an improvement in the tasks structure (workflows) and processes (Gunasekaran and Ichimura, 1997). The vehicles of BPR were the introduction of information technologies and restructuring of business processes. Introduction of new technologies in any context is a significant enabler for redesign of processes (Jansen-Vullers and Reijers 2005). Majority of the BPR projects would consider existing processes as a starting point. Jansen-Vullers and Reijers (2005), argues that process redesign for healthcare contexts, if implemented with care, can be beneficial.

Many studies have applied BPR in the health domain. Buchanan (1998) had conducted a study to apply BPR strategy to redesign the way in which a hospital scheduled patients to their operating theatres. The study was strengthened using process mapping, process value analysis and conducting interviews with the users and managers, to assess what processes are insufficient. Buchanan cautioned that it is crucial to know which processes are valued most among stakeholders, and to understand the impact of the changes on them. Mitchell and Zmud (1999) study elicited redesigned processes that improved when tightly coupled with information technology (IT) and work process strategies in health settings. Bliemel and Hassanaein (2004) also provided a framework that identified e-health technologies and processes to support effective process redesign in the health care environment.

Brand and Kolk (1995) offered four main dimensions of BPR measures: time (redesigning to decrease time required to do a task); cost (resigning to decreases the required cost of a business process); quality (redesigning to improve the services delivered); and flexibility (resigning the process to enable the business process to be more acceptable to variation). Jansen-Vullers and Reijers (2005) applied these measures to redesign existing scenarios/processes, and developed alternative scenarios that improved the process flows. From among a few alternatives, they chose the best-redesigned scenario. Snyder et al. (2005) who conducted a value mapping case study in a small health care network indicates that value stream mapping is a standardized way of documenting a process and applying a systematic method to analyze processes, to develop an improved plan.

Rosemann (2006:249) concurs that "process modelling is a widely used approach to achieve the required visibility for existing processes and future process scenarios as part of business process improvement projects". He indicates that the current generation of analysis prefers the term "process modelling as it claims more disciplined, standardised, consistent and overall more mature and scientific approach" (2006:250). While cautioning researchers to the 22 pitfalls in process modelling, Rosemann (2006) concludes that process modeling should be deployed, as required, in large organisations as it has been proved beneficial.

In the context of our research, we concurred that process redesign and modeling was well applicable for deployment of RFID in large hospitals. In the next section, we present the findings from the action research conducted in a group of hospitals, in Australia, in relation to RFID integration and process redesign, which lead us to the recommendations provided subsequently.

## FINDINGS AND DISCUSSION

Action research is an iterative process, with researchers and practitioners acting together, diagnosing problems, actively intervening to achieve enhancement and reflective learning (Susman, 1983). Some early citations (Avison et al., 1999) recommend action research as a means of making academic research relevant, in order to explore theories and assumptions with practitioners in real situations and real organisations. During the last few years, the method has been applied in health care settings, which often deploy innovative technologies. It has endorsed as a suitable method in health settings, as reported in academic journals (Hampshire 2000; Dick, 2006). Fraunholz (2001) purport that it draws from the synergy created by the co-operation of researchers and practitioners in particular settings.

The role of action research was demonstrated by the PRIDE project which developed, deployed and redesigned a technological innovation for use in primary health care setting of UK (Waterman et al., 2007). From their experiences, they uphold that: "action research can be employed successfully to diffuse innovations that need a high level of adaptation in each new setting or where there is high complexity and mismatch between groups of people in an organisation, providing there is an established need for researching the said innovation further (Waterman et al., 2007:380)". The participatory approach helped the researchers understanding the cultural context in which the innovation had to be developed, thus effectively helping them develop, test, redesign, and deploy the innovation.

Action research is a continuous cyclical approach (Susman, 1983) which involves the cycles of *situation diagnosis-action planning-action taking-evaluating-specifying learning*. The cycle continues until the researcher and practitioners are satisfied of the outcome of the project.

The first author of this chapter conducted an investigation post the pilot implementation of an RFID based real time location system integration, at a Private Hospital based in Australia (Unnithan, Smith, Fraunholz, 2009), supported by Intel, to track movable equipment such as wheel chairs, infusion pumps, and oxygen regulators. On the basis of the key learning from the pilot, the hospital had planned to implement RFID in the Public Hospital, which is part of the group of hospitals. The initial investigation revealed that this project lacked user involvement, required coordinated process redesign, hospital readiness and project management.

Specifically, when the action project was initiated, the first author of this chapter aimed to find out if RFID as a technology has been able to achieve its potential of being integrated into the processes of a hospital, and if process efficiencies were experienced. This was initiated via reviewing a report on a pilot implementation conducted at the private hospital for improving efficiencies in two departments. The review of the report revealed that the hospital found that the technology is useful post implementation. Nonetheless, the researcher found that the hospital had not subsequently taken up a full-scale implementation. Subsequently, interviews were conducted with users, project managers and technology implementers in two departments: the Sterilising Services Unit and Clinical Support Unit.

The Sterilising Services Unit had experienced major time savings as a result of the RFID pilot. According to the users, the time taken to search the equipment in particular has been reduced significantly. Most of the equipment are of high utilization nature, and need to be sterilized and reused continuously. Due to the high utility nature, these equipments would need to be loaned, or purchased and stocked in excess, to optimise staff time spend in tracing them. According to this set of users, the department has experienced better efficiencies in the process of day-to-day work, through time savings and "monetary saving" through better equipment recycling.

However, the user manager expressed that the tracking system must be made more efficient to detect smaller devices, which have high utilisation, but may get lost "under a patient bed" etc. Another concern was that the RFID tracking system was not yet integrated with the Clinical Support System, which meant that the users did have to understand/cope with a new interface, which caused some reluctance. And this was particularly due to staff being in shifts and part time, which meant that they were not interested in learning a new interface, rather than the one that was tested. Therefore, technology integration did emerge as a major factor for continued use of the tracking system, instead of manual tracking.

The Clinical Services users/user managers expressed that although the orderlies were advised to trial the system, the system was not being used effectively. The reason was that the orderlies usually received the order for equipment, with patient details on a pager. For using the RFID tracking system, they had to then look up a computer at the workstation. However, orderlies were staff always on the move, and may not be near a workstation. This meant that they had to find a closest workstation first, then spend time looking up the system for the equipment (such as a bariatric wheel chair, considered high value/scarce equipment). During this time, the orderlies found it easier to manually look for the equipment that may be available on a corridor and then transport the patient to the destination. On further investigations, it was revealed that due to the lack of integration of the tracking system, the orderlies also had to learn the new interface, which they were reluctant to do, in the time they were in the hospital – without disrupting their routine work. According to the set of users, the system would be potentially more efficient and effectively reshape their workflows, if the pager message also came with the "location of the equipment" as it already has the required equipment and patient location. Therefore, if the RFID deployment was fully integrated with the hospital information system, the users felt that it will definitely enhance their work flows, enhance quality of care for the patients, resulting in time and cost savings.

The technology implementers also felt that there were cost, time and efficiencies experienced. However, the interviews revealed that the technologists were supportive of the user view. They indicated that technology and not the users drove the implementation of the pilot. In such environments, users being the major catalysts of success, to effectively reshape processes, the take up of the tracking system effectively would mean that the user friendliness of the system needed improvement. This effectively could only be achieved on deployment of a full implementation covering all the hospitals, rather than some areas. The efficiency of tracking equipment and small devices, accurately from a location, was not possible until a full deployment was completed. In addition, the integration with the clinical resource support system that eliminated the need for users to learn another interface (particularly that the users are mainly part time and casual staff) was imperative for the continued use of RFID tracking system, which would then bring in significant time and cost savings and reshape the processes more efficiently. The technologists also revealed that there is potential for the RFID tracking system to be integrated into other areas such as bedside applications/monitoring and extending into remote monitoring in a large multi-hospital environment, where patients do tend to "wander away". The extension into patient monitoring and after care, support would bring in better efficiencies for the hospital.

The strategic project managers who were involved in the deployment of the pilot and those who were to be involved in the future implementation on a large scale (particularly emergency services), also felt that the pilot revealed significant potential of the technology in time and cost savings and process efficiencies. The constraints of non-integration with the clinical resources support system and having to educate the users on a new user interface were already noted. According to the strategic manager, the fullscale implementation was only possible after the potential was demonstrated/experienced to certain level. This objective was achieved. The emerging issues of technology integration (i.e. the integration with the hospital information system that will eliminate the need to educate users on another interface) and accuracy of location was already considered for the future full scale implementation. The strategic managers expressed that the technology does have potential to be deployed for tracking resources and patients in the future, which will definitely reshape the processes within the hospital, making it more efficient. The staff time would be recorded more efficiently, their work processed enhanced and result in time and cost savings.

Technological integration with the hospital information systems and user education were the major factors to be addressed for a complete and large scale implementation. The potential of integrating and expanding the technology into other areas, with the involvement of users/technologists and user managers was critical for maximising the benefits of RFID in this context. Based on this information, we planned for a process redesign in one of the areas which had already felt the maximum benefits from the pilot: the Sterilising Services Unit.

As a first step, a one-to-one interview was conducted with the users and managers of the unit, so as to map the processes involved in this department as it occurs now. The process map was then confirmed with the users/managers. Subsequently, in consultation with them, we redesigned the processes for integrating RFID where applicable (as indicated in Figure 1).

It was found that there are couple of process areas that need to be redesigned. As depicted in Figure 1, there is a collection point, where

*Figure 1. Process redesign with RFID intervention (barcoding is replaced by RFID)*

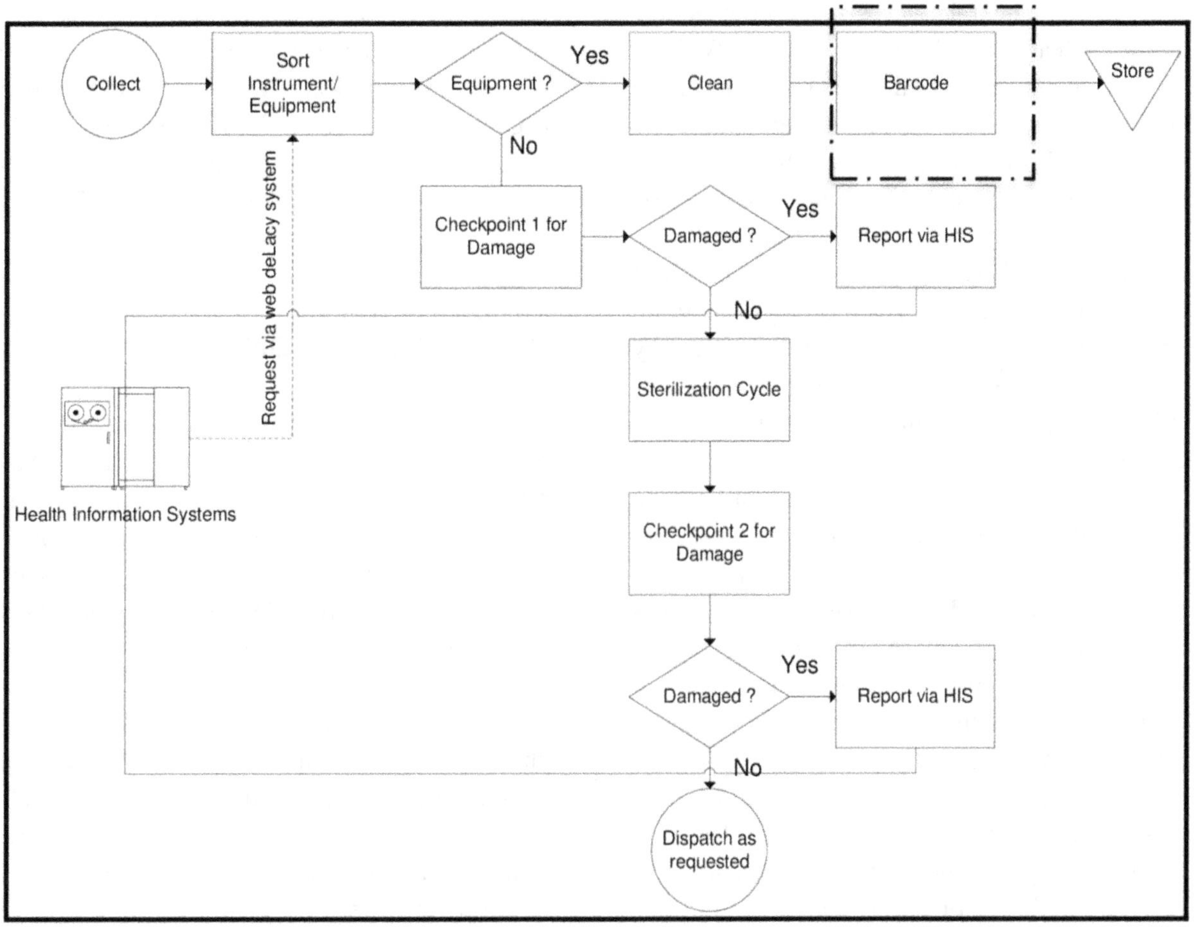


equipment and instruments are to be taken into the Sterilisation Unit, for undergoing the relevant processes of cleaning. The equipment and instruments are sorted separately and they go through different processes. For instruments, the cleaning process is simple, they are sorted, cleaned, and then bar code labelled. RFID tagging was recommended instead, so that these cleaned equipment, when then moves into their store (owned by the unit), can be traced quickly, when the equipment is requisitioned. The figure indicates the RFID intervention point. Conversely, if the sorting indicates these are instruments, they are sorted, arranged and placed in trays before sending into the next cycles of cleaning. All the sub processes of cleaning are not depicted in this diagram. Nonetheless, where RFID becomes relevant is the last cycle, when instruments are found to be damaged and therefore cannot be despatched as required for the relevant surgeries posted (which may be next day).

Specifically, the process works as follows. The requisitions for equipment and instruments come into the unit, via one of the sub-systems that are integrated into the Hospital's Information System (depicted as HIS in Figure 1). And the requisitions are addressed the same day. A print out is taken for the required equipment and these are gathered together, kept in an area for sending next day via an orderly or they are send out immediately via the person (orderly) who will collect them and take them to wherever required. However, if the requisitions come in towards end of the day, for a surgery posted next day, a set of instruments may go into a cleaning and sterilising cycle. When it finishes, they will be available at the end of the day. However, there is possibly no one at the time to check for damages. Therefore, when the orderly comes into collect the instruments next day morning, it may be found that the instruments may be damaged. Therefore, another set has to be sterilised and given. This causes a delay of anything between half hour to 2 hours, which can be very critical, if the patient is already under anaesthesia and on the operating table. Orderlies then search for alternatives, resulting in delays.

It was decided that the average incidents on delays in finding equipment will be documented, pre and post RFID integration, to study the efficiencies experienced. A redesign of the process was recommended, where the damage of equipment or instrument is reported via the Hospital Information System (HIS) the previous night, rather than waiting for the next day only to discover that there are critical instruments damaged causing delays. The integration of this redesigned process through the unit's information system and thereafter to the hospital information system was then planned. It is envisaged that this will reduce the delays in finding alternatives and enable rescheduling surgeries in advance. However, RFID systems are not "big brothers" in that they cannot monitor what is being done always. Nonetheless, RFID tracking within the cleaning cycles of the department, also cautions the staff to report any damage immediately, rather than leaving it for the next day.

At this juncture in the action research, two cycles were completed. At the end of the two cycles, the key learning indicated that no doubt, there is confidence in the ability of RFID as a technology for making processes efficient, when the user inputs were considered. Conversely, by initiating the deployment of RFID as a technology solution, the hospital was able to visualize the fragmented nature of its varied processes, resources that could be optimized and processes that could be made efficient, even without the RFID intervention at all levels. In the case of SSU, the intervention of RFID was the last mile, yet, it revealed many issues that could and need to be addressed for making processes efficient.

## SOLUTIONS AND RECOMMENDATIONS

As revealed in the literature as well as ongoing research investigation by first author in the Australian context, RFID implementation in hospitals seem to be an arbitrary process, often untimed, based on particular needs of a department/section, and often driven by vendors who would like to push the technology. We also find that many RFID implementations in hospitals require specific process changes within the departments, which are unique to them. Therefore, what is applicable in an emergency department may not be the same in an outpatient facility. A one size fits all integration approach cannot be envisaged, if the ultimate benefits have to outweigh costs of implementation. Therefore, we find the action research framework was useful for the iterative learning and informing another implementation.

Based on the learning from the action research, the researchers recommend RFID as a beneficial technology, to make processes efficient in large hospitals in concurrence with the literature synthesis presented in this chapter. Transcending this fact is the practical ability of the technology to become an analytical lens, to review existing processes within the hospital and the inconsistencies that can be addressed before any new technology is deployed. Based on this experience from the action research project, we recommend the approach that RFID as a technology is not simply plugged in, but, used as an analytical lens to review existing processes, so as to address existing inconsistencies, and then deployed where applicable – after redesigning processes suitably. This approach will help realise the full potential of the technology and help in evaluating its effectiveness to the context.

## FUTURE RESEARCH DIRECTIONS

Healthcare for average citizens have grown in importance, particularly in the western societies where significant expenditure occurs in this sector year after year. As the contemporary societies continue to demand better quality in health care facilities, hospitals continue to explore not only cost, but also time efficient approaches, that are now possible with emerging technologies. Among these wide ranging choices, the humble RFID technology which uses radio waves has emerged a winner in large hospitals, where this technology offers a cost efficient, uncomplicated solution for making processes efficient so as to enhance the quality of care. As this technology became widely accepted in hospitals, pilots and deployments proliferated, nonetheless, without considering its optimum benefits. While the technology can today be deployed for tracking high value assets in emergency settings, which reduces expenditure for hospitals, it can also be deployed for tracking patients and medical staff in emergencies. This is particularly useful in extending health care, by enhancing the efficiency in processes.

In alignment with the theme of this book, this chapter presented the technology, its emerging acceptance in hospitals, benefits experiences as well as issues that could be addressed. In addition, we introduce the readers to the opportunity that this technology presents i.e. to be utilized as an analytical lens as well as a technology solution in hospitals. The viability of this novel approach is already tested at one site, and is being progressively undertaken to validate it. In the domain of RFID and Business Process Management, this chapter offers a perspective to develop further research. As the research is based on real experience validation, it also offers researchers an opportunity to collaboratively develop this area with industry/practitioners.

## CONCLUSION AND CONTRIBUTIONS

Technologies to make processes efficient in hospitals are not a new paradigm. As technologies evolve, become cheaper, their utilization in healthcare and particularly large hospitals where resources are shared, is becoming rampant. However, many emergent technologies are deployed without user consultation and without reviewing existing processes completely so as to eliminate inconsistencies before the technology can realize its potential. RFID is such a technology, which has been accepted widely in hospitals, due to its relatively uncomplicated nature. Nonetheless, the deployment has often been capricious. Vendors have driven most of the deployments with vested interests. Nonetheless, there have been some failures and successes.

This chapter provided insights into the technology as it evolved, some key deployments worldwide followed by the role of business process redesign/management in the context. Subsequently, it discussed the findings from an action research in a setting where RFID was deployed, abandoned and then is being reconsidered again after the BPM approach has been used as a framework. The message of this chapter is that technologies as such must not be viewed in isolation, but rather in context. The result is that often the technology may have the potential to transcend its original expectation. In this instance, RFID has helped the hospital review its resources, inconsistencies in the processes and address them, such that process redesign for optimal utilization of technology was then possible.

The approach of utilizing RFID as a lens and a tool offers a new perspective in BPM research where the standard approach is to redesign processes to plug-in a technology, without reviewing the existing process. The new perspective offers collaborative research opportunities for academics and industry, to work together to develop this area and contribute to the body of knowledge.

## ACKNOWLEDGMENT

The authors would like to thank the anonymous reviewers and the editor for their insightful comments and suggestions.

## REFERENCES

Avison, D., Lau, F., Myers, M., & Nielsen, P. A. (1999). Action Research. *Communications of the ACM*, *42*(1), 94–97. doi:10.1145/291469.291479

Bacheldor, B. (2006, October). RFID Fills Security Gap at Psychiatric Ward. *RFID Journal*.

Bacheldor, B. (2007, August). RFID documents surgery at Huntsville hospital. *RFID Journal*.

Baldwin, G., & Larkin, M. (2008, January). Where did we put that wheelchair?. *Technology, HealthLeaders*, 33-34.

Bliernel, M., & Hassanein, K. (2004). E-health: applying business process reengineering principles to healthcare in Canada. *International Journal of Electronic Business*, *2*(6), 625–643. doi:10.1504/IJEB.2004.006129

Brand, N., & Kolk, H. V. D. (1995). *Workflow Analysis and Design*. Kluwer.

Buchanan, D. (1998). Representing process: the contribution of a re-engineering frame. *International Journal of Operations & Production Management*, *18*(12), 1163–1188. doi:10.1108/01443579810236610

Cavoukian, A. (2008). *RFID and Privacy - Guidance for Health Care Providers- A report*. January, Canada: Information Privacy Commissioner of Ontario and Hewlett Packard Company.

Chen, C. C., Wu, J., Su, Y. S., & Yang, S. C. (2008). Key drivers for the continued use of RFID technology in the emergency room. *Management Research News*, *31*(4), 273–288. doi:10.1108/01409170810851348

Collins, J. (2005, July). India adopts 865-867 MHz for RFID. *RFID Journal*.

Cox, J. (2008). RFID proving to be Rx for hospitals. *Network World*, *25*(33), 24.

Fisher, J. A., & Monahan, T. (2008). Tracking the social dimensions of RFID systems in hospitals. *International Journal of Medical Informatics*, *77*(3), 176–183. doi:10.1016/j.ijmedinf.2007.04.010 PMID:17544841

Fraunholz, B. (2001). Project Management in the German Trade Sector – A (preliminary) framework for computer assisted management of Projects in Small and Medium Sized Enterprises. In *Proceedings of Australasian Conference on Information Systems*. Academic Press.

Godinez, V. (2007). *RFID tracks hospitals devices: System improves heart facility's care, 29th April*. Dallas, TX: Dallas Morning News.

GOI. (2002). National Health Policy. Government of India, NIC, India.

Greene, J. (2005, September). Is your Hospital Ready for Radio Frequency Identification? Above Board Technology. *Trustee*, 30–32. PMID:16196403

Gunasekaran, A., & Ichimura, T. (1997). Business Process Reengineering: Modelling and Analysis. *International Journal of Production Economics*, *50*, 65–68. doi:10.1016/S0925-5273(97)00031-5

Hammer, M. (1990). Reengineering Work: Don't automate, obliterate. *Harvard Business Review*, *68*(4), 104–113.

Harrop, P. (2006). Rapid Adoption of RFID in Healthcare. *RFID in Healthcare 2006-2016, idtechex*.

HFM. (2006, August). RFID tracks ED overcrowding, Technology. *Health Facilities Management*, 8.

H&HN. (2004, May). Beyond Bar Codes, Technology, Inbox. *Hospitals and Health Networks Magazine*, 26.

H&HN. (2005, June). Behind the Hype, Technology, Inbox. *Hospitals and Health Networks Magazine*, 22-24.

Hoskins, R. (2006). *InfoLogix Announces HealthTrax RFID Asset Tracking Software for Hospital Mobile Assets Management*. Retrieved March 30, 2006 from http://www.bbwexchange.com/pubs/2006/02/11/page1395-98309.asp

Indulska, M., Recker, J., Rosemann, M., & Greene, P. (2009). Business process modelling: Current issues and future Challenges. In P. Van Eck, J. Gordijn, & R. Wierings (Eds.), CAiSE 2009, (LNCS) (vol. 5565, pp. 501–514). Berlin: Springer. doi:10.1007/978-3-642-02144-2_39

Jansen-Vullers, M.H., & Reijers, H.A. (2005). Business Process Redesign in HealthCare: Towards a structured approach. *INFOR - Journal of the Canadian Operational Research Society*, *43*(4), 321-339.

RFID Journal. (2005, August). A summary of RFID standards. *RFID Journal*.

Kahn, M. (2008, June). RFID in hospitals could pose risks. *PC Magazine Online*, 25.

Landt, J. (2001, October). *Shrouds of Time: The history of RFID*. Association for Automatic Identification and Mobility.

Lee, C. P., & Shim, J. P. (2007). An exploratory study of radio frequency identification (RFID) adoption in the healthcare industry. *European Journal of Information Systems*, *16*, 712–772. doi:10.1057/palgrave.ejis.3000716

Maillart, L.M., Kamrani, A., Norman B.A., Rajgopal, J., & Hawrylak, P.J. (2010). Optimizing RFID tag-inventorying algorithms. *IEEE Transactions*, (42), 690-702.

Mehrjerdi, Y. Z. (2008). RFID enabled systems: a brief review. *Assembly Automation*, *28*(3), 235–245. doi:10.1108/01445150810889493

Nagy, P., George, I., Bernstein, W., Caban, J., Klein, R., Mezrich, R., & Park, A. (2006). Radio Frequency Identification Systems Technology in the Surgical Setting. *Surgical Innovation*, *13*(1), 61–67. doi:10.1177/155335060601300110 PMID:16708157

Nahas, H. A., & Deogun, J. S. (2007). Radio Frequency Identification Applications in Smart Hospitals. In *Proceedings of the Twentieth IEEE International Symposium on Computer-Based Medical Systems (CBMS'07)*. IEEE.

O'Connor, M.C. (2005, August). Efficiencies Drive RFID adoption. *RFID Journal*.

O'Connor, M.C. (2006, November). Toronto area hospital kicks off asset tracking pilot. *RFID Journal*.

Page, L. (2007, August). Hospitals tap into RFID to track patients and equipment, Upfront, News and Trends. *Health Facilities Management*, 5–6.

Page L. (2007, May). Hospitals tune into RFID – Testing gives way to implementation. *Material Management in Health Care*, 18-20.

Pappu, M., Singhal, R., & Zoghi, B. (2004). *RFID in hospitals: Issues and Solutions*. A report from the Consortium for the Accelerated Deployment of RFID in Distribution.

Roark, D. C., & Miguel, K. (2006). Bar coding's replacement? *Nursing Management*, *37*(2), 29–31. doi:10.1097/00006247-200602000-00009 PMID:16452888

Rosemann, M. (2006). Potential Pitfalls in process modelling- Part 1. *Business Process Management Journal*, *12*(2), 249-254.

Simpson, G. (2007). Hospitals need RFID injection. *ZdNet Asia Communications.*

Snyder, K. D., Paulson, P., & McGrath, P. (2005). Improving processes in a small health care network: A value mapping case study. *Business Process Management Journal*, *2*(1), 87-99.

Thomas, K. (2008, May 30). Radio wrist tags that make for smoother operations: A technology for tracing consumer goods may help save lives and keep track of hospital equipment. *Financial Times*, p. 12.

Unnithan, C., Smith, R., & Fraunholz, B. (2009). Maximising the Benefits of Radio Frequency Identification Technology (RFID) Integration in Clinical Contexts: A Linear Conduit. In *Proceedings of HIC'09 Conference*. Canberra: Health Informatics Society of Australia.

Waterman, H., Marshall, M., Noble, J., Davies, H., Wakshe, K., Sheaff, R., & Elwyn, G. (2007). The role of action research in the investigation and diffusion of innovations in health care: The Pride Project. *Qualitative Health Research*, *17*(3), 373–381. doi:10.1177/1049732306298976 PMID:17301345

Wicks, A.M., & Visich, J.K., & Suhong, L. (2006). Radio Frequency Identification Applications in Hospital Environments. *Hospital Topics*, *84*(3), 3–8. doi:10.3200/HTPS.84.3.3-9 PMID:16913301

## ADDITIONAL READING

Chao, C. C., Yang, J. M., & Jen, W. Y. (2007) Determining technology trends and forecasts of RFID by a historical review and bibliometric analysis from 1991 to 2005, Technovation, Elsevier, 268-279.

Chung-Chih, L., Po-Kuan, L., Guan-Yu, H., Wei-Lun, L., & Ren-Guey, L. (2008). A Healthcare Integration System for Disease Assessment and Safety Monitoring of Dementia Patients. *IEEE Transactions on Information Technology in Biomedicine*, *12*(5), 579–586. doi:10.1109/TITB.2008.917914 PMID:18779072

Sun, P. R., Wang, B. H., & Wu, F. (2008). A New Method to Guard Inpatient Medication Safety by the Implementation of RFID. *Journal of Medical Systems*, *32*, 327–332. doi:10.1007/s10916-008-9137-9 PMID:18619096

## KEY TERMS AND DEFINITIONS

**Active RFID Tags:** Have an internal lithium battery power source that continuously receives and transmits signals on various different frequencies. The power source is used to run the microchip's circuitry and to broadcast a signal to a reader (the way a cell phone transmits to a base station. It uses a battery for both the chip and the transmission of data on the antenna. It has an internal data storage capability. Active tags have a limited life, are heavier and more expensive when compared to passive tags.

**BPR/BPM:** Business Process Redesign (BPR) is a process for assessing performance issues of a particular process and conducting radical redesign to the process, by redesigning the process itself and systems, policies or organizational structures. Business Process Management (BPM) is the method of managing the redesign and redeployment of business processes within a given situation and organization.

**Low-Frequency RFID Tags:** Read from a foot or less, High frequency RFID tags are read from about three feet and Ultra High Frequency (UHF) tags are read from 10 to 20 feet.

**Passive RFID Tags:** Those which react when the signal is received they are powered by an electronic reader and store small amount of data. They receive energy from a remote RFID reader. They have a 3 feet range of 3 feet approximately. Passive tags have no batteries, instead they draw power from the reader, which sends out electromagnetic waves that induce a current in the tag's antenna".

**RFID:** Radio Frequency Identification (RFID) is commonly defined as wireless technology for automatic identification of objects or people. It is an object recognition technology.

**Semi Passive RFID Tags:** Similar to passive tags except they have an internal power source that increases the storage capacity and the range. They use a small on board battery to power the chip.

**Semi-Active RFID Tags:** Use the battery for powering the antenna but the chip relies on the RF energy from the reader.

# Chapter 11
# Use and Reuse of Electronic Health Records:
## Building Information Systems for Improvement of Health Services

**Michele Ceruti**
*University of Turin, Italy*

**Silvio Geninatti**
*Catholic University "Sacro Cuore", Italy & Statistics and Epidemiological Research, Italy*

**Roberta Siliquini**
*University of Turin, Italy*

## ABSTRACT

*Electronic Health Record (EHR) is a term with several meanings, even if its very definition allows distinguishing it from other electronic records of healthcare interest, such as Electronic Medical Records (EMR) and Personal Health Records (PHR). EMR is the electronic evolution of paper-based medical records, while PHR is mainly the collection of health-related information of a single individual. All of these have many points in common, but the interchangeable use of the terms leads to several misunderstandings and may threaten the validity and reliability of EHR applications. EHRs are more structured and conform to interoperability standards, and include a huge quantity of data of very large populations. Thus, they have proven to be useful for both theoretical and practical purposes, especially for Public Health issues. In this chapter, the authors argue that the appropriate use of EHR requires a realistic comprehensive concept of e-health by all the involved professions. They also show that a change in the "thinking" of e-health is necessary in order to achieve tangible results of improvement in healthcare services through the use of EHR.*

DOI: 10.4018/978-1-4666-6316-9.ch011

## INTRODUCTION

Electronic records are being produced in several health contexts, mainly hospital, laboratory services, imaging services, insurance claims.

The aim of this chapter is to understand the nature of electronic health records, their subtypes, their expectations, the grey areas, those that need more clarification and disambiguation, the concerns about misuse and misinterpretation, highlighting the real potential for the ethical development of Information technology in healthcare.

As it has been stated (Habib, 2010), EHR technology is an important piece of health information technology infrastructure and is a cornerstone for reform health care systems across the world. EHR is an important tool for the improvement of health care quality, efficiency, and patient safety, diminishing research costs, decreasing the inefficiencies associated with paper based research and aligning research with implementation of new health technology devices. (Weiskopf & Weng, 2012).

Most countries are now focusing healthcare delivery through a health informatics strategy. EHR has been focused as the central power tool in most of the national e-health and HIT strategies, including telemedicine, personalized medicine, and large-scale genome analysis projects (Ruch, 2010).

## DEFINITION OF EHR

A semantic problem that researchers, engineers and developers in the field of Health Technology will encounter if they intend to extend the research on the topic both in Biomedical and in Engineering literature is the confusion between EHR and other electronic records. We believe that the core of the correct evolution of such a vision with the patient at the centre of care delivery needs a clear definition of what is and what is not an "electronic health record".

According to the current literature, the definition of EHR is evolving and still confusing (Hayrinen, Saranto & Nykanen, 2008). Electronic health records may include all health-related information on electronic support: Electronic medical record (EMR), Personal health record (PHR) and Electronic personal record (EPR). All these terms are often used interchangeably, although there are huge differences between each of them. This confusion has been propagated not only by the scientific community but by governments, consultants and vendors as well. (Healthcare Information and Management Systems Society [HIMSS] 2006).

It is conceivable to consider "widely" all these as health electronic records but scientists, developers and users are confused by these interchangeable meanings. Electronic health records need first of all to be defined as clearly as possible, in order to avoid any confusion in its interpretation and application. This is the reason for which we call the attention to the following definitions and clarifications.

In 2008 the US National Alliance for Health Information Technology defined EHR, EMR and PHR as separate concepts.

**Electronic Medical Record:** *An electronic record of health-related information on an individual that can be created, gathered, managed, and consulted by authorized clinicians and staff within one healthcare organization.*

**Electronic Health Record:** *An electronic record of health-related information on an individual that conforms to nationally recognized interoperability* *standards and that can be created, managed, and consulted by authorized clinicians and staff across more than one healthcare organization.*

**Personal Health Record:** *An electronic record of health-related information on an individual that conforms to nationally recognized interoperability standards and that can be drawn from multiple sources while being managed, shared, and controlled by the individual.*

*(National Alliance for Health Information Technology, 2008)*

This is the first official precision that allowed not only to distinguish EHR from other codified (or defined) concepts such as EMR and PHR but moreover to define clearly that EHR are not any medical mass of unstructured data stored without standards or rules from any clearinghouse around the world or from user-produced extractions of health data through the web.

Other important health information data, which may be collected as unstructured health records, are the ones directly produced and controlled by Internet users. These data are the information substratum of the so defined e-health 2.0. and are substantially separated from health information produced by technologies within the official care delivery organizations. They might, instead, be integrated within the framework of Health IT in a further evolution of the vision of personal health, care delivery and legal policy for all their challenging and potentially hazardous consequences. Indeed, health information research by Internet customers showed some evidence of measurable effects on health behaviors, such as drug consumption and access to healthcare providers (Siliquini et al., 2011). The comprehensive influence in health behaviors induced by the growing user-generated health information data with the health 2.0 is still uncertain and need further investigations. At moment, it is impossible to merge this health information with the severely structured and controlled data of the official EHRs.

## Disambiguation of EHR and EMR

Another important distinction to do in order to allow some clarity among electronic records related to health and health delivery is to clarify more precisely the differences between EHR and EMR.

In 2010, the Office of the National Coordinator for Health Information Technology (ONC) of the United States made an important distinction between the terms *EHR* and *EMR*.

"The EHR is the system that gives patients, physicians and other healthcare providers, employers, and payers or insurers access to a patient's medical records across facilities" (Garrett &Seidman, 2011), thus going beyond the restrictions and the geographical limitations, the mission of the healthcare provider and the possible fit-for-purpose health information technology system. It goes over the interpretation models applied within any single provider, allowing a more comprehensive patient history.

"The EMR is the legal patient record that is created in hospitals and ambulatory environments" (Garrett & Seidman, 2011). It is very important to note that EHR advances in quality, safety and accountability cannot be separated from the ones of EMR, as these are the main data source for EHR. Thus, the more EMR will be performing, well-built and predisposed to sharing, the more the portability and interoperability goals of EHR will be met, with higher quality accuracy of information gathered (The National Alliance for Health Information Technology, 2008). The collection from different EMRs is obviously enriching and depends on the policy of the national or regional EHR promoter.

As the term suggests in itself, EMR may be assumed as the electronic evolution of the "paper medical record". EMR may be unstructured, narrative, codified in several different ways according to the different services, uses and even habits. Clinicians, nurses, and administrative personnel produce EMRs. According to different countries it may be only a collection of clinical data or else a highly protected official legal document (but these differences are legally based on the different interpretation or use of the Medical records, electronic or not).

According to the Australian e-health Standards (2010), EHRs are information repositories that are "collected primarily to support the provision of integrated holistic healthcare to that individual but may also be used, subject to legislation and consent, for secondary purposes that benefit the health of the wider community".

The fundamental concept of a correct EHR is that it may be *sharable* and *comparable* with other collected health information. A further concept of EHR is *interoperability*. All these concepts are possible only if appropriate levels of standardization will be ensured.

EHR, according to official definitions that have been cited might be defined as any structured record that belongs to a official national or regional collector, through direct inputting or by extraction from medical databases. Specific rules must be followed, and data will be collected in information systems built according to official standards, and that may allow interoperability for further interpretation. (Habib, J. L., 2010)

The reason for which EHR models based on hospital information are much more prevalent across the world (rather than on primary care, ambulatory and laboratory settings) can be explained by the pre-existence of several structured EMR systems for hospitals. The transition from Paper Medical record, actually a medico-legal document that has been eminently recognized since a long time, has been much easier than the conception of the process care management taken by General Practitioners or by others health delivery actors. As for the management of in-patient data, formalized paper-based medical records are widely being used across the world, the shift to the electronic version has been less difficult. Actually, there are however quite a few complications that are directly connected with the construction of EHR. Conceptually EHR are indeed the electronic based evolution of a concept that is quite nearer to epidemiology databases and to health delivery management, but it is actually a tool primarily used for accountancy purposes, thus depleting it from its full potential (Hersh et al., 2013). A probable cause of this may be the need of a deeper underlying Public Health strategy. EHR may encourage the use of clinical decision support and for the use and evaluation of technologies. Vice versa the Health Technology Assessment Methodology may be enriched by EHR system.

While EMR models are expression of the health provider's policy or CDO's strategy, EHR seek to meet higher international semantic and architecture standards and aim to put the patient at the centre of data management. EHR data can be created, managed, and consulted by authorized providers across different health care organization. International aims are to build patient-centered EHR models in order to allow health data to move together with the patient whatever the health events he will come upon, such as medical encounters, hospitalization, home care delivery, nursing, etc. The international aspiration of EHR, such as it has been experienced in the US-India cooperation (Government Computer Based Patient Record Project [G-CPR], 1999) and in the EU, (epSOS - European Patients - Smart open Service), is to extend the *portability* (with all the standards concerning language, semantic, messaging, security, privacy) across different countries.

## EHR STANDARDS

Standard documentation must guarantee the unique identification of subjects, processes (or even subprocesses), providers, devices, codified diagnosis, treatment and potentially final outcomes.

Very often, clinicians are called to apply to recommendation ensuring all of these standards. Albeit, the compliance to such standard application is not the primarily mission of clinicians. Healthcare practitioners are indeed more and more suffering from an excess of constraining rules in the compilation of electronic records. As it has been suggested above, a frequent bias is that health care personnel is thought to be involved directly with EHR, whereas what there are filling are mainly "Electronic Medical records", more and more frequently through IT systems that may ensure completeness and easiness of compilation. Now it is interesting to note that EMR may not be the simple translation of a paper record to a digital support. There is instead the need of professional development among the involved human resources in order to enhance their own **flexibility** toward the "filling" of electronic records. By such a use, they are also called to be accustomed to a greater rigor in both the identification of concepts that must be filled or transcribed in the EMR, especially in the different phases of the process of care (intermediate diagnosis and procedures) as well as in the identification of the final outcome, that shall be "matching" with logical predetermined fields or checks in templates (final diagnosis, setting the follow-up, etc.). All these are essential competencies that cannot be mastered passively by only applying routine tasks, but need purpose-built vocational training programs. The enhancement of e-health in healthcare services will become crucial in the following years, involving all professionals, especially nurses and health technicians. The capacity building of all these professionals is a core component for an appropriate integration of all e-health applications within healthcare services. The promotion of a new way of thinking health is an essential step for a proper skill acquisition among all involved actors (i.e. health workers) for the approach, the utilization and the management of electronic health information.

In order to promote the *interoperability* of health informatics applications, many frameworks for health informatics standards have been proposed and have been made available. According to Sinha (2013) the essential ones are:

- Structural standards.
- Data content standards.
- Data exchange standards.
- Security standards.

EN 13606 European Standard is the first EU official "structural" proposal for a rigorous and stable *architecture* for the communication among partner and sharers of EHRs regarding any single subject of care. Through this standard, EHR building systems comprise two fundamental parts: a Root Architecture Component and a Record Component. The standards deal with Architecture, Domain Term Lists, Distribution Rules and Message for Information Exchange. The latter has been since 2006 the one that has influenced more deeply data exchange, through HL7 v3 standard, for the development of reliable and compatible paths for sharing information. This part of the EN 13606 explicitly focuses the possibility of rendering more easy the extraction of data from different environments, in observance of the ISO RM-ODP Information viewpoint for EHR Extract. This standards supports *interoperability* of different systems that need to transfer add or complete interchangeably without losing or overwriting previous messages, notes, preserving the privacy of attended by the health practitioner and the confidentiality of the patient towards data (see below for a WHO proposed distinction between privacy and confidentiality).

This standard is based also on the relatively new paradigm of "object" model for information sharing and does not restrict this modeling in the way the internal architecture and setting can be applied. The intention is to propose a guideline for designing or transforming EHR systems in a way that might not completely overwhelm the already existing health information systems through the building of a common set of external interfaces or communication procedures.

It is worth noting, however, that EN 13606 ignores ISO RM-ODP views towards behavioral aspects of EHR systems (Blobel, Engel & Pharow, 2006).

In the frame of HL7, *open*-EHR defines a method of querying based on archetypes, known as AQL (Archetype Querying Language). This is achieved by the innovation of 'multi-level modeling', whereby clinical content is standardized using a modeling layer known as 'archetypes' that is separate from the data standards layer. The openEHR foundation, integrating threads of R&D in Europe and Australia (openEHR, 2013), is an important example of such an application and implementation evolution of EN 13606. (Weiner, Fowles & Chan, 2012).

## APPLICATIONS OF EHR

Databases actually contain both structured and unstructured information such as patient gender, age, diagnosis and treatment or event features, hospital admission, length of stay and, furthermore, social conditions, eating and drinking habits.

Several Institutes and Official Boards have appointed the *reuse* of EHR as the future instrument for clinical research, health delivery management, quality assessment but also decision making for health policy. Research communities in the field of clinical engineering, epidemiology and health management have been actively searching new methodologies for enable secondary use of electronic data, enhancing accuracy and accountability (Hersh et al., 2013).

In the classification of research areas of EHR proposed by Najaftorkaman, Ghapanchi, Talaei-Khoei and Ray (2013), two topics are addressed to application research: impacts in terms of healthcare improvement and medical research.

### Healthcare Improvement

EHR for its very definition is already the output of a secondary use of EMR and of other electronic records. The concept that allows defining an EHR is actually the possibility of interoperability and reuse for any purpose. This reutilization may be interpreted both for profit and non-profit purposes.

In HIT (Health information technology) domain, reuse concerns the effort to optimize resources and investments particularly regarding software. High economic investments, performed technological research activities, sharing knowledge aims to support the necessity to assume reuse strategy.

Translating the concept of reuse, EHR availability enables a large opportunity for further interpretation and meta-interpretation in several scientific fields (Hripcsak, Albers, 2012). Health data reuse indeed has been focused as an e-government tool allowing both spending rationalization and more effective services supply (Blobel et al. 2006). Information is gathered in order to sustain adaptability of software development to customer needs, according to the fit-for use paradigm (Weiskopf & Weng, 2007; Hayrinen, Saranto & Nykanen 2008).

A topic that has led particular attention is the possibility to enhance the management and the monitoring of well-known and prevalent chronic diseases. In fact, during the last century the importance of chronic diseases has been expanding dramatically, especially in industrialized countries. Increased life expectancy, improved social and economic status, clinical care systems effective efforts to ensure better conditions, induces an increased risk for the general population to be affected from a chronic disease, thus inducing a continuous increase in health care spending for these conditions. Risk factors are quite known, mainly attributable to lifestyle like unhealthy diet, physical inactivity and tobacco and alcohol use. These causes do not work directly but through intermediate risk factors such as abnormal lipids level, raised blood pressure, impaired glucose levels and obesity. Still, others non-modifiable factors must be included like age and heredity. Moreover, a significant interaction between the major modifiable risk factors and the main chronic diseases has been observed in both low and high income countries and the impact of risk factors increases over the life course. All these information are potentially recordable in Health Information Systems. Acute or chronic complications and death associated to chronic diseases may be monitored through EHR. A valid support for monitoring hospitalization and follow-up of patients may be provided with information about the patient path within the hospital gathering main and secondary diagnoses, medical procedures or surgical interventions submission (according to ICD9-CM or ICD-10 classification according to different countries or to health delivery subset such as Medicare and Medicaid Program in the US).

Estimate occurrence, identify risk factors, evaluate potential determinants and precursors has began a core function of Public Health Institutions (Goldwater et al., 2013). Information related or perceived by patients such as health status, diet, tobacco and alcohol use, and physical activity may be gathered through electronic records together with evident clinical records such as blood pressure, body mass index (BMI), blood lipids level, and so on. Evidence based medicine approach implies the applications of effective procedures in diseases management. Guidelines collect recommendations about clinical management from best evidence based to provide health care through the application of diagnosis and therapeutic steps. EHR implementation may allow a better drug compliance of patients affected by hypertension or diabetes, the frequency of specific check-up, and a better appropriateness of healthcare services. Indeed, any clinical event may been recorded thus allowing the traceability of the whole disease history. Moreover EHR implementation for Public Health may allow the assessment of the impact of actions towards chronic disease monitoring and policies (Albu et al. 2013; Kudyakov et al., 2012; Maylahn, Fleming & Birkhead, 2013).

## Medical Research

The most important field of medical research that has been involving actively EHR in the last years is the Comparative Effectiveness Research (CER). Applying an Evidence Based Medicine (EBM) approach through EHR is not incongruous, as Hersh et al (2013) have pointed out. EHR information elaboration may be considered as observational data analysis. In contrast to RCTs and EBM projects designed to focus on specific aspects in selected samples, EHR-based research may much more reflective or real clinical world, because of the very large size of EHR, and much less expensive.

Use of EHR for Genomic information is under investigations. Several ethical (behavioral) and bioethical issues have been highlighted. Research may be profit of secondary use of existing EHR but it is obvious that fit for purpose model built especially and appropriately for the bimolecular and genomic research will be needed. Experts from the whole world are working together trying to merge all the methodology and the art in a unique apposite network (US eMERGE network -The Electronic Medical Records and Genomics Network).

Another interesting progress of e-health that will lead to evolutions in EHR applications is the implementation of Mobile Health (mHealth) systems, that will apply mobile communication technologies to healthcare delivery more efficiently (Zuehlke, Li, Talaei-Khoei & Ray, 2009). The convergence of progression of telemedicine, mHealth and other emerging health information technologies will make increasingly necessary the homogenization of electronic records both at coding and messaging levels.

## CONCERNS AND LIMITS OF EHR

There are albeit increasing concerns about the limits of EHR use (Bernat 2013; Steers 2013). EHR information use is already offering several benefits, but they can also foster errors that would not have been possible with paper based information use. This phenomenon has been termed e-iatrogenesis (Weiner, Kfuri, Chan & Fowles, 2007).

Burnum (1989) stated that the introduction of information technology for health data gathering has allowed disposing to a greater amount of bad data rather than to data of improved quality.

An important statement proposed by van der Lei (1991) is that "data shall be used only for purpose for which they were collected" in order to avoid misuse and misinterpretation. The core of most of this concern is the "processing" of data. Research orientation, epidemiology assumption and public health decision are all based on interpretation of available health information. If this interpretation is human based, it may content several biases. It is obvious, however, that research have always been based not only on information collected through purpose-built investigative systems but often through manual retrieval of useful health information of medical records, claims, registries and so on. For these purposes, the formation of the researcher was very important, as he was called to seize and grasp when and where information are congruent with targets and goals of the research. (Weiskopf et al. 2013; Roukema et al., 2006).

Medication ordering and monitoring seem to be very sensitive to errors (that may be of interest also for the promotion of telemedicine and telecare). Two kind of errors have been highlighted: 1) simple errors such as duplicate medication orders. 2) complex errors due to error in human-EHR interface, mainly errors in data recognition and cognitive errors (Institute of Medicine, 2012; Ash et al., 2011).

These topics are increasingly of interest for risk management in healthcare. The rise of simplicity of collect gather and retrieve data will be accompanied by an increase of the complexity of the "possible" errors as well of the complexity of algorithms, techniques and preventive measures against that risk.

In 1984, Horwitz and Yu reported three kinds of data-recording errors:

- Conflicting data in the source text;
- Information not transcribed;
- Transcription errors (i.e. errors during transcription).

This classification is clear and pragmatic, but is quite old as it does not take into account the possibility of the immediate filling of health records, bypassing the need for transcription to file.

Weiner, Fowles and Chan (2012) have proposed more recently three main electronic record related errors in their e-QM EHR quality measure:

- Incorrect medication ascribable to HIT-related errors in the CPOE/e-prescribing process;
- Erroneous sentinel event impacting in patient management;
- Not received automatically EHR system based e-notification resulting in patient harm.

There is another important distinction between error of omission (lack of completeness) and error of commission (lack of correctness)

As discussed by Weiskopf, Hripcsak, Swaminathan and Weng (2013) the complex issue of EHR completeness overtakes the statistical view of data missing. This is even more considerable because of the heterogeneity of EHR information source.

Lacks of EHRs related to a single patient during a period of time may be actually a error due to one of the following reasons:

1. There may be a lack in the information system of the EHR: for example the patient may have accessed a health provider that is connected with the EHR system.
2. The provider that should have collected the record has not accomplished correctly, partially or totally his mission.
3. There is the actual absence of medical encounter: this is known also as "extrinsic incompleteness" and may be due both to the actual healthy condition of the index subject (there is no reason for a medical encounter) or may be due to:
    a. Objective ignorance of the unhealthy condition;
    b. Subjective misperception of the unhealthy condition;
    c. Objective refusal, impossibility or renounce of the patient to access any health provider (this is possible in case of follow-up or secondary encounter).

This last possibility is much easier in countries where health services are paid for by third parts (Bernat, 2013).

Other dimensions of completeness have been investigated, (Blobel, 2006) but are specific objects of EMRs of healthcare providers, such as granular completeness and task-dependent completeness. As it has been highlighted, granularity and precision of electronic sources of EHRs are an important target for development of EHR consistency and reliability, however there are not specific feature that may be focused at that higher level.

Healthcare systems tend now especially in United Europe to develop platforms of cooperation and networks for which interoperability is highly necessary. EHR systems must meet first of all requirements of *flexibility* and *interoperability* through semantic integration.

The Governmental Computer-based patient Record (G-CPR) has been an important international effort concluded in 2003 that involved the US Department of Defense, the US Department of Veterans Affairs and the Indian Health Service trying to adhere to HL7 standards and to enable bi-directional secure sharing of patient health information among international participating agencies through the implementation of purpose built environments (GPCR, 2001). This is an example of fit for purpose EHR ideation, that has aimed to adhere to international standards and helped to the identification of critical points.

## ETHICAL ISSUES

Most of ethical issues raised by EHR use and in implementing strategies involving EMR and health delivery data management as well, were already seen with paper records. Therefore, ease of access, transmission and sharing have elicited more risk of violation of patient confidentiality, privacy and misuse of sharing (Bernat, 2013; Burnum, 1989). According to what stated by WHO in 2012, the concepts of privacy and confidentiality are defined referring to the way of relationship between the parts involved with a sensitive information.

In particular, EHR *privacy* reflects both the interest of the involved person as well of the public as a stakeholder to keep the information safe, away from any third party view.

EHR *confidentiality* concerns the degree to which the subject allows to share the information with relatives and other people with trusted relationship, as well as the government and application of such a rule, according to different laws and formalized codes.

Research models are focusing the attention on how to enhance patient-centered EHR evolution and amelioration keeping intact the standards improving reliability keeping confidentiality. Practical examples have been developed through problem-oriented approach aiming to a multi-professional electronic patient record (De Clercq, 2008).

In the field of EMR, "copying and pasting" issues have been illustrated by Thielke (2007) that provoked as well ambiguities of authorship with associated medico-legal concerns. There is no doubt that this problem has always existed, has been enlarged by first implementation of electronic records at hospital, primary care and other health providers and might have undermined derived EHR, but may be overcome by templates in which specification are mandatory and by second and third level quality controls. The challenging question is whether it is better to prefer a rigid template or a flexible format. This is the dilemma between *flexibility* and *uniformity* of data, that has been underpinned by Los, Ginneken, Roukema, Moll and van der Lei (2005): the advance of health data information availability may be accompanied by a lost in details, uniformity tending to lower quality data, too schematic and too synthetic with the hazard of artificial information.

Computerized Physician Order Entry (CPOE) users may not be satisfied by the possibility displayed, according to what found in the clinical findings; this issue is obviously more consistent for medical history and physical examination signs. Doctors and nurses may fill directly records of concluding judgment and to be inclined to prefer normal findings. In order to prevent this issue, it has been suggested (and already implemented) to separate rigidly findings from interpretations in separate format of the grid. (Los et al. 2005). Another problem is that checkboxes, very often associated for the filling the EMRs do not conceive all the degrees of subtlety of the clinical information. Indeed rigid templates may induce a more subjective derive and to avoid circumlocutory and bombastic language, not always associated to specific and distinguishable definition or feature. Another EMR-related pitfall is the presence of excess of rigidity built around the chief complaint that is an important voice for EHR. Indeed, some EMR allow automatically generated grid of questions from the selected chief complaint, potentially misleading the patient, especially in the case of multidisciplinary patient management (for example if a nurse or a trainee manage choices a misleading chief complaint according to symptoms and situation to specialty or to diagnostic services in hospitals as well as in primary care centers).

Threats in *pre populated data* have been raised (Bernat, 2005) as they can automatically be inserted, especially for laboratory or image reports if not validated by the health staff, may induce to automatically generated indication to further unnecessary in-depth examinations, exams or consultations or even handovers, sometimes hazardous.

The discharge summary may provide a clear understanding of exactly what has been done, why it has been done, the reasoning of the physicians leading to the formulation of conclusion and the proposal of the treatment plan or the follow-up. EHR purposes of interoperability, especially across countries might be set up, especially for trans-language classification or horizon scanning of archetype model implementation.

As it has been stressed, good EHR presume good EMR. But another limit of current electronic system in health provider, especially the most advanced in granularity, request much more time in front of the computer than in front of the patient. Patient-physician relationship, which is at the heart of good health delivery, may be suffering more deeply from this problem that might be increasing. Possible solutions may be to predispose the dedication of a health worker to the compilation of the Information Technology System (that may be aggregated into EHRs), possibly under dictation of the health practitioner (doctor, nurse or technician) performing the health action; another solution may be the development of advanced interpretation system of the unstructured field. This latter is actually under deep R&D actions, but has till now produced only unsatisfactory results (Weiner et al. 2012; Kahn, Raebel, Glanz, Riedlinger & Steiner, 2012; Spriggs, Arnold, Pearce & Fry, 2012).

It has been raised that attention to EHR may decrease attention to patients (Balka E, Tolar M, 2011). Indeed, well-built electronic records systems may help reminding the user in all the possible granularity, not to forget the parts of the medical history, of the physical examination and the collection of useful preventive medicine information, such as drugs, alcohol consumption, smoke etc (Burnum, 1989). As it was already emphasized, these features are particularly important for EHR-based healthcare improvement, especially for the management of chronic diseases.

There is finally the risk of a gradual evolutionof EMR and EHR from beinga tool for quality improvement and promotion to becoming a tool for a better compliance to national, mutual fund or assuring reimbursement goals (Bernat, 2013). In other words, a shift of EHR use from quality enhancement tool to performance monitoring tool. This may be a threatening deviance if such a use will not be balanced by a major attention to tempering the conflict between patient and policy regulatory interests, defending the paradigm of time for patients against time consumed in front of the technologies (computer and devices as such).

## FUTURE DIRECTIONS AND CONCLUSION

The ability to achieve a wide and correct use of EHR will become increasingly important in both developed and developing countries. (Legal frameworks for e-health, WHO, 2012). The target of a performing use in developed countries is to help with the provision of health through adequate tools for the growing old population, deals with the enhancement of connection with and through health providers, promoting the shift of health delivery outside the hospital, but outside the traditional General Practitioner setting as well, and through the integration of pre existing home-centered services, as support of realistic patient empowerment models, in order to chase in a sustainable way the goals of equity, safety and efficiency.

In developing countries, EHR are actually emerging, sometimes becoming the structural framework of health delivery and of the management of needs according to available resources and in which introduction of e-health solutions are increasingly successful.

Indeed EHR models are more and more connected with pay-for-performance programs, especially where these are more advanced such as in the US for Medicare and Medicaid Program (Health IT Gov, 2013), and in Australia (Australian e-health standards, 2010) where such EHR use is actually under discussion for General Practitioners.

There is wide agreement about the various and growing benefits of EHR for healthcare services, especially in terms of promotion of effectiveness, quality enhancement, and cost containment. Engineering, Informatics, Biostatics and Public Health Professionals should address these challenges together. An important advance in this direction is the evolving implementation of EHR information in Comparative effectiveness research (Hersh et al, 2013).

As it has been highlighted in the chapter, another very important question, both for theoretical and practical progress, is the consensus for coding and messaging EHR standards. This may facilitate the integration between the different forms of evolution of the e-health, as telemedicine, mHealth and the personalized genomic medicine.

A proper appraisal of the challenges of EHR and of all the electronic data requires a correct interpretation of the e-health. Thus, because of the evolving complexity of Informatics and Electronic applications for healthcare, this appraisal cannot be reached without the promotion of a change in the "thinking" of the e-health among all healthcare practitioners.

## ACKNOWLEDGMENT

The authors would like to thank the anonymous reviewers and the editor for their insightful comments and suggestions and are gratefully indebted with the Library of the Department of Public Health and Pediatrics of the University of Turin, for greatly contributing to retrieving bibliographic references for this work.

## REFERENCES

Albu, J., Sohler, N., Matti-Orozco, B., Sill, J., Baxter, D., Burke, G., & Young, E. (2013). Expansion of electronic health record-based screening, prevention, and management of diabetes in New York City. *Preventing Chronic Disease*, *10*, E13. doi:10.5888/pcd10.120148 PMID:23369766

Almond, H., Cummings, E., & Turner, P. (2013). Australia's personally controlled electronic health record and primary healthcare: Generating a framework for implementation and evaluation. *Studies in Health Technology and Informatics*, *188*, 1–6. PMID:23823280

Ash, J., Kilo, C. M., Shapiro, M., Wasserman, J., McMullen, C., & Hersh, W. (2011). *Roadmap for Provision of Safer Healthcare Information Systems: Preventing e-Iatrogenesis*. Institute of Medicine.

Australian e-health standards. (2010). *Electronic Health Record Interoperability*. Available at http://www.e-health.standards.org.au/IT014SubjectAreas/EHRInteroperability.aspx

Bernat, J. L. (2013). Ethical and quality pitfalls in electronic health records. *Neurology, 80*(11), 1057-61 doi: 10.1212/WNL.0b013e318287288c.

Blobel, B. (2005). Advances in secure and architectural EHR approaches. *International Journal of Medical Informatics*, *75*(3-4), 185–190. Epub 2005 Aug 19 doi:10.1016/j.ijmedinf.2005.07.017 PMID:16112891

Burnum, J. F. (1989). The misinformation era: The fall of the Medical Record. *Annals of Internal Medicine*, *110*, 482–484. doi:10.7326/0003-4819-110-6-482 PMID:2919852

*CEN. ISO 13606 standard. The EN 13606 Association*. (2009-2011). Retrieved September 29, 2013 from www.en13606.org

De Clerq, E. (2008). Problem-oriented patient record model as a conceptual foundation for a multi-professional electronic patient record. *International Journal of Medical Informatics*, *77*(9), 565–575. doi:10.1016/j.ijmedinf.2007.11.002 PMID:18248847

Garets, D., & Davis, M. (2006, January 26). *Electronic medical records vs. electronic health records: yes, there is a difference*. HIMSS Analytics. Retrieved 2013, September 28, from: http://www.himssanalytics.org/docs/wp_emr_ehr.pdf

Garrett, P., & Seidman, J. (2011). US Department of Health & Human Services. *EMR vs EHR – What is the Difference?* Retrieved 2013, September 28, from: http://www.healthit.gov/buzz-blog/electronic-health-and-medical-records/emr-vs-ehr-difference/

Gibbons, P. (2007). Health Level Seven EHR Interoperability Work Group. *Coming to terms: Scoping Interoperability for Health Care*. Retrieved 2013, October 2, from: http://www.hln.com/assets/pdf/Coming-to-Terms-February-2007.pdf

Goldwater, J.C., Kwon, N.J., Nathanson, A., Muckle, A.E., Brown, A., &Cornejo, K. (2013). Open source electronic health records and chronic disease management. *Journal of American Medical Informatics Association*. doi: 11367amiajnl-2013-001672

Habib, J. L. (2010). EHRs, meaningful use, and a model EMR. *Drug Benefit Trends*, *22*(4), 99–101.

Hayrinen, K., Saranto, K., & Nykanen, P. (2008). Definition, structure, content, use and impacts of electronic health records: A review of the research literature. *International Journal of Medical Informatics*, *77*, 291–304. doi:10.1016/j.ijmedinf.2007.09.001 PMID:17951106

Hersh, W. R., Cimino, J., Payne, P. R.O., Embi, P., Logan, J., Weiner, M., Bernstam, E. V., Lehmann, H., Hripcsak, G., Hartzog, T., & Saltz, J. (2013). Recommendations for the use of operational Electronic Health Record data in comparative effectiveness research. *eGEMs, 1*(1), Article 14. DOI: 10.13063/2327-9214.1018

Hripcsak, G., & Albers, D. J. (2012). Next-generation phenotyping of electronic health records. *Journal of the American Medical Informatics Association*, *0*, 1–5. doi: doi:10.1136/amiajnl-2012-001145 PMID:22955496

ICD-10. (2010). *International Classification of ICD*. Available at: http://www.who.int/classifications/icd/en/

ICD-9-CM. (2011). International Classification of Diseases, Ninth Revision, Clinical Modification. Available at http://www.cdc.gov/nchs/icd/icd9cm.htm#ftp

Institute of Medicine (IOM). (2012). *Health IT and Patient Safety: Building Safer Systems for Better Care*. Washington, DC: The National Academies Press.

ISO 18308 Conformance. (n.d.). *OpenEHR Foundation*. Retrieved September 29, 2013 from http://www.openehr.org

Joellenbeck, L. M., Russell, P. K., & Guze, S. B. (Eds.), *Strategies to Protect the Health of Deployed US Forces* (pp. 79–82). Washington, DC: National Academy Press.

Kahn, M. G., Raebel, M. A., Glanz, J. M., Riedlinger, K., & Steiner, J. F. (2012). A pragmatic framework for single-site and multisite data quality assessment in electronic health record-based clinical research. *Medical Care*, *50*, S21–S29. doi:10.1097/MLR.0b013e318257dd67 PMID:22692254

Kalra, D. (2006). Electronic Health Standards. *IMIA Yearbook of Medical Informatics*, *45*(Suppl1), S136–S144.

Kudyakov, R., Bowen, J., Ewen, E., West, S. l., Daoud, Y., Fleming, N., & Masica, A. (2012). Electronic health record use to classify patients with newly diagnosed versus preexisting type 2 diabetes: infrastructure for comparative effectiveness research and population health management. *Population Health Management*, *15*(1), 3–11. doi:10.1089/pop.2010.0084 PMID:21877923

Los, R. K., van Ginneken, A. M., Roukema, J., Moll, H. A., & van der Lei, J. (2005).. . *Medical Informatics and the Internet in Medicine*, *30*(4), 267–276. doi:10.1080/14639230500367563 PMID:16531353

Maylahn, C., Fleming, D., & Birkhead, G. (2013). Health departments in a brave new world. *Preventing Chronic Disease*, *10*, E41. doi:10.5888/pcd10.130003 PMID:23517584

*Medicare and Medicaid EHR Incentive Programs*. (2013). Available at http://www.healthit.gov/providers-professionals/ehr-incentive-programs

Najaftorkaman, M., Ghapanchi, A. H., Talaei-Khoei, A., & Ray, P. (2013). Recent research areas and grand challenges in Electronic Health Record: A Literature survey approach. *The International Technology Management Review*, *3*(1), 12–21. doi:10.2991/itmr.2013.3.1.2

Office of the National Coordinator for Health Information Technology (ONC). (2013). *Health IT Policy Committee: Recommendations to the National Coordinator for Health IT.* Retrieved September 12, 2013 from http://www.healthit.gov/policy-researchers-implementers/health-it-policy-committee-recommendations-national-coordinator-heal

Ruch, P. (2010). Section Editor for the IMIA Yearbook Section on Decision Support Systems. Findings from the yearbook 2010 section on decision support systems. *IMIA Yearbook of Medical Information*, *2010*, 55–57.

Siliquini, R. (2011). Surfing the internet for health information: an italian survey on use and population choices. *BMC Medical Informatics and Decision Making*, (11), 21. doi:10.1186/1472-6947-11-21 PMID:21470435

Sinha, P. K., Sunder, G., Bendale, P., Mantri, M. D., & Dande, A. C. (2013). *Electronic Health Record. Standards, Coding Systems, Frameworks, and Infrastructure. Wiley*. IEEE Press.

Steers, W. D. (2013). The Electronic Medical Record: How Not to Communicate. *The Journal of Urology*, *190*(5), 1636–1637. doi:10.1016/j.juro.2013.08.003 PMID:23933460

The National Alliance for Health Information Technology. (2008). *Report to the Office of the National Coordinator for Health Information Technology on Defining Key Health Information Technology Terms*. Retrieved September 12, 2013 at http://hitechanswers.wpengine.netdna-cdn.com/wp-content/uploads/2013/05/NAHIT-Definitions2008.pdf

*US eMERGE network The Electronic Medical Records and Genomics (eMERGE) Network*. (n.d.). Retrieved from http://emerge.mc.vanderbilt.edu/

Weiner, J. P., Fowles, J., & Chan, K. S. (2012). New paradigms for measuring clinical performance using electronic health records. *International Journal for Quality in Health Care*, *24*(3), 200–205. doi:10.1093/intqhc/mzs011 PMID:22490301

Weiskopf, N. G., Hripcsak, G., Swaminathan, S., & Weng, C. (2013). Defining and measuring completeness of electronic health records for secondary use. *Journal of Biomedical Informatics*, *46*, 830–836. doi:10.1016/j.jbi.2013.06.010 PMID:23820016

Weiskopf, N. G., & Weng, C. (2013). Methods and dimensions of electronic health record data quality assessment: enabling reuse for clinical research. *Journal of the American Medical Informatics Association*, *20*(1), 144–151. doi:10.1136/amiajnl-2011-000681 PMID:22733976

WHO. (2012). Legal frameworks for e-health. Global observatory for ehealth series – Vol.5.

Zuehlke, P., Li, J. H., Talaei-Khoei, A., & Ray, P. (2009). A functional specification for mobile eHealth (mHealth) systems. In *Proceedings of E-Health Networking, Applications and Services*. IEEE.

## KEY TERMS AND DEFINITIONS

**Data Reuse:** Use of data for purpose other than the one for which it was originally created.

**Electronic Health Record:** An electronic record of health-related information that conforms to interoperability standards allowing its creation, gathering and management across different healthcare organizations.

**Electronic Medical Record:** The electronic version of the paper-based medical record containing health information about a patient in one healthcare organization.

**Health Information Technology:** The technology for the creation, management and secure exchange of health information in an electronic environment across computerized systems for healthcare settings.

**Healthcare Services:** Services delivered to patients for the diagnosis and treatment of diseases and the maintenance of health.

**Interoperability:** The ability of a system to work together with other systems through a successful interpretation of the exchanged data.

**Medical Confidentiality:** The privacy and protection against unauthorized disclosure of information arising from any contact with healthcare services or professionals.

**Public Health:** The science and art of preventing diseases, promoting health and prolonging healthy life in a population through health education, directions for health policy and research.

# Chapter 12
# The E-Learning Experience in Medical School of Casablanca

**Ihssane Lembachar**
*Hassan II University, Morocco*

**Zineb Serhier**
*Hassan II University, Morocco*

**Samir Diouny**
*Chouaib Doukkali University, Morocco*

**Mohammed Bennani Othmani**
*Hassan II University, Morocco*

## ABSTRACT

*In recent years, higher education has witnessed significant growth. This unprecedented phenomenon can be attributed to distance education through the application of ICTs. The purpose of this chapter is to bring into focus the experience of e-learning implementation at Casablanca Medical School and investigate learners' attitudes towards e-learning strategy. Of particular relevance to this study are the implementation of two e-learning projects, namely the "Digital Environment Work" (DEW), which allows medical students, faculty, and administrators to access information and online services, and the "@U-PEL 2010 program," which was launched by Hassan II University in 2010 with a view to supporting holders of a comprehensive strategy for the development of e-learning institutions on the basis of clearly identified projects.*

## INTRODUCTION

Economic, social and technological forces have changed the global economy, and the way of life in the world. Specifically, these forces have revolutionized teaching and learning. Technology, the rapid obsolescence of knowledge and training, the need for just-in-time training delivery, and the search for cost-effective ways have redefined the processes that underlie design, development and delivery of training and education.

Over the past two decades, there has been a worldwide proliferation of information and communication technologies (ICT, henceforth) into the field of education. The global adoption of ICT into education has often been seen as a promising tool to revolutionize an outmoded educational system, better prepare students for the information age, and/or accelerate national development efforts (Albirini, 2006). Thioune (2003) notes that e- learning is one of the most rapidly growing fields of education, and its potential impact has

DOI: 10.4018/978-1-4666-6316-9.ch012

been greatly accentuated through the development of ICTs (Thioune). These technologies enhance the effectiveness and efficiency of the educational system through the transmission of different sorts of information required to facilitate the learning process and through adequate learning materials to meet users' needs (Bertea, 2009). In developing countries, the above promises have generated a national debate about the necessity of educational reforms that will accommodate the new tools (Pelgrum, 2001).

Today, medical education is facing challenges in terms of knowledge, skills and attitudes, resulting in less time for teaching than has previously been the case (Ozuah, 2002). Transition in sites of health care delivery from acute care institutions to community-based settings for chronic care has required adaptations in educational venues (Nair & Finucane, 2003). Therefore, to be considered competent to practice, medical students must cover new fields such as palliative care, geriatrics, genomics and complementary medicine while current medical school curricula is challenged to teach conventional materials (Ozuah, 2002). The traditional learner-centered model that puts learners in control of their own teaching has undergone a major shift toward competency-based curricula that emphasizes the learning outcome rather than the process of education (Leung, 2002). In this changing paradigm, educators are becoming facilitators of learning and assessors of competency; they no longer serve as the sole distributors of content (Ruiz, Michael, Mintzer & Leipzig, 2006).

E-learning gives medical educators the occasion to improve the efficiency and effectiveness of educational materials by providing them with a set of online resources to facilitate the learning process (Chodorow, 1996). Furthermore e-learning transforms the role of the teacher, allows learning to be individualized, and enhances learners' interactions with others, which seems to point toward a revolution in education (Ruiz, Michael, Mintzer & Leipzig, 2006).

An appropriate infrastructure to support e-learning within medical education namely repositories, allows clinicians to access a virtual database and get at the same time answers to clinical questions and the latest research information (Ruiz, Michael, Mintzer & Leipzig, 2006). E-learning also uses multimedia to assist with assimilation of medical content. A video clip that shows a child with a stridor, a ''flash'' animation that demonstrates a cellular process, a written case with pictures (a rash)/audio (heart sounds) to demonstrate a physical sign; the technology of such technologies allows medical students to practice away from the bedside or perhaps in areas where contact with certain pathologies is limited (Choules, 2007).

E-learning is defined as the acquisition and use of knowledge distributed and facilitated primarily by electronic means (Jansen, Hooven, Jägers & Steenbakkers, 2002). It may incorporate synchronous or asynchronous access and may be distributed geographically with varied limits of time. The learning is carried out either individually or on a small or large group basis and can be used as a hybrid to the face-to-face format, or exclusively in open and distance learning (ODL). As such, e-learning is not confined to the boundaries of the online format but also includes the offline format using any form of electronic media to facilitate the teaching and learning processes (Garrison & Anderson, 2003).

E-learning offers learners a number of advantages (Ruiz, Michael, Mintzer & Leipzig, 2006): Control over content, learning sequence, learning pace, and time allowing them to tailor their experiences to meet their personal learning objectives (p.207). In many contexts, students are very satisfied with e-learning compared to traditional learning (Gibbons & Fairweather, 2000; Chumley-Jones, Dobbie & Alford, 2002). However, students do not see e-learning as replacing traditional instructor-led training but as a complement to it, forming part of a blended-learning strategy (Gibbons & Fairweather; Chumley-Jones et al.). Such a strategy has allowed the shift from a teacher-centered approach to a learner's centered approach, where teachers are involved as facilitators of learning.

E-learning plays two main roles. First, it is seen as a learning environment. E-learning offers students more opportunity to engage in learning activities independently. Furthermore, e-learning makes it possible to offer the same learning content in various forms. Students themselves can then choose the form which suits them best. Through e-learning the content can be tailored to personal needs (Jansen, Hooven, Jägers, & Steenbakkers, 2002). Second, e-learning is viewed as a management environment; it can monitor, stimulate, and adjust the learning process by means of various testing, registration, administration and communication possibilities (Jansen et al.). In short, e-learning has a positive impact on the experience of learning (Laurillard, 2004); there is a cultural impact; students are comfortable with e-learning methods, because they are not different from the communications methods they use in their everyday lives; there is an intellectual impact, there is a technological interactivity that offers an online mode of involvement. There is a social impact; students take greater responsibility for their own learning. Lastly, there is a practical impact, e-learning offers the ability to manage quality at scale, and share resources across networks; its greater flexibility of provision in time and place makes it good for widening participation (Laurillard).

However, using e-learning does not necessarily lead to successful learning; an effective e-learning program depends on two main factors. The first one is the technology used: Finding an appropriate infrastructure is a real challenge when implementing e-learning in higher education institutions, especially in developing countries (Fares, 2007); also, technological obstacles may affect the adoption of this tool (Vencatachellum & Munusami, 2006). The second factor is the attitude towards this technology: A favorable attitude of learners indicates a greater probability that they will accept the new learning system (Bertea, 2009); therefore, understanding users' attitudes towards learning technology helps the development of adapted learning materials that meets the needs of students and instructors. Thus, Benzie (1995, p. 38) indicates that educational programs have been of limited success because they were not based on research. Initial stages, which require careful planning, are missing in the process of technology implementation (Albirini, 2006, p. 375).

It is important to note that distance education has long been solidly established in most Northern countries, and e-learning initiatives have been appearing for more than a decade. Most of these countries have seen real advances in the implementation of different types of e-learning applications; however, these advances have not, on the other hand, made a considerable impact in developing countries. For example, in Morocco, little progress has been registered in the field of e-learning whether in the area of academic studies, or research. In fact, using e-learning as a teaching tool in higher educational institutions is becoming consequently inevitable; modern day learning environments place many universities under pressure to integrate these aspects as a support to their classical learning (Al-adwane & Smedley, 2012). It is with the hope to promote this area of research that the present study aims to bring into focus the experience of e-learning implementation experience at Casablanca Medical School and investigate learners' attitudes towards e-learning strategy.

## LITERATURE REVIEW

E-learning refers to the use of Information and Communication Technologies (ICT) in education to support and enhance learning strategies (Al-adwane & Smedley, 2012). Developments in internet and multimedia technologies have promoted rich and interactive content for users and were the basic enabler of e-learning (Nagy,

2005). This learning tool is currently one of the most powerful solutions to the growing demand for education (Zhang, Zhao, Zhou, & Nunamaker, 2004).

Many arguments regarding the difference between traditional learning and e-learning have been reported in the literature, this include an interest in the learning outcomes for e-learners; a review of 355 comparative studies reveals no significant difference in grades or exam results between traditional and e-learning methods (Russell, 2001). Recent studies show that the effectiveness is similar in e-learning compared to face-to-face classroom instructions and that the combination of online and classical methods is the best strategy for learning (Hrastinski, 2008); nevertheless, e-learning offers ways which are not found in traditional learning such as applications and processes that deliver text, audio, images, animation and streaming videos (Tavangarian, Leypold, Nölting, & Röser, 2004); these tools help teachers to provide students with various supports of knowledge and to facilitate communication between teachers and learners (Krishnakumar & Rajesh Kumar, 2011).

With a view to bringing into focus the possible weaknesses and strengths of online and traditional face-to-face instruction (i.e. blended learning), Wuensch et al. (2008) conducted an investigation of students' satisfaction with online and traditional face-to-face instruction. The results showed that students were satisfied more with e-learning instruction than with face-to-face instruction in terms of convenience and in permitting self-pacing.

Providing a rigorous education has been and will remain the concern of any educational institution because training creates value not only for students but also for the establishment. In medical education, a vast collection of knowledge, skills and attitudes have to be considered; a mixture of lecturing, self-study and small group learning are needed to help learners achieve their objectives (Choules, 2007).

The adoption of an e-learning material goes through several stages, namely the development of the content, its' management, its' delivery and its' standardization (Ruiz, Mintzer, & Leipzig, 2006). In a digital environment, the content is represented by digital learning objects which consist of digital materials structured and tied to educational objectives (Smith, 2004). Based on instructional design and pedagogical principles, these objects are used to build larger educational materials; they are thereby grafted into lessons, modules or complete courses in order to meet the requirements of a specified curriculum (Littlejohn, 2003). To make content available to learners, management's content includes storing, indexing and cataloguing (Ruiz, Mintzer, & Leipzig). Many management internet-based softwares are available to medical educators such as Learning Management Systems (LMS) that operate as a repository for instructional resources, track learners' progress and automate administrative and supervisory tasks (Johnson, Hurtubise, Castrop, et al., 2004; Phelps & Michea, 2003).

There are basically two types of e-learning delivery: Synchronous and asynchronous. With synchronous delivery, learners take part in the learning process at the same time. A shared environment allows students and instructors to communicate directly as in teleconferencing and instant messaging. Apart from the constraints of time and place, asynchronous delivery creates on-demand student learning experience; interaction between the instructor and the students do not occur in real time, and communication is supported by e-mail or online bulletin boards.

Finally, the standardization of e-learning materials is a crucial step to promote compatibility across different computer systems (Ruiz, Mintzer, & Leipzig, 2006), the Sharable Content Object Reference Model (SCORM) is one example of standards that defines the inter-relationship of content objects and allows interaction between LMSs and e-learning materials.

Still, the integration of e-learning into existing medical curricula should be evaluated to justify the investment to administrators. Process or outcome evaluation should happen at all stages of the product to allow modifications.

Process evaluation explores the overall design and should meet the needs of the target audience, it also examines the ease of navigation and how learners can find their way around, the relevance of resources, the interactivity and its' suitability for the level of the learner. This type of evaluation needs a group testing to point out weaknesses and strengths of e-learning materials.

Outcome evaluation focuses on changes in learner's knowledge, skills and attitudes. An evaluation framework adapted to health care education (Barr, Freeth, Hammick, Koppel, Reeves, 2002) from Kirkpatrick (Kirkpatrick, 1998) in the 1950's is used to evaluate e-learning interventions (Horton, 2001). In his model, Kirkpatrick measures the outcome evaluation through four levels: Reaction of student, learning, change in learner's behaviour, and organizational change. First, the reaction evaluation assesses how the learners feel, and what they think about the learning materials. It attempts to answer questions regarding the trainees' perceptions - Did they enjoy it? Did they consider the training relevant? Secondly, teaching evaluation monitors the increase in knowledge or intellectual capability, measurement at this level is more difficult than in reaction evaluation; participants may take a pre-test and a post-test to check whether any learning has taken place. Thirdly, Behaviour evaluation is the most reliable of all measures since it examines the transfer that has occurred in learners' behaviour due to training. It tries to answer to questions such as: Were the skills and knowledge used? Were the learners able to transfer their learning to another person? And fourthly, results evaluation investigates the effect on the environment, this can be evaluated on the basis of performance of the learner, it measures the success of a program and represents the overall reason for a training program (Winfrey, 1999).

At last, even if all these measures help a meaningful evaluation of learning's material, a careful consideration should be given to the human factor training; to take advantage of e-learning in ways that benefit teaching, educational institutions need to opt for an e-solution that meets the learners' level of ability with information technologies, any other way will be frustrating (Link & Marz, 2006). Therefore, understanding students' attitudes towards e-learning facilitates the development of learning materials tailored to users' expectations.

## METHODOLOGY

To bring into focus the experience of e-learning implementation at Casablanca Medical School, two projects are described, namely the "Digital Environment Work" (DEW), which allows medical students, faculty and administrators to access information and online services, and the "@U-PEL 2010 program", which was launched by Hassan II University in 2010, with a view to supporting holders of a comprehensive strategy for the development of e-learning institutions on the basis of clearly identified projects. The organization of this program, its content, its method, the human and material resources and its outcomes are developed.

Determining users' attitude towards e-learning helps to predict the adoption of a certain behavior, therefore a cross-sectional study among 2010 internship medical students at Ibn Rochd Casablanca University Hospital was conducted. The questionnaire used contained variables which measured experience in computer use, involvement in distance courses and interest in online training.

## E-LEARNING IN MEDICAL SCHOOL OF CASABLANCA

Founded in 1975, the Medical School of Casablanca based at Hassan II University is located in the heart of the economic capital of Morocco. The Faculty extends over 6000 hectares and admits approximately 450 students each year. Medical studies lasts 7 years, including 5 years of theoretical courses at the Faculty and 2 years full-time internship at the University Hospital Ibn Rochd of Casablanca, at the end of which period, the student is granted a doctorate of general medicine.

Additionally, the Medical School of Casablanca offers postgraduate studies including certificates, diplomas, masters, and scientific doctorates. This diversity in trainings has prompted the Faculty of Medicine to integrate effective Information and Communication Technologies into teaching and learning strategies to improve students' outcomes.

The reason behind choosing e-learning is that it offers several advantages over traditional distance learning methods. Indeed, the Learning Management System (LMS) tools were developed in order to meet the growing demand for education and training while respecting educational standards. In addition, this new technology allowed better teachers-students and students-students interaction.

However, the implementing of e-Learning requires a perfect organization in scripting and structuring courses, compliance with educational standards, and mastery of the technical tool dedicated to this purpose; that is the e-learning platform.

The development of e-learning is, therefore, a comprehensive strategy of an institution; it allows institutions to offer more courses and meet the growing needs of their students more effectively. The success of an e-learning project cannot be achieved without the willingness of all institution's members and direct involvement of stakeholders involved in the educational process. The careful coordination of this project allows the combination of efforts in technical, pedagogical, and organizational fields.

To pursue the technological track in education, and recognize the challenge of the "information age", the Faculty of Medicine has recently adopted two projects, namely "The Digital Environment Work" (DEW) and the "@U-PEL 2010 program".

## THE DIGITAL ENVIRONMENT WORK (DEW)

Conscious of the advances in information technology, Hassan II University-Casablanca made considerable efforts to enhance the medical student learning experience through the implementation of a Digital Environment Work (DEW) that fits into the framework of a national project titled, "Computerization of University Digital Environments". The DEW is a protected digital space for students, teacher-researchers, and administrators; it allows access to information and services available online as shown in Figure 1. It provides its users with a range of personalized utilities according to their profiles through a login and a password, in compliance with the privacy policy (Fethi, 2010).

In addition, the DEW decompartmentalizes learning activities has helped remove many of the time and spatial constraints in traditional face-to-face courses, it helped students to study wherever they are, provided they have access to a computer and Internet. Thereby, the DEW is an ideal partner for students; it is especially useful to manage course administration online, such as creating a personalized agenda, finding out course information, and accessing directly to numerous electronic resources from library catalogues, national and international bibliographic databases. Information relating to students' activities is also available on the DEW; opportunities to join clubs and organizations, to get acquainted and interact with lot of new people help students to take an active part in campus life. Still, the successful

*Figure 1. Different services of the Digital Environment Work (DEW)*

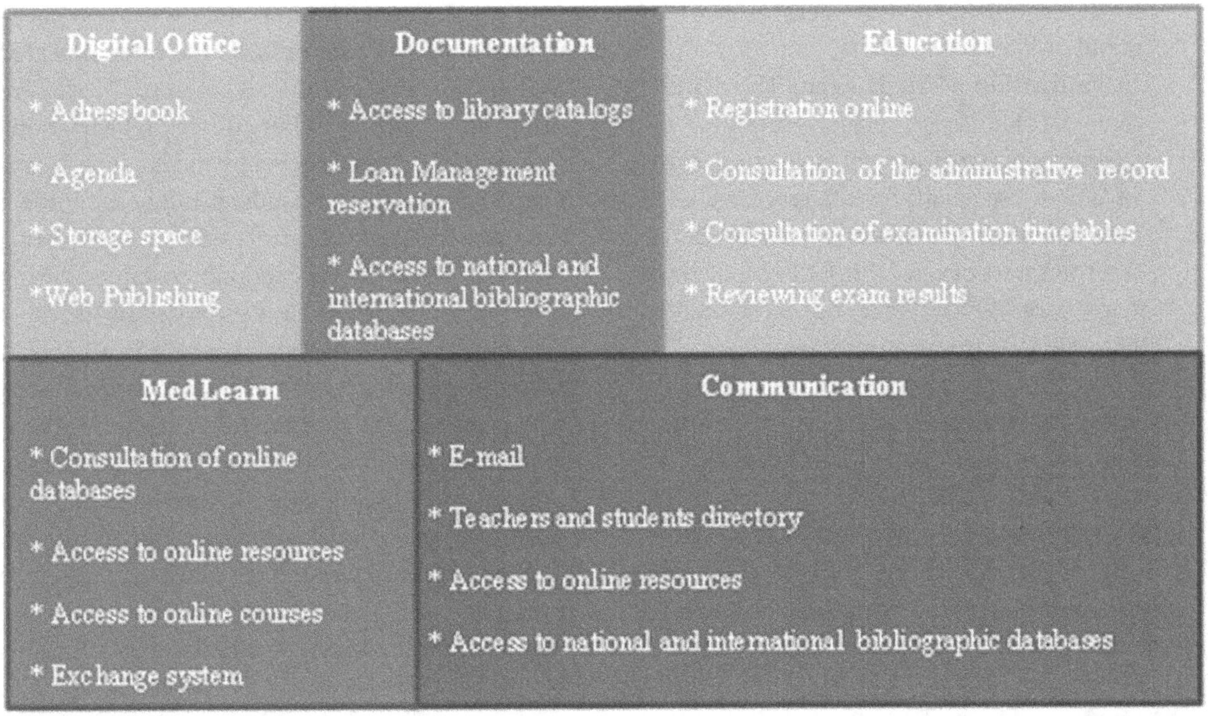


implementation of educational technologies depends largely on the attitudes of educators, who eventually determine how they are used. Bullock (2004) found that educators' attitudes are a major enabling/disabling factor in the adoption of technology. Similarly, Kersaint, Horton, Stohl, and Garofalo (2003) found that educators who have positive attitudes toward technology feel more comfortable with using it and usually incorporate it into their teaching. In fact, Woodrow (1992) asserts that any successful transformation in educational practice requires the development of positive user attitude toward the new technology.

The access speed and other technical aspects are of prime importance as well as access facilities (Esen, 2012). Thus, training and support are essential to ensure that all users can appropriate this tool; in our context, several workshops and seminars were organized to familiarize users with the DEW platform and to promote the implementation and production of distance education courses for medical students.

## THE @U-PEL 2010 PROGRAM

In 2010, Hassan II University-Casablanca launched the "@U-PEL 2010" e-learning program; its purpose was to support holders of a comprehensive strategy for the development of e-learning institutions on the basis of clearly identified projects. Casablanca Faculty of Medicine received funding for their project "MedLearn", the aim of which was to improve training and strengthen partnerships with other institutions.

1. **Description of MedLearn:** MedLearn is a pilot project presented by Casablanca Medical School at the "@U-PEL 2010"; it has two main components: Online courses with self-assessment exercises and E-trainings. While the objective of the first component was to ensure at least 30% of online courses (with self-assessment exercises); the second component's target was to promote distance education, the project

took into account the perceived needs of medical students practitioners; it involved about 10% of the teachers.

2. **Organization of MedLearn:** The deployment of MedLearn project required the implementation of internal procedures for the FMPC, consequently for online courses and a self-assessment component, correspondence with the participants' tutors and meetings with coordinators have been established with the E-learning committee.

Some organizational structures were involved in this project, namely, the editorial board of the Medical School website which validated online courses, the department of courses and exams, involved in communicating with students and the sub-committee of the Education Committee, responsible for the promotion of research and educational production.

A progress report of MedLearn was drafted by the e-learning committee; a compendium of half-yearly monitoring indicators of the project, and a quarterly report of the responsible pilot projects were submitted.

3. **Content:** Medical studies have a rich and varied program, requiring a combination of several teaching tools for a better understanding of the learning materials. Therefore, under the MedLearn project, the Faculty of Medicine of Casablanca is currently offering 37 online courses for medical students covering 4 subjects out of 9 (Anatomy, Biology, Histology-Embryology, Biophysics) and 48 online courses covering five graduate majors among 25 subjects (Pharmacology, Hematology, Pediatrics, Radiology, Internal Medicine). Furthermore, a number of self-assessment exercises, and a space for interaction with teachers are available for students.

The other component of MedLearn is represented by 6 e-trainings based on the following requirements: One need is about the fourth year medical students who must follow several classroom courses, which reduces the time allocated to their practical training. Therefore, MedLearn offers an e-training in Functional and Metabolic Imaging [E-T1] conducted by the Nuclear Medicine Department. Also, students in the seventh year are required to take a clinical examination knowing that they receive no academic coaching during this year; thus, MedLearn proposes for them an e-training in Radiology during this period [E-T2]. In addition, teachers of the Faculty of Medicine of Casablanca are required to supervise residents in their medical practice; however, as the number of residents is going up each year, the quality of practical training is getting increasingly mediocre. Then, MedLearn recommends two e-trainings in Pediatrics [E-T3] and Gastroenterology [E-T4]. Another e-training in "Methods of Exploration of the Nervous System" [E-T5] is dedicated to students enrolled in the Master of Neuroscience. Finally, as part of continuing education and in order to meet the increasing needs in research methodology training, MedLearn proposes a remote University Degree in Biostatistics and Measurement of Perceptual Health [E-T6]. (Figure 2)

4. **Method:** To ensure the proper functioning of MedLearn's components, a secure connection allowing students to access online courses was established as well as a space dedicated to Questions and Answers, giving students the opportunity to interact with each other and with their teachers. The Digital Environment Work was used to access the different distance learning components.
5. **Human and Material Resources:** A total number of 32 participants took part in the MedLearn project; these participants were drawn from different pools: 5 full professors, 6 associate professors, 11 assistant professors, 6 residents, 1 specialist in radiology, 1 radio-physicist, 2 technicians, and 1 pedagogical assistant. A theoretical training in

*Figure 2. Components of MedLean project*

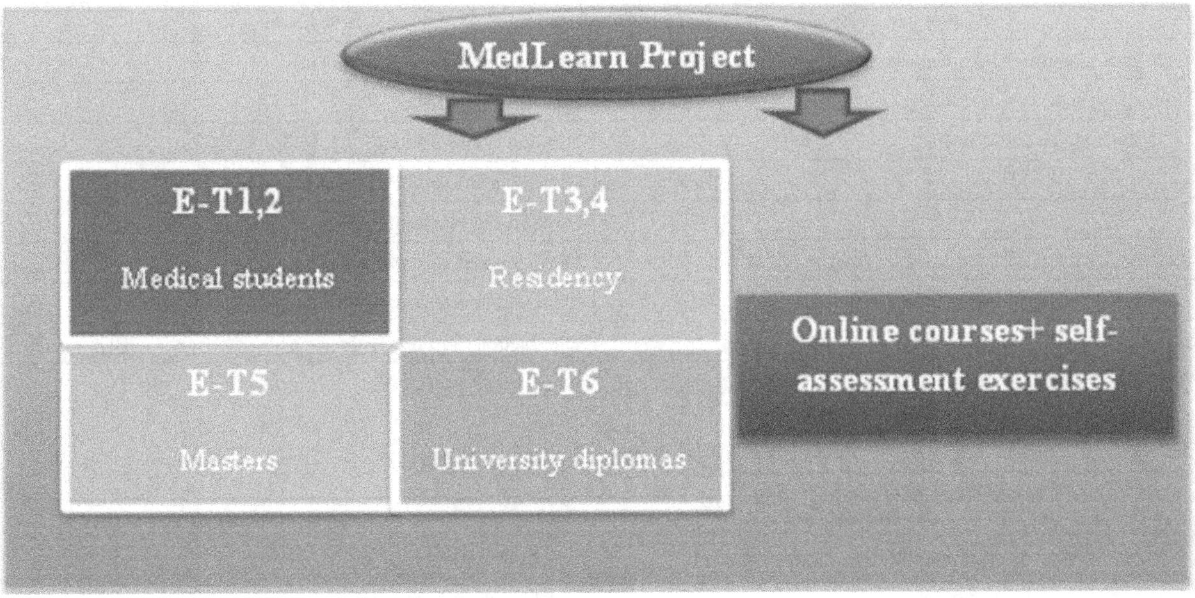


e-learning and workshops in many software solutions required to integrate learning materials were organized for the e-learning team (see Table 1).

The material resources allocated to the MedLearn project included both equipment (microcomputers, scanners, printers…) and software products; furthermore, an e-learning room was designed to accommodate the e-learning production sessions.

6. **Outcomes:** The main expected results of the MedLearn project were to develop learner autonomy and skills training, as well as to diversify teaching methods. Moreover, MedLearn was initiated to develop mutual courses in accordance with our national and international partners. In order to evaluate the project's progress, six indicators were established to monitor MedLearn as shown in Table 2.

## CHALLENGES TO USERS

Like any other educational innovation, there are pitfalls and barriers confronting the implementation of e-learning. These barriers pose as challenges. The success of an e-learning program is obviously linked to the adoption at a user level; reluctance to use new technologies has been reported in the literature especially among seniors (Buabeng-Andoh, 2012). The major restrictions identified were the lack of confidence in ICT classes, and the perceived lack of access to quality resources including hardware and software (Jones, 2012).

In our case, the experience of MedLearn showed two categories of participants: Those teachers who were aware of the e-learning environments and those who were motivated, but had no ICT familiarity. After their first-hand experience, both categories had a favorable attitude towards the project; hence, it is safe to conclude that encouraging seniors to adopt e-learning strategies

*Table 1. Training program of the e-learning team*

| Theoretical Training | Workshops |
|---|---|
| Pedagogical approach in e-learning | Introduction to Moodle platform |
| Role of the tutor in E-learning | Essential office tools |
| Script writing an online course | Editorial chain: Scenari |
| | Create Questions on Hot Potatos |
| | Macromedia Flash: Animation |
| | Medical image processing in Photoshop |
| | Exploitation and manipulation of DICOM file format |
| | Introduction to Adobe presenter |

*Table 2. Progress indicators of MedLearn Project*

| Indicator | Means of Measuring |
|---|---|
| Number of online courses and self-assessment exercises | Census website |
| Number of specialties involved | Census website |
| Number of downloads | Counter flow computer |
| Number of access to the portal FAQ | Counter flow computer |
| Number of accesses per course | Counter flow computer |
| Student Satisfaction | Satisfaction questionnaire, online survey |

by assisting and supporting them can play a vital role in developing a positive attitude towards e-learning.

Unlike seniors, young learners are often first adopters of new technologies (Halewood & Kenny, 2008), many studies noted that youth have more access to ICT and struggle less than older users (Selwyn, Gorard, Furlong, & Madden, 2003). In order to illustrate that, we ran a cross-sectional study among 43 internship medical students at Ibn Rochd Casablanca University Hospital to investigate their perceptions; 54% of the participants were females, aged 24 to 26. The results showed that the majority had computers with internet connection. The experience of computer use was "average" in 54.8% of the cases, "high" in 29% of the cases and "limited" in 16.2% of the cases. 9.8% of the participants have been involved in distance courses and 63% have used discussion forums; approximately 73.8% were interested in online training. However, young users have other challenges regarding e-learning, related fundamentally to the content of this new form of learning; students may have a positive attitude if e-learning content fits their needs; otherwise, they may not adapt to the new system (Bertea, 2009). Another major challenge to take into consideration is the level of dedication that is required to follow an online course; some e-courses can induce a certain discipline of work for students such as establishing rules, meeting deadlines, and evaluating systems throughout the whole period of learning; in this case, students with low motivation may not follow the study conditions because of the absence of a real face to face contact between students and tutors (Alonso Díaz & Blázquez Entonado, 2009).

## CONCLUSION

To conclude, the use of e-learning as a support to traditional classrooms has offered to Casablanca Medical School more flexibility in delivering learning information and improving the efficiency and effectiveness of medical students' learning process; the implementation of e-learning environments have changed the method of teaching and benefited students in terms of time and space.

The "MedLearn" project was the first step that enabled Hassan II University-Casablanca and the Faculty of Medicine to appreciate the current situation of e-learning in higher education in Morocco; the positive attitude of users encouraged these institutions to implement other initiatives in order to cater for the needs of the majority of users.

Based on our experience, the success of online learning in higher education may be attributed to the following factors: the awareness of the importance of e-learning tools, the motivation of both teachers and students, and the adequation of e-learning content to the users' needs.

Still, more efforts have to be made to improve teacher's ICT skills and to encourage them to integrate e-learning tools in their daily activities, by providing them with ICT facilities and assisting them when producing their own courses. However, for students, e-learning is an opportunity to be independent and responsible for their own learning process, provided that they are motivated and that the content meets their needs. Finally, the implementation of e-learning is a strategy that institutions should adhere to. The success of e-learning projects depends on the degree of involvement of all parties involved (management, faculty, tutors, students, etc.).

## ACKNOWLEDGMENT

The authors would like to thank the anonymous reviewers and the editor for their insightful comments and suggestions.

## REFERENCES

Al-adwane, A., & Smedley, J. (2012). Implementing e-learning in the Jordanian Higher Education System: Factors affecting impact. *International Journal of Education and Development using Information and Communication Technology, 8*(1), 121-135.

Albirini, A. (2006). Teachers' Attitudes toward Information and Communication Technology: The case of Syrian EFL Teachers. *Computers & Education, 47*(4), 373–398. doi:10.1016/j.compedu.2004.10.013

Alonso Díaz, L., & Blázquez Entonado, F. (2009). Are the Functions of Teachers in e-Learning and Face-to-Face Learning Environments Really Different? *Journal of Educational Technology & Society, 12*(4), 331–343.

Barr, H., Freeth, D., Hammick, M., Koppel, I., & Reeves, S. (2002). *Evaluating interprofessional education: a United Kingdom review of health and social care*. London, UK: Centre for the Advancement of Interprofessional Education.

Benzie, D. (1995). IFIP Working group 3.5: Using computers to support young learners. In J.D. Tinsley & T.J. van Weert (Eds.), *World Conference on Computers in Education VI: WCCE' 95 Liberating the Learner* (pp. 35-42). Chapman & Hall.

Bertea, P. (2009). Measuring students' attitude towards e-learning: A case study. In *Proceedings of 5th International Scientific Conference*. Elearning and Software for Education.

Buabeng-Andoh, C. (2012). Factors influencing teachers' adoption and integration of information and communication technology into teaching: A review of the literature. *International Journal of Education and Development using Information and Communication Technology, 8*(1), 136-155.

Bullock, D. (2004). Moving from theory to practice: An examination of the factors that pre-service teachers encounter as they attempt to gain experience teaching with technology during field placement experiences. *Journal of Technology and Teacher Education*, *12*(2), 221–237.

Chodorow, S. (1996). Educators must take the electronic revolution seriously. *Academic Medicine*, *71*, 221–226. doi:10.1097/00001888-199603000-00009 PMID:8607916

Choules, A. P. (2007). The use of e-learning in medical education: a review of the current situation. *Postgraduate Medical Journal*, *83*, 212–216. doi:10.1136/pgmj.2006.054189 PMID:17403945

Chumley-Jones, H. S., Dobbie, A., & Alford, C. L. (2002). Web-based learning: sound educational method or hype? A review of the evaluation literature. *Academic Medicine*, *77*(10), 86–93. doi:10.1097/00001888-200210001-00028 PMID:12377715

Ecole supérieure de l'éducation nationale de l'enseignement supérieur et de la recherché. (2012). *ENT-Espace Numérique de Travail*. Retrieved November 24, 2013 from http://www.esen.education.fr/index.php?id=79&a=102&cHash=fa2c3c0948

Fares, A. (2007). *ICT Infrastructure, Applications, Society, and Education*. Nairobi: Strathmore University.

Fethi, A. (2010). L'Environnement Numérique de Travail (ENT). *Bulletin de l'Université*, *24*, 22.

Garrison, D., & Anderson, T. (2003). *E-learning in the 21st Century*. London: Routledge Falmer. doi:10.4324/9780203166093

Gibbons, A., & Fairweather, P. (2000). Computer-based instruction. In S. Tobias, & J. Fletcher (Eds.), *Training & Retraining: A Handbook for Business* (pp. 410–442). Macmillan Reference.

Halewood, N., & Kenny, C. (2008). Young people and ICTs in Developing Countries. *Information Technology for Development Journal, 14*.

Horton, W. (2001). *Evaluating E-learning*. Alexandria, VA: American Society for Training and Development.

Hrastinski, S. (2008). Asynchronous and synchronous e-learning. *EDUCAUSE Quarterly*, *31*(4), 51–55.

Jansen, W., & Hooven, H.M. v.d., Jägers, M., & Steenbakkers, J. (2002). The added value of e-learning. *Informing Science*.

Johnson, C. E., Hurtubise, L. C., & Castrop, J. et al. (2004). Learning management systems: technology to measure the medical knowledge competency of the ACGME. *Medical Education*, *38*, 599–608. doi:10.1111/j.1365-2929.2004.01792.x PMID:15189256

Jones, A. (2012). Teacher perceptions and use of ICT in unfamiliar classroom situations. In *Proceedings of International Conference on Information Communication Technologies in Education*, (pp. 314-322). Academic Press.

Keegan, D. (2004). *The impact of new technologies on distance learning students*. Distance Education International.

Kersaint, G., Horton, B., Stohl, H., & Garofalo, J. (2003). Technology beliefs and practices of mathematics education faculty. *Journal of Technology and Teacher Education*, *11*(4), 549–577.

Kirkpatrick, D. (1998). *Evaluating Training Programs* (2nd ed.). San Francisco: Berrett-Koehler.

Krishnakumar, R., & Rajesh Kumar, M. (2011). Attitude of teachers' of higher education towards e-learning. *Journal of Education and Practice*, *2*(4), 48–53.

Laurillard, D. (2004). E-Learning in higher education. In P. Ashwin (Ed.), *Changing higher education*. London: Routledge Falmer.

Leung, W. C. (2002). Competency based medical training [review]. *BMJ (Clinical Research Ed.), 325*, 693–696. doi:10.1136/bmj.325.7366.693 PMID:12351364

Link, T. M., & Marz, R. (2006). Computer literacy and attitudes towards e-learning among first medical students. *BMC Medical Education, 6*(34). PMID:16784524

Littlejohn, A. (2003). Issues in reusing online resources. In A. Littlejohn (Ed.), *Reusing online resources: A Sustainable Approach to eLearning* (pp. 1–6). London: Creative Print and Design.

Nagy, A. (2005). The Impact of E-Learning. In P. A. Bruck, A. Buchholz, Z. Karssen, & A. Zerfass (Eds.), *E-Content: Technologies and Perspectives for the European Market* (pp. 79–96). Berlin: Springer-Verlag. doi:10.1007/3-540-26387-X_4

Nair, B. R., & Finucane, P. M. (2003). Reforming medical education to enhance the management of chronic disease. *The Medical Journal of Australia, 179*, 257–259. PMID:12924974

Ozuah, P. O. (2002). Undergraduate medical education: thoughts on future challenges. *BMC Medical Education, 2*, 8–10. doi:10.1186/1472-6920-2-8 PMID:12149136

Pelgrum, W. J. (2001). Obstacles to the integration of ICT in education: results from a worldwide educational assessment. *Computers & Education, 37*, 163–178. doi:10.1016/S0360-1315(01)00045-8

Phelps, C., & Michea, Y. F. (2003). Learning management systems' evaluation focuses on technology not learning. In *Proceedings of AMIA Annual Symposium*. AMIA.

Rashty, D. (2003). *Traditional learning vs. e-learning*. Retrieved August 02, 2013 from http://www.researchtrail.com/articles/Traditional_Learning_vs_eLearning.pdf

Ruiz, J. G., Mintzer, M. J., & Leipzig, R. M. (2006). The Impact of E-Learning in Medical Education. *Academic Medicine, 81*(3), 207–212. doi:10.1097/00001888-200603000-00002 PMID:16501260

Russell, T. L. (2001). *The no significant difference phenomenon* (5th ed.). Montgomery, AL: International Distance Education Certification Center.

Selwyn, N., Gorard, S., Furlong, J., & Madden, L. (2003). Older adults' use of information and communications technology in everyday life. *Ageing and Society, 23*, 561–582. doi:10.1017/S0144686X03001302

Smith, R. (2004). *Guidelines for Authors of Learning Objects*. Retrieved November 26, 2013 from http://archive2.nmc.org/guidelines/NMC%20LO%20Guidelines.pdf

Tavangarian, D., Leypold, M., Nölting, K., & Röser, M. (2004). Is e-learning the Solution for Individual Learning?. *Journal of e-Learning*.

Thioune, R.M.C. (2003). *Information and communication technologies for development in Africa: Opportunities and challenges for community development*. Retrieved October 28, 2013 from http://www.idrc.ca

Vencatachellum, I., & Munusami, V. (2006). *Barriers to effective corporate e-learning in Mauritius*. Retrieved August 04, 2013 from http://www.ufhrd.co.uk/wordpress/wp-content/uploads/2008/06/1-1_vencatachellum_munusami.pdf

Winfrey, E. C. (1999). Kirkpatrick's Four Levels of Evaluation. In B. Hoffman (Ed.), *Encyclopedia of Educational Technology*. Retrieved November 26, 2013, from http://www.4cleanair.org/Kirkpatrick.pdf

Woodrow, J. E. (1992). The influence of programming traininig on the computer literacy and attitudes of pre-service teachers. *Journal of Research on Computing in Education*, *25*(2), 200–219.

Wuensch, K., Aziz, S., Ozan, E., Kishore, M., & Tabrizi, M. H. (2008). Pedagogical characteristics of online and face-to-face classes. *International Journal on E-Learning*, *3*(7), 523–532.

Zhang, D., Zhao, J. L., Zhou, L., & Nunamaker, J. F. Jr. (2004). Can e-learning replace classroom learning? *Communications of the ACM*, *47*(5), 75–79. doi:10.1145/986213.986216

## KEY TERMS AND DEFINITIONS

**Complementary Medicine:** A mode of delivering of health care that combines conventional medicine to alternative medicine. An example of a complementary therapy is using acupuncture and herbal medicine.

**DICOM:** Digital Imaging and Communications in Medicine (DICOM) is a standard of medical imaging that allows handling, storing, and transmitting information.

**Hot Potatoes:** Is a software suite that holds applications for creating exercises on the World Wide Web.

**Learning Management System (LMS):** Is a software application or Web-based technology used to implement, administer and deliver e-learning education courses or training programs.

**Resident:** A person who has received a medical degree and practices medicine usually in a hospital or clinic.

**Sharable Object Content Reference Model (SCORM):** Is a set of technical standards and specifications for e-learning software products; it is used to define and access information about learning objects so they can be easily shared among different learning management systems.

**Stridor:** Is an abnormal musical breathing sound resulting from a blockage in the larynx or throat.

# Chapter 13
# Knowledge Discovery and Data Mining Applications in the Healthcare Industry:
## A Comprehensive Study

**Iman Barazandeh**
*Iran University of Science and Technology, Iran & Islamic Azad University, Mahshahr Branch, Iran*

**Mohammad Reza Gholamian**
*Iran University of Science and Technology, Iran*

## ABSTRACT

*The healthcare industry is one of the most attractive domains to realize the actionable knowledge discovery objectives. This chapter studies recent researches on knowledge discovery and data mining applications in the healthcare industry and proposes a new classification of these applications. Studies show that knowledge discovery and data mining applications in the healthcare industry can be classified to three major classes, namely patient view, market view, and system view. Patient view includes papers that performed pure data mining on healthcare industry data. Market view includes papers that saw the patients as customers. System view includes papers that developed a decision support system. The goal of this classification is identifying research opportunities and gaps for researchers interested in this context.*

## INTRODUCTION

Since human learned to inscribe his thinks in the world out of his/her mind, Data has been created and started to growing and its growing accelerates through continuous advances in storing technology during the years and recent years are explosion age of data. Large and valuable volume of data is accumulated in databases and data warehouses in all domains. Online stores store sale details and customer information and interests in their databases. In banking industry account information and transactions are stored. In healthcare industry general patient information and his/her point of care information are stored in databases. These days information is stored either digital or

DOI: 10.4018/978-1-4666-6316-9.ch013

manual because it is proved that information and knowledge are the main success driver in every domain and industry.

However, what we can do with this large volume of data and how we can extract high level knowledge from low level and raw data. It is obvious that we can mine the data to find new and valuable relations and patterns. Pattern is an expression in some language describing a subset of the data or a model applicable to the subset and we can consider a pattern to be knowledge if it exceeds some interestingness threshold that is depends on domain and user definition (Fayyad, Piatetsky-Shapiro & Smyth, 1996). Extracted knowledge can be used to make more effective decisions.

For long years, statisticians used classical statistic methods for pattern identification. Statistics, especially as taught in most statistics texts, might be described as being characterized by data sets which are small and clean, which permit straightforward answers via intensive analysis of single data sets, which are static, which were sampled in an iid manner, which were often collected to answer the particular problem being addressed, and which are solely numeric. None of these apply in the data mining context (Hand, 1998). Data mining technology is presented to pass the constraints of statistic methods. Data mining is a technology that blends traditional data analysis methods with sophisticated algorithms for processing large volumes of data. It has also opened up exciting opportunities for exploring and analyzing new types of data (Tan, Steinbach & Kumar, 2005). Brossette and Hymel (2008) believe that the main tenet of data mining is that the models and patterns contain insights that were previously unsuspected. For that reason alone, data mining is not an exercise in hypothesis-driven exploratory statistics, or hypothesis-driven statistical model building, because "hypothesis-driven" implies previously suspected. Data mining is a new discipline lying at the interface of statistics, database technology, pattern recognition, machine learning, and other areas (Hand, 1998).

There are several definitions for data mining, but all of these definitions have a same understating of underlying concept and there are keywords that are common in all of them. Tan et al. (2005) define data mining as the process of automatically discovering useful information in large data repositories. From Fayyad et al. (1996) point of view knowledge discovery in databases (KDD) is the overall process of discovering useful knowledge from data, and data mining refers to a particular step in this process that is the application of specific algorithms for extracting patterns from data. Usefulness is depends to domain of problem and user definition. Data mining is always associated with analysis. Everywhere that analysis of a small or large data set is needed, data mining can be useful.

Healthcare industry is one of the most interesting areas in which data mining may have an important practical impact. In healthcare, data mining is becoming increasingly popular for several reasons: the extremely large amounts of data; the need for organizations to make decisions based on the analysis of clinical and financial data; and the power to generate information that is fundamentally useful to all parties involved in the healthcare industry (Santos, Malheiros, Cavalheiro & Parente de Oliveira, 2013). Databases are growing in hospitals, clinics, medical research centers, pharmaceutical companies and other related businesses. Researchers and practitioners of this industry seek for solutions to enable them using hidden patterns of data, to extract valid knowledge for more accurate and timely diagnosis, effective genetic data analysis, more effective care, drug discovery, drug repositioning, more effective monitoring and evaluating system, outlier detection, reducing errors, improving decision making for physicians and personnel performance, improving customer relationship management in hospitals and clinics, healthcare tourism and also better understanding of characteristics of care processes. To the best of our knowledge there is not a survey that investigates general applications of knowledge discovery and data mining in healthcare industry. Thus, this chapter proposes a new classification of applications of knowledge discovery and data mining in healthcare industry through studying of recent five years researches. Studies show that knowledge discovery and data mining applications in healthcare industry can be classified to three major classes named patient view, market view and system view. Patient view includes papers that performed pure data mining on healthcare industry data. Market view includes papers that saw the patients as customers. System view includes papers that developed a decision support system.

The rest of chapter organized in two main sections. First section introduces knowledge discovery in databases, data mining and its main techniques, and also domain driving data mining ($D^3M$) methodology in short. Second section discusses data mining in healthcare industry, healthcare data set characteristics and challenges of applying domain driving data mining in this industry. Proposed classification is presented and chapter is concluded finally.

## KNOWLEDGE DISCOVERY AND DATA MINING

### Data Mining Tasks

Data mining tasks can be generally classified into two tasks of predictive and descriptive tasks (Tan et al, 2005). Predictive tasks predict the value of a particular attribute based on the values of other attributes. Classification, regression and anomaly detection are three types of predictive tasks. Descriptive tasks find human-interpretable patterns and relations that describe particular characteristics in data. Clustering, association rule mining and sequential pattern discovery are three types of descriptive tasks. These tasks are briefly explained in following.

- **Classification:** It is used for building predictive models for discrete target variables. In classification objects are assigned to one of several predefined categories. Decision tree classifiers, rule-based classifiers, neural networks, support vector machines and naïve Bayes classifiers are of this type. Each technique employs learning algorithm to identify a model that best fits the relationship between the attribute set and class label of input data. Obviously these techniques use supervised learning algorithm.
- **Regression:** It is used for building predictive models for continuous target variables assuming a linear or nonlinear model of dependency. Regression is greatly studied and discussed in statistics and neural networks. Regression uses supervised learning algorithm like classification.
- **Anomaly Detection:** It is the task of identifying observation known as anomalies or outliers whose characteristics are significantly different from the rest of the data. Applications like detection of fraud and unusual patterns of disease are of this type.
- **Clustering:** It seeks to find groups of closely related observation so that observations that belong to the same cluster are more similar to each other than observations that belong to other clusters. The greater the similarity (or homogeneity) within a group and the greater the difference between groups, the better or more distinct the clustering. There are not predefined class labels in clustering problems.
- **Association Rule Mining:** It is used to discover patterns in the form of implication rules or feature subsets that describe

strongly associated features in the data. Association analysis includes two main parts. First part is discovering patterns from a large data set and second is selecting interesting patterns from the set of all possible patterns.

- **Sequential Pattern Discovery:** It is used to find rules that predict strong sequential dependencies among different events. It is applicable on databases that consist of sequences of ordered elements or events, recorded with or without a concrete notion of time.

## DOMAIN DRIVEN DATA MINING (D³M)

Cao and his colleagues (Cao, Yu, Zhang & Zhao, 2010; Cao, 2010) has presented a methodology that emphasis on the importance of actionability of the knowledge presented in academic researches. They try to warn the existing big gap between academic objectives and what business managers needs for decision making in real world problems and situations. Actionable knowledge discovery aims to deliver knowledge that is business friendly, and which can be taken over by business people for seamless decision making. They believe that the process of data mining should not stop at pattern identification and building a model and satisfying technical significances, but also it should be able to solve real world problems.

Domain driven data mining has been proposed to engage the relevant aspects in actionable knowledge discovery. On top of the data-driven framework, domain driven data mining aims to develop proper methodologies and techniques for integrating domain knowledge, human roles and interaction, as well as actionability measures into the KDD process to discover and deliver actionable knowledge in the constrained environment. Furthermore, it aims to ensure the delivery of actionable and dependable knowledge that can be taken over by business people for direct decision-making and business operation purposes. Table 1 compares major dimensions of the traditional data-centered data mining and domain driven data mining (Cao, Yu, Zhang & Zhao, 2010).

*Figure 1. The gap between academic and business objectives*

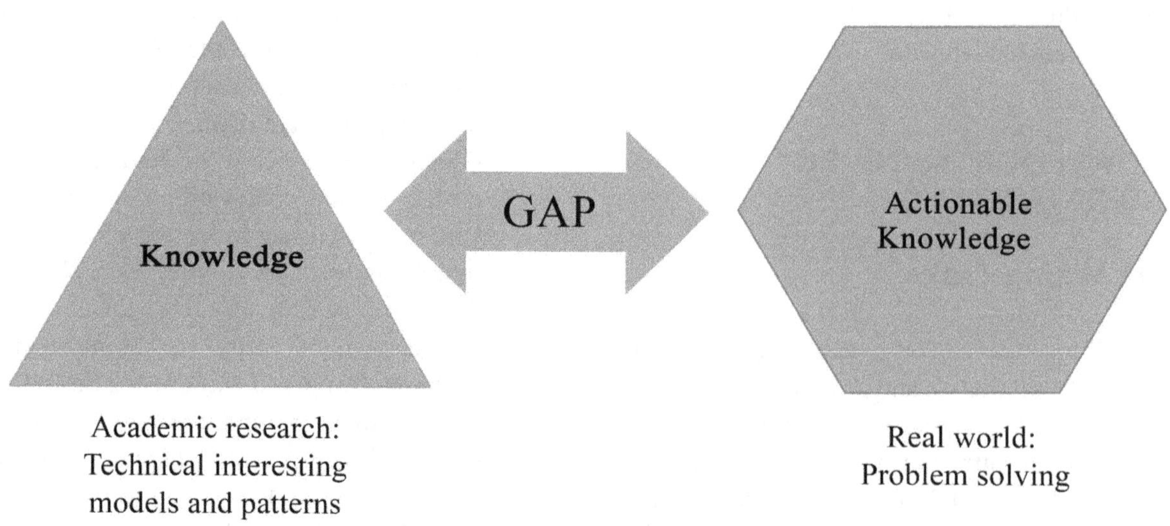

*Table 1. Data-centered vs. domain driven data mining*

| Domain Driven | Traditional Data-Centered | Dimensions |
|---|---|---|
| Solving business problems | Developing innovative approaches | Aims |
| Let data and domain knowledge Tell hidden story in business; discovering actionable knowledge to satisfy real user needs | Let data create/verify research innovation; Demonstrate and push the use of novel algorithms discovering knowledge of interest technically | Goals |
| Problem-solving is the target | Algorithms are the focus | Objectives |
| Data and domain-oriented factors tell the story | Data tells the story | Object mined |
| Mining constrained real-life data | Mining abstract and refined datasets | Datasets |
| Ad-hoc, running-time and personalized model customization | Predefined | Models and methods |
| Human is in the circle of data mining process | Data mining is an automated process | Process |
| Technical and business aspects such as actionability | Technical sides such as accuracy and computational aspects | Performance |
| Business says "yes" or "no" | Evaluation based on technical metrics | Evaluation |
| Operationalizable business rules | Hidden patterns | Deliverables |

## KNOWLEDGE DISCOVERY IN HEALTHCARE INDUSTRY

### Data Analysis in Healthcare Industry

Data mining is effectively nowadays employed in various industries like insurance, marketing, banking, agriculture, customer relationship management, genetic, human right and other sciences. The World Health Organization (WHO) identified the potential of data mining for improving the problems in the medical domain as early as 1997. In the WHO research, emphasis was placed on the usefulness of knowledge detection from medical data repositories that could benefit medical diagnosis and prediction, patient health planning and progress, healthcare system monitoring and assessment, hospital and health services management, and disease prevention (Nahar, Imam, Tickle, & Chen, 2013). Researchers believe that data analysis in healthcare industry is different from other industries because of its heavy relying to background knowledge (Fig. 2). Bellazzi et al. (2011) reports the reasons as safety critical aspect of medical decision making, hardly reproducibility of data, affection of data by several sources of uncertainty and etc. Yeh, Wu and Tsao (2011) explain that Medical data analysis includes data gathering, preprocessing, result evaluation, favorable interaction, and discussions with clinicians for correct analytic results. Lavrac et al. (2007) believe that Healthcare are a knowledge-intensive domain, in which neither data gathering nor data analysis can be successful without using knowledge about both the problem domain and the data analysis process.

## HEALTHCARE DATA SETS CHARACTERISTICS

Data sets in healthcare industry have unique characteristics. Harrison (2008) and Cios and Moore (2002) comprehensively investigate these characteristics and some of them are explained at following. Raw medical data are voluminous and heterogeneous. Medical data may be collected from various images, interviews with the patient,

*Figure 2. All of the KDD steps need domain knowledge to be effective*

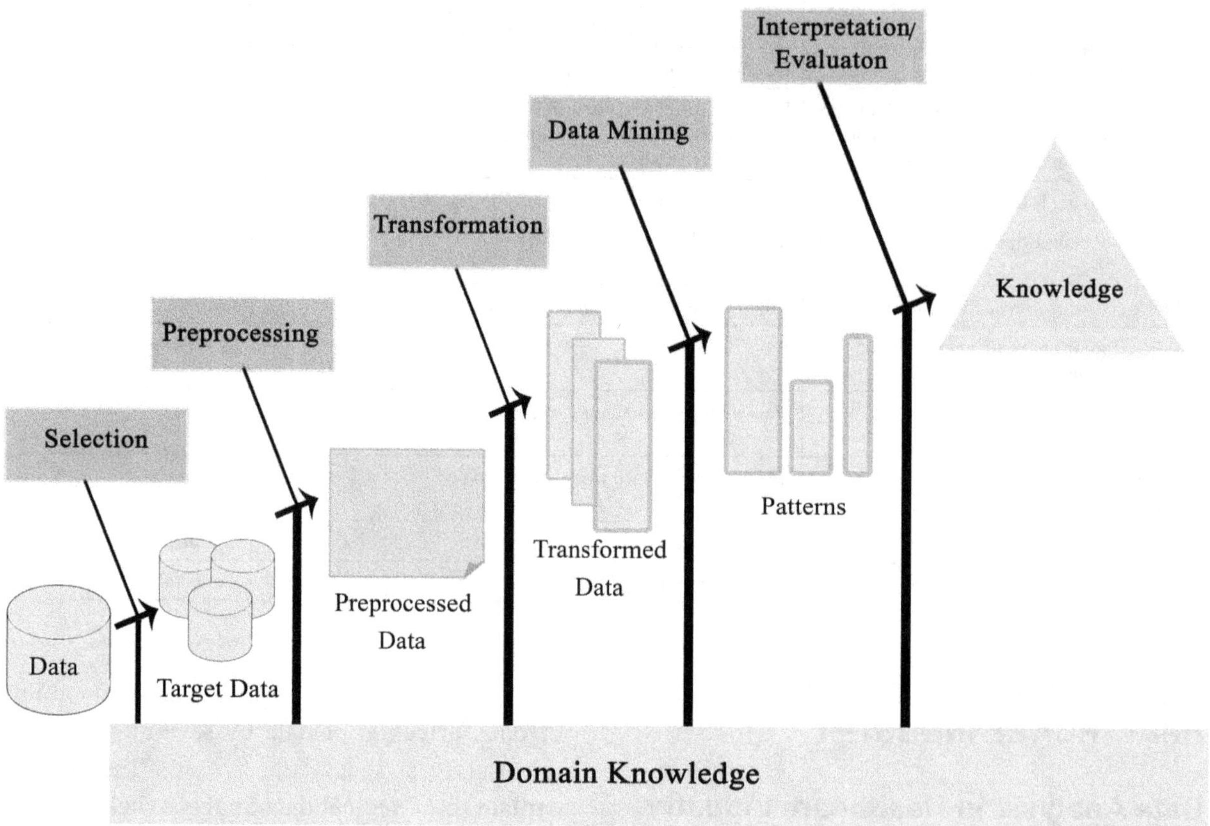


laboratory data, and the physician's observations and interpretations. All these components may bear upon the diagnosis, prognosis, and treatment of the patient, and cannot be ignored. Each record may includes many different data elements, each representing a dimension that can vary in type and value, characterize an item of interest, such as a patient, disease, or specimen. Thus, high dimensionality is one the main characteristics of healthcare data. Diagnoses and other summary data in medical records are generally human interpretations of aggregates of observations and objective data values. Interpretations by different individuals may differ or even conflict.

Data elements in clinical records may not be meaningful outside of a particular temporal context. This phenomenon is particularly true for laboratory databases, which are largely composed of time sequences. So, temporal structure of data should be considered in analysis. Another issue is that data mining methods themselves, especially statistics, and the basic assumptions underlying these methods, may be fundamentally different for medical data and these differences should be considered before analysis. Finally, because medical data are collected on human subjects, there is an enormous ethical and legal tradition designed to prevent the abuse of patients and misuse of their data. Thus for working on such a data all of these constraints should be considered.

Many of data analysis constraint are resolved if data stored in an integrated and standard manner. This is caused data analysis gets more and more simple and precise and extracted knowledge will be more useful in practice. From a research perspective, integrated patient data constitute a computable collection of fine-grained longitudinal phenotypic profiles, facilitating cohort-wide investigations and knowledge discovery on an unprecedented scale (Jensen, Jensen & Brunak, 2012). The Electronic Health Records (EHR) offers the hope for such improved access to patient-specific information and should provide a major benefit both for the quality of care and for the quality of life for clinicians in practice (Shortliffe & Cimino, 2006). Jensen et al. (2012) believe that EHRs capture and integrate data on all aspects of care over time, with the data being represented according to relevant controlled vocabularies. EHR data comprise various data types, from structured information such as drug prescription data consisting of dates and dosages that are captured through a standardized ePrescription system, to unstructured data such as clinical narratives that describe the medical reasoning behind the prescription. This range of different data types highlights the challenge in EHR integration. However, knowledge discovery and data mining in EHRs make delivering personalized and stratified medicine, discovering disease comorbidities and adverse drug events, predicting future patient outcomes, genotype– phenotype association studies and other important applications of data mining in healthcare industry more simple and precise.

## CLASSIFICATION OF KNOWLEDGE DISCOVERY AND DATA MINING APPLICATIONS IN HEALTHCARE INDUSTRY

### Method

Figure 3 describes the analysis process of conducted survey. The main objective is to create a road map that clearly represents current research trends in this domain. Reviewed papers are mostly of recent five years, from 2008 to mid-2013 and are results of searching "data mining" keyword next to other keywords like "health", "clinic", "patient", "medicine" or "decision support systems" in several online databases include Elsevier, IEEE, ACM, Wiley and Springer. These keywords are generally key components of healthcare industry and can be found in title, keyword indices or abstract of papers in surveyed domain. Selected

*Figure 3. Analysis process*

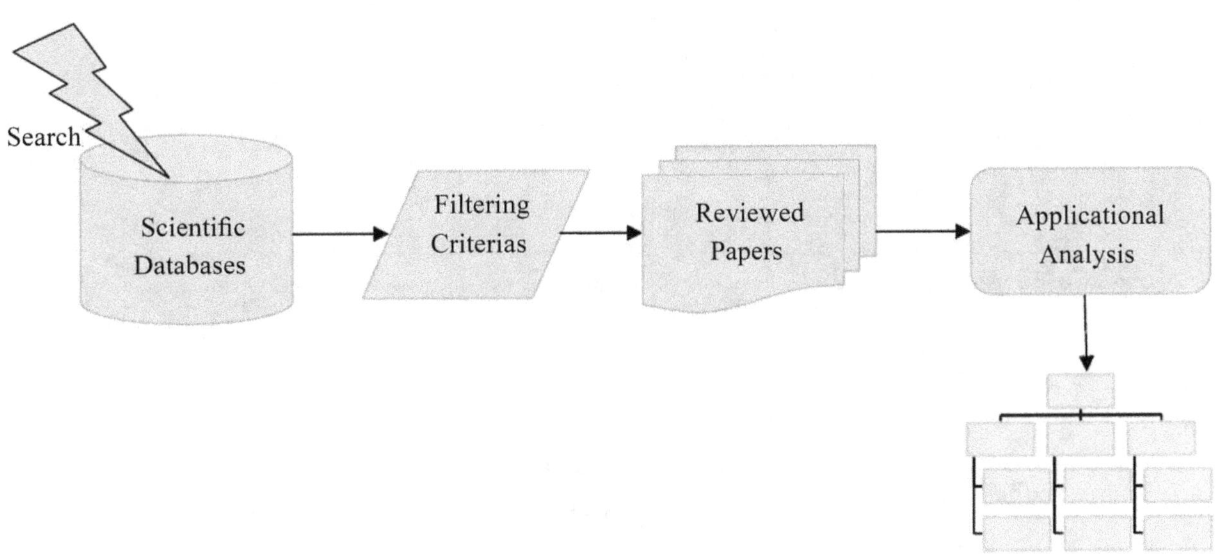

papers add some knowledge to healthcare industry and those that solely use health data sets for evaluating their algorithms were not considered. Also text mining papers were not considered. This filtering reduced the number of search results to 60 papers, from 24 journals and one proceeding, which were closely related to the survey objectives. The number of papers published in this domain is enormous and it is impossible to consider all of them. So, these papers are not covered all papers in this domain but in researchers belief other existing papers certainly lie in one of the classes of the proposed classification.

## Classification

This section classifies knowledge discovery and data mining applications in healthcare industry. The proposed classification is based on main healthcare industry pillars. These pillars can be patient as most important pillar, information and knowledge of healthcare activities, practitioners include managers, physicians, nurses and other personnel, and business issues that cause the industry survive and establish the relationship between all pillars. Patients need high quality services and these services are based on high quality knowledge. Practitioners that deliver these services need high quality and available information and knowledge that enable them to make best decisions. Thus, they need systems and tools that at proper time and intelligently provide them latest and up-to-date knowledge. Healthcare businesses need customer acquisition and retention to increase their revenue and profit and automatically it cases businesses to improve their service quality. Thus, as it is shown in Figure 4 and Table 2, based on these pillars and reviewed papers,

*Figure 4. The proposed classification*

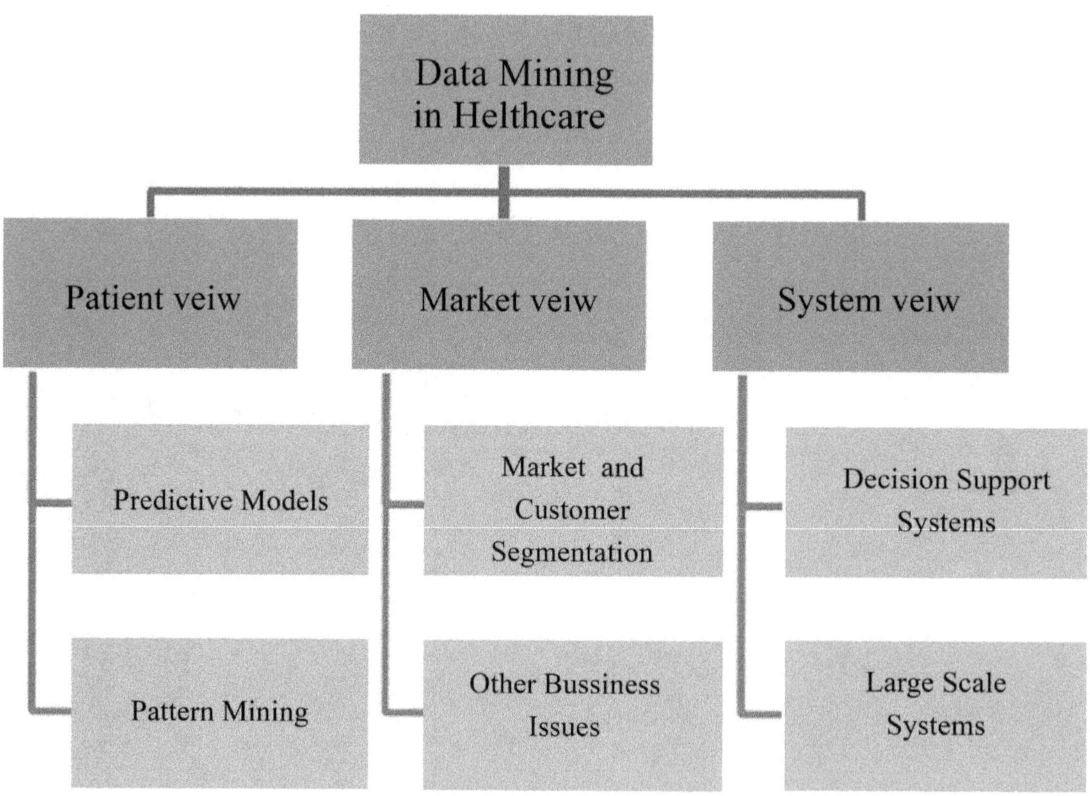

*Table 2. The proposed classification including reviewed papers*

| Percent | Number | References | Group | Class |
|---|---|---|---|---|
| **42%** | **25** | (Bellazzi et al, 2008), (Moon et al, 2012), (Rahman et al, 2011), (Gregori et al, 2011), (Meng et al, 2013), (Marcano-Cedeno et al, 2013), (Yang et al, 2009), (Ghazavi et al, 2008), (Parhizi et al, 2013), (Alizadehsani et al, 2013), (Lehman et al, 2005), (Gil & Johnsson, 2010), (Chi et al, 2010), (Yan et al, 2009), (Zayed et al, 2013), (Roham et al, 2012), (Delen et al, 2009), (Kandula et al, 2011), (Zhao & Weng, 2011), (Bennett et al, 2012), (Hauskrecht et al, 2013), (Lee et al, 2011), (Bellazzi et al, 2011), (Chen et al, 2011), (Shimada et al, 2008) | **Predictive Models** | **Patient view** |
| **18%** | **11** | (Nahar et al, 2013), (Guerrero et al, 2012), (Lazarou et al, 2012), (Kakilehto et al, 2009), (Tai & Chiu, 2009), (Ou-Yang et al, 2013), (Cruz, 2013), (Semenova, 2004), (Yao et al, 2011), (Lee & Giraud-Carrier, 2013), (Lavrac et al,2007) | **Pattern Mining** | |
| **8%** | **5** | (Chen et al, 2012), (Lee & Shih, 2009), (Wei et al, 2012), (Jo et al, 2010), (Hung et al, 2010) | **Market and Customer Segmentation** | **Market view** |
| **5%** | **3** | (Lee et al, 2008), (Orentlicher, 2010), (Shanmugam, 2012) | **Other Business Issues** | |
| **20%** | **12** | (Chae et al, 2003), (Chi et al, 2008), (Yeh et al, 2011), (Alonso et al, 2002), (Kumar et al, 2010), (Da Silva et al, 2011), (Aral et al, 2012), (Ting et al, 2011), (Tenorio et al, 2011), (Cho et al, 2013), (Brossette& Hymel, 2008), (Tartarisco et al, 2012) | **Decision Support Systems** | **System view** |
| **7%** | **4** | (Santos et al, 2013), (El-Sappagh & El-Masri, 2013), (Yan et al, 2004), (Vicente et al, 2004) | **Large Scale Systems** | |
| | **60** | | | |

knowledge discovery and data mining applications in healthcare industry can be classified to three major classes named patient view, market view and system view. Patient view includes papers that their goal is discovering knowledge for improving patient care and treatment. Market view includes papers that their goal is discovering knowledge for improving healthcare businesses revenue. System view includes papers that their goals is discovering knowledge and make it available to healthcare practitioners in an intelligent manner.

## Patient View

Patient view includes papers that purely mined clinical data sets to derive models and discovered patterns. Patient view is divided to predictive models and pattern mining groups. Predictive models include papers that mine records of patients with specific diseases or characteristics to derive a predictive model for in time diagnosis, therapy and trial outcome prediction, determining risk factors of a disease and improving monitoring tasks. Some papers worked on administrative data of hospitals and clinics to improve services and reduce errors. As it can be seen in Table 3 almost 42 percent of the reviewed papers are in this group. Apparently predictive models group are most investigated field in this context. Building predictive models can be simple or complicated based on adopted data sets and techniques. Decision tree is one of the simplest techniques for implementation from technical perspective and for interpreting from a domain expert perspective. Moon, Kang, Jitpitaklert & Kim (2012) have used Classification and regression trees (CART) to characterize smoking behavior among older adults by assessing the psychological distress, physical health status, alcohol use, and demographic variables in relations to the current smoking. Parhizi, Steege and Pasupathy (2013) have used a tree-based Chi-Square Automatic Interaction Detection (CHAID) to identify relationships between multiple psychosocial factors and dimensions of fatigue using data mining classification methods. Kumar et al. (2010) believe that people typically use decision trees because they are easy to explain the classification to domain experts. Often, this comprehensibility comes at the expense of accuracy. Artificial Neural Networks (ANNs) are black box artificial intelligence-based algorithms that have been until recently quite popular in clinical medicine, although they are prone to overfitting (Bellazzi et al, 2011). Accuracy and performance of ANN based models are mostly depends on domain, selected features, data set and mining software. In Marcano-Cedeno et al. (2013) in contrast to most of studies that are focused in determining survival, predicting disability or the recovery of patients, and looking for the factors that are better at predicting the patient's condition after suffering an acquired brain injury (ABI), the purpose was the novel application of data mining to predict the outcomes of the cognitive rehabilitation of patients with ABI. They used decision tree, multilayer perceptron and general regression neural network to construct the prediction models. In Delen, Fuller, McCann & Ray (2009) the healthcare coverage of individuals has been examined by applying artificial neural network and decision tree on a wide-variety of predictive factors and they claimed that experimental results indicated that the most accurate classifier for this phenomenon was the multi-layer perceptron type artificial neural network model. A more robust approach, grounded in statistical learning theory, is provided by support vector machine (SVM), which may handle both linear and nonlinear decision boundaries. Although the learned classifiers may be difficult to interpret, the classification performance can be quite high (Bellazzi et al, 2011). In Kandula, Zeng-Treitler, Chen, Salomon & Bray (2011) proposed a bootstrapping method that supplements ICD-9 codes with lab results, medications, etc. to build classification models that can be used to identify cohorts more accurately. The proposed method does not require prior information about the true class of the patients. They used SVM to build the models. Probabilistic classifiers, such as Naive Bayes classifiers and Bayesian networks are also exploited in the medical literature, although less frequently (Bellazzi et al, 2011). In Zhao & Weng (2011) a novel method have been proposed that combines PubMed knowledge and Electronic Health Records to develop a weighted Bayesian Network Inference (BNI) model for pancreatic cancer prediction. They claimed that in an evaluation using a case-control dataset, the weighted BNI model significantly outperformed the conventional BNI and k-Nearest Neighbor (KNN) and SVM. Anomaly or outlier detection is another predictive data mining task that is exploited in the literature, although less frequently. Hauskrecht et al. (2013) have developed and evaluated a data-driven approach for detecting unusual (anomalous) patient-management decisions using past patient cases stored in electronic health records (EHRs). Their hypothesis was that a patient-management decision that is unusual with respect to past patient care may be due to an error and that it is worthwhile to generate an alert if such a decision is encountered. They used SVM to build their model. Bennett, Doub and Selove (2012) believe that next version of predictive models in future are the patient personalized ones and it is possible through combining mixing genetic and clinical indicators, rather than using one or the other.

Second group of patient view is pattern mining. Papers in this group investigates mining hidden relations, dependencies and interesting patterns, finding useful and meaningful groups, determining effective and key factors in patients data with a specific disease and also in administrative data sets. Patterns embedded in large volumes of clinical data may provide important insights into the characteristics of patients or care delivery processes, but may be difficult to identify by traditional means (Rahman & Hasan, 2011). Almost 18 percent of the reviewed papers are in this group. In this context, association rule discovery is the most popular descriptive technique. In contrast to other data mining techniques, association rule is not driven from statistics. In Healthcare, association rules are considered to be quite useful as they offer the possibility to conduct intelligent diagnosis and extract invaluable information and build important knowledge bases quickly and automatically (Rahman & Hasan, 2011). Nahar, Imam, Tickle and Chen (2013) investigate the sick and healthy factors which contribute to heart disease for males and females. Association rule mining, a computational intelligence approach, is used to identify these factors. In Tai & Chiu (2009) association rule mining has been applied to explore the labyrinthian network of Attention Deficit/Hyperactivity Disorder (ADHD) comorbidity, and to examine the practicality of association rule mining in comorbidity studies using clinic databases. Clustering is also used frequently in this context especially in business related issues. Self organizing map (SOM) is a type of artificial neural network that because it produces a low-dimensional (typically two-dimensional), discretized representation of the high dimensional input space that is one of the main characteristics of clinical data sets, called a map, is one of the most popular clustering techniques in this context. SOMs are different from other artificial neural networks in the sense that they use a neighborhood function to preserve the topological properties of the input space (Wikipedia, Self-organizing map, n. d.). Guerrero et al. (2012) have used SOM to detect a residual area of low satisfaction in dialysis patients. Lee and Giraud-Carrier (2013) have adapted and extended association rule mining and clustering algorithms to extract useful knowledge regarding diabetes and high blood pressure from mined data set and to demonstrate how data mining techniques may be used to support evidence-based medicine.

## Market View

One of the interesting issues for businesses in every industry is customer relationship management (CRM) for better customer acquisition and retention. Improving quality of care and customer satisfaction are the key business drivers in healthcare industry (Hung, Hung, Tsai & Jiang, 2010). The effective and efficient utilization of IT is a method for implementing a successful CRM strategy to understand customer needs, satisfy customer demands, mine for valuable customer information, identify target and potential customers, realize the maximum customer value, increase customer loyalty, and finally maximize profits (Chen, Cheng, Lai, Hsu & Syu, 2012). Market view includes papers that look at the patient as a potential customer. These papers are 13 percent of all the reviewed papers and divide to market and customer segmentation, and other business related issues groups. Market and customer segmentation through data mining are one of the most popular research fields in CRM context. The health care industry is one of the world's largest and fastest-growing industries (Wikipedia, Healthcare industry, n. d.). As the competition increased in this industry, related businesses like hospitals, clinics, pharmaceutical companies and others needed to identify their core competencies and increase their competitive advantages. CRM can be the most valuable core competency that a business can have especially in health related business as people care about their health more than anything else. However, apparently market view is the smallest research area in this context and it can be because of difficulties of accessing to financial data for researches and also constraints that exist because of ethical and legal issues. But definitely like other industries, businesses in healthcare industry can use data mining for market analysis, discovering customer behavior patterns and designing effective marketing strategies. Papers in market and customer segmentation group mostly mine customer and market data to find the profitable segments of customers and maximize the profit through developing targeted effective marketing strategies. Chen et al. (2012) propose a two-stage clustering-classification model through initially integrating the RFM attribute and K-means algorithm for clustering the target customer segment (TCS) patients and then integrating the global discretization method and the rough set theory for classifying hospitalized departments and optimizing healthcare services. Wei, Lin, Weng and Wu (2012) develop an extended RFM (recency, frequency, and monetary) model, namely LRFM (length, recency, frequency, and monetary) model, by adopting SOM technique for a children's dental clinic to segment its dental patients. Second group in market view include papers in others business related issues like hospital selection, health tourism and pharmaceutical marketing. Shanmugam, (2012) explains that mainly for the sake of affordability, many patients in much advanced nations, often voluntarily, seek medical services in far less underdeveloped nations. He applies a data mining approach to compute and interpret economic indices and portray the economic booming in the hosting nations which render the medical treatments to the patients who emanate from the guest nations.

## System View

Clinical decision support systems (CDSS) are systems that support clinician to make effective decisions in diagnosis, prognosis, therapy and prescription and also used for preventing medical errors, especially diagnostic errors, reducing cost, and improving patient safety (Mitchell et al, 2011). System view is divided into two groups of decision support systems and large scale systems. Former includes papers that explicitly propose an algorithm, information flow diagram, application or architecture for decision support systems. Yeh et al. (2011) have combined temporal abstraction with data mining techniques for analyzing dialysis patients' biochemical data to develop a decision support system. The mined temporal patterns are helpful for clinicians to predict hospitalization of hemodialysis patients and to suggest immediate treatments to avoid hospitalization. Chi, Street and Katz (2010) have proposed a machine learning based expert system approach, called optimal decision path finder (ODPF), to dynamically determine the test that is most likely to be informative in terms of diagnostic accuracy while minimizing the time and money spent on diagnostic testing. Tartarisco et al. (2012) have proposed an automatic simple, compact, wireless, personalized and cost efficient pervasive architecture for the evaluation of the stress state of individual subjects suitable for prolonged stress monitoring during normal activity. It used SOM to cluster the received bio-signals from a wearable device. Papers propose architecture or systems that can perform or have potential to perform knowledge discovery and data mining in a large scale manner are in the large scale system group. Santos et al. (2013) have described that the large-scale adoption of data mining has been limited thus far because it is difficult to use, especially for non-expert users and one way to facilitate data mining by non-expert users is to automate the process. They presented an automated data mining system that allows public health decision makers that probably do not have any knowledge about data mining techniques and tools, to access analytical information regarding brain tumors. The difference between previous data mining approaches and the approach proposed in their study is that the proposed approach is concept-centric; the reports stem from concepts selected by users from the domain ontology. In addition, the approach does not require users to select input parameters; instead, they only select the concepts to be analyzed. System view includes the considerable number of reviewed papers, about 20 percent. It is considerable because developing a decision support system in small or large scale, have their own complexity and challenges in addition of all of common challenges of applying knowledge discovery and data mining in healthcare industry. Mitchell et al. (2011) believe that these challenges are of three major types. The first is domain challenges that related to large number of interacting and complicating conditions or factors that is usually involved in clinical decisions; relevant information and available options are incomplete, uncertain, and often changing with the progression of the disease(s), the genetic makeup of the patients, and the outcome of the actions. Second challenge is system challenges that related to the constantly varying clinical workflows, rapidly changing information technology platforms, and exponentially accumulating information and data of various forms that render many subsystems or processes incompatible or obsolete very quickly. These in turn complicate the proper encoding, maintenance, and integration of the information and knowledge needed to support cost-effective decision making; and the third challenge is usage challenges that related to existing of different users with vastly different backgrounds, different objectives, and even different preferences in their decision making approaches for the same system and difficulty of fulfilling their needs.

## DISCUSSION

According to the united nation International Standard Industrial Classification (ISIC) definition, the healthcare industry generally consist of three major activities include hospital activities, medical and dental practice activities, and other human health activities (Wikipedia, Healthcare industry, n. d.). Knowledge discovery and data mining have powerful capability to discover hidden patterns in data related to all of these activities. Wherever significant volume of stored data are accessible, knowledge discovery and data mining can effectively improve system performance or enhance the knowledge related to mined data. Discovered patterns and derived models help practitioners to make the right, effective and timely decisions and lead to better services.

Knowledge discovery and data mining in healthcare industry is much more knowledge intensive in compared to other industries and this should be considered in all of KDD steps from feature selection to choosing the data mining techniques and evaluation and interpretation of results. Problem and data set characteristics and analyzing goals should be considered in choosing every techniques used in KDD steps. Because for example selecting an unrelated feature or ignoring an important feature can heavily affect final results or can lead to incorrect results. Also an analysis that does not solve the healthcare practitioner problems is not useful even if it satisfies technical measures. That is why the synergy between technical and healthcare domain experts to recognize data characteristics, to determine significance and effectivity of every feature and to choose the most effective techniques for all steps of data analysis is the key success factor in KDD. If we determine the criteria of success assessment rigidly the ability of extracted knowledge to solve real world problems, the necessity and importance of existence of this synergy will be much more. Lack or incompleteness of both sides leads to poor problem definition and analysis and therefore results to less valuable or worthless knowledge.

Each data mining techniques include classification or clustering or association rules mining has specific characteristics and analyze the data in a different manner. If these characteristics and extracted knowledge of these techniques used to complete each other rather than using them in a divergence manner, final results will be more valuable. However, data mining techniques are not without imperfections. Being imperfect for any reason, intrinsic or data set, other techniques such as statistical techniques and algorithms, case based reasoning, rule-based methods, evolutionary algorithms and machine learning techniques can help to improve data analysis.

One of the advantages of research in patient view class is its variety of research areas. Literature review shows that available data sets of large number of diseases including mortal ones such as heart disease and cancer to less mortal ones like children's obesity or urological dysfunctions are investigated. Each data set can be inspiration for new models and patterns. Wherever patients data set with a specific disease are available, it can be used to build predictive models and discovered valuable patterns. These models and patterns can be related to final state or trial and rehabilitation activities results of patients.

Wherever the aim of data miner is discovering hidden relationships between data elements, there is no technique more applicable than association rule mining. Healthcare industry is not an exception too. These elements in the healthcare are disease symptoms, trials, medications, prescription and reaction. These elements along with demographic and psychographic data are almost fixed in most data sets. Mining association rules elegantly discover hidden relationships between these elements and lead to producing new knowledge, improving care processes and reducing care and service errors. Clustering in this domain in most cases is used as a supplement for mining association rules.

Competition among businesses in healthcare industry has grown like other industries. Knowledge about customers and market to create competitive advantage and implement powerful CRM is the most important assets of a business. In order to manage customers better, organizations need to classify their customers. Among the customers that organizations deal with them, few ones are most profitable. These are customers that an organization try to continue its relationship with them. Additionally, segmenting customers to separate groups in which all members are similar in many characteristics, allowing the organization to design marketing strategies tailored to the needs and desires of each group. Most of researches on market view area were somehow related to CRM and it reflects the importance of this issue in healthcare industry businesses.

The development of decision support systems is a step forward to solve real world problems, where uncertainty and high dimensionality cause decision making be a difficult task. It causes extracted knowledge be applicable for managers, physicians in care environment, and individuals outside of care environment through personal health systems. Heart of a decision support system is the knowledge that it uses to make decision. The challenges facing researchers interested in developing decision support systems are getting the data and processing them automatically or semi-automatically and efficiently, optimal knowledge updatability and dynamic learning of system, efficient result evaluation and presentation. It seems that one of the limitations in developing of decision support systems is automating preprocessing step. However, research shows that the role of the user in this step should still remain strong. Technically it is not simply possible, but the standard and structured data storages like electronic health records is a step towards improving data sets structure and optimizing preprocessing step. Also, systems must be able to be compatible with multi-class decision making problems, because most of real world problems in this industry deal with several complicated conditions that are even unknown in worst case. For this reason the main criticism that can make on several number researches is oversimplification of problems. Ongoing advances in computer networks and distributed systems as well as powerful software architectures provide interesting research areas in designing and implementing large-scale systems to improve collaboration and resource sharing.

Several numbers of papers explicitly or implicitly considered D$^3$M methodology and could get close to real world problem solving without exorbitance problem simplification. However, there is a long way to realize all the specifications of D³M methodology in healthcare industry as it is described in Cao et al. (2010). Wide research areas, different approaches in diagnosis, prognosis, therapy and other car processes, continuous developments in information technology and medicine cause that presenting comprehensive solutions harder. However, there are researches (Sebastian and Then, 2011; Kuo, Lonie, Sonenberg and Paizis, 2007; Santos et al, 2013) that make well considerable progression toward realizing D³M visions.

The main limitations of our research were dependency of knowledge discovery and data mining in healthcare industry to background knowledge and also its variety of applications. Analyzing models and parameters used to build the models, evaluating discovered pattern and derived models and generally presented results are affected by mentioned limitations. On the other hand, dependency of data mining in healthcare industry to context and data makes accurate comparing of data mining techniques difficult.

According to our research's applicational perspective, the ideas at macro level to improve using knowledge discovery in healthcare industry can be as following:

- Using domain driven data mining in healthcare industry to enhance the actionability of extracting knowledge.
- Defining the problem, designing and conducting knowledge discovery toward solving real world problems in healthcare industry.
- Designing a healthcare driven data mining (HD²M) framework in all dimensions.
- Proposing customized KDD techniques according to general characteristics of healthcare data.

These four ideas stress on D³M primary objective that is reducing the gap exists between research and real world problem solving. Here the domain is healthcare, so we seek for healthcare specific data mining problem definition and design, techniques and frameworks, or in other words, healthcare driven data mining (HD²M). The aim is making extracted knowledge or models and pattern more useful and executable and somehow easier to understand and to use for healthcare industry practitioners.

- Making discovered patterns and derived models usable for healthcare industry practitioners through developing decision support systems to help them for making better decisions.
- Proposing large scale and distributed architectures for decision support systems using novel technologies to enhance system availability.

As discussed before, one of the main ways of making extracted knowledge from knowledge discovery and data mining easier to use and also executable for practitioners is providing it in small and large scale decision support systems. Developing intelligent decision support systems that their knowledge is provided through knowledge discovery and data mining engine is another major research area.

- Proposing large scale and distributed architectures for decision support systems that consider knowledge integration after KDD.

The world contains a vast array of complex and diverse data, but locating and connecting the information are difficult (Cases et al, 2013). One of the ways to overcome these problems is developing a framework to connect and integrate different data mining processes and extracted knowledge without completely integrating original data sets.

- Proposing real time data analysis frameworks to use KDD in real time healthcare applications.

Another research idea can be developing decision support systems that use data mining for analyzing instant patient data in real time situations that timely decision making is very crucial such as operating room, intensive care unit (ICU) or emergency department to help practitioners make vital decisions better and quicker.

- Proposing methods and approaches for mining EHRs more efficient.
- Discovering analysis opportunities to improve CRM in healthcare industry businesses with respect to the ethical and legal constraints.

## CONCLUSION

This chapter has reviewed recent studies on knowledge discovery applications in healthcare industry and proposes a new classification of these applications. Studies has shown that knowledge discovery and data mining applications in healthcare industry can be classified to three major classes named patient view, market view and system view. Patient view includes papers that performed pure data mining on healthcare industry data. Market view includes papers that saw the patients as customers. System view includes papers that developed a decision support system. The goal of this classification was identifying research opportunities and gaps for researchers are interested to this context.

## ACKNOWLEDGMENT

The authors would like to thank the anonymous reviewers and the editor for their insightful comments and suggestions.

## REFERENCES

Alizadehsani, et al. (2013). A data mining approach for diagnosis of coronary artery disease. *Computer Methods and Programs in Biomedicine*, *111*(1), 52–61. doi:10.1016/j.cmpb.2013.03.004 PMID:23537611

Alonso, F., Caraca-Valente, P. J., Gonzalez, A. L., & Montes, C. (2002). Combining expert knowledge and data mining in a medical diagnosis domain. *Expert Systems with Applications*, *23*(4), 367–375. doi:10.1016/S0957-4174(02)00072-6

Aral, K. D., Guvenir, H. A., Sabuncuoglu, I., & Akar, A. R. (2012). A prescription fraud detection model. *Computer Methods and Programs in Biomedicine*, *106*(1), 37–46. doi:10.1016/j.cmpb.2011.09.003 PMID:22088866

Bellazzi, R., Ferrazzi, F., & Sacchi, L. (2011). Predictive data mining in clinical medicine: a focus on selected methods and applications. *WIREs Data Mining and Knowledge Discovery*, *1*(5), 416–430. doi:10.1002/widm.23

Bellazzi, R., & Zupan, B. (2008). Predictive data mining in clinical medicine: Current issues and guidelines. *International Journal of Medical Informatics*, *77*(2), 81–97. doi:10.1016/j.ijmedinf.2006.11.006 PMID:17188928

Bennett, C. C., Doub, T. W., & Selove, R. (2012). EHRs connect research and practice: Where predictive modeling, artificial intelligence, and clinical decision support intersect. *Health Policy and Technology*, *1*(2), 105–114. doi:10.1016/j.hlpt.2012.03.001

Brossette, S. E., Hymel P. A. (2008). Data mining and infection control. *Clinics in Laboratory Medicine*, *28*(1), 119–126.

Cao, L. (2010). Domain-driven data mining: challenges and prospects. *IEEE Transactions on Knowledge and Data Engineering*, *22*(6), 755–769. doi:10.1109/TKDE.2010.32

Cao, L., Yu, S. P., Zhang, C., & Zhao, Y. (2010). *Domain driven data mining*. Springer. doi:10.1007/978-1-4419-5737-5

Cases, et al. (2013). Improving data and knowledge management to better integrate health care and research. *Journal of Internal Medicine*, *274*(4), 321–328. doi:10.1111/joim.12105 PMID:23808970

Chae, Y., Kim, H., Tark, H., Park, H., & Ho, S. (2003). Analysis of healthcare quality indicator using data mining and decision support system. *Expert Systems with Applications*, *24*(2), 167–172. doi:10.1016/S0957-4174(02)00139-2

Chen, H. Y., Chuang, C. H., Yang, Y. J., & Wu, T. P. (2011). Exploring the risk factors of preterm birth using data mining. *Expert Systems with Applications*, *38*(5), 5384–5387. doi:10.1016/j.eswa.2010.10.017

Chen, Y. S., Cheng, C. H., Lai, C. J., Hsu, C. Y., & Syu, H. J. (2012). Identifying patients in target customer segments using a two-stage clustering-classification approach: A hospital-based assessment. *Computers in Biology and Medicine*, *42*(2), 213–221. doi:10.1016/j.compbiomed.2011.11.010 PMID:22177941

Chi, C. L., Street, W. N., & Katz, D. A. (2010). A decision support system for cost-effective diagnosis. *Artificial Intelligence in Medicine*, *50*(3), 149–161. doi:10.1016/j.artmed.2010.08.001 PMID:20933375

Chi, C. L., Street, W. N., & Ward, M. M. (2008). Building a hospital referral expert system with a prediction and optimization-based decision support system algorithm. *Journal of Biomedical Informatics*, *41*(2), 371–386. doi:10.1016/j.jbi.2007.10.002 PMID:18054523

Cho, I., Park, I., Kim, E., Lee, E., & Bates, D. W. (2013). Using EHR data to predict hospital-acquired pressure ulcers: A prospective study of a bayesian network model. *International Journal of Medical Informatics*, *82*(11), 1059–1067. doi:10.1016/j.ijmedinf.2013.06.012 PMID:23891086

Cios, K., & Moore, G. W. (2002). Uniqueness of medical data mining. *Artificial Intelligence in Medicine*, *26*(1-2), 1–24. doi:10.1016/S0933-3657(02)00049-0 PMID:12234714

Cruz, A. M. (2013). Evaluating record history of medical devices using association discovery and clustering techniques. *Expert Systems with Applications*, *40*(13), 5292–5305. doi:10.1016/j.eswa.2013.03.034

Da Silva, S. F., Ribeiro, M. X., Batista Neto, J. D. E. S., Traina-Jr, C., & Traina, A. J. M. (2011). Improving the ranking quality of medical image retrieval using a genetic feature selection method. *Decision Support Systems*, *51*(4), 810–820. doi:10.1016/j.dss.2011.01.015

Delen, D., Fuller, C., McCann, C., & Ray, D. (2009). Analysis of healthcare coverage: A data mining approach. *Expert Systems with Applications*, *36*(2), 995–1003. doi:10.1016/j.eswa.2007.10.041

El-Sappagh, S. H., & El-Masri, S. (2013). A distributed clinical decision support system architecture. *Journal of King Saud University-Computer and Information Sciences*, *26*(1), 69–78. doi:10.1016/j.jksuci.2013.03.005

Fayyad, U., Piatetsky-Shapiro, G., & Smyth, P. (1996). From Data Mining to Knowledge Discovery in Databases. *AI Magazine*, *17*(3), 37–54.

Garrett, P., & Seidman, P. (2011). *EMR vs EHR – What is the Difference?*. Retrieved August 10, 2013, from http://www.healthit.gov/buzz-blog/electronic-health-and-medical-records/emr-vs-ehr-difference/

Ghazavi, S. N., & Liao, T. W. (2008). Medical data mining by fuzzy modeling with selected features. *Artificial Intelligence in Medicine*, *43*(3), 195–206. doi:10.1016/j.artmed.2008.04.004 PMID:18534831

Gil, D., & Johnsson, M. (2010). Using support vector machines in diagnoses of urological dysfunctions. *Expert Systems with Applications*, *37*(6), 4713–4718. doi:10.1016/j.eswa.2009.12.055

Gregori, D., Petrinco, M., Bo, S., Rosato, R., Pagano, E., Berchialla, P., & Merletti, F. (2011). Using data mining techniques in monitoring diabetes care. The simpler the better? *Journal of Medical Systems*, *35*(2), 277–281. doi:10.1007/s10916-009-9363-9 PMID:20703563

Guerrero, et al. (2012). Self-Organising Maps: A new way to screen the level of satisfaction of dialysis patients. *Expert Systems with Applications*, *39*(10), 8793–8798. doi:10.1016/j.eswa.2012.02.001

Hand, D. J. (1998). Data mining: statistics and more? *American Statistical Association*, *52*, 112–118.

Harrison, J. H. (2008). Introduction to the mining of clinical data. *Clinics in Laboratory Medicine*, *28*(1), 1–7. doi:10.1016/j.cll.2007.10.001 PMID:18194715

Hauskrecht, M., Batal, I., Valko, M., Visweswaran, S., Cooper, G. F., & Clermont, G. (2013). Outlier detection for patient monitoring and alerting. *Journal of Biomedical Informatics*, *46*(1), 47–55. doi:10.1016/j.jbi.2012.08.004 PMID:22944172

Healthcare Industry. (n.d.). In *Wikipedia*. Retrieved Sep 17, 2013, from http://en.wikipedia.org/wiki/Health_care_industry

Hung, S. Y., Hung, W. H., Tsai, C. A., & Jiang, S. C. (2010). Critical factors of hospital adoption on CRM system: Organizational and information system perspectives. *Decision Support Systems*, *48*(4), 592–603. doi:10.1016/j.dss.2009.11.009

Jensen, P. B., & Jensen, L, J, Brunak, S. (2012). Mining electronic health records: towards better research applications and clinical care. *Nature Reviews. Transactional Genetics*, *13*(6), 395–405.

Jo, H. S., Hwang, M. S., & Lee, H. (2010). Market segmentation of health information use on the Internet in Korea. *International Journal of Medical Informatics*, *79*(10), 707–715. doi:10.1016/j.ijmedinf.2010.07.006 PMID:20810307

Kakilehto, T., Salo, S., & Larmas, M. (2009). Data mining of clinical oral health documents for analysis of the longevity of different restorative materials in Finland. *International Journal of Medical Informatics*, *78*(12), e68–e74. doi:10.1016/j.ijmedinf.2009.04.004 PMID:19428290

Kandula, S., Zeng-Treitler, Q., Chen, L., Salomon, W. L., & Bray, B. E. (2011). A bootstrapping algorithm to improve cohort identification using structured data. *Journal of Biomedical Informatics*, *44*(1), S63–S68. doi:10.1016/j.jbi.2011.10.013 PMID:22079803

Kumar, M., Ghani, R., & Mei, Z. S. (2010). Data mining to predict and prevent errors in health insurance claims processing. In *Proceedings of the 16th ACM SIGKDD International Conference on Knowledge Discovery and Data Mining* (pp. 65-74). ACM.

Kuo, Y. T., Lonie, A., Sonenberg, L., & Paizis, K. (2007). Domain Ontology Driven Data Mining. In *Proceedings of the 2007 international Workshop on Domain Driven Data Mining* (pp 11-17). Academic Press.

Lavrac, N., Bohanec, M., Pur, A., Cestnik, B., Debeljak, M., & Kobler, A. (2007). Data mining and visualization for decision support and modeling of public health-care resources. *Journal of Biomedical Informatics*, *40*(4), 438–447. doi:10.1016/j.jbi.2006.10.003 PMID:17157076

Lazarou, C., Karaolis, M., Matalas, A. L., & Panagiotakos, D. B. (2012). Dietary patterns analysis using data mining method. An application to data from the CYKIDS study. *Computer Methods and Programs in Biomedicine*, *108*(2), 706–714. doi:10.1016/j.cmpb.2011.12.011 PMID:22296977

Lee, J. W., & Giraud-Carrier, C. (2013). Results on mining NHANES data: A case study in evidence-based medicine. *Computers in Biology and Medicine*, *43*(5), 493–503. doi:10.1016/j.compbiomed.2013.02.018 PMID:23566395

Lee, T. T., Liu, C. Y., Kuo, Y. H., Mills, M. E., Fong, J. G., & Hung, C. (2011). Application of data mining to the identification of critical factors in patient falls using a web-based reporting system. *International Journal of Medical Informatics*, *80*(2), 141–150. doi:10.1016/j.ijmedinf.2010.10.009 PMID:21115393

Lee, W., & Shih, B. (2009). Application of neural networks to recognize profitable customers for dental services marketing-a case of dental clinics in Taiwan. *Expert Systems with Applications*, *36*(1), 199–208. doi:10.1016/j.eswa.2007.09.028

Lee, W., Shih, B., & Chung, Y. S. (2008). The exploration of consumers' behavior in choosing hospital by the application of neural network. *Expert Systems with Applications*, *34*(2), 806–816. doi:10.1016/j.eswa.2006.10.020

Lehman, T. M., Guld, M. O., Deselaers, T., Keysers, D., Schubert, H., & Spitzer, K. et al. (2005). Automatic categorization of medical images for content-based retrieval and data mining. *Computerized Medical Imaging and Graphics*, *29*(2-3), 143–155. doi:10.1016/j.compmedimag.2004.09.010 PMID:15755534

Liao, S. H., Chu, P. H., & Hsiao, P. Y. (2012). Data mining techniques and applications – A decade review from 2000 to 2011. *Expert Systems with Applications*, *39*(12), 11303–11311. doi:10.1016/j.eswa.2012.02.063

Marcano-Cedeno, A., Chausa, P., Garcia, A., Caceres, C., Tormos, J. M., & Gomez, E. J. (2013). Data mining applied to the cognitive rehabilitation of patients with acquired brain injury. *Expert Systems with Applications*, *40*(4), 1054–1060. doi:10.1016/j.eswa.2012.08.034

Meng, X. H., Huang, Y. X., Rao, D. P., Zhang, Q., & Liu, Q. (2013). Comparison of three data mining models for predicting diabetes or prediabetes by risk factors. *The Kaohsiung Journal of Medical Sciences*, *29*(2), 93–99. doi:10.1016/j.kjms.2012.08.016 PMID:23347811

Mitchell, et al. (2011). 50 Years of Informatics Research on Decision Support: What's Next. *Methods of Information in Medicine*, *50*, 525–535. doi:10.3414/ME11-06-0004 PMID:22146915

Moon, S. S., Kang, S. Y., Jitpitaklert, W., & Kim, S. B. (2012). Decision tree models for characterizing smoking patterns of older adults. *Expert Systems with Applications*, *39*(1), 445–451. doi:10.1016/j.eswa.2011.07.035

Nahar, J., Imam, T., Tickle, K. S., & Chen, Y. P. (2013). Association rule mining to detect factors which contribute to heart disease in males and females. *Expert Systems with Applications*, *40*(4), 1086–1093. doi:10.1016/j.eswa.2012.08.028

Orentlicher, D. (2010). Prescription data mining and the protection of patients' interests. *The Journal of Law, Medicine & Ethics*, *38*(1), 74–84. doi:10.1111/j.1748-720X.2010.00468.x PMID:20446986

Ou-Yang, C., Agustianty, S., & Wang, H. C. (2013). Developing a data mining approach to investigate association between physician prescription and patient outcome – A study on re-hospitalization in Stevens–Johnson Syndrome. *Computer Methods and Programs in Biomedicine*, *112*(1), 84–91. doi:10.1016/j.cmpb.2013.07.004 PMID:23910224

Parhizi, S., Steege, L. S., & Pasupathy, K. S. (2013). Mining the relationships between psychosocial factors and fatigue dimensions among registered nurses. *International Journal of Industrial Ergonomics*, *43*(1), 82–90. doi:10.1016/j.ergon.2012.11.010

Patel, et al. (2009). The coming of age of artificial intelligence in medicine. *Artificial Intelligence in Medicine*, *46*(1), 5–17. doi:10.1016/j.artmed.2008.07.017 PMID:18790621

Rahman, R. M., & Hasan, F. R. M. (2011). Using and comparing different decision tree classification techniques for mining ICDDR,B Hospital Surveillance data. *Expert Systems with Applications*, *38*(9), 11421–11436. doi:10.1016/j.eswa.2011.03.015

Roham, M., & Gabrielyan, A, R., Archer, N. P. (2012). Predicting the impact of hospital health information technology adoption on patient satisfaction. *Artificial Intelligence in Medicine*, *56*(2), 123–135. doi:10.1016/j.artmed.2012.08.001 PMID:22964161

Santos, R. S., Malheiros, S. M. F., Cavalheiro, S., & Parente de Oliveira, J. M. (2013). A data mining system for providing analytical information on brain tumors to public health decision makers. *Computer Methods and Programs in Biomedicine*, *109*(3), 269–282. doi:10.1016/j.cmpb.2012.10.010 PMID:23122302

Sebastian, Y., & Then, P. H. H. (2011). Domain-driven KDD for mining functionally novel rules and linking disjoint medical hypotheses. *Knowledge-Based Systems*, *24*(5), 609–620. doi:10.1016/j.knosys.2011.01.008

Self-Organizing Map. (n.d.). In *Wikipedia*. Retrieved Sep 10, 2013, from http://en.wikipedia.org/wiki/Self-organizing_map

Semenova, T. (2004). Discovering patterns of medical practice in large administrative health databases. *Data & Knowledge Engineering*, *51*(2), 149–160. doi:10.1016/j.datak.2004.02.001

Shanmugam, R. (2012). Booming medical tourism and economic indices. *International Journal of Research in Nursing*, *3*(2), 38–47. doi:10.3844/ijrnsp.2012.38.47

Shimada, K., Wang, R., Hirasawa, K., & Furuzuki, T. (2008). Medical association rule mining using genetic network programming. *Electronics and Communications in Japan*, *91*(2), 46–54. doi:10.1002/ecj.10022

Shortlife, E. H., & Cimino, J. J. (2006). Biomedical informatics: Computer applications in health care and biomedicine (3rd ed.). New York: Springer.

Shortliffe, E. H. (1993). The adolescence of AI in medicine: will the field come of age in the 90s? *Artificial Intelligence in Medicine*, *5*(2), 93–106. doi:10.1016/0933-3657(93)90011-Q PMID:8358494

Tai, Y. M., & Chiu, H. W. (2009). Comorbidity study of ADHD: Applying association rule mining (ARM) to National Health Insurance Database of Taiwan. *International Journal of Medical Informatics*, *78*(12), e75–e83. doi:10.1016/j.ijmedinf.2009.09.005 PMID:19853501

Tan, P. N., Steinbach, M., & Kumar, V. (2005). *Introduction to data mining*. Pearson Addison-Wesley.

Tartarisco, G., Baldus, G., Corda, D., Raso, R., Arnao, A., & Ferro, M. et al. (2012). Personal Health System architecture for stress monitoring and support to clinical decisions. *Computer Communications*, *35*(11), 1296–1305. doi:10.1016/j.comcom.2011.11.015

Tenorio, J. M., Hummel, A. D., Cohrs, F. M., Sdepanian, V. L., Pisa, I. T., & Marin, H. D. F. (2011). Artificial intelligence techniques applied to the development of a decision–support system for diagnosing celiac disease. *International Journal of Medical Informatics*, *80*(11), 793–802. doi:10.1016/j.ijmedinf.2011.08.001 PMID:21917512

Ting, S. L., Kwok, S. K., Tsang, A. H. C., & Lee, W. B. (2011). A hybrid knowledge-based approach to supporting the medical prescription for general practitioners: Real case in a Hong Kong medical center. *Knowledge-Based Systems*, *24*(3), 444–456. doi:10.1016/j.knosys.2010.12.011

Vicente, J., Garcia-Gomez, J. M., Vidal, C., Marti-Bonmati, L., Arco, A. D., & Robles, M. (2004). SOC: A Distributed Decision Support Architecture for Clinical Diagnosis. *Biological and Medical Data Analysis*. *Lecture Notes in Computer Science*, *3337*, 96–104. doi:10.1007/978-3-540-30547-7_11

Wei, J., Lin, S., Weng, C., & Wu, H. (2012). A case study of applying LRFM model in market segmentation of a children's dental clinic. *Expert Systems with Applications*, *39*(5), 5529–5533. doi:10.1016/j.eswa.2011.11.066

Yan, H., Jiang, Y., & Zheng, J., Fu, B., Xiao, S., & Peng, C. (2004). The internet-based knowledge acquisition and management method to construct large-scale distributed medical expert systems. *Computer Methods and Programs in Biomedicine*, *74*(1), 1–10. doi:10.1016/S0169-2607(03)00076-2 PMID:14992822

Yan, Q., Yan, H., Han, F., Wei, X., & Zhu, T. (2009). SVM-based decision support system for clinic aided tracheal intubation predication with multiple features. *Expert Systems with Applications*, *36*(3), 6588–6592. doi:10.1016/j.eswa.2008.07.076

Yang, C. C., Lin, W. T., Chen, H. M., & Shi, Y. H. (2009). Improving scheduling of emergency physicians using data mining analysis. *Expert Systems with Applications*, *36*(2), 3378–3387. doi:10.1016/j.eswa.2008.02.069

Yao, L., Zhang, Y., Li, Y., Sanseau, P., & Agarwal, P. (2011). Electronic health records: Implications for drug discovery. *Drug Discovery Today*, *16*(13/14), 594–599. doi:10.1016/j.drudis.2011.05.009 PMID:21624499

Yeh, J. Y., Wu, T. H., & Tsao, C. W. (2011). Using data mining techniques to predict hospitalization of hemodialysis patients. *Decision Support Systems*, *50*(2), 439–448. doi:10.1016/j.dss.2010.11.001

Zayed, N., Awad, A. B., El-Akel, W., Doss, W., Awad, T., Radwan, A., & Mabrouk, M. (2013). The assessment of data mining for the prediction of therapeutic outcome in 3719 Egyptian patients with chronic hepatitis C. *Clinics and Research in Hepatology and Gastroenterology*, *37*(3), 254–261. doi:10.1016/j.clinre.2012.09.005 PMID:23141214

Zhao, D., & Weng, C. (2011). Combining PubMed knowledge and EHR data to develop a weighted Bayesian network for pancreatic cancer prediction. *Journal of Biomedical Informatics*, *44*(5), 859–868. doi:10.1016/j.jbi.2011.05.004 PMID:21642013

## KEY TERMS AND DEFINITIONS

**Actionable Knowledge Discovery:** Actionable knowledge discovery aims to deliver knowledge that is business friendly, and which can be taken over by business people for seamless decision making.

**Data Mining:** Tan et al. (2005) define data mining as the process of automatically discovering useful information in large data repositories.

**Healthcare Industry:** According to the united nation International Standard Industrial Classification (ISIC) definition, the healthcare industry generally consist of three major activities include hospital activities, medical and dental practice activities, and other human health activities (Wikipedia, Healthcare industry, n. d.).

**Knowledge Discovery:** From Fayyad et al. (1996) point of view knowledge discovery in databases (KDD) is the overall process of discovering useful knowledge from data, and data mining refers to a particular step in this process that is the application of specific algorithms for extracting patterns from data.

**Market View:** Market view is one of the proposed classification groups. Market view includes papers that look at the patient as a potential customer. Most of researches on market view area were somehow related to CRM and it reflects the importance of this issue in healthcare industry businesses.

**Patient View:** Patient view is one of the proposed classification groups. It includes papers that purely mined clinical data sets to derive models and discovered patterns. Patient view is divided to predictive models and pattern mining groups.

**System View:** System view is one of the proposed classification groups. It includes papers that explicitly propose an algorithm, information flow diagram, application or architecture for decision support systems and also papers that propose architecture or systems that can perform or have potential to perform knowledge discovery and data mining in a large scale manner.

# Section 4
# Applications of Informatics for Aged Care and Chronic Diseases

# Chapter 14
# Using Narrative with Avatars and Robots to Enhance Elder Care

**Lundy Lewis**
*Southern New Hampshire University, USA*

## ABSTRACT

*Elderly care is of increasing global concern. The aging population is expected to increase two-fold by 2050. It is anticipated that there will not be enough caregivers to assist the elderly very soon, and thus, researchers are looking at various technologies and potential applications that will help alleviate the problem of elderly care. This chapter examines one such assistive technology: conversational agents in the form of avatars or robots as an aid to decrease loneliness and depression among the elderly and increase the cognitive function and quality of life. The authors discuss the state-of-the-science of research prototypes and commercial off-the-shelf systems. They propose a novel concept and design, and the authors discuss the ethical ramifications of senior citizens possibly bonding with inanimate objects as if they were human companions.*

## INTRODUCTION

Socialization through narrative and story-telling is important for elder care and quality of life. The elderly enjoy reminiscing and communicating. They enjoy being reminded of past experiences and having conversations with other interested parties such as family and friends about their life history or particular life events. However, there are common reports of frustration that caregivers who are around on a daily basis do not know the elderly person in the way that families do and thus cannot engage in such meaningful conversation. Further, with staff turnover, it is difficult for a single staff member to get to know the patient well enough to provide meaningful conversations about the older person's life history or to generally bond with the patient. And further, due to advances in healthcare, a better understanding of living healthy, and birthing trends, in the next few decades there is expected to be a large number of elderly patients but fewer professional caregivers, thus reducing the amount of time that caregivers can spend with individual patients beyond the

DOI: 10.4018/978-1-4666-6316-9.ch014

provision of essential services. This prediction holds for all developed countries, most notably for Japan.

To make matters worse, young students in psychology, sociology, nursing, and related disciplines are less interested in elder care than in areas such as child development and disability management. For these reasons, a current interest among researchers and entrepreneurs is to develop ways to allow the elderly patient to enjoy narrative, conversation, and reminiscing without requiring human accompaniment but yet without diminishing the quality of conversation, e.g. by using avatars or robots rather than human caregivers. The idea is worthy of pursuit, but it is a hard problem. A good resource that explores how avatars and robots will be used in the next ten to fifteen years is (Robots+Avatars, 2014). In particular, the resource (Robot-Era, 2014) provides information on research in robotic systems and intelligent environments for the aging population.

Many people will argue that human touch is essential and indispensable for elderly care, where by "human touch" we mean proximity and sympathy with another human being. Others will argue that even if one were able to substitute human touch with some technological device, it would be unethical to do so.

This chapter will explore socialization through narrative from perspectives of both technological possibility and ethical ramifications. In particular, this chapter discusses the possibilities of technologies such as avatars and robots to provide the service of narrative and human touch effectively, i.e. to provide an experience that is at least as acceptable, albeit not identical, to traditional family-oriented conversation.

A challenging question from a technology perspective is how to structure personal knowledge regarding the patient's interests and experiences into an avatar or robot, called *knowledge representation* in the Artificial Intelligence community. A second challenge is how to extract knowledge and insert it into the structure, called *knowledge acquisition*. Clearly, the apparatus must know about some of the patient's history and local or global events occurring during the patient's lifetime and be able to converse interactively with the patient about them. A possible approach is that the elderly person or her/his family could work though exercises in which participants answer questions regarding past experiences. This could be assisted by family, care staff, or students on placement. Answers to the questions could be compiled into a composite view of the person's experiences.

A benefit of this approach to knowledge acquisition is that the process itself may enhance family involvement and personalized care that does not require additional resources or specialized skills. In addition, the same knowledge could be inserted into a humanoid robot whereby the robot converses with the elder person, laying aside for now the question of whether the approach is ethical.

Beyond the knowledge of personal experiences, there could be a standard, public ontology for various geographical locations, events, or time periods that the patient would know about, and to which the avatar could appeal when engaging the patient in conversation. As an example, for a patient in the United States, an ontology describing basic facts about the assassination of President John F. Kennedy and the appointment of Lyndon B. Johnson to the presidency could be a standard ontology or knowledge store. Or, an ontology that contained geographical and temporal facts and relationships about Atlanta Georgia might be useful. An avatar could then use this knowledge to converse with the elderly person in a meaningful way.

Consider a possible embodiment of the avatar to be a cyber-relative of the patient. The patient would be interacting with a representation of a cyber-relative in the form of an avatar, where the avatar has the appearance of the real relative and has knowledge to converse about things relevant to the patient. However, the approach raises ethical concerns, e.g. is the patient being deceived and if so, is it morally right? Do we have a moral obligation not to deceive humans? Does the answer to this question depend on culture? On the other hand, if it can be shown that the technology does indeed increase an elder person's quality of life, does that make it morally correct?

In this chapter we examine several contemporary approaches to the problem of engaging the elderly in narrative, story-telling, and meaningful conversation when family members and friends may not be available and caregivers do not have sufficient resources to get to know the patient. We consider it our social responsibility to maintain and increase the quality of life of the elderly as well as the peace of mind of the elder's family. We are especially interested in the efficacy of using avatars or robots to engage older people in meaningful conversations about their past and the ethical ramifications thereof.

The chapter considers the following essential issues regarding the narrative and conversation for the elderly:

1. What technologies currently exist that tackle the problem of narrative and conversation for the elderly?
2. What technologies show promise for further development?
3. How does one extract knowledge and represent it in a cyber-companion such that meaningful conversation is possible?
4. What is the methodology by which to populate the knowledge-base of a cyber-companion?
5. To what extent will elderly patients adopt or accept a cyber-companion?
6. Are certain technologies better suited for elderly patients in certain conditions or certain stages of elderly life?
7. Does the approach increase the quality of life of the elderly?
8. What are the ethical ramifications of the approach?

In order to address these essential issues, we first examine the literature in order to compare the approach discussed in this chapter with other approaches. A thorough analysis of research on the adoption of assistive technologies for aged care is reported in (Vichitvanichphong et al, 2013). The authors discovered eight categories of technologies that have been used as assistive care for the elderly:

1. General purpose technologies such as computers, mobile phones, the Internet, and email are being used by some seniors to cope with the transition period or life style change after retirement or to communicate with family, friends and caregivers.
2. Social media is used by some to stay in touch with people, establish social networks, gain information, and share thoughts and experiences.
3. Video games are used by some for therapy, entertainment, relaxation, and socialization.
4. Robots are used by some seniors in their domestic environments; however, research has found that for seniors to adopt robots in their daily lives, building long term relationship with the robots is necessary.
5. On-line information services are used by some, e.g. using online services to seek and update health information and electronic health records.
6. Smart homes are used to help seniors balance safety and independence through remote monitoring, motion detecting sensors, and alerting technology.
7. Remote care or tele-care has been used for balancing safety and independence, and providing support for seniors who have dementia.
8. Supportive devices such as medicine reminder services, hearing assistance technology, and rehabilitation assistive devices are used by some seniors in order to improve their functional capability.

A useful theoretical model by which to explain or predict the adoption of a particular technology is the Technology Acceptance Model (TAM) in which two variables are determinants of technology adoption: (i) perceived usefulness, i.e. the degree to which a person believes that using a particular system will enhance job performance and (ii) perceived ease-of-use, i.e. the degree to which a person believes the use of a particular would be free of effort (Davis, 89). The TAM suggests that, all else being equal, an application that is higher in perceived ease-of-use is more likely to be accepted by users. Although the TAM has been applied mainly to job performance in industry, it is straightforward to apply the model to technologies for the elderly by considering the enhancement of quality of life instead of job performance. As we examine current trends in using narrative for elderly care in the next section, it is useful to keep the TAM in mind. In particular, we are interested in the extent to which socially assistive technologies may be adopted by elders, by caregivers, and by the elder's family (Heerink et al, 2006; Heerink et al, 2009).

## CURRENT TRENDS IN NARRATIVE FOR ELDERLY CARE

Consider the common way that a family interacts with the elderly, be it in the patient's home or in a nursing home. The family typically gathers around the elderly person and simply talks. The topic may be what's currently going on with family members, neighborhood gossip, perhaps politics, and the like. Often a family member will bring along a traditional photo album with items such as pictures, newspaper clippings, memos, even dried flowers or other items that spark memories in the elderly patient. Home videos and music are popular as well but the elderly really enjoy the human interaction.

Let us consider various technical vehicles for duplicating this kind of experience in order of increased technical difficulty and challenge. We are concerned with the difficulty of implementing the approach, the degree to which the elderly patient will take advantage or adapt to the approach, and the extent to which to approach maintains or increases the patient's quality of life.

### Electronic Multi-Media Photo Albums

Tablet computers and touchscreen interfaces are for the most part useable by today's elderly patients. Of course, each successive generation of the elderly will be more comfortable with the use of computers so the problem of technical difficulty will become less problematic in the next few decades. Thus, the first and perhaps simplest approach to our problem is to provide the patient with a tablet computer that simply duplicates the photo album. The leaves of the album could be enhanced with recorded voice or music that will be familiar to the patient. Let us call this the "electronic multi-media photo album" (EMPA) approach. There are many commercial applications that will allow non-technical family members to create such EPMAs for the elderly.

The problems with the EMPA approach are fairly obvious. It gets boring after repeated use. It is static. It isn't in real time and doesn't solve the problem of human touch when relatives and friends are not present. Nonetheless, the EMPA approach could be a reasonable, inexpensive method for complementary care, e.g. a device that the elderly patient could use for comfort in the middle of a sleepless night.

Importantly, one can imagine several enhancements of the EMPA approach that could alleviate some of its drawbacks. First, consider the static problem. There are several social networking applications that allow one to set up a dynamic site such that family members can add to the site at will. New photos, videos, or voice can be added to site. One can imagine an elderly patient looking forward to bedtime, knowing that a new video will be there from a family member. Second, one could add VoIP to the site such that the patient can talk to the family member in real time whenever both parties are available. Still, however, these enhancements do not address the problem of the lack of human touch.

Another enhancement is to transform the EMPA into a general engagement platform (Andrews, 2013). See Figure 1.

The platform includes several cognitive tasks that can be tailored to the needs and desires of individual seniors so than seniors can have a unique experience. Low-functioning seniors would have a set of cognitive tasks different than those of more high-functioning seniors. Such tasks include various brain games to exercise brain activity, staying connected to family members via video conferencing, watching videos or taking courses of interest to the senior, e.g. how technology works, viewing a life performance of a favorite artist, or taking a virtual trip.

In general, this enhancement of the EMPA seeks to apply recent advances in networking, applications, and content to applications that can be enjoyed by seniors. Voice-to-text is such an application that can be quite helpful to seniors. Typically, however, a caregiver is required to de-

*Figure 1. An engagement platform using well-known technologies*

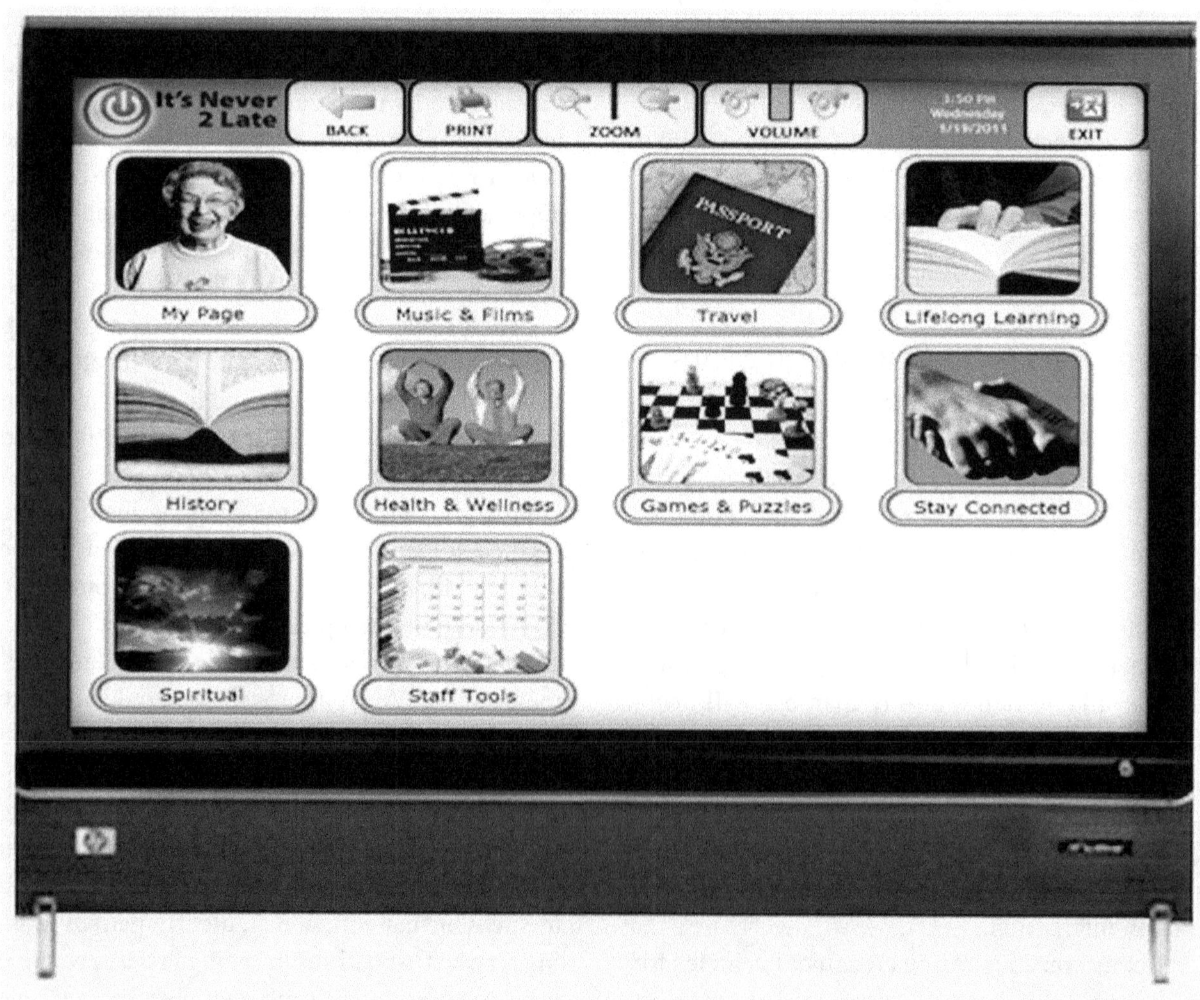

velop a configuration of applications especially suited for an elderly patient. The approach is often called "engagement-based therapy" for seniors.

## Avatars as Social Companions

A more complex approach is to develop an avatar as the on-screen companion of the elderly patient (González et al, 2007). Many applications exist by which an avatar can be constructed to represent an advice-giver in some domain of interest. However, to date, avatars have not been considered as the actual companion of the elderly – someone who can take the place of the human relative. Most current avatars are similar to cartoon characters or are rather stiff human-like characters. Increasingly, however, researchers are trying to develop avatars with realistic facial expressions and gestures that accompany real conversations.

If avatars could be developed such that an elderly patient is comfortable interacting with it, then we have a candidate solution loosely approximating human touch. However, two problems need to be overcome with this approach: (i) the look and feel of the avatar and (ii) the ability of the avatar to have meaningful conversations. A recent commercial approach to the problem of elderly care combines the EMPA approach and the avatar approach as an attempt to resolve these problems (GeriJoy, 2014). See Figure 2.

The approach includes an animaloid avatar who communicates with the patient in real time. The screen can be divided such that the avatar is in the top portion of the screen and an EMPA is on the bottom portion of the screen. The avatar can flip through the pages of the EMPA whilst carrying on an intelligent conversation with the patient. Pet therapy is well-known to benefit the elderly's quality of life, and likewise in this approach the avatar with whom the patient interacts is usually a puppy or a kitten.

The avatar is responsive to touch and can verbalize accordingly while being guided by a remote operator. Note that the remote operator can maintain an intelligent conversation with the patient in the moment but the operator typically is not familiar with the background of the patient. Thus, conversation about past history and life events is not likely with this approach.

## Tele-Presence Robots

Another approach to providing socialization for elderly patients is to use robotic tele-presence.

*Figure 2. Electronic multi-media photo album with an avatar*

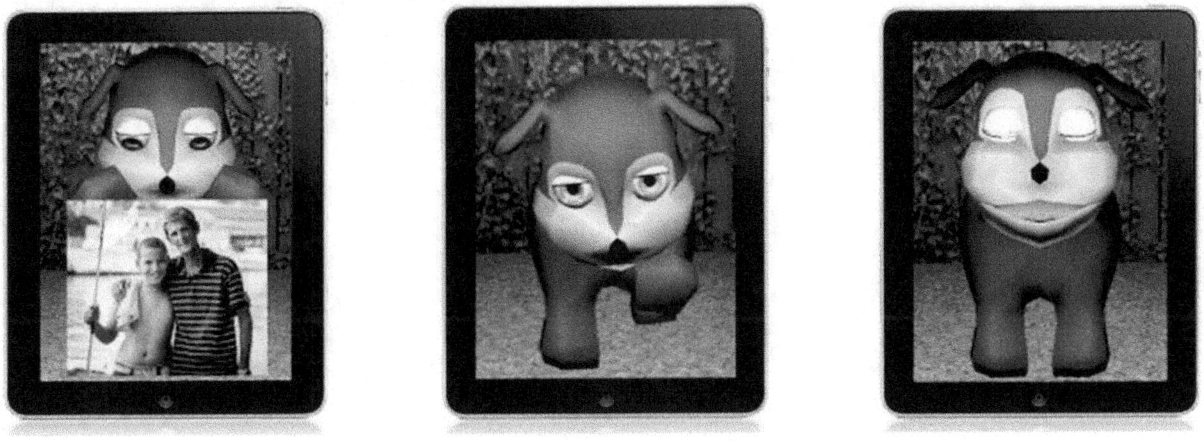

Figure 3 shows an example of a commercial tele-presence robot. A good source that compares commercial tele-presence robots is (Tele-Presence Robots, 2014).

A tele-presence robot is driven remotely by a user, say a family member, and allows the patient to converse with another party remotely. One can imagine the robot starting up upon a command by a remote user, traveling to the bedside of the patient or finding the patient in a room, and beginning a chat with the patient. An outstanding question, however, is the extent to which an elderly patient will feel comfortable with this approach and the extent to which it will substitute for real human touch. Also, this approach requires participation from the other party and thus only partially addresses the problem of busy life-schedules of family members.

Note that this approach does not use avatars or autonomous robots. Rather, the robot is tethered through common network communication methods. Internet connectivity is required for most commercial tele-presence robots. It is easy to see how this approach could be combined with the EPMA approach.

## Autonomous Robots as Social Companions

A commercial robot that has been reported to have positive effects with elderly is an animaloid robot seal named Paro (Paro, 2014). See figure 4. Paro is noted primarily for its cuteness and cuddliness. It responds non-verbally to touch, wiggles on one's lap, and exhibits facial expressions. There are reports that elderly patients are content interact-

*Figure 3. A tele-presence robot*

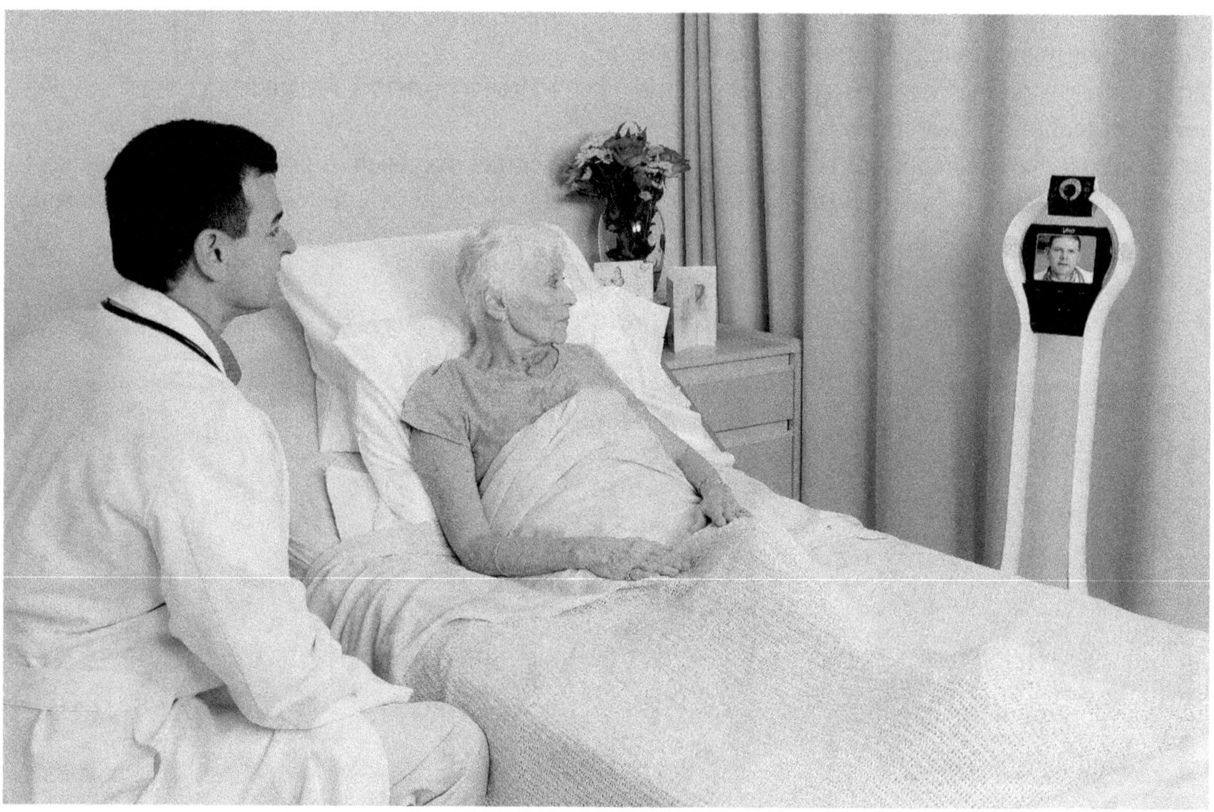

*Figure 4. Paro the seal robot*

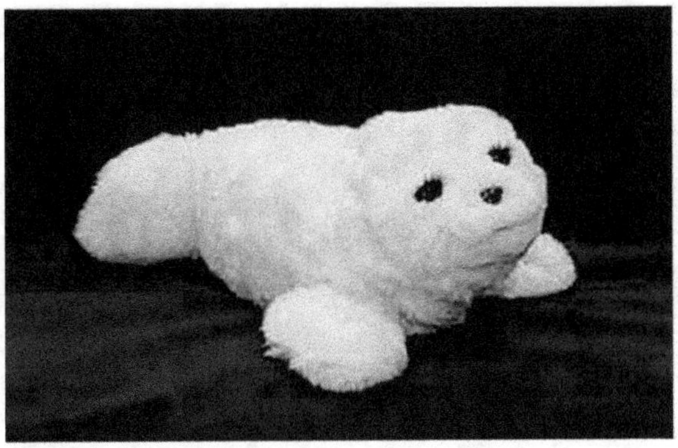

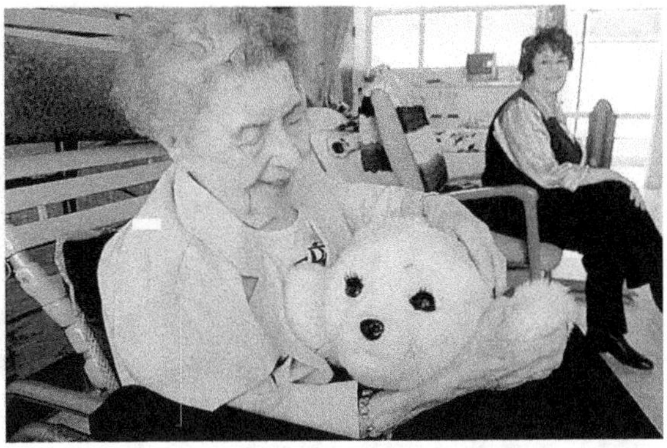

ing with Paro. In some cases, the interaction with Paro causes the patient to remember and talk about past life experiences. Note that this robot does not attempt to mimic a human being but rather simply offers a kind of artificial pet therapy.

Given the natural evolution in our review of current technologies, it is logical to make the final jump to a humanoid robot that resembles a relative or friend of the patient. We may undergo a thought experiment: What would it be like for a patient to interact with an artificial human being? What about an artificial human being that resembles a person whom the patient knows and cherishes – say a child, a grandchild, a close friend, or perhaps a deceased sibling or spouse? On the other hand, what would it be like to introduce the patient to a stranger robot, albeit a stranger who's familiar with the patient's past, and then let the patient bond with the stranger robot and development a new relationship, much like the patient would develop a new relationship with a new potential friend?

From a technical point of view, the approach of building a humanoid robot who exhibits both intelligence, looks, and personality, and who would substitute for such a human being is the goal of several researchers. See Figure 5.

For example, researchers in Vermont USA guide their work by two bold hypotheses (Lifenaut, 2014):

1. By combining detailed data about a person, future AI software will be able to reanimate the person's consciousness. The database, called a mindfile, will contain the person's unique and essential characteristics made up of memories, photos, videos, documents, conversation logs, and personality test results.
2. A person's mindfile may be downloaded into a robotic, nanotechnological or biolocial body to provide life experiences comparable to those of a typical human.

With a realistic appearance as illustrated in Figure 5, and the possibility of at least coming close to fulfilling the above two hypotheses, then there is a good possibility that eventually one will able to create a substitute for a human who can share in conversation with an elderly patient. The success and practicality of this approach would seem to be several decades into the future. One can perform thought experiments now, however, as to what it would be like to have a humanoid robot and the ethical ramifications of using the robot for elderly care. One issue might be the phenomenon of the "uncanny valley" for some cultures, i.e. the fact that when an artifact such as a game, avatar, or robot comes too close to resembling real humans, then the artifact is not accepted and interactive conversation becomes impossibly. As

*Figure 5. Humanoid robot with a realistic appearance*

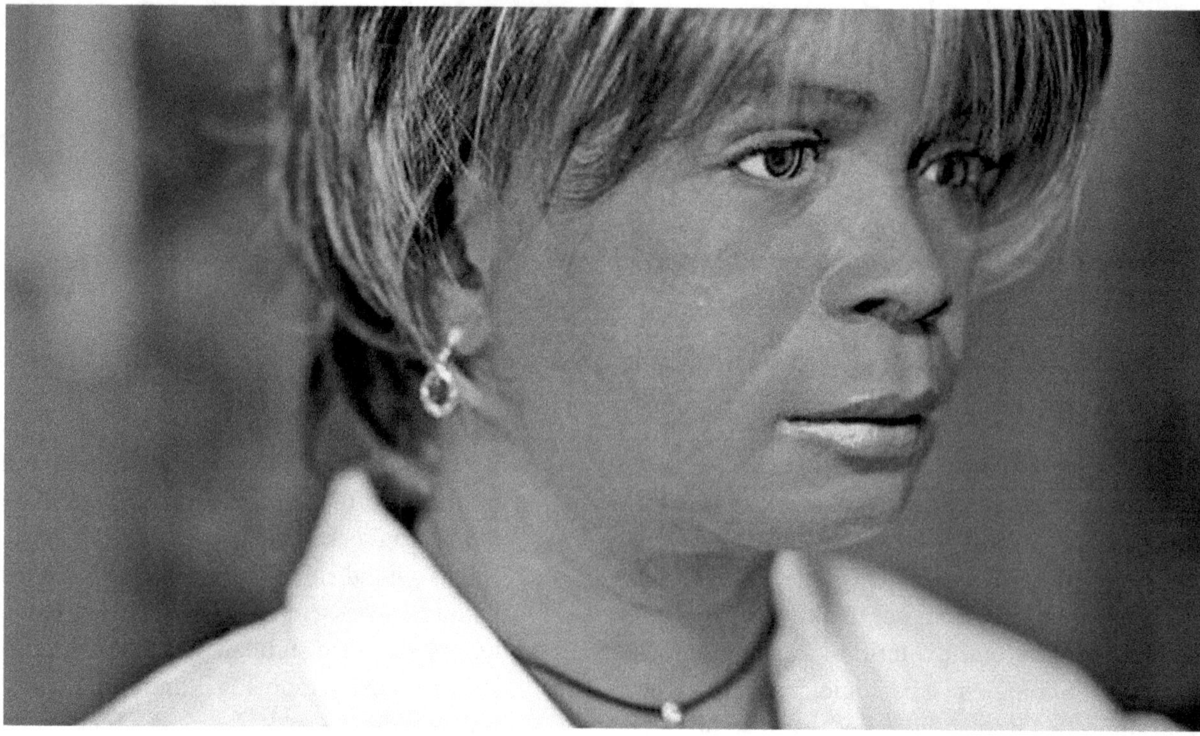

an example, the uncanny valley phenomenon is more of a problem in the Unites States than it is in Japan because of different attitudes towards animate and inanimate objects.

A further issue with the approach of humanoid robots is the ethical question mentioned earlier. Let us assume that we can build a practical humanoid robot from a technical point of view. Assume that the uncanny valley is not an issue, and that indeed many elderly persons spend many precious hours conversing and reminiscing with a robot relative or companion. What are our moral feelings about this? One might be ambivalent about the issue. If the elderly patient is deriving pleasure and peace of mind having a robot companion, then all is right and there is no ethical concern. On the other hand, the fact that the elderly patient is deceived into thinking the robot is a real human, or perhaps not deceived but doesn't care that her best friend is a robot, might cause a pain of moral guilt. For some cultures it is a classic ethical dilemma, but for other cultures there may be no problem at all. If one holds to moral relativism, then one would examine the background culture to answer the question of whether a robot companion is a morally correct thing to allow happen.

## Discussion

In this section we focus on a current problem that is anticipated to be a huge problem in the next several decades -- that of providing companionship for elderly patients for ordinary conversation and story-telling. The problem would not be so severe if there were plenty of caregivers available to spend time learning about and bonding with elderly patients. Thus, one current trend in elderly healthcare is to find ways to provide such companionship without the use of humans. Since the elderly really enjoy story-telling and reminiscing about old times, most current approaches to the problem use avatars, while other forward-looking approaches aim to develop robots for the purpose.

The approaches described in this section aim to provide solutions or at least partial solutions to the problem. We group avatars and autonomous robots together under the category "knowledge-based approaches." In those approaches, knowledge of the patient's past experiences is needed in order to maintain a meaningful conversation with the patient. This is a hard technical problem. The next sections will examine several knowledge representation techniques for representing the kind of knowledge needed to carry on interactive conversations with elderly patients.

Before proceeding, let us note that elderly care certainly involves more than socialization through narrative and story-telling, e.g. the elderly need reminders of things such as exercise, walking, taking medicine and the like. Further, the elderly need to be watched in case a patient begins to act strangely or fall. These tasks are not the subject here; however, it is not hard to see that if one is successful in representing the knowledge required for conversation, then one should be able to add new knowledge such that the avatar or robot could indeed work into the conversation reminders for exercising and taking medicine (Fasola and Matarić, 2013).

A robot application for Japan's space program is quite similar to the challenge here. The problem there is that astronauts are quite lonely in outer space, much like the elderly can be lonely in a nursing home. The Toyota Company has built a small robot named Kirobo, as shown in Figure 6, designed to carry out conversation with a space commander (Robot Astronaut, 2013). That is its sole function.

*Figure 6. The astronaut robot Kirobo*

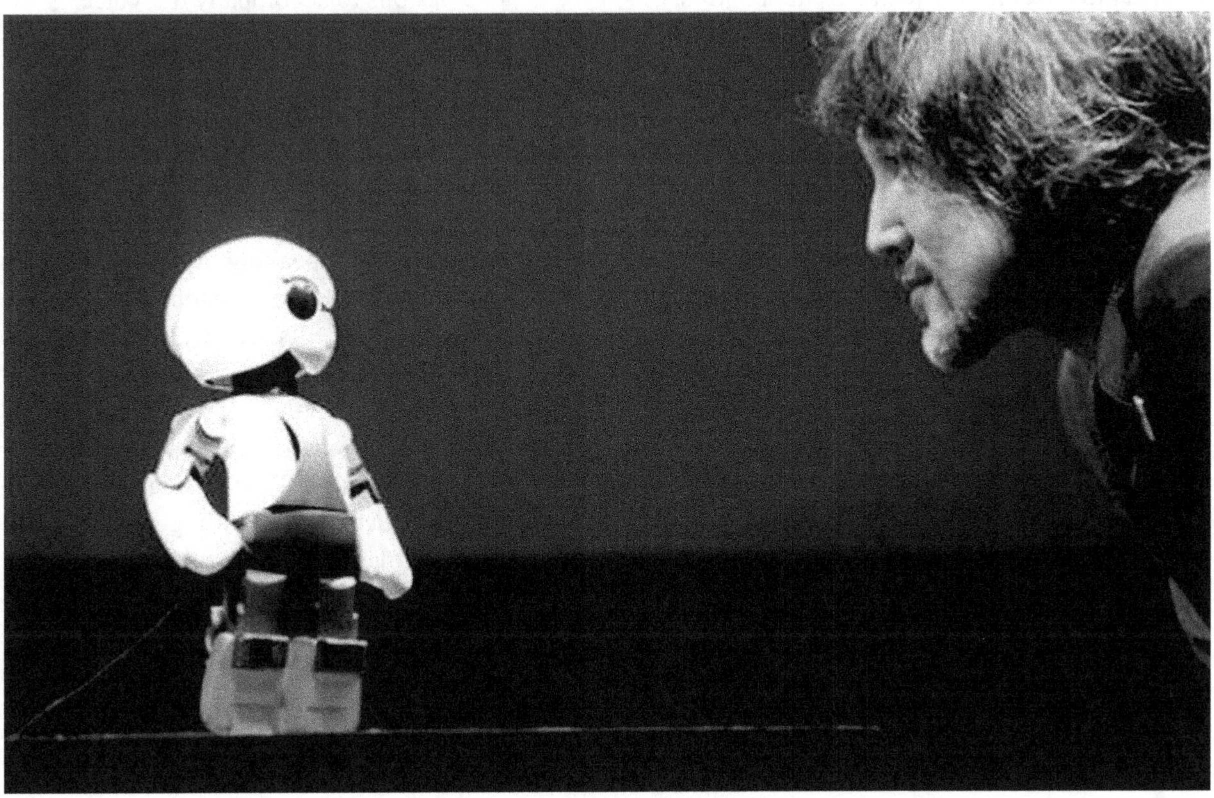

The robot includes voice recognition, facial recognition, and natural language processing in order to have an ability to converse with the commander. It has the ability also to relay messages back to a command station and provide transcripts of conversations. It is not a stiff one-on-one question and answer system seen in many avatar and robot applications. It is designed to accompany its conversational input with gestures and emotions such as kindness and sympathy in order to engage the interest of the commander. The technology and lessons learned from this robot could be used to design and develop partner robots for the elderly.

## KNOWLEDGE STRUCTURES FOR CONVERSATIONAL AVATARS AND ROBOTS

In this section we wish to concentrate on the kind of knowledge representation best suited for holding information about a patient and then using that information to converse with the patient. Most of the current avatars use a rather stiff question-and-answer method, where answers to questions are hardcoded and non-flexible. One can see many good examples of avatars and interact with them at the Virtual Agent/Chatbots Directory (Chatbots, 2014). (Note that "avatar" as used in this chapter may be interchanged with other synonyms such as Virtual Human, Virtual Assistant, Chatbot, and Conversational Agent). A competition, The Loebner Prize in Artificial Intelligence, was set up in 1990 to encourage researchers and scientists to develop avatars that engage in conversation that is indistinguishable or is more realistic than conversation with humans (Loebner, 2014). This work concentrates on realistic conversation rather than specifically engaging seniors in conversations about themselves and their history, but nonetheless the techniques are useful for understanding advances in natural language processing. Here, we are concerned with the kind of knowledge structure needed to support story-telling and reminiscing with seniors.

### Stories, Reminiscing, and Artificial Intelligence

One can imagine what is involved in an ordinary conversation among two people. At a high level of abstraction, the steps in a unit of story-telling and reminiscing are the following:

Repeat

1. Translate patient voice to text.
2. Parse the text to retrieve salient concepts and relations.
3. Retrieve stories and knowledge based on the parsing of the text.
4. Determine what to say next based on the retrieval.
5. Translate text to voice.
6. Determine intonation, gestures, and/or facial expressions to accompany the voice.
7. Deliver saying with intonation, facial expressions, and gestures.
8. Wait until detection of patient voice.

There are at least two other things related to these steps that happen during a conversation. First, while the patient is speaking, a listener exhibits some gestures and facial expression that insures the patient that the listener is actually listening, e.g. a nod of the head or looking away and then back at the speaker. Second, although we have described a unit of conversation, it is clear that the speaker and listener maintain a kind of mental log as to how the conversation is unfolding. Often people make a mental marker of a particular concept in the unfolding of a conversation with a mental note to go back to it when the time is right or when there is a lag in the conversation. For now, however, we wish to focus on steps 3 and 4.

Most people who use smartphones are impressed with today's capabilities in translating voice to text (step 1), and there are several applications that are pretty good at finding salient concepts and relations in text (step 2). The output from step 2 then is the input for step 3, and that is our focus. Also, applications that translate text to voice are rather common and are getting increasingly better at the nuances of speech.

One can try out prototype avatars at the University of Southern California's Institute for Creative Technologies at (USC-ICT, 2014). The goal of the research at USC is to create avatars that do indeed exhibit realistic behaviors required in steps 1, 2, 5, and 7, especially with respect to intonation, facial expressions, and gestures. A Virtual Human Toolkit is also available whereby one can experiment with building additional applications. An example of a deployed avatar that converses with veterans who might be suffering from Post-Traumatic Stress Syndrome can be seen at (BraveHeart, 2014) although the conversation is text-based rather than voice based (Figure 7). While this application is impressive, one will note the limitations, e.g. the conversation lacks naturalness and can become repetitive over time. One will likely note that the avatar does not seem to be too intelligent although the visual representation is rather realistic.

Our goal then is to come up with a structure of knowledge that will decrease repetitiveness and increase the possibility of a more natural experience. The AI community over the last fifty years or so has developed several types of knowledge structures that are candidates for the kind of knowledge an avatar may appeal to while conversing with a senior. For example, rule-based reasoning (RBR) is a knowledge structure in which the unit of knowledge is a simple if-then rule. A set of rules may be developed that captures the knowledge of an expert in some domain as she goes about finding a solution to a problem. Many expert systems have been developed that use RBR. However, RBR is not good at capturing stories and history of a patient. Note that a RBR system would be a good choice to guide the dispensation of medicine or provide other reminders to the patient, but it is not the best choice to support a conversation. RBR would also be a good choice for implementing standard question-and-answer systems where the if-part of the rule is the question and the then-part is the answer.

Other knowledge structures, a.k.a. AI paradigms, include fuzzy reasoning, constraint-based reasoning, case-based reasoning, frame-based reasoning, analogical reasoning, and other representations. A good source for reviewing various knowledge structures for various kinds of tasks is the Representation and Reasoning section of AI Topics at the Association for the Advancement of Artificial Intelligence (AI Topics, 2014). A good source that describes intelligent technology for an aging population is (Pollack, 2005).

## Case-Based Reasoning and Ontologies

A particular knowledge representation that stands out for our purposes is Case-Based Reasoning (CBR) (Kolodner, 1993). The unit of knowledge in CBR is a case, where a case holds a particular experience or a story, unlike RBR. A case library holds a collection of experiences. For example, a case describing an experience with a problem will hold three different sections: (i) a section describing the surrounding circumstances of a problem, (2) a section describing the problem at hand, and (3) a section describing the past solution to a problem. Given input to a CBR system, a matching function is performed whereby a particular case is retrieved that best matches the input, much like the adage "That reminds me of a story." In most commercial and prototype CBR systems, the retrieved case is used for solving a particular problem.

A commonsense example is as follows: A parent contacts a professor at a university and says that his son is not happy with the major he has

*Figure 7. An avatar for veterans*

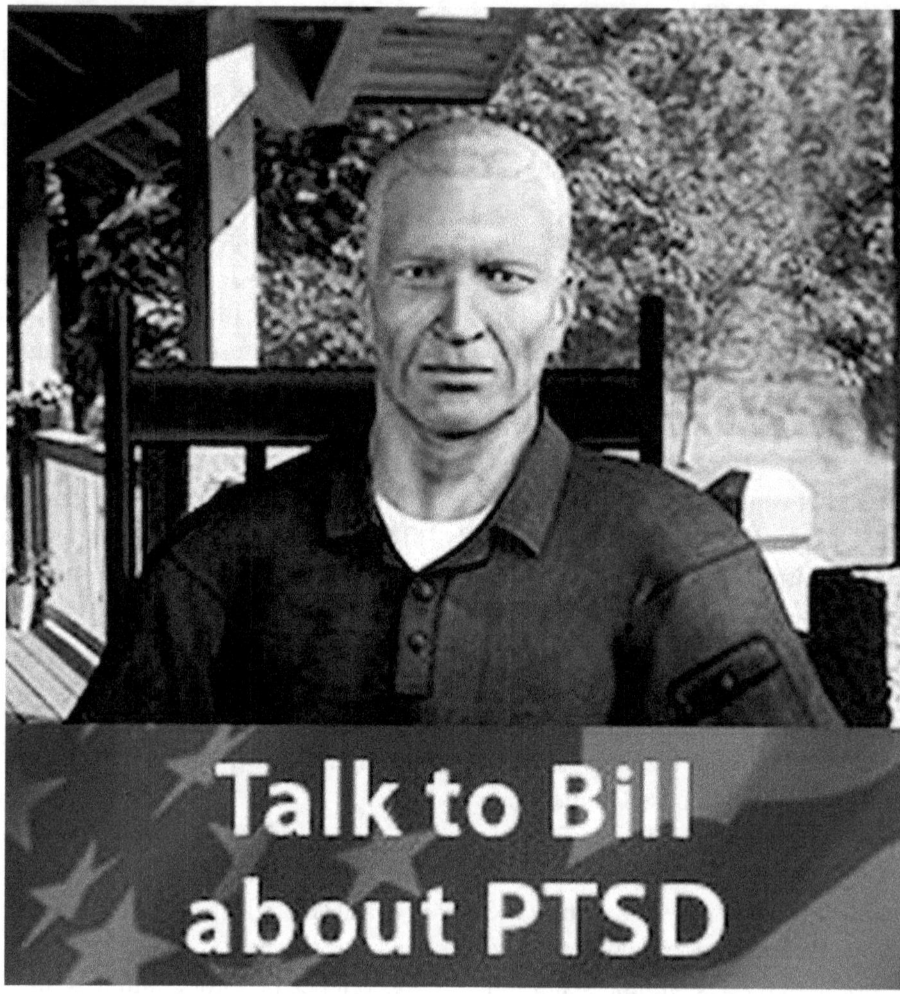


chosen. The father wants some advice from the professor. The professor is reminded of a similar past experience in which the professor sat down to chat with a father and his son. In the past situation, the student was having trouble selecting a major. The student had tried IT but did not like it, and then tried Game Design and did not like that either. The professor asked the student: "Have you had a course at the university you really enjoyed?" The student replied that he really liked his marketing course. The professor then introduced the student to a marketing professor. Ultimately the student switched majors to marketing and his been happy ever since. So, the professor plans to ask the new student the same question: Have you had a course that you really enjoyed? The professor does not know that this course of action will work, but it is worth a try based on past experience.

Here is a commercial example in industry: All companies have a trouble ticketing system through which employees submit problems with IT. A trouble ticket is an ordinary electronic form which has slots for information, (e.g., name, date, location, type of computer, type of operating system, an application, and the problem). An IT support person reviews the trouble ticket and appeals to experience to try to diagnose the problem. The IT support person might do a search over all past trouble tickets to try to find a ticket that had a similar problem in similar circumstances and was resolved successfully. The support person then tries the same solution. If it works, the solution is strengthened. If not, the support person eventually finds a solution, closes the ticket, and the ticket is entered back into the ticket database and may be used in future situations.

This last example illustrates a hallmark of CBR: learning from experience. The outcome of a new experience is entered back into the sum total of experiences and may be used in the future. In this way, one can say that a CBR system gets better and more knowledgeable over time as new experiences are resolved. The case library becomes increasingly fine-tuned and complete. Further, the knowledge in the case library can change as the domain changes.

On a historical note, the name "case-based reasoning" came from case law in the legal domain. When an attorney defends a client, the attorney may appeal to past cases in which the circumstances are similar. One can imagine an attorney studying volumes of past legal cases in a law library trying to find a case that is similar to the client's case. The argument to a judge and jury goes this way: "This case is identical in all essential aspects to a case that was resolved ten years ago and the verdict was not guilty. One can save money and time by mapping the not guilty verdict to the current case."

The overall operation of a CBR system is shown in Figure 8. The sum total of knowledge in some domain is contained in a case library. When a new situation comes to the fore, one compares the data in the new situation to the cases in the library to find a case that is most similar to the new situation. This is called case retrieval. Now, it is hardly ever true the new situation will be exactly like the prior case, so the prior case and solution may have to

*Figure 8. Components of case-based reasoning systems*

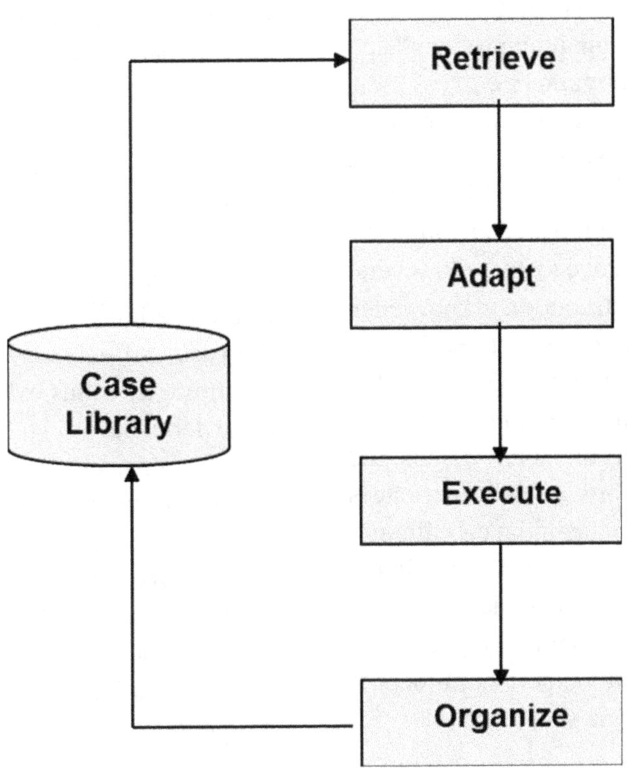

be adapted to fit the new situation. This is called case adaptation. The adapted solution is tried for the new situation. This is called case execution. The results of the execution are entered back into the case library for use in the future. In this way, CBR systems learn from experience.

There are several different approaches for each step in CBR. For example, there are several approaches to comparing two cases to derive a similarity metric in the Retrieve step. The simplest approach is key-term matching. The most complex approach is analogy based matching in which one sees a structural similarity between items in quite separate domains.

For our purposes, we are not too interested in problem-solving and more interested in guiding a gentle conversation with a patient. Nonetheless, we can use certain features of an overall CBR system to an advantage. The first challenge is the structure of a case for a particular domain. We want a case to hold experiences of the patient. Once a structure is agreed upon, a second challenge is to embed knowledge of the patient's past experiences into the structure. This latter challenge is called the "knowledge acquisition problem" and is well-known in the AI community.

For most applications, a knowledge engineer is required who understands knowledge structure and also understand the domain of interest, in this case the experiences of the patient. Often the knowledge engineer will have to undergo several iterations over attempts at structure and knowledge acquisition to settle upon a good structure of a case. Of course, the engineer cannot depend upon the patient in this regard, but the engineer can have several sessions with family members, friends, and the patient in order to record several experiences of the patient to enter into the initial case library. A common method of the formal representation of case structure suitable for algorithmic processing is predicate logic and logic programming. One can imagine a case for a patient's experience proceeding through development as shown in Box 1.

*Box 1.*

```
case_name(trip_to_rome).
date(september_43).
city(florence).
person(henry).
person(jane).
person(tom).
spouse(henry, jane).
son(tom, henry).
event(florence_museum).
event(missed_plane).
```

Now, during conversation with the patient, the output from steps 1 and 2 above (Translate patient voice to text, Parse the text to retrieve salient concepts and relations), the retrieval algorithm may select the case that best matches the concepts by using one of the retrieval methods, and appeal to other elements of the case to continue the conversation. Alternatively, an avatar or robot may select a case randomly to begin a conversation. A very difficult challenge is to gauge the patient's interest in the selected experience and decide whether to continue the line of conversation or move to another selected experience. This challenge will require a kind of feedback mechanism, e.g. simple reticence or indications of annoyance or unsettledness. Interestingly, the determination of the usefulness of a case could be recorded in the case and entered back into the case library for future use, thus exhibiting a kind of learning by experience.

An enhancement of this basic approach to conversational intelligence is to couple the CBR system with various ontologies that are likely to be shared by several patients. An ontology is a body of facts and relations about a particular concept where the concept could be a process, an event, a location, or the like. The development of ontologies for particular domains have become useful in science and engineering. One can view a list of public domain technologies at Stanford University's Protégé wiki at (Protégé Ontology Library, 2014). One will see ontologies for concepts as mundane as pizza to more complex ontologies such as financial instruments. In the example above, there could be a basic ontology for Italy, Florence, the Florence Museum, and the year 1943 to which the avatar or robot could appeal when conversing with a patient. Further, there could be meta-ontologies for countries, cities, museums which could guide specific ontologies. Such ontologies have not been worked through completely to date. It should be expected that more and more standard, public-domain ontologies will be developed in the future that can be used across applications.

## Discussion

We have outlined an approach to a knowledge structure that seems to show promise for capturing life events and history of an elderly patient, where an avatar or robot appeals to the knowledge when conversing with the patient. The approach has not been realized in commercial applications such as those discussed at the beginning of the chapter. There is much work to be done to develop the approach and to provide experimental results. However, given the trends in population growth, life expectancy, and the circumstances surrounding caregivers and the elderly, it is inevitable that the approach or some similar approach will be developed and commercialized within the next decade or so.

Interestingly, a 2012 popular movie "Robert and Frank" is about robots caring for the elderly and has been described as a sci-fi film that is not so far-fetched (Robert & Frank, 2012). In addition to being an engaging movie, it raises questions of ethics, technology, and human-robot interaction. The movie is good inspiration for researchers wishing to take up the challenges discussed in this chapter.

# ETHICAL CONSIDERATIONS

An influential paper on technology and ethics is (Berdichevsky and Neuenschwander, 1999). The paper establishes a framework for thinking about the ethics of persuasive technologies. The authors view "persuasion" as an intentional effort to change attitudes or behavior and they view "technology" as the directed application of abstract ideas. The framework includes three primary items: (i) a designer with motivations for creating a technology, (ii) the technology that employs methods of persuasion, and (iii) the person who is persuaded.

Clearly, the topic of this chapter fits into this framework, and thus we start here to consider the ethics of avatars and robots for elderly care. We wish to increase the quality of life of the elderly by providing an experience that results in contentment and well-being. Further, we wish to influence the attitudes of the elderly's family members by providing them peace of mind.

The authors provide eight ethical principles of persuasive technology design as listed below.

1. The intended outcome of any persuasive technology should never be one that would be deemed unethical if the persuasion were undertaken without the technology or if the outcome occurred independently of persuasion.
2. The motivations behind the creation of a persuasive technology should never be such that they would be deemed unethical if they led to more traditional persuasion.
3. The creators of a persuasive technology must consider, contend with, and assume responsibility for all reasonably predictable outcomes of its use.
4. The creators of a persuasive technology must ensure that it regards the privacy of users with at least as much respect as they regard their own privacy.

5. Persuasive technologies relaying personal information about a user to a third party must be closely scrutinized for privacy concerns.
6. The creators of a persuasive technology should disclose their motivations, methods, and intended outcomes, except when such disclosure would significantly undermine an otherwise ethical goal.
7. Persuasive technologies must not misinform in order to achieve their persuasive end.
8. **The Golden Rule of Persuasion:** The creators of a persuasive technology should never seek to persuade a person or persons of something they themselves would not consent to be persuaded to do.

Principles 1 and 2 are straightforward and do not violate the aims of our concept. In fact, the concept is to complement caregivers with technology devices that achieve similar results.

Principle 3, 4, 5, and 7 are problematic and require more reflection and research. One can imagine many possible scenarios in which there is an undesirable outcome of the approach, or where the patient's privacy is violated, or where personal information leaks to undesirable third parties, or where the technology might misinform the patient. A simple example will suffice: Suppose the knowledge of the patient includes reminders about taking medicine. If an irresponsible person enters the knowledge into the system incorrectly, then the outcome could be quite undesirable. Further, if the avatar or robot presses a line of conversation which makes the patient uncomfortable, then the goals of the approach are somewhat defeated. The approach would need a feedback mechanism form patient to device in order to know when this is happening and to steer the conversation in more comfortable directions. In sum, much more consideration is needed to satisfy consumers that the approach is useful.

Principle 6 is straightforward. As designers, our motivations, methods, and intended outcomes are clear.

Principle 8 is quite problematic and controversial. It is related to the problem of deception mentioned earlier in the chapter. Suppose that the patient begins to believe that the avatar or humanoid robot is a real entity. Is it morally responsible to let the patient hold this belief, or rather to correct the patient? A possible approach to this problem is to make it clear to consumers that the technology is an assistive and complementary therapy for caregivers. Nonetheless, it remains possible that an elderly person will begin to see the technology otherwise.

A thought experiment may shed light on Principle 8. An elderly patient may not be as clear-headed as a younger person. Thus, younger people may ask themselves: As an older person, would I want myself to be comforted by a human-like entity that I do not know is unreal? If my contentment and quality of life in increased, am I ok with bonding with a technical companion such as a robot? These are hard questions to answer and they will likely depend upon the culture in which the therapy takes place. Some cultures view inanimate objects differently that other cultures.

As an alternative approach, (Feil-Seifer and Matarić, 2011) examines the ethical challenges of socially assistive robotics from three points of view (user, caregiver, peer) using core principles from medical ethics (autonomy, beneficence, non-maleficence, justice) to determine how intended and unintended effects of a SAR can impact the delivery of care.

In sum, it is clear that there is a need to develop new ways to help manage the elderly. One can see current trends in which designers are using technology in various ways to try to solve the problem of an increased population of the elderly and a decreased population of caregivers.

Several approaches to solutions are available as commercial products already, and researchers are busy trying to perfect those solutions or come up with new solutions. As the technology for a solution progresses during the next decade, one is advised to consider the ethical ramifications of the solutions as well.

## CONCLUSION AND FUTURE RESEARCH DIRECTIONS

There are several research dimensions to consider in using narrative with avatars and robots to enhance elder care: the technical dimension, the adoption dimension, and the ethical dimension. Each of these dimensions require much more research and experimentation. In this chapter we examined and critiqued state-of-the-science research prototypes and off-the-shelf applications. We proposed a concept and an initial design for a conversational structure that can be embedded in avatars and robots.

At the time of this writing, plans are underway by the author, another roboticist, and two professorial nurses to create a conversational robot for experiments in a retirement home. The robot is the humanoid robot NAO developed by Aldebaran Robotics in France (Vital, 2013; NAO, 2014). The plan is to program a set of interactive, conversational behaviors into the robot. The experiment will include separate sessions with two groups of people: (i) a group of elderly people with acceptable cognitive abilities and (ii) a younger generation of users. The methodology of the Technology Adoption Model (TAM) will be used to compare the adoption attitudes of each group of users. One of the behaviors is a popular game in the USA named *Jeopardy!* in which the humanoid robot will play the part of the host and the contestants will be members of the groups (Jeopardy, 2014). All people in the USA are familiar with this game, and most all seniors in the USA watch it on television and play along with it pretending to be contestants. These experiments should inform our research with respect to each of the three dimensions above: technology, adoption, and ethics.

## ACKNOWLEDGMENT

The author acknowledges the generous support of Christos and Mary Papoutsy for sponsorship of the Distinguished Chair in Ethics and Social Responsibility at Southern New Hampshire University in the USA. The author would like to thank the anonymous reviewers and the editor for their insightful comments and suggestions.

## REFERENCES

Andrews, J. (2013). Seniors on the move: As media technology has advanced, so have programs for seniors' improved well-being. Assisted Living, 11(5).

Berdichevsky, D., & Neuenschwander, E. (1999). Toward an Ethics of Persuasive Technology. *Communications of the ACM*, *42*(5).

*BraveHeart*. (2014). Retrieved February 28, 2014 from http://braveheartveterans.org/

*Chatbots*. (2014). Retrieved February 28, 2014 from http://www.chatbots.org/

Davis, F. (1989, September). Perceived Usefulness, Perceived Ease Of Use, and User Acceptance of Information Technology. *Management Information Systems Quarterly*.

Fasola, J., & Matarić, M. (2013). Socially Assistive Robot Exercise Coach: Motivating Older Adults to Engage in Physical Exercise. *Springer Tracts in Advanced Robotics*, *88*, 463–479. doi:10.1007/978-3-319-00065-7_32

Feil-Seifer, D., & Matarić, M. (2011). Ethical Principles for Socially Assistive Robotics. *IEEE Robotics & Automation Magazine*, *18*(1), 24-31.

*Gerijoy*. (2014). Retrieved February 28, 2014 from http://www.gerijoy.com/

González, M., Buiza, C., Etxeberria, I., Yanguas, J., Ortiz, A., & Carretero, M. et al. (2007). *The Effect of an Avatar in Natural Interaction. IOS Press Ebooks* (Vol. 20). Challenges for Assistive Technology.

Heerink, M., Krose, B., Evers, V., & Wielinga, B. (2006). The Influence of a Robot's Social Abilities on Acceptance by Elderly Users. In *Proceedings of 15th IEEE International Symposium on Robot and Human Interactive Communication*. IEEE.

Heerink, M., Krose, B., Evers, V., & Wielinga, B. (2009). Measuring acceptance of an assistive social robot: a suggested toolkit. In *Proceedings of 18th IEEE International Symposium on Robot and Human Interactive Communication*. IEEE.

*Jeopardy*. (2014). Retrieved February 28, 2014 from http://www.youtube.com/watch?v=vsUDWSEp_6o

Kolodner, J. (1993). Case-Based Reasoning. Morgan Kaufmann Publishers.

*Lifenaut*. (2014). Retrieved February 28, 2014 from https://www.lifenaut.com/bina48/

*Loebner*. (2014). Retrieved February 28, 2014 from http://loebner.net/Prizef/loebner-prize.html

*NAO*. (2014). Retrieved February 25th 2014 from http://www.aldebaran-robotics.com/en/

*Paro*. (2014). Retrieved February 28, 2014 from http://www.parorobots.com/

Pollack, N. (2005). Intelligent Technology for an Aging Population: The Use of AI to Assist Elders with Cognitive Impairment. *AI Magazine*, *26*(2).

*Protégé Ontology Library*. (2014). Retrieved February 28, 2014 from http://protegewiki.stanford.edu/wiki/Protege_Ontology_Library

*Robert & Frank*. (2012). Retrieved February 28, 2014 from http://www.imdb.com/title/tt1990314/news

*Robot Astronaut*. (2013). Retrieved February 28, 2014 from http://www2.toyota.co.jp/en/news/13/09/0905.pdf

*Robot-Era*. (2014). Retrieved February 28, 2014 from http://www.robot-era.eu/robotera/

*Robots+Avatars*. (2014). Retrieved February 28, 2014 from http://www.robotsandavatars.net/

*Tele-Presence Robots*. (2014). Retrieved February 28, 2014 from http://telepresencerobots.com/

*AI Topics*. (2014). Retrieved February 28, 2014 from http://aitopics.org/

*USC-ICT*. (2014). Retrieved February 28, 2014 from http://ict.usc.edu/

Vichitvanichphong, S., Kerr, D., Talaei-Khoei, A., & Ghapanchi, A. (2013). Analysis of Research in Adoption of Assistive Technologies for Aged Care. In *Proceedings of 24th Australasian Conference on Information Systems*. Melbourne: Academic Press.

Vital, J., Couceiro, M., Rodrigues, N., Figueiredo, C., & Ferreira, N. (2013). Fostering the NAO platform as an elderly care robot. In *Proceedings of IEEE 2nd International Conference on Serious Games and Applications for Health* (SeGAH). IEEE.

## KEY TERMS AND DEFINITIONS

**Avatar:** An electronic visual representation of a character, often substituting for a real human, which performs tasks such as answering question, providing advice, having conversations, etc.

**Elder Care:** The processes and methods of maintaining and nurturing persons in later stages of life, especially with a concern for the person's quality of life.

**Ethical Ramifications:** The consideration of a process or invention with respect to some definition of good and evil, and a measure of the process or invention accordingly, often couched in terms of unforeseen consequences.

**Knowledge Acquisition:** The process of extracting knowledge about a particular domain from a domain expert, usually through interviews, and inserting the knowledge into a well-defined structure for knowledge representation, e.g. rule-based reasoning. See Knowledge Representation.

**Knowledge Representation:** A particular, well-defined structure for holding computerized knowledge, e.g. rule-based reasoning, case-based reasoning, fuzzy logic, et al. See Knowledge Acquisition.

**Narrative:** A story, often a reminiscence, typically accompanied by verbal interaction and conversation among two or more living entities.

**Ontology:** A list of terms and relations that describe a particular domain of interest, e.g. an ontology for Vienna or an ontology for American football.

**Ontology:** A list of terms and relations that describe a particular domain of interest, e.g. an ontology for Vienna or an ontology for American football.

**Quality of Life:** A measure of the state of a living entity, which can be objective or subjective, and which may be provided by the entity or inferred by another entity, where such measures may include degrees of happiness, pain and pleasure, anxiety, depression, awareness, motor control, etc.

**Robot:** (a) A *humanoid* robot is a robot that has likeness to a human, e.g. with torso, arms, and legs that usually has sensors for object recognition, voice recognition, and speech, and is designed to be autonomous; (b) A *tele-presence* robot is a robot that is operated remotely by a human, usually lacking autonomy, where the human is able to see, hear, navigate, and talk from a distance. Other kinds of robots include those that have a likeness to animals, those used exclusively for manufacturing, or those that do not resemble any sort of living entity such as a vacuum cleaner robot. A socially assistive robot is one that engages in common social behaviors such as conversation and playing.

# Chapter 15
# The Role of Knowledge Management (KM) in Aged Care Informatics:
## Crafting the Knowledge Organization

**Margee Hume**
*University of Southern Queensland, Australia*

**Paul Johnston**
*Care Systems Pty Ltd, Australia*

**Craig Hume**
*Griffith University, Australia*

**Jeffrey Soar**
*University of Southern Queensland, Australia*

**Jon Whitty**
*University of Southern Queensland, Australia*

## ABSTRACT

*Aged care is projected to be the fastest-growing sector within the health and community care industries (Reynolds, 2009). Strengthening the care-giving workforce, compliance, delivery, and technology is not only vital to our social infrastructure and improving the quality of care, but also has the potential to drive long-term economic growth and contribute to the Gross Domestic Product (GDP). This chapter examines the role of Knowledge Management (KM) in aged care organizations to assist in the delivery of aged care. With limited research related to KM in aged care, this chapter advances knowledge and offers a unique view of KM from the perspective of 22 aged care stakeholders. Using in-depth interviewing, this chapter explores the definition of knowledge in aged care facilities, the importance of knowledge planning, capture, and diffusion for accreditation purposes, and offers recommendations for the development of sustainable knowledge management practice and development.*

## INTRODUCTION

Key to responding to this pressure is increased empowerment and capability of leadership and management within the aged care workforce and offsetting practices through advance technological developments and knowledge creation. Aged care is becoming more diverse and complex advancing from residential care to incorporate community directed care. As a result, "aged care knowledge" is becoming increasingly heterogeneous which puts more emphasis on the need for

DOI: 10.4018/978-1-4666-6316-9.ch015

better Knowledge Management (KM) including its creation, access and diffusion to ensure an appropriate/fit for purpose level of care. It other words, one size does not fit all and while there might be some commonalities there will also be substantial differences.

Health informatics is a field of growing interest, popularity and research. It deals with the resources, ICT (information computer technology), and methods required to facilitate the acquisition, storage, retrieval, and use of information in the health sector. Tools include computers, formal medical terminologies and information and communication systems, with knowledge management systems at the forefront of thought in health (Murray & Carter, 2005). This chapter embraces the important area of knowledge generation and informatics in aged care healthcare. This chapter focuses on informing the development of an analytics - driven operational systems and advanced KM hub for aged care management and patient care services. Analytics is focused on communication and decision-making based on meaningful patterns in data gained from a methodological analysis. The chapter introduces the concepts of knowledge management, decision support systems and big data management in aged care and focuses on the importance of diffusion of knowledge to those in need.

This chapter focuses on the important area of aged care services as a national priority with this a priority for many countries worldwide (Cartwright, Sankaran, Kelly, 2008) and adopts a case study approach with the Australian aged care sector as the basis of analysis. The Australian aged care system is seen as innovative globally and provides the benchmark for many countries developing reforms and strategies for aged care. Many countries including Australia are burdened with an ageing population (Venturato & Drew, 2010). This burden has created the need for policy reform and the introduction of new programs to improve the quality of life of senior citizens (Department of Health and Ageing, 2013). The changing industry needs are driven by a combination of changing demographics, changing care needs, increased funding for community care and restructuring by service providers to meet government reforms and initiatives. The reform and accreditation process has created the need to exploit new information and knowledge to ensure innovative delivery. This need and the increased complexity of the information required encourage the need to be innovative in the management of knowledge ((Bailey & Clarke, 2001; Binney, 2000; Blair, 2002; Wiig, 1997) There is no doubt that the sector manages some types of knowledge efficiently such as patient medical records, funding reporting and basic accreditation records however there is much data available that can enable better work practice that is not being accessed (Venturato & Drew, 2010; Sankaran, Cartwright, Kelly, Shaw, Soar, 2010).

## THE AUSTRALIAN AGED CARE SECTOR

The aged sector needs are driven by a combination of demographics, changing care needs, increased funding for community care and restructuring by service providers to meet government reforms and initiatives. With 84% of community care packages and approximately 60% of residential aged care services, provided by not-for-profit (NFP) organizations (Productivity Commission, 2011) it is vital to assist and inform leadership, decision making and productivity improvements through advanced leadership techniques and decision making support such as KM (Bailey &Clarke, 2001; Binney, 2000; Blair, 2002) . The notion of effective leadership warrants continued investigation with focus on skilling governance bodies of NFPs to solve complex business challenges including financial, legal, property, service delivery, ethical and management issues. Previous work (Jeon, Merlyn, & Chenoweth, 2010; Cartwright, Sankaran & Kelly, 2008) identified that NFP aged care leaders require improved and supported decision making and knowledge support for leadership and performance was identified as an essential part (Riege, 2005). Knowledge supporting the accreditation process and ability to meet compliance expectation and standards was the primary focus of this knowledge. While some KM systems and knowledge hubs have been developed in health they have failed to meet the needs of the sector related to knowledge creation, information management, diffusion and the offered preparation for the leadership needed for the sector (Pinnington, 2011; Hume and Hume 2008; Hume, Pope & Hume 2012; Hume Clarke & Hume, 2012).

It is proposed that this is because of the following:

- They are not context specific to aged care;
- Are business cases for profit firms and insufficiently flexible for use in NFP organizations and in particular health and faith based firms;
- Fail to embrace the aged care sector diversity, complexities and requirements of accreditation and quality of care; and
- Do not encompass the emergence of increased reporting requirements, client demand and flexibility required to deliver end to end aged care and community directed care.

Examining the role of knowledge management and advancing the understanding of the requirements will assist in developing rigorous corporate system to support the sector.

The Australian Bureau Statistic (ABS) has projected growth of the number of Australians aged 65 years or over to increase from the current 15 per cent to 21 per cent by 2026 and 28 per cent by 2056 (ABS 2012). This trend towards an ageing population poses social and economic challenges which are being responded to by the Australian Government through its *Living Longer Living Better* reform package (DOHA: Department of Health and Ageing, 2013). The 2011 Productivity Commission report, *Caring for Older Australians* and the Commonwealth Department of Health and Ageing 2012 *Living Longer, Living Better,* aged care reform package, will be implemented between 2013 and 2022. The NFP providers in aged care sector employ nearly 900,000 staff, with support from 4.6 million volunteers (Productivity Commission 2010 and face continued funding and regulatory constraints, workforce shortages (Palmer, 2012), increasing frailty of clients and a rapidly increasing demand for complex professional and health services. These have been heralded major changes in the aged care sector (Comondor, Devereaux, Zhou, Stone, Busse, Ravindran, Burns, Haines, Stringer, Cook, Walter, Sullivan, Berwanger, Bhandari, Banglawala, Lavis, Petrisor, Schünemann, Walsh, Bhatnagar, Guyatt, 2009). These changes include an expansion of home care services and the introduction of a dementia supplement to support people with dementia receiving care at home and in residential care. In addition, recent changes to the Aged Care Funding Instrument (ACFI) for residential care aims to embed consumer-directed care principles into mainstream aged care program delivery and ensure the sustainability of facilities in regional, rural and remote areas. The reforms combine income and assets tests into a means-testing arrangement and introduced a lifetime cap on care fees (AIHW 2012). This reform package aims to deliver systems that provide older Australians with more choice, control and easier access to a full range of services, when and where they require it.

With these reforms come advanced management, leadership and business applications requirements for providers to meet the challenges and requirements of the future and comply with government legislation. The management of knowledge in aged care sectors is currently erratic and inconsistent and firms are suggested to be low on the capability maturity index KM considers the requirements and current practice of knowledge capture, storage, retrieval and diffusion (Davenport & Prusak, 2000) and the system assists current aged care providers in meeting the compliance and reporting needs of reforms and government legislation. A KM system also assists in creating flexibility catering for these and other imminent reforms and changes. Better management of knowledge and business intelligence will enable aged care providers in improved and streamlined patient management and service delivery (Lettieri, Borga, Savoldelli, 2004). The aged care sector is growing in most OECD countries; cost pressures and challenges of access and affordability are commonly reported. With baby-boomers now entering their late-60s, it is critical to incorporate technology-enabled solutions to facilitate the delivery of cost-effective aged care and address many of the challenges of managing this sector.

## AGED CARE AND KM

KM is a foundation practice in the organization and informs what is valued as knowledge, capture and diffusion of it. Embracing knowledge management and decision support mechanism ensure improved productivity and efficiency (Vestal, 2005). Knowledge management (KM) is increasingly being discussed as a cornerstone of an organisation's ability to compete (Treleaven & Sykes, 2005). Despite the increasing recognition of the benefits of KM, a number of significant implementation challenges exist for consideration by both practitioners and academics especially in not for profits (NFPs) and sectors with low capability maturity for technological innovations and practices such as KM. Identifying the current KM needs and practices to inform the development of KM for future implementation and compliance is vital. This chapter presents and collates current knowledge capture, storage, retrieval and diffusion and builds the business case for the data needed to advance decision-making in the aged care industry. Vichitvanichphong, Kerr Talaei-Khoei and Hossein Ghapanchi, (2013) have explored and collated the extent literature examining the role of technologies in aged care. Although this work focused primarily on assistive technologies adopted by the elderly it strongly highlights the limited amount or research conducted on general purpose information technology and online information services in this sector. This supports the need for research into knowledge management in this sector.

Many aged care organisations are being driven to adopt more commercial practices in order to improve their ability to effectively provide End to end care and delivery quality patient outcomes. Knowledge Management (KM) is one such "corporate" practice being explored to address the increasingly competitive environment, competitor intelligence and strategic intelligence (Haggie & Kingston, 2003). Although the concept of knowledge management may be basically understood researchers and managers are yet to explore and fully understand the complex inter-relationships of big data management, informatics, organizational culture, ICT, internal marketing, employee engagement and performance management as collective enablers on the capture, co-ordination, diffusion and renewal of knowledge in the aged care environment. This chapter will present research into the relationship of KM with those enabling elements and will offer a conceptual framework and implementation model to assist in planning and sustaining KM activity from integrated organizational and knowledge worker perspectives in aged care. The chapter will emphasize an enduring integrated approach to aged care industry KM to drive and sustain the knowledge capture and renewal continuum. The chapter will provide an important contribution on *how to* do KM in aged care and propose the need for interactive and Web 2.0 enabled knowledge hubs.

Aged care providers require leadership and innovation in Informatics and KM for Ageing and Aged-care to ensure productivity, innovation and growth and the ability to manage the imminent growth in the sector. Moreover, industry and consumer peak bodies have become more structured and planned in raising their concerns about aged care services (Reynolds 2009) and supporting and advising aged care providers. Aged care services are currently provided to more than 1 million people in Australia every year, through residential, community and flexible care services (Kane, 2003; Jeong & Keatinge, 2004). By 2050, it is expected that the number of Australians needing aged care services will increase to 3.5 million (Productivity Commission, 2011). As Australia's population ages at 20% per year with a predicted number of retirees by 2020 and the number of people reaching retirement doubling by 2030 and tripling by 2050, the aged care sector is under increasing pressure to ensure that quality aged care. Supporting providers, industry and consumer peak bodies with knowledge and data management frameworks will assist in moving them successfully into a new era of aged care. Many reports on ageing and the age (AIHW, 2012) identify the significant shortage in the current workforce trained to care for the needs of our nation's older adults, community care services and residential places. These places are predicted to grow explosively as the Baby Boomers retire and residential aged services will need to grow, evolve and innovate their service provision. Capital investment and allocation of capital is becoming increasingly hard for aged care providers and any measure which will assist in cost savings, improved service provision and efficiency such as KM is welcomed.

Managing the new advent of big data for known and sought knowledge and also having the ability to search for relevant but unknown sources will assist with industry transformation to improve productivity and enhance consumer directed care in the aged care services sector (AIHW 2012). Management of big data, knowledge, analytics and informatics are suggested to build services efficiency, improve quality of service and business profitability in many sectors especially knowledge intensive sectors like aged care and health (Hillmer, Wodchis, Gill Anderson Rochon, 2005; Tsai, Chien-Tzu, & Pao-Long, Chang, 2005; Vestal, 2005). It is widely believed that the use of information technology can reduce the cost of healthcare while improving quality and delivery (Manyika, Chui, Brown, Bughin, Dobbs, Roxburgh, and Hung Byers, 2011). The main issue with informatics and data management in this sector is the embryonic understanding of the data needed the ability to access the data, the storing of data, technology efficacy and how to use and integrate data and knowledge into the service delivery to improve service provision and patient outcomes. These are reinforced by the case of the Australian aged care sector.

## DATA AND METHOD

The purpose of this research is to examine how KM and knowledge in operating in the aged care sector in Australia, what practices are required and preferred and provide a validation of the need for KM in an aged care NFP setting. This research reports qualitative findings from a 22 in-depth interviews of NFP managers, senior full time staff. See Table 1 for a breakdown of survey respondents' roles.

A qualitative exploration and orientation study (Patton, 1990) was adopted for this research using in depth interviews with each of the aged care employees and is used to reflect the aged care sector. The advantage of using qualitative methods

*Table 1. Distribution of subjects*

| Job Role | Frequency |
|---|---|
| Ceo | 5 |
| Facility manager | 5 |
| Chief information officer | 4 |
| Operational staff | 6 |
| Professional contractor | 2 |
| TOTAL | 22 |

is the ability to extract rich and thick data and use inductive strategies for theory development (Patton, 1990). As recommended by Eisenhardt (1989), the qualitative research sample consisted of more than six (6) case subjects with sampling continuing until theoretical saturation. These studies complete 22 interview subjects to ensure a consistent and complete set of responses. The sample consisted of a good coverage of all role types with these depicted in Table 1.

The interviews selected subjects ranging from NFPs senior managers to operational staff. This reflected the leadership structure in the facilities accessed. These facilities were accessed using snowballing technique. Interestingly, in many facilities it was operational staff operation leading the facility on a regular basis. For the interviews all NFPs aged care managers, senior and operational were purposively selected to ensure full assessment of current behavior and needs of line staff in aged care facilities and also to explore opinion of managerial level workers in the aged care sector. The interviews were conducted onsite and took approximately 2 hours to complete. Each interview was recorded and transcribed with emergent themes highlighted. The scope of questions followed previous research knowledge management to focus topic areas. Probing questions were used to gather thick and deep descriptions of opinions and attitudes.

Open ended question were used and allowed for free flowing comments from subjects related to knowledge needs and the aged care sector. An open ended approach provides a forum for data variation from subjects, the collection of in depth scripts and ultimate theoretical saturation as recommended by Glaser and Strauss (1967), Eisenhardt (1989), Eisenhardt and Graebner (2007) and Perry (1998). The questions, based on previous KM research, were used to lead the interview and bring focus to KM and the aged care sector. They focused on the following areas:

- Do aged care NFP employees think KM assists in improving the understanding and management of information and knowledge in an aged care setting?
- Do aged care NFP organizations currently try manage the capture collection and diffusion of knowledge effectively using a KM system?
- How do you define knowledge; what is data in your sector what is known and what is recognized but not known?
- Do you have a KM Collection, Implementation and Diffusion Strategy?
- What is you perception of leadership style,
- Is knowledge performance management practiced?
- What is the culture and the culture of change?
- How do you leverage ICT and are you "technology enabled"?

A sample of 22 created a usable set of answer scripts enabling rigorous inductive analysis. As the sampling method was non-random, generalizability inferences of findings to the overall population are restricted, making the findings indicative to the population tested. However, these indicative findings contribute to the development of our understanding of KM in aged care NFPs. A set of transcripts were created verbatim from each of the respondents and were coded and organized using sequential incident analysis. A content analysis was undertaken resulting in the findings with this process consistent with the method outlined by Eisenhardt (1989). These findings identified the emergent themes and behaviors of KM in an aged care context. Further, inductive analysis was undertaken based on understanding of the extant literature and narratives were drawn from the scripts. Each of the question areas lead to specific response with some leading to advanced discussions in the topic areas.

## PROBLEMS IDENTIFIED

The interviews responses were coded and analyzed through logical deduction by experts in the field. These identified the following problems.

**Problem 1:** Lack of leadership and expertise in management of Knowledge: Current leadership in the sector is suggested to have little expertise in how to implement efficient KM strategies. This is compounded by a high turnover of staff, low technical efficacy and low capability maturity with these specifically hindering the adoption and implementation of KM strategies. The majority of subjects suggested that the understanding of the current capabilities and developing training strategies would assist in better knowledge definition, capture, storage and use. With this offering a real benefit to the sector.

**Problem 2:** The subjects suggested a lack of capability of current KM systems to meet the needs for efficient knowledge systems: Current KM/information support systems rely heavily on informal socialization and paper based systems with limited consistent document capture and storage, and limited formal engagement of staff. Many ICT systems lack the ability to manage knowledge and intelligence with very little understanding to date of Cloud technology and other virtual storage mediums. Improving the capability of accessing, storing massive amounts of data in its various forms would aid in providing efficiency and cost reductions for delivery. It was also identified that staff had relatively low technological efficacy, especially with more complex administration technology. Coupled with the informal nature of interactions and paper based recording KM was at a very embryonic stage with much tacit knowledge lost and much repetition with collection.

**Problem 3:** limited comprehensive understanding of what is knowledge, what needs to be stored and who are the key players in the knowledge process. Many subjects knew that they needed knowledge and that it was required for accreditation purposes however the specifics of who, what, where, when and why was overlooked.

**Problem 4:** The subjects identified some specific types of data that they collected and they knew was relevant. These have been identified as MUST. These were related to patient data and medical practice. The understanding of knowledge related to organizational systems, continuous improvement, (an essential component of accreditation) and specific needs for funding we found to be rudimentary. The foundation factors were known yet more complex and advanced knowledge were unknown and unrecognized. The areas have been clustered based on current standards requirements (ACSAA http://www.accreditation.org.au/accreditation/accreditationstandards/).

Table 2 depicts the data identified by the subjects as known and with further questioning and discussion, subjects discussed data they were not considering and were not aware of. Interestingly, the most unknown data was management and service data especially ICT tools and data management factors that may assist in accreditation and continuous improvement capability. There was little patient data that the subjects were not aware of or did not recognize. This supports the need for stronger managerial training and leadership in the sector with clinical training for registered staff, satisfactory.

**Problem 5:** Subjects identified there were problems with where to find the knowledge. Subject suggested knowledge hubs were poorly defined, advertised and accessible. They suggested that many of the organi-

*Table 2. Data known and unknown*

| | Known Data Sources Must | | Unknown Data Sources | |
|---|---|---|---|---|
| | **Patient** | **Firm** | **Patient** | **Firm** |
| Mgt. systems, staffing and organization development | residential care service's needs clinical indication regulatory requirements in general pain palliation and specialist care needs | service quality goals Information systems manuals Inventory and equipment Payroll | KM /ICT system specs External CDC services Complaints board regulatory requirements advanced Big data meta-analysis ICT data management tools how to use data in decision making –and the impact on clients (for residents) – increased life expectancy from increased quality of life (enjoyment/fulfillment/ mobility), decreased complaints; | KM systems specs External service providers Alternate food providers CI processes HR retention methods training alternatives Big data meta-analysis definitions and coding CI techniques for documentation business recording method of CI Benefits –can /how can you quantify the benefits of building ICT services like the knowledge hub? - ie. Improved Quality of Care (for staff) form increased staff satisfaction, reduced staff turnover |
| Health and personal care | Medications Carer details Sleep patterns Sensory needs Dental care Continence Morbidity and mortality data Falls | Documentation for funding level Insurance | Service providers and CDC | How to track this in home care |
| Resident lifestyle | Mobility Cognizance Nutrition and self-care Cultural and spiritual life needs Individual interests, customs, beliefs and cultural and Ethnic backgrounds Self-Choice and decision-making Resident security | Entertainment local and onsite | Service providers and CDC Quality of life measures | Best practice Way to capture data from in home care Staff satisfaction and turnover |
| Physical environment and safe systems | Level of care required Mental capacity Self-care documents Personal, civic, legal Education and staff development Independence Privacy and dignity Leisure interests and activities | Hazards and occupation health goals and practices Physical environment and safe systems Living environment Occupational health and safety Fire, security and other emergencies Infection control Catering, cleaning and laundry services | Service providers and CDC | Hospitality services and channel alternatives |

zations and support service functioned in silos and applied the information from their perspective. Some providers suggested this was often confusing, very time consuming to access and they rarely knew what they were looking for. They suggested these hubs needed to be more collaborative, relevant and interactive.

## RECOMMENDATIONS AND CONTRIBUTIONS

**Consideration 1:** Recognize knowledge and discover knowledge leaders. A key element of this project is that there is currently a wide gap between the potential of managing known information, acquiring information using big data and accessible data, analyzing the knowledge and its realization into business service provision and profits in aged care services. One of the hardest decisions is to know what data and information is of value to decision making and should be acquired and stored and what information should be discarded. Data and information can come from many sources as identified in Table 2 and can be tacit and or explicit and as such, the volume of data in the knowledge era is extensive. Figure one identifies many of the areas where data can be gathered and proposed that as KM is better understood that each of these areas has a specific strategy for the capture and creation of knowledge in aged care.

The problems of knowledge acquisition commence immediately with deciding what data to keep and what to discard. The next challenge is how to store what we keep reliably with the right metadata or filing system. Meta data refers to a set of data that describes and gives information about other data (www.techterms.com/definition/metadata). Exploiting vast new flows of big data captured from all paths of the internet and information can radically improve your company's performance, if managers can locate it easily and use it to measure and inform problem solving. This forms the basis of what we call analytics. Analytics is the science of logical analysis including identifying patterns in data that can inform decisions. Firms that capture and store data well know radically more about their businesses and directly translate that knowledge into improved decision making and performance. These firms have strategies and practices to transform big data such as KM and have a decision-making culture constructed on evidence based data. Clever KM systems have the ability to embrace the velocity and speed at which new data and information is entering the market with no question that technology enablement assists in the collection and storage of data and knowledge. Less consideration has been given to technology enablement for diffusion and the push of knowledge. A push knowledge strategy is the solution for unfamiliarity with knowledge especially known unknown data and unknown-unknown data . This strategy needs knowledge champions (Jones, Herschel, & Moesel, 2003) and needs knowledge leaders (Wenger &Snyder, 2000). Knowledge leaders in the sector need to create and disseminate knowledge through hubs and identify the key areas of core business, external legislation and accreditation, industry metrics and practices, consumer metrics like satisfaction and quality and organizational successes and failures. Knowledge champions disseminate this in the organization and encourage others to engage with knowledge creation. They promote that essential data is available and where to find it and what to do with. Currently in the aged care sector this is limited.

Figure 1 is not conclusive for all areas of data required in the sector however it introduces conceptually the areas identified by the subjects and shows how the capture, creation and diffusion is a feedback link for improved organizational performance and is the data flower. These are in essence the known areas of data with the unknown needs requiring push dissemination. Knowledge champions work to support technology enablement and the practice of KM in the firm whilst also championing the role of knowledge in lessons learnt (Zuber-Skerritt, 2001) and improving performance.

**Consideration 2:** The future of knowledge- interactive hubs.A feature of globally competitive knowledge-based economies is that governments, universities, consumers and industry work together in these economies to create regional 'knowledge hubs'. Recent advances in the role of big data are topical and it proved very effective. Interactive big data capture and diffusion is now moving to real time and constant sourcing. Developing Knowledge hubs with real time collaboration via "subscribed" knowledge groups with constant pull and push. Creating knowledge networks is a solution to the support the leadership and decision making issues in the age care sector (Venturato, & Drew, 2010). Many facilities are managed by clinically trained staff that lack managerial and administrative training and knowledge supports systems would support the deficit (Salipante & Aram, 2003, O'Sullivan & McKimm, 2011). To create world best practice and position the Australian aged care system as the benchmark for global aged care knowl-

*Figure 1. The big data flower*

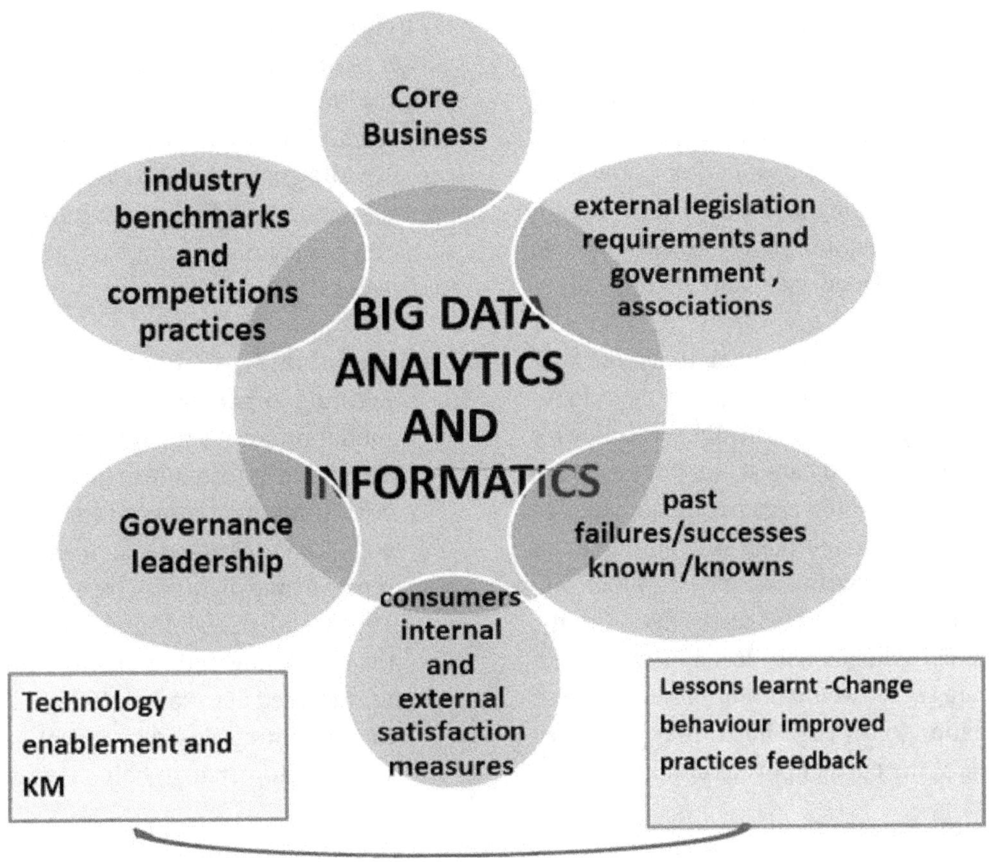

edge sharing and diffusion of knowledge through a collaborative, inclusive aged care knowledge hub is vital. Improving diffusion through using social media and interactive web 2.0 platforms will improve access to known and unknown data.

Currently knowledge hubs are static and focused. They have been suggested to have three major functions: to generate knowledge; to transfer and apply knowledge; and to transmit knowledge to others in the community through education and training. Knowledge hubs have generated new and basic knowledge of relevance for many industries, both old and new and the knowledge-users provide a focus for knowledge-generation, transmission and diffusion. The early generations of knowledge hubs have captured and stored knowledge systematically with this knowledge accessed by a pull strategy i.e. the knowledge must be found and accessed by the user. Ideally a well-designed hub will link and portal all available knowledge foci. Unfortunately in many sectors and particular to the aged care sector, competing knowledge hubs have been created from different stakeholder perspectives simulating knowledge and creating competing knowledge hub "silos". These hubs are often disconnected with those in need ie "the knowledge user" and are difficult to find and navigate.

Exploring the notion of interactivity and web 2.0 enabled knowledge hubs supporting a diffusion push strategy would radically revolutionize current KM in the aged care sector (. The notion of a push strategy would channel the knowledge to those in need through push web strategies of email, social media, webinars, forums, blogs discussion, alerts, pokes and rss feeds. Specifically, leadership, compliance and decision-making in the aged care sector would be supported by these next generation knowledge hubs. Irrespective of the existent of the current portals and knowledge hubs problems still exist based on the nature of the knowledge tacit or explicit. Explicit knowledge is knowledge that has been articulated, codified, and stored in a certain retrieval media. It can be readily transmitted to others. Conversely tacit knowledge is knowledge, people are not often aware of the knowledge they possess nor how it can be valuable to others. Effective transfer of tacit knowledge generally requires extensive personal contact, regular interaction and trust as creation.

In the traditional setting, the transmission function of a knowledge hub takes place through educational institutions such as universities and schools but also through life-long learning processes that involve firms, community based institutions and a variety of government agencies and services including hospitals, clinics and professional associations. Users must be aware of these channels. Social media is underutilised and provides a stronger diffusive and viral mechanism for knowledge distribution. The aims are to maximse cooperation coordination, collaboration and conservation. Identifying the factors that influence the knowledge needs of aged care providers, advocates and associations, when considering and providing care, and the extent to which these preferences are met by current knowledge based services, is essential to capturing tacit and explicit knowledge.

**Consideration 3:** A Conceptual Model for the learning organization in aged care. The model proposed for KM for aged care services that informs and innovate aged care KM implementation framework: knowledge identification, acquisition, capture, retrieval and diffusion(Nonaka,&Takeuchi, 1995) and decision-making and supports the development of a learning organization for the aged care sector. Figure 2 suggested that adopting lessons learnt philosophy will develop change behaviour and organisational rewiring. The importance of this is the involvement of people and the role that people play in generating and creating knowledge. Figure 2 depicts the development of learning organisations and improved performance through informed workforce leadership and efficiency in decision making, organisational knowledge capture, Knowledge leaders, knowledge champions and application of aged care health informatics (Senge, 1990; Senge, Roberts, Ross, Smith, and Kleinter, 1994). This figure proposes the use of technology enabled analytics (KM) and infrastructure in aged care services improving leadership, social interactions and innovation in processes and availability and delivery through knowledge and lessons learnt. This framework suggests improved access to knowledge, analytics and use of data [for reporting compliance and funding] is required and that developing a feedback system will manifestly improve decision making resulting in a learning organisation. The framework also considers aspects of culture, performance management and education as vital inputs for success. Finally, the recommendations for management include the needs to address the four Management Challenges of KM implementation.

Finally, the recommendations for management include the needs to address the four Management Challenges of KM implementation.

Companies won't reap the full benefits of a transition to using big data, KM and Knowledge hubs unless they're able to manage change effectively and embrace lessons learnt philosophy. Four areas are particularly important in that process.

1. **Leadership:** Companies succeed in the KM and big data era due to leadership teams that set clear goals, define what success

*Figure 2. Organisational learning model and knowledge*

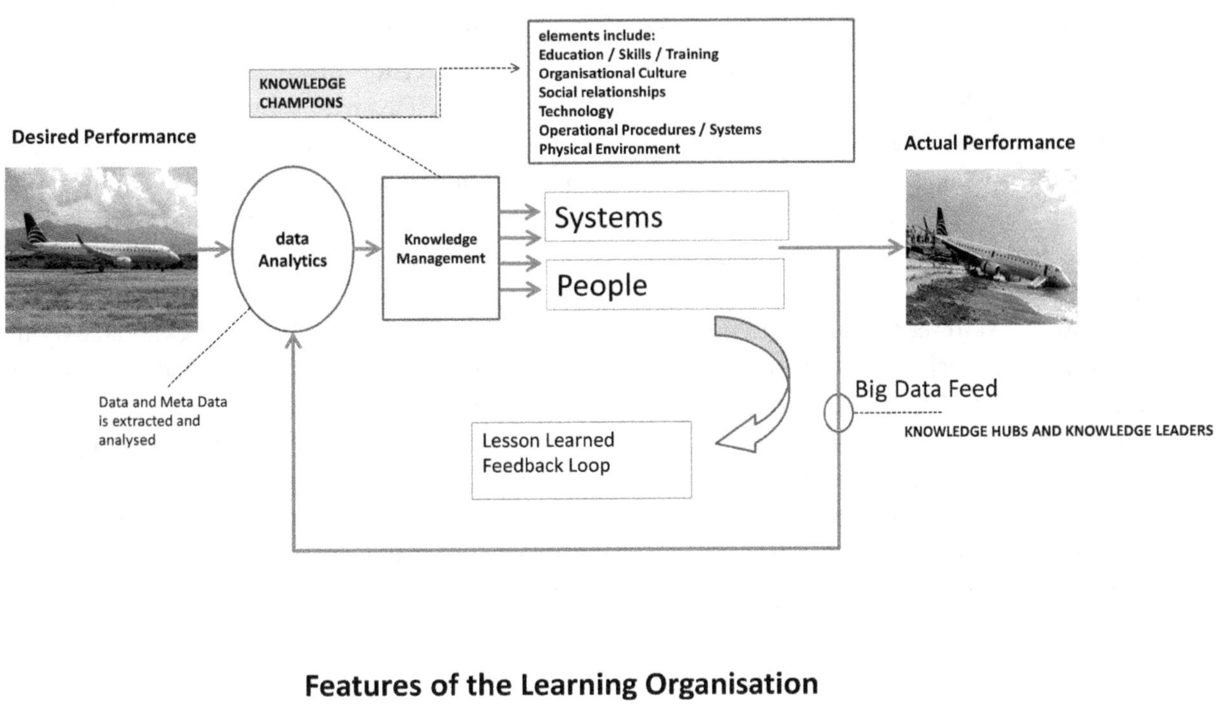

looks like, and identify the correct needs. These leaders have vision and recognize opportunity and understand how the sector as a whole is developing. The customer orientation and internal marketing (Martinsons, & Hosley, 1993; Ballantyne, 2000) . This includes employees and other stakeholders. The successful participants in the aged care sector will be those with the ability to be flexible in changing the way their organizations make many decisions and develop a decision-making culture.

2. **Knowledge Leaders, Data Experts, and Champions:** As data becomes easily accessible and of low cost, the data experts and knowledge workers are of greater demand (Chong, 2005). Experts skilled in working with data are needed if the role of data and analytics is going to be incorporated in the business. The most valuable data experts will be those that can link the needs of the sector, the firm, data and design ways in which data can be used. These will be our knowledge leaders and champions.
3. **Information and Communications Technology (ICT):** The tools available to handle the volume, velocity, and variety of big data have advanced substantially in recent times (Chong, 2005). There are many inexpensive, open source libraries that can aid the technologically minded in setting up a system. However, these technologies do require a skill set that is new to most IT departments, which will need to work hard to integrate all the relevant internal and external sources of data. In the aged care sector this skill set is at a lower capability so sourcing expert staff will be a priority
4. **Evidence Based Decision Making Culture:** Effective and performance oriented firms use evidence to make decisions. People who understand the problems need to be brought together with the right data, but also with the people who have problem solving techniques that can effectively exploit them.

## CONCLUDE FUTURE RESEARCH AND IMPLEMENTATION CONSIDERATIONS

This chapter has introduced the concepts of KM in aged care. The chapter has reported the findings of qualitative work that highlighted the current problems and the need for KM, KM champions and an easy and effective way to access knowledge. The chapter has offered the following considerations and recommendations and these are vital for the Australian aged care system to be globally innovative and be the benchmark for many countries developing reforms and strategies for aged care.

The chapter suggested that the theoretical understanding of knowledge creation needs to be advanced in the ACC sector with particular reference to knowledge storage, retrieval and diffusion needs for decision-making for accreditation and compliance. This will better manage information and knowledge and equip leaders with KM support for informed decisions, service innovations, staffing and training for current and future change and intensifying pressures.

Finally, testing and refining the elements of a dynamic, interactive KM framework and satisfying the knowledge and information needs of the sector are essential for productivity. Developing a specific business cases for organisations and testing these in organizational settings using action research interventions and reflection will confirm the need and specifications of each system. For the sector to advance into the future further empirical work would advance understanding of the knowledge needs and creation and the successful development and adoption of knowledge hubs in the aged care sector. The Benefits of building the knowledge hub including improved Quality of Care (for staff) increase staff satisfaction, reduced staff turnover and improved consistency and quality (for residents) and decreased complaints should all be examined to support the business case.

## REFERENCES

Australian Institute of Health and Welfare (AIHW). (2012). *Residential aged care in Australia 2010-11: a statistical overview, Aged care statistics series no. 36, Cat. No. AGE 68*. Canberra: AIHW.

Bailey, C., & Clarke, M. (2001). Managing knowledge for personal and organizational benefit. *Journal of Knowledge Management*, *5*(1), 58. doi:10.1108/13673270110384400

Ballantyne, D. (2000). Internal relationship marketing: A strategy for knowledge renewal. *International Journal of Bank Marketing*, *18*(6), 274. doi:10.1108/02652320010358698

Binney, D. (2000). The knowledge management spectrum-understanding the KM landscape. *Journal of Knowledge Management*, *5*(1), 21–32.

Blair, D. C. (2002). Knowledge Management: Hype, Hope or Help? *Journal of the American Society for Information Science and Technology*, *53*(12), 1019. doi:10.1002/asi.10113

Cartwright, C., Sankaran, S., & Kelly, J. (2008). *Developing a New Leadership Framework for Not-For-Profit Health and Community Care Organisations in Australia*. Lismore, Australia: Southern Cross University.

Chong, C. S. (2005, June). Critical factors in the successful implementation of Knowledge Management. *Journal of Knowledge Management*, 21–42.

Productivity Commision. (2010). Contribution of the Not-for-Profit Sector (Research Report). Canberra: Author.

Comondore, V. R., Devereaux, P. J., Zhou, Q., Stone, S. B., Busse, J. W., & Ravindran, N. C. et al. (2009). Quality of care in for-profit and not-for-profit nursing homes: systematic review and meta-analysis. *BMJ (Clinical Research Ed.)*, *339*, b2732. doi:10.1136/bmj.b2732 PMID:19654184

Davenport, T. H., & Prusak, L. (2000). Working Knowledge: How Organisations Manage What They Know. Harvard Business School Press.

Department of Health and Ageing (Australian Government) (DoHA). (2012). Living Longer: Living Better. DoHA.

Eisenhardt, K. (1989). Building theories from case study research. *Academy of Management Review*, *14*(4), 532-550

Eisenhardt, K., & Graebner, M. E. (2007). Theory building from cases: Opportunities and Challenges. *Academy of Management Journal*, *50*(1), 25–32. doi:10.5465/AMJ.2007.24160888

Glaser, B., & Strauss, A. (1967). *The Discovery of Grounded Theory: Strategies for Qualitative Research*. Chicago, IL: Aldine Publishing Company.

Haggie, J. K., & Kingston, J. (2003, June). Choosing a knowledge management strategy. *Journal of Knowledge Management*, 33–56.

Haggie, K., & Kingston, J. (2003). Choosing your knowledge management strategy. *Journal of Knowledge Management Practice*, 1 – 20.

Hall, R. (2003). *Knowledge Management in the New Business Environment (A report prepared for the Australian Business Foundation)*. Sydney: ACIRRT, University of Sydney.

Hall, R. (2003). *"Knowledge Management in the New Business Environment", A report prepared for the Australian Business Foundation, ACCIRT.* University of Sydney.

Hillmer, M. P., Wodchis, W. P., Gill, S. S., Anderson, G. M., & Rochon, P. A. (2005). Nursing home profit status and quality of care: Is there any evidence of an association? *Medical Care Research and Review*, *62*(2), 139–166. doi:10.1177/1077558704273769 PMID:15750174

Hume, C., Clarke, P., & Hume, M. (2012). The role of knowledge management in the large non profit firm: building a framework for KM success. *International Journal of Organisational Behaviour*, *17*(3), 82–104.

Hume, C., & Hume, M. (2008). The strategic role of knowledge management in nonprofit organizations. *International Journal of Nonprofit and Voluntary Sector Marketing*, *13*(2), 129–140.

Hume, C., Pope, N., & Hume, M. (2012). KM 100: Introductory knowledge management for not-for-profit organizations. *International Journal of Organisational Behaviour*, *17*(2), 56.

James, M., Chui, M., Brown, B., Bughin, J., Dobbs, R., Roxburgh, C., & Byers, A. H. (2011, May). Big data: The next frontier for innovation, competition, and productivity. *Harvard Business Review*, 59–69.

Jeon, Y. H., Merlyn, T., & Chenoweth, L. (2010). Leadership and management in the aged care sector: a narrative synthesis. *Australasian Journal on Ageing*, *29*(2), 54–60. doi:10.1111/j.1741-6612.2010.00426.x PMID:20553534

Jeong, S., & Keatinge, D. (2004). Innovative leadership and management in a nursing home. *Journal of Nursing Management*, *12*, 445–451. doi:10.1111/j.1365-2834.2004.00451.x PMID:15509274

Jones, N. B., Herschel, R. T., & Moesel, D. D. (2003). Using knowledge champions to facilitate knowledge management. *Journal of Knowledge Management*, *7*(1), 49. doi:10.1108/13673270310463617

Kane, R. (2003). Definition, Measurement, and Correlates of Quality of Life in Nursing Homes: Toward a Reasonable Practice, Research, and Policy Agenda. *The Gerontologist*, *43*, 28–36. doi:10.1093/geront/43.suppl_2.28 PMID:12711722

Lettieri, E., Borga, F., & Savoldelli, A. (2004). Knowledge Management in Nonprofit Organizations. *Journal of Knowledge Management*, *8*(6), 16. doi:10.1108/13673270410567602

Lettieri, E., Borga, F., & Savoldelli, A. (2004). Knowledge Management in non-profit organizations. *Journal of Knowledge Management*, *8*(6), 16–30. doi:10.1108/13673270410567602

Martinsons, M., & Hosley, S. (1993). Planning a strategic information system for a market-oriented non-profit organization. *Journal of Systems Management*, *44*(2), 14.

Miles, M. B., & Huberman, A. M. (1994). *An Expanded Sourcebook: Qualitative Data Analysis* (2nd ed.). Sage Publications International.

Murray, P., & Carter, L. (2005). Improving marketing intelligence through learning systems and knowledge communities in not-for-profit workplaces. *Journal of Workplace Learning*, *17*(7), 421–435. doi:10.1108/13665620510620016

Murray, P., & Carter, L. (2005). Improving marketing intelligence through learning systems and knowledge communities in not-for-profit workplaces. *Journal of Workplace Learning*, *17*(7/8), 421–435. doi:10.1108/13665620510620016

Nonaka, I., & Takeuchi, H. (1995). The Knowledge Creating Company. Oxford University Press.

Nonaka, I., & Takeuchi, H. (1995). The Knowledge Creating Company. Oxford University Press.

O'Sullivan, H., & McKimm, J. (2011). Doctor as professional and doctor as leader: same attributes, attitudes and values? *British Journal of Hospital Medicine*, *72*, 463–466. doi:10.12968/hmed.2011.72.8.463 PMID:21841592

Oliver, S., & Kandadi, K. R. (2006). How to develop knowledge culture in organizations? A multiple case study of large distributed organizations. *Journal of Knowledge Management*, *10*(4), 6–24. doi:10.1108/13673270610679336

Palmer, E., & Eveline, J. (2012). Sustaining low pay in aged care work. *Gender, Work and Organization*, *19*, 254–275.

Patton, Q. M. (1990). *Qualitative Evaluation and Research Methods* (2nd ed.). Sage Publications.

Pinnington, A. (2011). Leadership Development: Applying the same leadership theories and development practices to different contexts? *Leadership*, *7*, 335. doi:10.1177/1742715011407388

Productivity Commission. (2011). *Caring for Older Australians, Report No. 53, Final Inquiry Report*. Canberra: Author.

Raymond, L. (1985). Organizational characteristics and MIS success in the context of small business. *Management Information Systems Quarterly*, *9*(1), 37–52.

Reynolds, A. (2009). *The Myer Foundation 2020: A Vision for Aged Care in Australia*. Fitzroy, Australia: Outcomes Review, Brotherhood of St Laurence.

Riege, A. (2005). Three dozen knowledge sharing barriers managers must consider. *Journal of Knowledge Management*, *9*(3), 18–35. doi:10.1108/13673270510602746

Salipante, P., & Aram, J. D. (2003). Managers as knowledgeable generators: The nature of practitioner-scholar research in the non-profit sector. *Nonprofit Management & Leadership*, *14*(2), 129–150. doi:10.1002/nml.26

Sankaran, S., Cartwright, C., Kelly, J., Shaw, K., & Soar, J. (2010). Leadership of non-profit organisations in the aged care sector in Australia. In *Proceedings of the 54th Meeting of the International Society for the Systems Sciences*. Academic Press.

Senge, P. M. (1990). *The Fifth Dimension - The Art and Patience of The Learning Organisation*. New York: Doubleday.

Senge, P. M., Roberts, C., Ross, R. B., Smith, B. J., & Kleinter, A. (1994). *The Fifth Discipline Field Book: Strategies and Tools for Building a Learning Organisation*. New York: Doubleday.

Treleaven, L., & Sykes, C. (2005). Loss of organizational knowledge: From supporting clients to serving head office. *Journal of Organizational Change Management*, *18*(4), 353–368. doi:10.1108/09534810510607056

Tsai, C.-T., & Chang, P.-L. (2005). An integration framework of innovation assessment for the knowledge-intensive service industry. *International Journal of Technology Management*, *30*(1-2), 85-104.

Vasconcelos, J., Seixas, P., Kimble, C., & Lemos, P. (2005). Knowledge management in non-government organisations: A partnership for the future. In *Proceedings of the 7th International Conference on Enterprise Information Systems* (ICEIS 2005). ICEIS.

Venturato, L., & Drew, L. (2010). Beyond'doing': Supporting clinical leadership and nursing practice in aged care through innovative models of care. *Contemporary Nurse, 35*(2), 157–170. doi:10.5172/conu.2010.35.2.157 PMID:20950197

Vestal, W. (2005). Making sense of KM costs. *KM World, 14*(7), 8–11.

Vichitvanichphong, S., Kerr, D. T.-K. A., & Amir, H. G. (2013). *Analysis of Research in Adoption of Assistive Technologies for Aged Care*. Paper presented at the 24th Australasian Conference on Information Systems. Melbourne, Australia.

Wenger, E. C., & Snyder, W. M. (2000). Communities of practice: The organizational frontier. *Harvard Business Review, 78*(1), 139–145. PMID:11184968

Wiig, K. M. (1997). Integrating intellectual capital and knowledge management. *Long Range Planning, 30*(3), 399–405. doi:10.1016/S0024-6301(97)90256-9

Zuber-Skerritt, O. (2001). *Action Learning and action research: paradigm, praxis and programs. Effective change management using action research and action learning: Concepts, frameworks, process and applications*. Lismore, Australia: Southern Cross University Press.

## KEY TERMS AND DEFINITIONS

**Aged Care:** Elderly care, or simply eldercare, is the fulfilment of the special needs and requirements that are unique to the led rely. This broad term encompasses such services as assisted living, adult day care, long term care, nursing homes, hospice care, and home care.

**Content and Document Management Systems:** Represent the convergence of full-text retrieval, document management, and publishing applications.

**Data Marts:** Represent specific database systems on a much smaller scale representing a structured, searchable database system, which is organised according to the user's needs.

**Data Repository:** A database used primarily as an information storage facility, with minimal analysis or querying functionality.

**Data Warehouses:** The main component of KM infrastructure and stores data in a number of databases. It organizes data and provides meaningful knowledge to the business, which can be accessed for future reference.

**Health Informatics:** A discipline at the intersection of information science, computer science, and health care. It deals with the resources, devices, and methods required to optimize the acquisition, storage, retrieval, and use of information in health and biomedicine.

**Knowledge Capture:** A variety of techniques used to elicit facets of an individual's technical knowledge such that insights, experiences, social networks.

**Knowledge Diffusion:** The movement of useful ideas between organizations.

**Knowledge Management:** The process of capturing, distributing, and effectively using knowledge.

**Knowledge Storage:** Includes data warehouses, data marts, content management systems and data repositories.

## APPENDIX

### List of Abbreviations

**ABS:** Australian Bureau Statistic.
**ACC:** Aged Care Community (Sector).
**ACFI:** Aged Care Funding Instrument.
**DOHA:** Department of Health and Ageing.
**GDP:** Gross Domestic Product.
**ICT:** Information computer technology.
**KM:** Knowledge Management.
**NFP:** Not-for-profit organization.
**OECD:** The Organization for Economic Co-operation and Development.

# Chapter 16
# Ontology for Data Quality and Chronic Disease Management:
## A Literature Review

**Alireza Rahimi**
*University of New South Wales, Australia & Isfahan University of Medical Sciences, Iran*

**Pradeep Kumar Ray**
*University of New South Wales, Australia*

**Siaw-Teng Liaw**
*University of New South Wales, Australia*

**Jane Taggart**
*University of New South Wales, Australia*

**Hairong Yu**
*University of New South Wales, Australia*

## ABSTRACT

*Improved Data Quality (DQ) can improve the quality of decisions and lead to better policy in health organizations. Ontologies can support automated tools to assess DQ. This chapter examines ontology-based approaches to conceptualization and specification of DQ based on "fitness for purpose" within the health context. English language studies that addressed DQ, fitness for purpose, ontology-based approaches, and implementations were included. The authors screened 315 papers; excluded 36 duplicates, 182 on abstract review, and 46 on full-text review; leaving 52 papers. These were appraised with a realist "context-mechanism-impacts/outcomes" template. The authors found a lack of consensus frameworks or definitions for DQ and comprehensive ontological approaches to DQ or fitness for purpose. The majority of papers described the processes of the development of DQ tools. Some assessed the impact of implementing ontology-based specifications for DQ. There were few evaluative studies of the performance of DQ assessment tools developed; none compared ontological with non-ontological approaches.*

DOI: 10.4018/978-1-4666-6316-9.ch016

## INTRODUCTION

The growing use of electronic health records (EHRs) raises issues of semantic interoperability and the quality management/improvement of large datasets derived from multiple EHRs. Improved data quality in EHRs can improve the quality of decisions and lead to better policy that actually meet needs, strategies, evidence-based care and patient outcomes.

The acceptable level of data quality is not fixed in the system. Rather health professionals can provide it at different times and data users need to assess that quality contextually, based on the fitness for research, audit and quality assurance purposes (Devillers, Bedard, Jeansoulin, & Moulin, 2007). It is important to take a user view point of quality because it is the end user who evaluate whether or not data is fit for use. A focus is the quality of patient or disease registers derived from EHRs to support policy and practice. Patients registers need to have a level of completeness and the information contained, need a level of correctness and consistency to be useful for clinical, quality improvement and research purposes (S. Liaw, Taggart, Dennis, & Yeo, 2011).

DQ was conceptualised in terms of its "fitness for purpose/use" in a few papers (R. Wang, 1998; R. Y. Wang, D. M. Strong, & L. M. Guarascio, 1996). DQ can be described from two perspectives: (1) intrinsic quality of data elements and set of data elements (data set) and (2) how the set meets the user's needs i.e. fitness for purpose. The commonly approved definition of DQ has been epitomized in the International Standards Organisation definition: "the totality of features and characteristics of an entity that bears on its ability to satisfy stated and implied needs" (ISO 8402-1986, Quality Vocabulary). DQ also can be specified in terms of its "fitness for purpose/use" (R. Wang, 1998; R. Y. Wang, 1998; R. Y. Wang, et al., 1996).

Intrinsic DQ refers to the extent that data is free of defects as measured by specific DQ dimensions, including "accuracy, perfection, freshness and uniformity" (Redman, 2005) and "completeness, unambiguity, meaningless and correctness" (Choquet et al., 2010; Orme, Yao, & Etzkorn, 2007; Wand & Wang, 1996; Yao, Orme, & Etzkorn, 2005). The Canadian Institute for Health Information recommendations were the basis for an information quality framework comprising 69 quality criteria grouped into 24 quality characteristics, which was further grouped into 6 quality dimensions: accuracy, timeliness, comparability, usability, relevance and privacy & security (K. Kerr, A. Norris, & R. Stockdale, 2007). Research in DQ has tended to focus on the identification of generic quality characteristics such as accuracy, currency and completeness (Orme, et al., 2007; R. Wang, D. Strong, & L. Guarascio, 1996) or completeness, correctness, consistency and timeliness (S. Liaw, et al., 2011) as core dimensions of DQ that are relevant across application domains. However, a pervious review shows there is a lack of consensus conceptual framework and definition for DQ (S. T. Liaw et al., 2013).

Many studies regularly report a range of deficiencies in the collected information for professionals practice (Devillers, et al., 2007; B. K. Kahn, Strong, & Wang, 2002), clinical (Azaouagh & Stausberg, 2008; de Lusignan et al., 2010; Mitchell & Westerduin, 2008; Moro & Morsillo, 2004) and health promotion (Gillies, 2000b) purposes. Similar deficiencies exist with information in geographic (Devillers, et al., 2007; Ivanova, Morales, de By, Beshe, & Gebresilassie, 2013), hospital and general practice (ST Liaw et al., 2011) information systems, where the lack of coding rules meant that much of the data are often incomplete or in relatively inaccessible text format. The evidence is more encouraging for data for administrative purposes (Lain, Roberts,

Hadfield, Bell, & Morris, 2008; Quan et al., 2008). Hybrid record keeping systems in primary care are believed to be more complete than computer-only or paper-only systems (Hamilton, Round, Sharp, & Peters, 2003).

Relational database models have been prevalent in last few decades, enabling information to be efficiently stored and required within a hierarchical database architecture. On the other hand, ontologies, usually with non-hierarchical databases, have been used in applications that required more flexibility in capturing more semantic meanings. However, there is no well-documented evidence or experiments that suggest that one is better than the other in terms of outputs, data quality and fitness for purpose.

This literature review extended a previous literature (S. T. Liaw, et al., 2013) to include references from 2000-13 (previous was 2001-11) and focused on the conceptualization of data quality on the "fitness for purpose" paradigm, including methodologies to specify data quality for implementation, ontology-based approaches to develop data quality and semantic interoperability.

This systematic review of the domain will examine the breadth and depth of research into the conceptualization of data quality based on the "fitness for purpose" paradigm, methodologies to specify data quality for implementation, some advantages of ontology-based approaches to develop data quality, and semantic interoperability. We built on a pervious literature review (S. T. Liaw, et al., 2013) to address the following questions:

- How is data quality being conceptualized within the "fitness for purpose" definition for a range of uses?
- What specification methodologies are being used to specify data quality for implementation?
- What ontology-specified implementations are being used and how do they compare with other methods?
- How is the impact of implementing ontology-based specifications for data quality in chronic disease management being measured and evaluated?

## METHODS

A literature review was conducted of all English language studies, from January 2000-March 2013, which addressed data/information quality, fitness for purpose, used ontology-based approaches and involved healthcare/chronic disease. Inclusion criteria were: (a) conceptualises data quality based on "fitness for purpose"; (b) formal methodologies used to specify data quality for implementation; (c) involved some form of data models and ontologies to improve quality of clinical data in EHRs and patient registers; and (d) used data models and ontology-based approaches in CDM. These papers were screened by title and abstract content for inclusion. The references of the included papers were hand-searched for other eligible papers.

Included papers were critically appraised with a "context-mechanism-impacts/outcomes" framework. Appraised papers were summarized using specifically developed templates and discussed to achieve the final consensus on how it addressed the review questions. The conceptual framework developed for the literature review included:

- **Context:** Integrated CDM, evidence based practice, evidence-based policy patient or disease registers;
- **Mechanisms:** Methods to assess and manage quality of the register/EHR and data

quality based on "fitness for purpose", ontology-based approaches;
- **Impacts/Outcomes:** Measurable impacts outcomes based on improved quality of the register, data quality, "fitness for purpose".

The search strategy and keywords were organised around the three broad concepts:

- **Context:** Diseases (chronic diseases, chronic illnesses, chronic disease management, chronic illness management, electronic health records (EHRs), registers);
- **Mechanisms:** Data models and ontology (ontological based models, ontology approaches, ontology based multi agent systems (OBMAS), and ontological framework);
- **Impacts:** Data Quality (data quality, information quality, data quality management, data quality assessment, quality of register, fitness for purpose).

The search was repeated three times with the following phrases:

(data quality OR information quality) AND ("fitness for purpose" OR "fitness for use") AND (quality of register* OR quality of electronic health records) in Title, Abstract or Keywords, Subject or MESH

(ontology OR data model*) in Title, Abstract or Keywords, Subject or MESH AND (data quality OR information quality OR quality of register) in Title, Abstract or Keywords, Subject or MESH AND (fitness for purpose OR fitness for use) in Title, Abstract or Keywords, Subject or MESH

((ontology AND traditional data model*) in Title, Abstract or Keywords, Subject or MESH OR (ontology AND SQL) in Title, Abstract or Keywords, Subject or MESH) AND (chronic diseases OR chronic illnesses) in Title, Abstract or Keywords, Subject or MESH AND (data quality OR information quality OR quality of register) in Title, Abstract or Keywords, Subject or MESH.

The initial screening of the articles was based on their abstracts. AR read all abstracts independently and studies without electronic abstracts were excluded. Selection of relevant articles was based on the information obtained from the abstracts and was agreed upon in discussion with co-authors. In the case of differences, the original paper was obtained and agreement was achieved after it was read. We hand-searched the references of the included papers to ensure completeness of the search. Papers that satisfied the inclusion criteria were independently examined by authors and any disagreements resolved by consensus.

A specific template (Figure 1) was used to keep the extracted information consistent and focused on the analysis and synthesis of the literature review by study types, methods, tools, outputs and impacts. The quality appraisal uses traditional methods of critical appraisal for validity (internal and external), reliability, generalizability and relevance of the research methods, tools and measurements. We also classified a paper as having addressed "fitness for purpose" if it a) defined a purpose for the project or dataset and b) assessed whether the data or dataset was fit for the specified purpose.

AR appraised all 52 papers using our extraction template based on the realist "context-mechanism-impacts/outcomes" approach (Figure 1). The literature was analysed by study types, methods, tools, outputs and impacts in terms of: requirements analysis, design and tools development, implementation, deployment and testing, evaluation (descriptive evaluation, comparative and/or contemporary control). The summarised appraisals were then distributed among all co-authors (TL, PR, JT and HY) to discuss and achieve final consensus and synthesis of the findings.

*Figure 1. Specific template to analytical review of papers*

**Template: Systematic review of ontological approaches to creating patient registers and assessing their quality**

**Research questions:**

1. How data quality is being conceptualized within the "fitness for use" definition for a range of uses?
2. What specification methodologies are being used to specify data quality for implementation?
3. What ontology-specified implementation are being used and how they compare with other methods?
4. How the impact of implementing ontology-based specifications for data quality in chronic disease management is being measured and evaluated?

| | Author / title / reference | Study type[1] | Context & Population studied | Aims of project being reported on | Details of terminology, DQ models & ontology | Methods / Tools used in project | Results / Outputs of project | Critical Appraisal: 1. quality[2] of methods & tools 2. relevance to review questions |
|---|---|---|---|---|---|---|---|---|
| 1 | | | | | | | | |

[1] This classification of study types has been developed to cover the pattern of R&D in this multidisciplinary field. There are 5 types broadly based on the stage in the development lifecycle:

1. Requirements analysis e.g. literature reviews, qualitative research, etc
2. Design and tools development: data/information models and ontologies
3. Implementation, deployment and testing of information systems
4. Evaluation: descriptive evaluation
5. Evaluation: comparative (e.g. pre and post, time series, etc) with/without contemporary control (e.g. RCT)

This matrix (study types X current column headings) will focus the analysis and synthesis of the literature review e.g. by study types, methods, tools, outputs and impacts.

[2] The quality appraisal will include traditional methods of critical appraisal: validity (internal and external), reliability, generalizability, relevance, etc of the research methods, tools and measurements

## RESULTS

Both medical and computer sciences online databases were searched: MEDLINE (67 papers), the Cochrane Library (18 papers), ISI Web of Knowledge (35 papers), Science Direct (75 papers), Scopus (76 papers), IEEE Xplore (25 papers) and Springer (19 papers). Table 1 summarised the source of the 315 papers found.

In the first iteration, searches using a combination of keywords and controlled vocabulary term searches (specifically in Titles and Subjects fields of all papers) were conducted. The application of Titles and Subjects fields in a user's search strategy and search limitation in each database has been shown to increase relevance, precision and recall (McJunkin, 1995). We screened 315 papers, excluded 36 duplicates, 182 on abstract review and a 46 on full-text review; leaving 52 papers for critical appraisal. Of these 6 papers conceptualized data quality within the fitness for purpose definition for a range of uses, 16 used a defined process to specify data quality for implementation, 2 papers used the ontology-specified implementation in DQ improvement compare with other non-ontological approaches, and 28 demonstrated how the impact of implementing ontology-based specifications for data quality in chronic disease management is being measured and evaluated.

Table 1 showed 85 papers (26.98%) in the medicine and health domains and 44 papers (13.97%) in computer and IT sciences domains; 186 papers (59.05%) were multi-disciplinary which is by far the most prevalent. This reflects the multidisciplinary nature of the research.

Figure 2 shows how other eligible papers were included in the second iteration using hand-searching process. The references were retrieved from the papers included in the first iteration.

*Table 1. Online databases and the relevant papers*

| Database | Subjects | Field | Document Type | # Papers |
|---|---|---|---|---|
| Pubmed | Medicine, Health Science, Medical Informatics and Bioinformatics | Title, Mesh and Abstract | Journal articles and Proceeding | 67 |
| Cochrane Central Databases | Medicine and Health Science | Title, Mesh and Abstract | Journal articles | 18 |
| ISI Web of Sciences | Computer Science, Information Technology, Medical Informatics, Bioinformatics and Health Science | Title, Subject and Abstract | Journal articles | 35 |
| ScienceDirect | Computer Science, Medical Informatics, Engineering, Decision Science, Engineering, Mathematics, Psychology, Social Sciences, and Medicine | All fields | Journal articles | 75 |
| Scopus | Computer Science, Health Science, Medical Informatics, Bioinformatics, Information Technology, Psychology, Social and Behavioural Sciences | Al fields | Journal articles | 76 |
| IEEE Xplore | Computing and Processing, Medical Informatics, Bioinformatics, Communication Networking and Cybernetics | Title, Subject and Abstract | Journal articles | 25 |
| SpringerLink | Computer Science, Medical Informatics, Bioinformatics, information science and Engineering | Title, Subject and Abstract | Journal articles | 19 |
| Total | | | | 315 |

*Figure 2. Selection process*

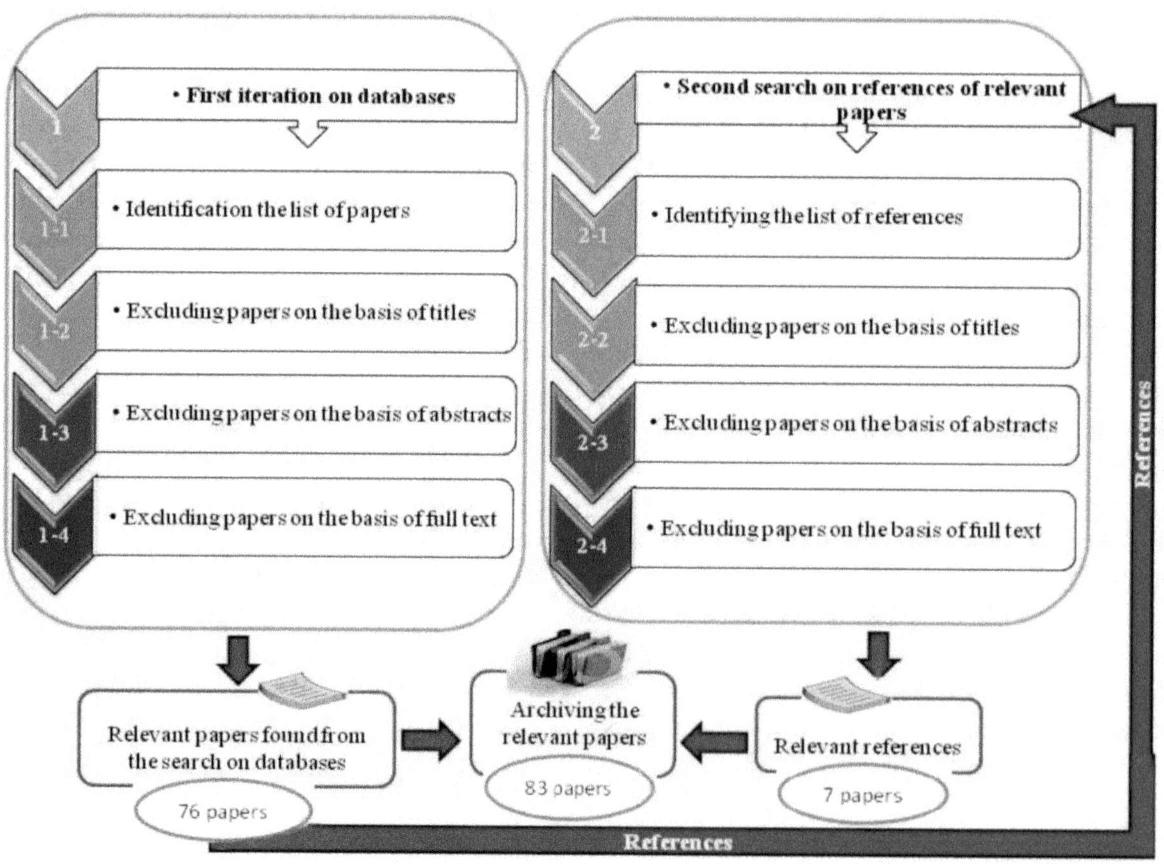

The keywords of references that matched with the search keywords were chosen. Based on their title, keywords, abstract and full text, 7 papers were included from the hand-searching.

It can be seen from the data in Table 2 that most of the papers (54%) show the various roles and impacts of ontology based approaches in CDM and how those approaches can be evaluated.

Table 3 presents the analysis of papers by study type and how they contributed to the review questions. The majority (83%) of studies involved design and tools development; 38% implemented/deployed and tested implementations; and 20% conducted a descriptive evaluation. A considerable number of studies (42 papers) demonstrate that the ontological approach was used to address semantic interoperability, data linkage, data integration, remote patient monitoring and reduce complexity of information models and networks. The majority of ontology-specified implementations in this category did not compare the performances and processes between ontology and non-ontology approaches. There were few attempts to conceptualize data quality based on "fitness for purpose" definition in a range of uses and purposes.

Figure 3 shows an increase in papers addressing ontologies for CDM and DQ from 2001, accelerating from 2005.

Figure 4 shows an increase in papers on ontology in CDM and DQ from 2006. There is an increase in studies reporting on the use of "fitness for purpose" when dealing with data quality from 2010 (probably stared with the small spike in 2007). This suggests that researchers may be

*Table 2. Distribution of papers by contribution review questions (Total papers >52 because each paper may be classified as two or more study types, or may address two or more review questions)*

| Research Questions | Number | % |
|---|---|---|
| 1. How is data quality being conceptualized within the "fitness for purpose" definition for a range of uses? | 6 | 12% |
| 2. What specification methodologies are being used to specify data quality for implementation? | 16 | 31% |
| 3. What ontology-specified implementations are being used and how do they compare with other methods? | 2 | 4% |
| 4. How is the impact of implementing ontology-based specifications for data quality in chronic disease management being measured and evaluated? | 28 | 54% |

*Table 3. Distribution of papers by study types and research questions*

| Study Type | Study Type | | Review Questions | | | | | | | |
|---|---|---|---|---|---|---|---|---|---|---|
| | | | Q1 | | Q2 | | Q3 | | Q4 | |
| | n | % | n | % | n | % | n | % | n | % |
| 1. Formal Requirements Analysis e.g. literature reviews, qualitative research. | 29 | 34% | 4 | 5% | 10 | 12% | 9 | 11% | 36 | 43% |
| 2. Design & tools development: including data/information models & ontologies. | 69 | 83% | 4 | 5% | 4 | 5% | 13 | 15.5% | 41 | 49% |
| 3. Implementation, deployment and testing of information systems. | 32 | 38% | 2 | 2.5% | 3 | 3.5% | 5 | 6% | 22 | 26.5% |
| 4. Evaluation: descriptive evaluation of DQ or ontology in health area. | 17 | 20% | 1 | 1% | 2 | 2.5% | 2 | 2.5% | 12 | 14.5% |
| 5. Evaluation: comparative +/- contemporary control (e.g. RCT). | 2 | 2.5% | 0 | 0 | 0 | 0 | 1 | 1% | 1 | 1% |

*Figure 3. The year distribution of studies in general*

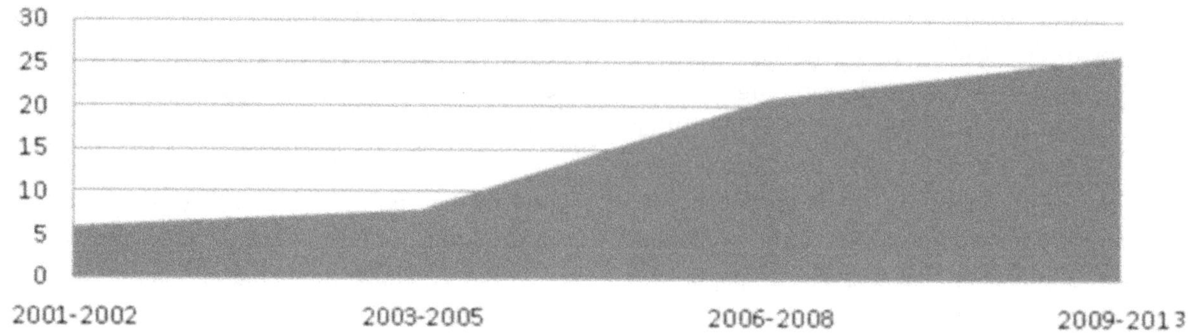


*Figure 4.The year distribution of the papers related to each category*

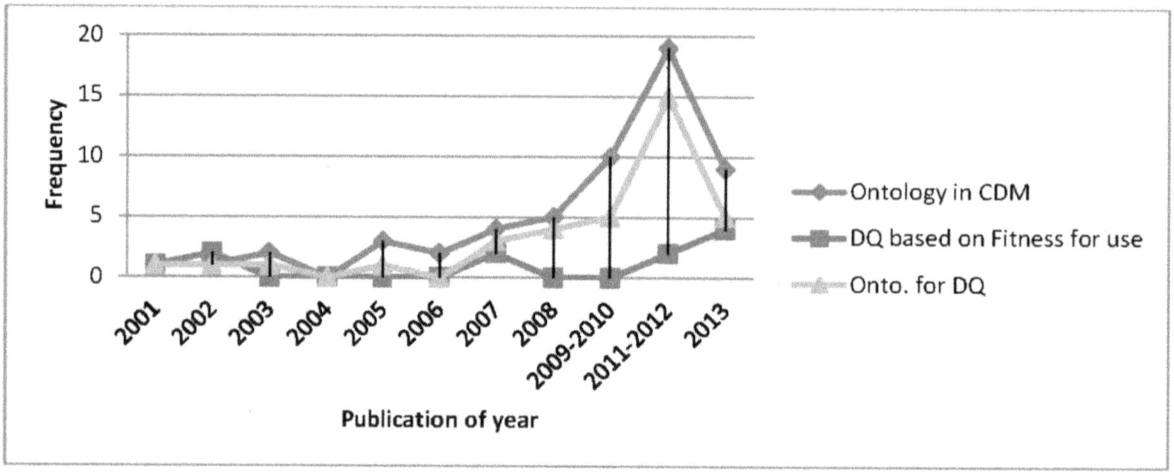


starting to take a more realistic approach to the quality of "big data": the intrinsic data quality is important but it does not need to be prefect to be "fit for purpose".

The Figure 5 gives a breakdown of the frequency of the studies conducted in different continents 2006 based on the setting of the studies. Europe is the most profile with 42.6% of the authors affiliated with European universities and institutions. North America is next with 21.3% of the studies followed by Oceania (18%), Asia (13.1%), South America (3.3%) and Africa with 1.7%. Although a paper being affiliated to a particular university in a country does not necessarily mean that the context under study has been in the same country or even continent, it might provide insights to a limited extent. For example, data quality research and ontological frameworks proposed seem to be much higher in the European countries. That might be because of a greater concern with DQ and/or ontologies in Europe. North America, Oceania and Asia stand in the second, third and fourth spot after Europe in terms of the number of studies that have been conducted. South America and Africa have a relatively lower rate of papers than the other continents, which is consistent with the general trends. The distribution of papers by continent might suggest that the topic has grabbed the attention of academics as well as health professionals as a major concern for patients registers.

The drivers of ontological approaches for DQ and/or CDM include better software for: (1)

*Figure 5. Distribution of papers found by continent*

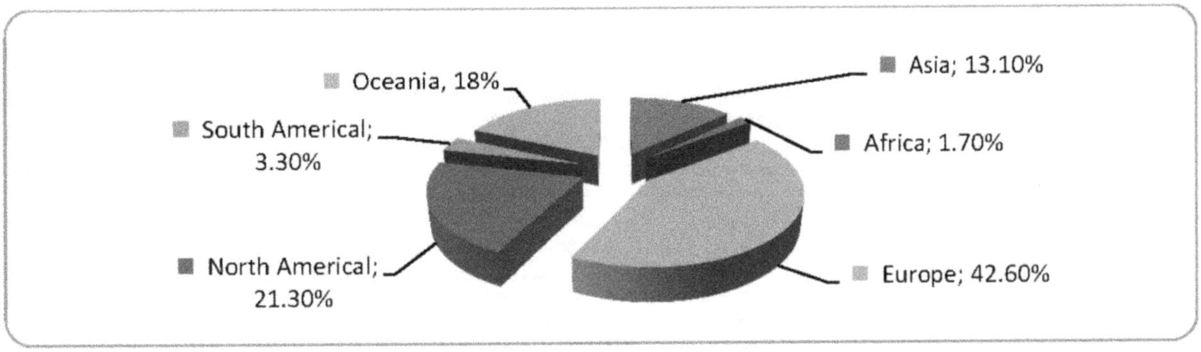


quality of care and/or health care issues and (2) the description, assessment and management of DQ in health (e.g. role of clinical guidelines in DQ, effects of quality of information in CISs and networking, defining and describing various attributes of DQ) as well as individual dimensions of DQ (e.g. accuracy, completeness, correctness, and consistency).

## Conceptualization of Data Quality within the "Fitness for Purpose" Paradigm

Table 4 shows a few studies have conceptualized and implemented data quality based on the "fitness for purpose" definition in their data models for a range of uses in health and non-health areas including improved searches for spatial data resources, including in languages other than English (Ivanova, et al., 2013), support expert users in the assessment of the fitness for purpose of a given dataset (Devillers, et al., 2007), better decision making (F. H. Chen, 2009), support analyses in comparative effectiveness research (M. G. Kahn, Batson, & Schilling, 2012), support agentd to choose how much information to gather (F. H. Chen, 2009), and for research and clinical purposes (S. Liaw, et al., 2011).

Many studies regularly report a range of deficiencies in the collected information for professionals requirements (Devillers, et al., 2007; B. K. Kahn, et al., 2002), clinical (Azaouagh & Stausberg, 2008; de Lusignan, et al., 2010; Mitchell & Westerduin, 2008; Moro & Morsillo, 2004) and health promotion (Gillies, 2000b) purposes. Similar deficiencies exist with information data in geographic (Devillers, et al., 2007; Ivanova, et al., 2013), hospital and general practice information systems (ST Liaw, et al., 2011), where the lack of coding rules meant that much of the data are often incomplete or in relatively inaccessible text format. The evidence is more encouraging for data for administrative purposes (Lain, et al., 2008; Quan, et al., 2008). Hybrid record keeping systems in primary care are believed to be more complete than computer-only or paper-only systems (Hamilton, et al., 2003).

## Methodologies to Specify Data Quality for Implementation

Table 5 shows that the majority of studies (81%) reported the design and development of tools to specify data quality for implementation; requirements analysis e.g. literature reviews and qualitative research methodologies (75%); system implementation, deployment and testing of information systems (25%), and descriptive evaluation (12%). There were no outcomes or comparative evaluation of the methodologies used.

Various qualitative methods such as interview and reports analysis, usually interpreted using

*Table 4. Data quality conceptualized within fitness for purpose*

| Author Reference | Context | Aims of Project | Methods/Tools Used in Project | Results |
|---|---|---|---|---|
| (Ivanova, et al., 2013) | Geo-spatial datasets in the national geo-information repositories in Netherlands | To suggest a system for guided search for spatial data resources called GUESS | • Use of popular search engines like OpenSearch to help in assessing fitness for purpose.<br>• Use metadata (information that helps users to assess the usefulness of a dataset relative to their problem) as a tool to evaluate fitness for purpose of datasets.<br>• Their approach is based on a 3-part data model (user profile, spatial data profiles and interaction profiles).<br>• Theoretical discussion on accuracy and completeness of data. | Defined fitness for purpose of data based on users (experts and non-experts in geo-informatics) satisfaction from search results<br>Allowed users without specific expertise to conduct free form search requests in their own language |
| (Devillers, et al., 2007) | Spatial On-Line Analytical Processing (SOLAP) as a GIS data repository | To manage heterogeneous data quality and provide functions to support expert users in the assessment of the fitness for purpose of a given dataset | • Use the Quality Information Management Model = QIMM.<br>• Focus on intrinsic data quality indicators such as completeness, correctness and accuracy underpins a prototype.<br>• Apply data quality analysis tool which is the Multidimensional User Manual (MUM) prototype.<br>• Validate the QUMM of through demonstrations of the prototype to different users (GIS scientists, specialists in data quality issues, consultants in GIS, data producers, governmental agencies, typical GIS users, etc.). | Defined fitness for purpose as the closeness of the agreement between data characteristics and the explicit and/or implicit needs of a user for a given application in a given area<br>Researchers attempt to provide data quality indicators to help users determine a dataset's fitness for purpose and better assess the fitness of data based on quality indicators/ experts in GIS |
| (M. G. Kahn, et al., 2012) | Clinical dataset in US | To develop the efficacy of their data model in three large healthcare organizations | • Use a two-by-two conceptual model (PSP/IQ) for describing IQ.<br>• Focus on 8 dimensions of data quality (completeness, correctness, flexibility, etc.).<br>• Surveyed 45 professionals to determine which IQ dimensions belong in each quadrant of the model.<br>• Use case study method in 3 healthcare organizations that 75 people in each organization completed a 70-item questionnaire for assessing the quality of their patients information on the IQ dimensions. | This is a well-grounded, logical approach and a case study to indicate health organizations need to use "fitness of use" to determine IQ (specifically soundness, dependable, useful and usable information) for analytical purposes<br>This assessment of DQ provides a reasonable baseline for determining what improvements should be made in DQ based on fitness for purpose for analytical purposes |
| (F. H. Chen, 2009) | Infectious diseases dataset in US | To investigate the effect of 'quality' of information and 'amount' of information are used in the health behaviour | • Use mathematical modelling of infectious disease transmission, seeks to analyse how the amount of information about disease prevalence affects individuals' incentives.<br>• More focus on data timeliness.<br>• Use of mathematics software. | Demonstrated "fitness for purpose" of data for agents to choose how much information to gather from others (personal communication from an anonymous reviewer)<br>This is a theoretical paper using several mathematical models to show that information quality affects health behaviour i.e better information leads to better decision making |

*continued on following page*

*Table 4. Continued*

| Author Reference | Context | Aims of Project | Methods/Tools Used in Project | Results |
|---|---|---|---|---|
| (S. Liaw, et al., 2011) | An electronic Practice Based Research Network (ePBRN) with a data repository of routinely data from multiple EHRs | To develop a matrix for assessment and management the quality of data | Their methods include 3 phases: (1) requirements specification based on the conceptual framework, (2) design and establishment of the ePBRN, and (3) evaluation of the data quality and fitness for research. • Use Microsoft Structured Query Language (SQL) to manage the extracted data and SAS used for data cleansing and analysis. • Focus on correctness, completeness and consistency of clinical data. | They used a well-designed framework to describe the intrinsic DQ (correctness and consistency) and fitness for purpose (completeness) for research and clinical purposes This study raised the theoretical dependence of the SQL/SAS approach on the lack of a transparent and explicit data model, metadata and process within proprietary EHRs |
| (Hamilton, et al., 2003) | Eighteen general practices in the Exeter Primary Care Trust in UK | To compare computer-only record keeping to paper-only and hybrid systems | • Use case control study of cancer patients aged over 40 years. • Classify records as paper, computer, or hybrid, depending on which medium stored the clinical information from consultations by descriptive statistics. • Focus on completeness of data. | Define more completeness of data as a fitness for consolation in primary care Hybrid systems of primary care record keeping document higher numbers of consultations than computer-only or paper-only systems |

*Table 5. The following methodologies to specify data quality for implementation*

| Study Types / Reference | 1 | 2 | 3 | 4 | 5 | Summary and Results of Methodologies | Contexts |
|---|---|---|---|---|---|---|---|
| (Gillies, 2000a) | | √ | | | | Represent a tool to assist with continuous improvement of the use of information systems in general practice based on their requirements which is accurate information Shows how the model can be practically used to improving the use of coding (external consistency of data) and accurate information (data correctness) within a general practice in a systematic way | Health information |
| (M. G. Kahn, et al., 2012) | √ | √ | | | | This is a well-grounded, logical approach and a case study to indicate health organizations need sound, dependable, useful and usable information for analytical purposes. However, there is need to some details of their participants, sampling and why focus on only 16 dimensions of Information Quality (IQ). This approach could be applicable way for the assessment of DQ in CDM because such an assessment provides a reasonable baseline for determining what improvements should be made in DQ based on fitness for purpose for analytical purposes | Clinical data |
| (S. Liaw, et al., 2011) | √ | √ | √ | | | They used a well-designed framework to describe the intrinsic DQ (correctness and consistency) and fitness for purpose (completeness) for research and clinical purposes However, this study raised the theoretical dependence of the SQL/ SAS approach on the lack of a transparent and explicit data model, metadata and process within proprietary EHRs | Clinical data |
| (D. G. Arts, Bosman, de Jonge, Joore, & de Keizer, 2003) | √ | √ | | | | Their approach demonstrates that after physicians' training, completeness, correctness and adherence to data definitions increased in ICUs significantly | Clinical data |

*continued on following page*

*Table 5. Continued*

| Study Types / Reference | 1 | 2 | 3 | 4 | 5 | Summary and Results of Methodologies | Contexts |
|---|---|---|---|---|---|---|---|
| (D. G. Arts, De Keizer, & Scheffer, 2002) | √ | √ | | | | Demonstrate a list of procedures for high data quality assurance in medical registry based on causes of insufficient data quality | Health information |
| (D. Arts, de Keizer, Scheffer, & de Jonge, 2002) | √ | √ | √ | | | Show that the overall DQ of medical registries has good quality (focusing on accuracy and completeness) and also explain their positive results as compared with earlier reports from the literature.<br>However, they did not compare data quality before and after the implementation of procedures to improve the accuracy of data | Clinical data |
| (Stvilia, et al., 2009) | √ | √ | | | | Use a mixed methodology with multiple data sources: 1. The analysis of 150 Web pages and related web sites identified the major approaches the providers use to define their IQ criteria set: a. centrally defined, b. community constructed, and c. outsourced to third-party raters. 2. The researchers surveyed a convenience sample of 108 healthcare information consumers to gain better insight into the health IQ evaluation behaviour of consumers. 3. Semi structured in-depth interviews with a sample of 20 survey participants<br>Results show that consumers may lack the motivation or literacy skills to evaluate the information quality of health | Health web pages |
| (B. K. Kahn, et al., 2002) | √ | | | | | Developing a two-by-two conceptual model for describing IQ (PSP/IQ)<br>Mapping the 16 IQ dimensions into their model<br>Provide a reasonable baseline for determining what improvements should be made in DQ (soundness, dependable useful and usable information) based on fitness for purpose for professionals analytical purposes. | Health information |
| (Britt, et al., 2007) | √ | √ | | | | Use statistical methods to manage data quality using SAS as a computer program in statistical package<br>Measure representativeness, reliability, validity and accuracy of BEACH data e.g. Reliability of coding of reasons for encounters and issues validity of ICPC to categorizing data. Accuracy of problem labels recorded by GPs (About 1000 GPs participate yearly) | Clinical data |
| (F. H. Chen, 2009) | √ | √ | | | | Focus on a full mathematical analysis (mathematical software)<br>Investigate the effect of quality of information and amount of information are used interchangeably in the health behaviour e.g. decision making | Infectious diseases |
| (Choquet, et al., 2010) | | √ | | | | Use Talend Open Studio open source software as well as developed stored procedures in SQL for the object quality criteria<br>Propose methods and measures to assess data quality (focus on data accuracy)<br>Propose 3 dimensions to classify the quality measures proposed (objects, concepts, and terms) as vertexes of their model Information Quality Triangle=IQT)<br>Measure the distance between standardized information models and reference terminologies against its CIS<br>Present that controlled vocabularies are a necessity to share data | Hospital dataset |

*continued on following page*

*Table 5. Continued*

| Study Types / Reference | 1 | 2 | 3 | 4 | 5 | Summary and Results of Methodologies | Contexts |
|---|---|---|---|---|---|---|---|
| (Cunningham-Myrie, Reid, & Forrester, 2008) | | | | √ | | Use ICD-10 for coding various collected data and to facilitate comparability of standardized data<br>Use Two broad categories of information were sought: a) epidemiological data and b) health service utilization data<br>Show that data management systems in hospitals were not linked to facilitate generation of cost-effectiveness estimates and other information required to compare options for health investment<br>Show methodological way for improvement health information quality for the economic analysis | Health information |
| (Huaman, et al., 2009) | √ | √ | | | | Timeliness and data quality were assessed by calculating the percentage of reports sent on time and percentage of errors per total number of reports, respectively<br>Use training program: 12 week prospective study with training program for reporting personnel.<br>Randomised selection to phone, visit or control for their supervisions<br>The training improved report timeliness but did not have such impact on data quality. | Infectious disease surveillance |
| (Kiragga, et al., 2011) | √ | √ | √ | | | Use the Research Cohort database as the reference "gold standard" for the assessment of data accuracy<br>Use statistical test e.g.: Categorical variables were compared using Chi-square test, the Mann-Whitney test was used for the continuous variables<br>Compare 2 databases, one from a clinic and one from a research team to assess the quality of data (completeness and accuracy)<br>Their findings have important implications for the use and interpretation of data derived from routine HIV observational databases for research and audit, and they highlight the need for ongoing regular validation of key data items in these databases | Infectious diseases |
| (Lima, Novais, Costa, Cruz, & Neves, 2010) | | √ | √ | | | Use a decision support example around a hypothetical patient called John who experiences an exacerbation of his COPD<br>Use the Clinical Guideline for COPD that there are 16 criteria that suggest the patient should be admitted and the model takes into account answers to each criterion<br>Present a model for the prediction and evaluation of quality of information to a multi criteria decision making process<br>Model describes a decision support tool for use in the management of COPD | Clinical Guidelines (CG) for COPD |

1. Requirements analysis e.g. literature reviews, qualitative research, etc.
2. Design and tools development: data/information models and ontologies.
3. Implementation, deployment and testing of information systems.
4. **Evaluation:** Descriptive evaluation.
5. **Evaluation:** Comparative (e.g. pre and post, time series, etc) with/without contemporary control (e.g. RCT).

grounded theory have been implemented to evaluate Usability (K. Kerr, T. Norris, & R. Stockdale, 2007), privacy (Stvilia, Mon, & Yi, 2009), comparability (K. Kerr, et al., 2007) and relevance (K. Kerr, et al., 2007). Consistency (W. L. Chen, Zhang, Gao, & Ieee Computer, 2009) of data has been assessed with concept mapping in non-health contexts. Timeliness (currency) (Huaman et al., 2009; K. Kerr, et al., 2007), accuracy (precision) (Stvilia, et al., 2009), reliability (Britt, Miller, & Bayrarn, 2007), representativeness (Britt, et al., 2007), correctness (Gillies, 2000a) and completeness (Kiragga, Castelnuovo, Schaefer, Muwonge, & Easterbrook, 2011) were assessed with quantitative statistical methods.

## Ontology-Specified Implementation to Develop Data Quality and Compare with Other Models

Table 6 shows two papers found that used ontological and non-ontological approaches to DQ in clinical information systems (CIS). Both papers suggested that ontology-based models had more advantages than other data models in the health domain. For example, Mabotuana and Warren (2009) showed the ontology driven approach to determining patients who needed a follow-up in hypertension management provided more advantages than SQL. They listed the limitations of the traditional SQL-based approach as i) lack of abstract, domain-level query support; ii) lack of the notion of a hierarchy and iii) nature of temporal SQL queries (Mabotuwana & Warren, 2009). They used SWRL rules which allow user to write rules to reason about individuals and to infer new knowledge about these individuals. The ontology based approach was sufficiently flexible to enable new audit criteria to be easily added as required, easy visualization of the knowledge base and standardized ways of querying the knowledge based. However, the paper was not explicit about whether was a formal outcome-based comparison of ontological and non-ontological approaches.

Maragoudakis and others (2008) develop an ontology with 5 domains for a clinical Decision Support System (CDSS) for management of Chronic Obstruction Pulmonary Disease (COPD). The ontology, based on hierarchical Bayesian networks, encoded a domain (COPD) and compared the predictive accuracy of this ontology-based hierarchical Bayesian network method with linear programming and artificial neural network methods (Maragoudakis, Lymberopoulos, Fakotakis, Spiropoulos, & Ieee, 2008).

By using 10-fold cross validation and precision and recall metrics, they concluded that the Hierarchical Bayesian method is comparable to Artificial Neural Network (ANN) and far more accurate than linear programming approaches. In addition, their ontology can be easily updated with new elements, while using ANN to do this would be a painstaking laborious process. The most important advantage of such an approach, however, is the ability to shift this model to other domains, incorporating new mobile network appliances - such as GPS - and new hospitals and other health institutes, in an attempt to effectively monitor a patient in different locations.

*Table 6. The comparative studies between the implemented ontologies and other data models*

| References | Research Findings | Results of Ontology Implemented for Data Quality | Compare with Non-Ontology | Context |
|---|---|---|---|---|
| (Maragoudakis, et al., 2008) | A tool in hierarchical Bayesian networks which can encode a domain and make prediction | Data mining classification No DQ | By using precision and recall metrics, show ontology approach is more accurate than Linear Programming in the monitoring of patients | COPD |
| (Mabotuwana & Warren, 2009) | Enhance and facilitate temporal querying requirements in general practice medicine | Facilitate temporal querying requirements | Represent only some limitations of traditional SQL-based approach to show flexibility of ontology in easily add any requirement in ontology queries. | CVD (hypertension) |

## The Impact of Ontologies for Data Quality in CDM and Their Evaluation

As Table 7 shows, a large number of studies have been published on the application of ontologies in both health and non-health areas. However, none compared ontologies with other non-ontological or data model approaches. Studies to demonstrate the impact of ontology-based implementations included clinical decision support systems (Brüggemann & Grüning, 2009; Min et al., 2009; Topalis et al., 2011) for information management (O'Donoghue, Herbert, O'Reilly, & Sammon, 2009; Young et al., 2009), diagnosis (Nimmagadda, Nimmagadda, Dreher, & Ieee, 2008), clinical data analysis and management (H. C. Li & Ko, 2007),. A few studies examined ontology-based approaches to support data consistency (Esposito, 2008a) and accuracy. However, we found no reports on any systematic and comprehensive ontological approaches to DQ issues or evaluation in the various contexts.

The application of ontological approaches to data quality management addressed the following issues: data quality problems and errors (Brüggemann & Grüning, 2009), data heterogeneity problem (Min, et al., 2009), semantic decision making (Lee, et al., 2009), efficient services (H. C. Li & Ko, 2007), procedures concerning the acquisition of data (Nimmagadda, et al., 2008), classification and identification of specific patients types (Lee, et al., 2009; Wang, Lee, Li, & Ko, 2007), data collection, data sharing and data integration (Min, et al., 2009; O'Donoghue, et al., 2009; Perez-Rey, et al., 2006; Young, et al., 2009). There were no studies that examined efficiency or effectiveness of ontology-based models in DQ management.

As Table 8 shows, there are less publications on the use of domain ontologies for the assessment of data quality in the querying requirements (Mabotuwana & Warren, 2009), extracting knowledge from natural language documents (Valencia-Garcia, Fernandez-Breis, Ruiz-Martinez, Garcia-Sanchez, & Martinez-Bejar, 2008), and data expression (Preece, Missier, Ernbury, Jin, & Greenwood, 2008). The majority of these studies used precision and recall as metrics to assess the accuracy and validate the ontological approaches (Brank, Grobelnik, & D., 2005; Brewster, Alani, Dasmahapatra, & Wilks, 2004; Euzenat, 2007; Gangemi, Catenacci, Ciaramita, & Lehmann, 2006; Z. Li, 2010; Min, et al., 2009; Pathak, Kiefer, Bielinski, & Chute, 2012; Pathak, Kiefer, & Chute, 2012; Spasic & Ananiadou, 2005; Stvilia, et al., 2009; Valencia-Garcia, et al., 2008; Wang, et al., 2007).

Despite a growing body of literature on ontology-based approaches in assessing the accuracy of the retrieval of clinical data, none of them have attempted to compare the performance between ontology-based and other (non-ontological) approaches. Most studies have used precision and sensitivity (recall) to assess the accuracy of ontology-based approaches in health domains (Brewster, et al., 2004; Euzenat, 2007; Gangemi, et al., 2006; McGarry, Garfield, & Wermter, 2007; Min, et al., 2009; Pathak, Kiefer, Bielinski, et al., 2012; Pathak, Kiefer, & Chute, 2012; Spasic & Ananiadou, 2005; Stvilia, et al., 2009; Valencia-Garcia, et al., 2008; Wang, et al., 2007).

Table 9 illustrates various definitions to identify the most common criteria to assess validity of ontologies and data models. Studies have attempted to define criteria such as Flexibility, Reusability, Cohesiveness, Precision, and Recall. However, there are less coordinated attempts to define other criteria such as Scalability, Completeness, Correctness, Extensibility, and Adaptability.

There are overlaps in the definition of criteria such as Flexibility, Scalability, Completeness, Correctness, Extensibility, and Adaptability in both ontological and non-ontological approaches. There were no guidance on the definition and scope of Reusability, Cohesiveness, Precision, and Recall in the data model approaches in the literature. Standardising these metrics can help to standardise the specification of ontologies and data models. This can then standardise the comparison of ontology and non-ontology approaches.

*Table 7. The impact of implemented ontologies for the management of data quality in non-comparative studies*

| Ontology functions | References | Defined Purpose | Assessed of Fitness for Purpose using DQ and Findings | Context |
|---|---|---|---|---|
| **Management** *(9 papers)* | (H. C. Li & Ko, 2007) | To develop automated ontology approach to manage nutrients in a diabetes diet care knowledge management | • Used expert opinions to decide which are the important nutrients to include in the diabetes diet and therefore the ontology.<br>• This is face validity and consistency of the data.<br>• Authors suggested that there is a further step using ontology approach for more efficient diet knowledge management. | Diabetes diet care in Taiwan |
| | (Esposito, 2008a) | To detect abnormalities and malformations due to heart diseases | • Use as an ontology approach and rules to perform the instance and consistency checking and verifies that patient information violates the normal cardiovascular model loaded based on the SNOMED vocabulary.<br>• Theoretical discussion on data consistency.<br>• Researchers show applicability of ontology to define either the anatomy of the cardiovascular system in normal patients or the anatomy characterized by malformations or abnormalities in CHD patients to support cardiologist in the identification of diseases. | Congenital Heart Disease (CHD) dataset in Italy |
| | (Nimmagadda, et al., 2008) | To provide a solution to problems around handling increasing amounts of clinical information and solves some issues related to managing large | • Simulate human body disorders into metadata through ontology based data warehouse modeling.<br>• Theoretical discussion on managing accuracy and correctness of data.<br>• Authors states ontology can facilitate logic processes and semantics for data quality management and decision support for health care providers and clinicians. | Human body anatomy and pathology dataset in Australia |
| | (Min, et al., 2009) | To collect/retrieve information intelligently and address the semantic heterogeneity problem from the integration of data from multiple information resources | • Apply ontology mapped with medical thesaurus to integrate and retrieve the data from two independent database systems.<br>• Theoretical discussion about data consistency.<br>• Authors state that ontology can solve the semantic heterogeneity problem from the integration of two databases by recognition of inconsistence data. | 3000 records registered for the prostate cancer patients and Tumour Registry in US |
| | (Brüggemann & Grüning, 2009) | To improve the outcome of data quality management (DQM) | • Use an algorithm and data model for consistency checking, an algorithm for detecting duplicates and give three examples of DQM-specific metadata tasks (data provenance, data quality annotations at schema and instance level and an ontology for the DQM domain).<br>• Authors mentioned the usefulness of their ontology approach to define a shared vocabulary for improved interoperability, and performing DQM include consistency checking, data duplicate detecting and metadata management. | Cancer registries in Germany |

*continued on following page*

*Table 7. Continued*

| Ontology functions | References | Defined Purpose | Assessed of Fitness for Purpose using DQ and Findings | Context |
|---|---|---|---|---|
| | (Topalis, et al., 2011) | To retrieve data and information extraction | • Use ontology based model to integrate and capture the right terms (variables) and the relationships between such concepts in a disease map.<br>• Theoretical discussion about data accuracy in multiple information sources.<br>• Authors demonstrate the importance of capturing the right terms in ontologies to use both in the development of specific databases and, in the construction of decision support systems to control diseases for biologists, and epidemiologists. | Neurological disease, malaria, vector-borne diseases in Greece |
| | (Perez-Rey et al., 2006) | To develop a method and tool for database integration from remote sources | • Test the implemented ontology on eight different private databases with biomedical data stored in different database management packages such as MySQL, PointBase, Access, and others and provide integrated access to their data.<br>• Use case study to retrieve information in three sources using queries and theoretical discussion on data consistency.<br>• Authors believe that ontologies are the most suitable representation formalism for schemas in database integration system. | Public genomic and clinical databases in Spain |
| | (Lee et al., 2009) | To classify a person as a diabetic patient | • Represent new ontology methods for fuzzy medical relationship using taxonomical knowledge.<br>• Manage accuracy of data.<br>• Authors state that fuzzy ontology can effectively develop semantic decision making and reduce uncertainty (inaccurate data) to classify patients for medical staffs. | Diabetes domain in Taiwan |
| | (O'Donoghue, et al., 2009) | To demonstrate the data quality benefits of integrating remote patient monitoring solutions | • Use a Body Area Network (BAN) datasets within patient EHR solutions.<br>• Use Jade Content Ontology classes for their the Medical Knowledge Base agent.<br>• Use 2 experiments (with/without knowledge base) for effect on risk prediction accuracy.<br>• Focus on data accuracy and correctness.<br>• Authors states that ontology can improve patient management through the reduction of false alarm generations and facilitate the categorisation of the data to indicate risk categories for decision support. | Three patient types are identified 1) Non-Athletic Adult, 2) Athletic Adult and 3) Child from Ireland |

*Table 8. The impact of implemented ontologies for the assessment of data quality in non-comparative studies*

| Ontology functions | References | Defined Purpose | Assessed of Fitness for Purpose using DQ | Context |
|---|---|---|---|---|
| **Assessment** ***(7 papers)*** | (Christian Jacquelinet et al., 2003) | To develop semantic data interoperability | • Apply an ontological tool to develop semantic data interoperability through domain terminologies using quantitative analysis of the existing coding information system and a qualitative analysis checking completeness, consistency, ambiguity and implicitness of terms.<br>• Represent DQ factors such as completeness of data, appropriated terms, structured thesaurus, and terminology standard.<br>• Authors state usefulness of ontology based approach to support the processing of texts, and extending a terminological basis for medical experts. | Failure, dialysis and transplant datasets from National information system in France |
| | (Maragoudakis, et al., 2008) | To develop decision support system | • Use 25 patients records from various networking appliances such as mobile phones and wireless medical sensors to establish a ubiquitous environment for medical treatment of pulmonary diseases.<br>• Use ontology approach based on hierarchical Bayesian networks which can encode a domain and make prediction.<br>• Focus on data timeliness.<br>• Authors states the importance of ontology based model as an ubiquitous platform to improve patient monitoring and health services in real time treatment decision. | Mobile sensor data from 25 patients in Artificial Neural Network (ANN) in GREECE |
| | (Wang, et al., 2007) | To classify diabetic patients | • Use measuring precision and recall of results to show accuracy of clinical data achieved from an ontology-based fuzzy inference agent, including a fuzzy inference engine, and a fuzzy rule base, for diabetes classification<br>• Authors state that ontology approach can classify effectively classify a person as a diabetic patient for medical staff | Retrieve 392 cases from the Pima Indians diabetes database in US |
| | (Valencia-Garcia, et al., 2008) | To develop retrieval and extract clinical information | • Represent multiple semantic relationships among concepts with UMLS ancestors through MESH descriptors in the ontology to enrich the ontology extracted from the text.<br>• Use an experiment (4 PhD students were asked to use the system with a Spanish corpus) to analyse a software tool by measuring precision and recall of the result (accuracy of data).<br>• Solve semantic clinical data issues and develop accuracy of retrieval information through ontologies. | Use breast cancer domain in the system with a Spanish corpus of 8649 words in Spain |
| | (Mabotuwana & Warren, 2009) | To identify hypertensive patients database in the context of quality use of medicines in the management | • Use the querying capabilities of one GP database in the context of quality use of medications in the management of hypertension over time.<br>• Use 8 criteria and 4 scenarios to identify hypertensive patients.<br>• Focus on semantic interoperability and also data completeness and timeliness, consistency.<br>• Authors show the importance of ontology based approach to enhance temporal querying requirements and identify patient data, semantically. | CVD in practice management system in NZ |

*continued on following page*

Table 8. Continued

| Ontology functions | References | Defined Purpose | Assessed of Fitness for Purpose using DQ | Context |
|---|---|---|---|---|
| | (Young, et al., 2009) | To develop semantic data collection and integration | • Use the modelling of terms to conform to and extend the existing ontologies development framework.<br>• Theoretical discussion on completeness of data, data availability and accessibility.<br>• Authors state that ontology help to extract, query, integrate and federate data for clinical researcher. | Data on Autism in the National Database for Autism Research in US |
| | (Preece, et al., 2008) | To manage information quality (IQ) in a real-life example of gene expression research | • Implication of viewing high IQ as 'fitness for purpose' for providers and consumers, in which users state their quality requirements in terms of domain concepts (such as accuracy, currency and completeness).<br>• Guide the development and use of metrics to measure the complexity and cohesion of ontologies.<br>• Authors state that ontology helps to allow a practical division of the work between providers and consumers, in order to minimize the costs to all concerned. | Gene expression data which involve the use of microarrays in UK |

## DISCUSSION

1. *How is data quality being conceptualized within the "fitness for purpose" definition for a range of uses?* We found few papers on DQ used within the definition of fitness for purpose. There are more studies on the ontologies for management of DQ (26 papers) and assessment of DQ in all contexts (11 papers). These findings support the current perception of DQ as a complex concept with many dimensions, often overlapping conceptually (Wand & Wang, 1996). Liaw and others (2010) developed a conceptual framework for DQ that include intrinsic DQ (correctness and consistency) of data elements and fitness for purpose (completeness) of data set for research and clinical purpose.
2. *What specification methodologies are being used to specify data quality for implementation?* The literature on the specification of data quality for implementation is fragmentary and there is not a comprehensive approach. The findings of the current study are consistent with our previous review (S. T. Liaw, et al., 2013) that the ontological approach to develop DQ is poorly evaluated. However, most agreed that DQ is a multidimensional construct (Devillers, et al., 2007; Nimmagadda, et al., 2008); with completeness, accuracy, correctness, consistency and timeliness being the most commonly used dimensions. A few studies examined ontology-based approaches to support data consistency and accuracy. However, no research was found that formally and systematically assessed the association between ontologies for DQ and fitness for purpose in various contexts.
3. *What ontology-specified implementations are being used and how do they compare with other methods?* There were few comparative and evaluative studies on assessment of data quality or compared ontological and

*Table 9. Definition for metrics to evaluate ontology and data model*

| Criteria | Definitions for Ontology Evaluation | References | Definitions for Traditional Data Model evaluation | References |
|---|---|---|---|---|
| **Flexibility** | An ontology that can be easily adapted to multiple views in terms of some parameters such as modularity, partitioning, context-boundedness | (Gangemi, et al., 2006) | Does the data model deal with changes in business and/or regulatory change? | (Moody & Shanks, 2003) |
| | Ability of ontology to accept input of new data from various research groups and disciplines | (Gilbert & Ddembe, 2008) | Can new data elements and relationships be added if project scope or if regulatory rules (eg, patient identification) change? | (M. G. Kahn, et al., 2012) |
| | the user can easily re-define the extraction procedure logics and adapt it to his needs | (Pannarale et al., 2012) | Some criteria to evaluate the flexibility of data models include "extensibility", "scalability" and "adaptability". | (M. G. Kahn, et al., 2012) |
| | allows to easily manage the changes of the database schema or of the ontology | (Pannarale, et al., 2012) | | |
| **Reusability** | Ability of ontology to integrate data useful to different users and disciplines | (Gilbert & Ddembe, 2008) | | |
| | Ontology can match user requirements across different disciplines | (Pinto, 2004) | | |
| **Scalability** | | | Can data model be sized in smaller or larger data sets? | (M. G. Kahn, et al., 2012) |
| **Completeness** | | | Does the data model contain all user requirements? | (Moody & Shanks, 2003) |
| | | | Can the data model store and retrieve data to meet investigator needs? | (M. G. Kahn, et al., 2012) |
| **Correctness** | | | Does the data model conform to the rules of the data modelling techniques? | (Moody & Shanks, 2003) |
| | | | Does the model conform to good data modelling practices such as limited data storage redundancy? | (M. G. Kahn, et al., 2012) |
| **Extensibility** | | | Ability of data model to expand data elements, data types and new data domains. | (M. G. Kahn, et al., 2012) |
| **Adaptability** | | | Ability of data model to model a broad data domain. | (M. G. Kahn, et al., 2012) |
| **Cohesiveness** | measure separation of responsibilities and independence of components of ontologies | (Yao, et al., 2005) | | |
| **Precision** | reflect the amount of knowledge correctly identified in the ontology with respect to the whole knowledge available in the ontology | (Brewster, et al., 2004) | | |

*continued on following page*

*Table 9. Continued*

| Criteria | Definitions for Ontology Evaluation | References | Definitions for Traditional Data Model evaluation | References |
|---|---|---|---|---|
| **Recall** | reflect the amount of knowledge correctly identified with respect to all the knowledge that it should identify | (Brewster, et al., 2004) | | |
| **Cohesiveness** | measure separation of responsibilities and independence of components of ontologies | (Yao, et al., 2005) | | |

non-ontological approaches to representing knowledge in clinical information systems. This literature review suggests that, compared to non-hierarchical data models, there may be more advantages and benefits in the use of ontologies to solve semantic clinical data quality issues and improve the validity and reliability of data retrieval, collection, storage, extraction and linkage algorithms and tools. Formal ontological approaches enable the systematic development of automated, valid and reliable methods to assess and manage the DQ and semantic interoperability issues (Lee, et al., 2009; Valencia-Garcia, et al., 2008; Verma et al., 2009; Verma, Kasabov, Rush, & Song, 2008). The expressiveness of ontology based models can facilitate accuracy and precision compared to non-ontology models and approaches (Esposito, 2008a, 2008b; Preece, et al., 2008).

Current ontological approaches have limited evaluation. There are little studies comparing to addressing chronic disease management and even less examining data quality. The challenges to the development and validation of an ontology-based model to the assessment and management of DQ include methodological immaturity, an immature knowledge base, and a lack of tools to support ontology-based design of information systems, evaluation of ontological approaches, and engagement of users in design and implementations. There are insufficient studies to define ontology evaluation metrics comprehensively and show practical techniques to evaluate ontological approaches in terms of flexibility, scalability and reusability versus non-ontology based models.

4. *How is the impact of implementing ontology-based specifications for data quality in chronic disease management being measured and evaluated?* Current evidence demonstrates there is a lack of valid and reliable data quality assurance (D. G. Arts, et al., 2003; D. G. Arts, et al., 2002) to ensure fitness for a range of uses by consumers, patients, health providers and professionals. This study has added to our understanding of ontology-based approaches to improve the quality of the data so it is useful for the various purposes such as clinical research, teaching, audit and evaluation. (e.g. quality assurance and clinical decision making). This study found that, despite an increasing amount of papers on ontology of chronic diseases, there were little on ontological approaches for data quality based on the "fitness for purpose" specifically or in health generally. This gap needs to be addressed.

The main advantages of building ontologies for data quality in health are to automate the extraction of data from EHRs into clinical data warehouses;

assessment and management of the intrinsic and extrinsic quality of this "big data" so that they are fit for purposes such as research, quality improvement and health information exchange and sharing; management of controlled vocabularies and optimising semantic interoperability; curation of data for use by human users and applications such as electronic decision support systems; mining of data to discover relationships between the concepts; discovery of new knowledge; and reuse of knowledge in the management of chronic diseases (Abidi, 2011; Buranarach, Chalortham, Chatvorawit, Thein, & Supnithi, 2009; Gedzelman et al., 2005; Gupta, Ludäscher, Grethe, & Martone, 2003; Jara, Blaya, Zamora, Skarmeta, & Ieee, 2009).

## LIMITATION OF THE REVIEW

While we are confident that our search strategy was comprehensive and robust with use of synonyms and valid operators, there is always the possibility that we may not have identified all eligible studies. The major limitation was that we did not search the grey literature, an important source in this relatively immature field. However, there were also limitations of access to proprietary materials. The majority of studies involved design and tools development for data models and ontologies in health area and chronic diseases rather than implementation, deployment and evaluation of the relevant procedures. The trends are encouraging for ontological approaches. However, there are no formal large scale studies to systematically compare the quality of outputs of ontological to non-ontological approaches to the assessment and management of data quality and fitness for purpose of the implementations.

Also, the large number of studies which were used data quality in the health area made individual analysis of the measurement of accuracy of their results. The use of concepts search related to the ontology part to overcome the limitations of the choice of keyword search has been put forward as one of the motivations of the semantic web.

## CONCLUSION

The understanding of data quality, as a multidimensional concept applied to the data elements (intrinsic DQ) and the set of data elements (extrinsic DQ), is progressing. However, data quality needs to be contextual. Our review found that many studies on data quality either did not consider the purpose or intended use as part of the definition or considered it implicitly. This approach needs to be changed.

Ontological approaches are emerging and theoretically important to address the complex relationships among overlapping concepts in this complex area. This review has described the small but emerging published literature in this domain. As the field matures, it would be useful to systematically examine the strengths and weaknesses of the ontological approaches as compared to the more traditional data model approaches to examine "big data" from multiple EHRs. Ontology-based applications could support automated processes to address DQ and semantic interoperability in the large datasets.

## ACKNOWLEDGMENT

The authors would like to thank the reviewers for their thoughtful review and suggestions to extend our paper to make more explicit the relationship to health informatics.

## REFERENCES


Abidi, S. R. (2011). *Ontology-based knowledge modeling to provide decision support for comorbid diseases*. Paper presented at the 19th European Conference in Artificial Intelligence. Retrieved from http://www.scopus.com/inward/record.url?eid=2-s2.0-79952016090&partnerID=40&md5=d6e8e7441e3e9118fa395e5fc0b77b95

Arts, D., de Keizer, N., Scheffer, G. J., & de Jonge, E. (2002). Quality of data collected for severity of illness scores in the Dutch National Intensive Care Evaluation (NICE) registry. *Intensive Care Medicine*, *28*(5), 656–659. doi:10.1007/s00134-002-1272-z PMID:12029418

Arts, D. G., Bosman, R. J., de Jonge, E., Joore, J. C., & de Keizer, N. F. (2003). Training in data definitions improves quality of intensive care data. *Critical Care (London, England)*, *7*(2), 179–184. doi:10.1186/cc1886 PMID:12720565

Arts, D. G., De Keizer, N. F., & Scheffer, G. J. (2002). Defining and improving data quality in medical registries: a literature review, case study, and generic framework. *Journal of the American Medical Informatics Association*, *9*(6), 600–611. doi:10.1197/jamia.M1087 PMID:12386111

Azaouagh, A., & Stausberg, J. (2008). Frequency of hospital-acquired pneumonia--comparison between electronic and paper-based patient records. *Pneumologie (Stuttgart, Germany)*, *62*(5), 273–278. doi:10.1055/s-2008-1038099 PMID:18270924

Barchini, G., Álvarez, M., & Herrera, S. (2006). Sistemas de informaci6n: Nuevos escenarios basados en ontologías/information systems: New ontology-based scenarios. *Journal of Information Systems and Technology Management*, *3*(1), 2–18. doi:10.4301/S1807-17752006000100001

Brank, J., Grobelnik, M., & D., M. (2005). *A survey of ontology evaluation techniques*. Paper presented at the 8th Int. Multi-Conf. Information Society. New York, NY.

Brewster, C., Alani, H., Dasmahapatra, S., & Wilks, Y. (2004). *Data Driven Ontology Evaluation*. Paper presented at the International Conference on Language Resources and Evaluation. Retrieved from http://eprints.soton.ac.uk/259062/

Britt, H., Miller, G., & Bayrarn, C. (2007). The quality of data on general practice - A discussion of BEACH reliability and validity. *Australian Family Physician*, *36*(1-2), 36–40. PMID:17252082

Brüggemann, S., & Grüning, F. (2009). Using ontologies providing domain knowledge for data quality management. *Studies in Computational Intelligence*, *221*, 187–203. doi:10.1007/978-3-642-02184-8_13

Buranarach, M., Chalortham, N., Chatvorawit, P., Thein, Y., & Supnithi, T. (2009). *An Ontology-based Framework for Development of Clinical Reminder System to Support Chronic Disease Healthcare*. Retrieved from http://text.hlt.nectec.or.th/ontology/sites/default/files/reminder_is-bme09_cr_0.pdf

Chen, F. H. (2009). Modeling the effect of information quality on risk behavior change and the transmission of infectious diseases. *Mathematical Biosciences, 217*(2), 125–133. doi:10.1016/j.mbs.2008.11.005 PMID:19059272

Chen, W. L., Zhang, S. D., & Gao, X. (2009). *Anchoring the Consistency Dimension of Data Quality Using Ontology in Data Integration*. IEEE.

Choquet, R., Qouiyd, S., Ouagne, D., Pasche, E., Daniel, C., Boussaïd, O., et al. (2010). *The information quality triangle: A methodology to assess clinical information quality.* Paper presented at the 13th World Congress on Medical and Health Informatics, Medinfo 2010. Cape Town, South Africa.

Cunningham-Myrie, C., Reid, M., & Forrester, T. E. (2008). A comparative study of the quality and availability of health information used to facilitate cost burden analysis of diabetes and hypertension in the Caribbean. *The West Indian Medical Journal, 57*(4), 383–392. PMID:19566021

de Lusignan, S., Khunti, K., Belsey, J., Hattersley, A., van Vlymen, J., & Gallagher, H. et al. (2010). A method of identifying and correcting miscoding, misclassification and misdiagnosis in diabetes: a pilot and validation study of routinely collected data. *Diabetic Medicine, 27,* 203–209. doi:10.1111/j.1464-5491.2009.02917.x PMID:20546265

Devillers, R., Bedard, Y., Jeansoulin, R., & Moulin, B. (2007). Towards spatial data quality information analysis tools for experts assessing the fitness for use of spatial data. *International Journal of Geographical Information Science, 21*(3), 261–282. doi:10.1080/13658810600911879

Esposito, M. (2008a). Congenital Heart Disease: An ontology-based approach for the examination of the cardiovascular system. In I. Lovrek (Ed.), *Knowledge - Based Intelligent Information and Engineering Systems* (Vol. 5177, pp. 509–516). doi:10.1007/978-3-540-85563-7_65

Esposito, M. (2008b). *An ontological and non-monotonic rule-based approach to label medical images.* Los Alamitos, CA: IEEE Computer Soc.

Euzenat, J. (2007). *Semantic Precision and Recall for Ontology Alignment Evaluation.* Paper presented at the Twentieth International Joint Conference on Artificial Intelligence (IJCAI-07). New York, NY.

Gangemi, A., Catenacci, C., Ciaramita, M., & Lehmann, J. (2006). *Modelling ontology evaluation and validation.* Paper presented at the 3rd European Conference on the Semantic Web: Research and Applications. New York, NY.

Gedzelman, S., Simonet, M., Bernhard, D., Diallo, G., & Palmer, P. (2005). Building an ontology of cardio-vascular diseases for concept-based information retrieval. In *Proceedings of Computers in Cardiology 2005,* (Vol. 32, pp. 255-258). New York: IEEE.

Gilbert, M., & Ddembe, W. (2008). A Flexible Approach for User Evaluation of Biomedical Ontologies. *International Journal of Computing and ICT Research,* 2(2), 62–74.

Gillies, A. (2000a). Assessing and improving the quality of information for health evaluation and promotion. *Methods of Information in Medicine, 39*(3), 4. PMID:10992745

Gillies, A. (2000b). Assessing and improving the quality of information for health evaluation and promotion. *Methods of Information in Medicine, 39*(3), 208–212. PMID:10992745

Gupta, A., Ludäscher, B., Grethe, J. S., & Martone, M. E. (2003). Towards a formalization of disease-specific ontologies for neuroinformatics. *Neural Networks, 16*(9), 1277–1292. doi:10.1016/j.neunet.2003.07.008 PMID:14622884

Hadzic, M., & Chang, E. (2005, Dec 11 2005). *Ontology-based multi-agent systems support human disease study and control.* Paper presented at the International Conference on Self Organization and Adaptation of Multi-Agent and Grid Systems (SOAS). Glasgow, UK.

Hamilton, W. T., Round, A. P., Sharp, D., & Peters, T. J. (2003). The quality of record keeping in primary care: a comparison of computerised, paper and hybrid systems. *The British Journal of General Practice, 53*(497), 929–933, discussion 933. PMID:14960216

Huaman, M. A., Araujo-Castillo, R. V., Soto, G., Neyra, J. M., Quispe, J. A., & Fernandez, M. F. et al. (2009). Impact of two interventions on timeliness and data quality of an electronic disease surveillance system in a resource limited setting (Peru): a prospective evaluation. *BMC Medical Informatics and Decision Making*, 9. PMID:19183479

Ivanova, I., Morales, J., de By, R. A., Beshe, T. S., & Gebresilassie, M. A. (2013). Searching for spatial data resources by fitness for use. *Journal of Spatial Science, 58*(1), 15–28. doi:10.1080/14498596.2012.759087

Jacquelinet, C., Burgun, A., Delamarre, D., Strang, N., Boutin, B., & Le Beux, P. (2001). Building an ontology for end-stage diseases and organ failure in the context of transplantation and dialysis. In V. L. Patel, R. Rogers, & R. Haux (Eds.), *Medinfo 2001: Proceedings of the 10th World Congress on Medical Informatics, Pts 1 and 2* (Vol. 84, pp. 297-297). Amsterdam: I O S Press.

Jacquelinet, C., Burgun, A., Delamarre, D., Strang, N., Djabbour, S., Boutin, B., et al. (2003). Developing the ontological foundations of a terminological system for end-stage diseases, organ failure, dialysis and transplantation. *International Journal of Medical Informatics, 70*(2-3), 317-328. doi: 10.1016/S1386-5056(03)00046-7

Jara, A. J., Blaya, F. J., Zamora, M. A., & Skarmeta, A. F. G. (2009). *An Ontology and Rule Based Intelligent Information System to Detect and Predict Myocardial Diseases*. New York: IEEE.

Kahn, B. K., Strong, D. M., & Wang, R. Y. (2002). Information quality benchmarks: product and service performance. *Communications of the ACM, 45*(4), 8. doi:10.1145/505248.506007

Kahn, M. G., Batson, D., & Schilling, L. M. (2012). Data model considerations for clinical effectiveness researchers. *Medical Care, 50*(Suppl), S60–S67. doi:10.1097/MLR.0b013e318259bff4 PMID:22692260

Kerr, K., Norris, A., & Stockdale, R. (2007). *Data quality, information and decision making: A healthcare case study.* Paper presented at the 18th Australasian Conference on Information Systems. Toowoomba, Australia.

Kerr, K., Norris, T., & Stockdale, R. (2007). *Data Quality Information and Decision Making: A Healthcare Case Study*. Paper presented at the 18th Australasian Conference on Information Systems. New York, NY.

Kiragga, A. N., Castelnuovo, B., Schaefer, P., Muwonge, T., & Easterbrook, P. J. (2011). Quality of data collection in a large HIV observational clinic database in sub-Saharan Africa: Implications for clinical research and audit of care. *Journal of the International AIDS Society*, *14*(1). doi:10.1186/1758-2652-14-3 PMID:21251327

Lain, S. J., Roberts, C. L., Hadfield, R. M., Bell, J. C., & Morris, J. M. (2008). How accurate is the reporting of obstetric haemorrhage in hospital discharge data? A validation study. *Australian and New Zealand Journal of Obstetrics and Gynaecology*, *48*(5), 481–484. doi:10.1111/j.1479-828X.2008.00910.x PMID:19032664

Lee, C. S., Wang, M. H., Acampora, G., Loia, V., & Hsu, C. Y. (2009). *Ontology-based Intelligent Fuzzy Agent for Diabetes Application*. New York: IEEE.

Li, H. C., & Ko, W. M. (2007). *Automated food ontology construction mechanism for diabetes diet care*. New York: IEEE. doi:10.1109/ICMLC.2007.4370653

Li, Z. (2010). *An ontology-driven concept-based information retrieveal approach for Web documents*. Edmonton, Canada: University of Alberta.

Liaw, S., Chen, H., Maneze, D., Taggart, J., Dennis, S., & Vagholkar, S. et al. (2011). Health reform: is current electronic information fit for purpose? *Emergency Medicine Australasia*. PMID:22313561

Liaw, S., Taggart, J., Dennis, S., & Yeo, A. (2011). *Data quality and fitness for purpose of routinely collected data – A general practice case study from an electronic Practice-Based Research Network (ePBRN)*. Paper presented at the AMIA 2011 Annual Symposium Improving Health: Informatics and IT Changing the World. New York, NY.

Liaw, S. T., Rahimi, A., Ray, P., Taggart, J., Dennis, S., & de Lusignan, S. et al. (2013). Towards an ontology for data quality in integrated chronic disease management: A realist review of the literature. *International Journal of Medical Informatics*, *82*(2), 139. doi:10.1016/j.ijmedinf.2012.12.007 PMID:23122633

Lima, L., Novais, P., Costa, R., Cruz, J., & Neves, J. (2010). Decision Making Based on Quality-of-Information a Clinical Guideline for Chronic Obstructive Pulmonary Disease Scenario. In A. de Leon F. de Carvalho, S. Rodríguez-González, J. De Paz Santana & J. Rodríguez (Eds.), Distributed Computing and Artificial Intelligence (Vol. 79, pp. 417-424). Springer.

Mabotuwana, T., & Warren, J. (2009). An ontology-based approach to enhance querying capabilities of general practice medicine for better management of hypertension. *Artificial Intelligence in Medicine*, *47*(2), 87–103. doi:10.1016/j.artmed.2009.07.001 PMID:19709865

Maragoudakis, M., Lymberopoulos, D., Fakotakis, N., & Spiropoulos, K. (2008). A Hierarchical, Ontology-Driven Bayesian Concept for Ubiquitous Medical Environments- A Case Study for Pulmonary Diseases. In *Proceedings of 2008 30th Annual International Conference of the Ieee Engineering in Medicine and Biology Society,* (pp. 3807-3810). New York: IEEE.

McGarry, K., Garfield, S., & Wermter, S. (2007). Auto-extraction, representation and integration of a diabetes ontology using Bayesian networks. In P. Kokol, V. Podgorelec, D. MiceticTurk, M. Zorman & M. Verlic (Eds.), In *Proceedings of Twentieth IEEE International Symposium on Computer-Based Medical Systems,* (pp. 612-617). IEEE.

McJunkin, M. C. (1995). Precision and recall in title keyword searches. *Information Technology and Libraries*, *14*(3), 161–171.

Min, H., Manion, F. J., Goralczyk, E., Wong, Y. N., Ross, E., & Beck, J. R. (2009). Integration of prostate cancer clinical data using an ontology. *Journal of Biomedical Informatics*, *42*(6), 1035–1045. doi:10.1016/j.jbi.2009.05.007 PMID:19497389

Mitchell, J., & Westerduin, F. (2008). Emergency department information system diagnosis: how accurate is it? *Emergency Medicine Journal*, *25*(11), 784. doi:10.1136/emj.2007.050104 PMID:18955631

Moody, D. L., & Shanks, G. G. (2003). Improving the quality of data models: empirical validation of a quality management framework. *Information Systems*, *28*(6), 619–650. doi:10.1016/S0306-4379(02)00043-1

Moro, M. L., & Morsillo, F. (2004). Can hospital discharge diagnoses be used for surveillance of surgical-site infections? *The Journal of Hospital Infection*, *56*(3), 239–241. doi:10.1016/j.jhin.2003.12.022 PMID:15003675

Nimmagadda, S. L., Nimmagadda, S. K., & Dreher, H. (2008). Ontology based data warehouse modeling and managing ecology of human body for disease and drug prescription management. In *Proceedings of 2008 2nd IEEE International Conference on Digital Ecosystems and Technologies* (pp. 465-473). IEEE.

O'Donoghue, J., Herbert, J., O'Reilly, P., & Sammon, D. (2009). Towards Improved Information Quality: The Integration of Body Area Network Data within Electronic Health Records. In M. Mokhtari, I. Khalil, J. Bauchet, D. Zhang, & C. Nugent (Eds.), *Ambient Assistive Health and Wellness Management in the Heart of the City* (Vol. 5597, pp. 299–302). doi:10.1007/978-3-642-02868-7_46

Orme, A. M., Yao, H., & Etzkorn, L. H. (2007). Indicating ontology data quality, stability, and completeness throughout ontology evolution. *Journal of Software Maintenance and Evolution-Research and Practice*, *19*(1), 49–75. doi:10.1002/smr.341

Pannarale, P., Catalano, D., De Caro, G., Grillo, G., Leo, P., & Pappada, G. et al. (2012). GIDL: A rule based expert system for GenBank Intelligent Data Loading into the Molecular Biodiversity Database. *BMC Bioinformatics*, *13*(Suppl 4), S4. doi:10.1186/1471-2105-13-S4-S4 PMID:22536971

Pathak, J., Kiefer, R. C., Bielinski, S. J., & Chute, C. G. (2012). Mining the human phenome using semantic web technologies: a case study for Type 2 Diabetes. In Proceedings of *AMIA ... Annual Symposium Proceedings*, (pp. 699–708). AMIA. PMID:23304343

Pathak, J., Kiefer, R. C., & Chute, C. G. (2012). Using semantic web technologies for cohort identification from electronic health records for clinical research. *AMIA Summits Transl Sci Proc*, *2012*, 10–19. PMID:22779040

Perez-Rey, D., Maojo, V., Garcia-Remesal, M., Alonso-Calvo, R., Billhardt, H., & Martin-Sanchez, F. et al. (2006). ONTOFUSION: Ontology-based integration of genomic and clinical databases. *Computers in Biology and Medicine*, *36*(7-8), 712–730. doi:10.1016/j.compbiomed.2005.02.004 PMID:16144697

Pinto, H. S. (2004). Ontologies: How can They be Built? *Knowledge and Information Systems*, *6*(4), 441–464. doi:10.1007/s10115-003-0138-1

Preece, A., Missier, P., Ernbury, S., Jin, B., & Greenwood, M. (2008). An ontology-based approach to handling information quality in e-Science. *Concurrency and Computation*, *20*(3), 253–264. doi:10.1002/cpe.1195

Quan, H., Li, B., Saunders, L. D., Parsons, G. A., Nilsson, C. I., & Alibhai, A. et al. (2008). Assessing validity of ICD-9-CM and ICD-10 administrative data in recording clinical conditions in a unique dually coded database. *Health Services Research*, *43*(4), 1424–1441. doi:10.1111/j.1475-6773.2007.00822.x PMID:18756617

Redman, T. (2005). Measuring data accuracy. In W. Rea (Ed.), *Information Quality* (p. 21). Armonk, NY: ME Sharpe Inc.

Spasic, I., & Ananiadou, S. (2005). A flexible measure of contextual similarity for biomedical terms. *Pacific Symposium on Biocomputing. Pacific Symposium on Biocomputing*, 197–208. PMID:15759626

Stvilia, B., Mon, L., & Yi, Y. J. (2009). A Model for Online Consumer Health Information Quality. *Journal of the American Society for Information Science and Technology*, *60*(9), 1781–1791. doi:10.1002/asi.21115

Topalis, P., Dialynas, E., Mitraka, E., Deligianni, E., Siden-Kiamos, I., & Louis, C. (2011). A set of ontologies to drive tools for the control of vector-borne diseases. *Journal of Biomedical Informatics*, *44*(1), 42–47. doi:10.1016/j.jbi.2010.03.012 PMID:20363364

Valencia-Garcia, R., Fernandez-Breis, J. T., Ruiz-Martinez, J. M., Garcia-Sanchez, F., & Martinez-Bejar, R. (2008). A knowledge acquisition methodology to ontology construction for information retrieval from medical documents. *Expert Systems: International Journal of Knowledge Engineering and Neural Networks*, *25*(3), 314–334. doi:10.1111/j.1468-0394.2008.00464.x

Verma, A., Fiasché, M., Cuzzola, M., Iacopino, P., Morabito, P., & Kasabov, N. (2009). Ontology based personalized modeling for type 2 diabetes risk analysis: An Investigated Approach. In C. S. Leung, M. Lee, & J. H. Chan (Eds.), *ICONIP 2009, Part II* (pp. 360–366). Berlin: Springer-Verlag.

Verma, A., Kasabov, N., Rush, A., & Song, Q. (2008, 2008). *Ontology based personalized modeling for chronic disease risk analysis: an integrated approach.* Paper presented at the 15th International Conference on Advances in Neuro-Information Processing. New York, NY.

Wand, Y., & Wang, Y. (1996). Anchoring Data Quality Dimensions in Ontological Foundations. *Communications of the ACM*, *36*(11), 86–95. doi:10.1145/240455.240479

Wang, M. H., Lee, C. S., Li, H. C., & Ko, W. M. (2007). *Ontology-based fuzzy inference agent for diabetes classification*. New York: IEEE. doi:10.1109/NAFIPS.2007.383815

Wang, R. (1998). A product perspective on total data quality management. *Communications of the ACM*, *41*(2), 58–65. doi:10.1145/269012.269022

Wang, R., Strong, D., & Guarascio, L. (1996). Beyond accuracy: What data quality means to data consumers. *Journal of Management Information Systems*, *12*(4), 5–33.

Wang, R. Y. (1998). A product perspective on total data quality management. *Communications of the ACM*, *41*(2), 58–65. doi:10.1145/269012.269022

Wang, R. Y., Strong, D. M., & Guarascio, L. M. (1996). Beyond accuracy: What data quality means to data consumers. *Journal of Management Information Systems*, *12*(4), 5–33.

Yao, H., Orme, A., & Etzkorn, L. H. (2005). Cohesion metrics for ontology design and application. *Journal of Computer Science*, *1*(1), 107–113. doi:10.3844/jcssp.2005.107.113

Young, L., Tu, S. W., Tennakoon, L., Vismer, D., Astakhov, V., Gupta, A., et al. (2009). Ontology Driven Data Integration for Autism Research. In *Proceedings of 2009 22nd IEEE International Symposium on Computer-Based Medical Systems* (pp. 54-60). New York: IEEE.

## KEY TERMS AND DEFINITIONS

**Chronic Diseases:** Long term diseases that are rarely cured and require ongoing treatment and control.

**Data Model:** A data model organizes the data types, attributes, rules and relationships between data items.

**Data Quality:** Is an assessment of the fitness of data for a specific purpose or context and can be expressed in terms such as completeness, correctness and consistency of data.

**Fitness for Purpose:** "Something that is fit for purpose is good enough to do the job it was designed to do" (Macmillan Dictionary).

**Ontology Development Methodology:** A systematic plan of activities to design, create and evaluate an ontology based model.

**Ontology:** In information science, an ontology is a semantic data model using a hierarchical construct to represent the types, properties and interrelationships of the concepts within a domain.

**Primary Health Care:** Essential health care; based on practical, scientifically sound, and socially acceptable method and technology; universally accessible to all in the community through their full participation; at an affordable cost; and geared toward self-reliance and self-determination (WHO & UNICEF, 1978).

# Chapter 17
# A Reconfigurable Supporting Connected Health Environment for People with Chronic Diseases

**Abbes Amira**
*University of the West of Scotland, UK & Qatar University, Qatar*

**Naeem Ramzan**
*University of the West of Scotland, UK*

**Christos Grecos**
*University of the West of Scotland, UK*

**Qi Wang**
*University of the West of Scotland, UK*

**Pablo Casaseca-de-la-Higuera**
*University of the West of Scotland, UK*

**Zeeshan Pervez**
*University of the West of Scotland, UK*

**Xinheng Wang**
*University of the West of Scotland, UK*

**Chunbo Luo**
*University of the West of Scotland, UK*

## ABSTRACT

*Digital healthcare is becoming increasingly important as the ageing population and the number of people diagnosed with chronic diseases is increasing. The face of healthcare delivery has changed radically and at its core is a digital and customer revolution. Connected health is the convergence of medical devices, security devices, and communication technologies. It enables patients to be monitored and treated remotely from their home or primary care facility rather than attend outpatient clinics or be admitted to hospital. This chapter discusses the recent advances in connected health technologies and applications. The authors investigate a reconfigurable supporting connected health solution for people with chronic diseases using reconfigurable hardware and intelligent data interpretation and analysis. In addition, a thorough review of the existing information and communications technologies and challenges in the area of connected health including embedded medical devices, sensors, social networking, knowledge management, data fusion, and cloud computing is presented in this chapter. Finally, future directions and ongoing research in the area of connected health are presented.*

DOI: 10.4018/978-1-4666-6316-9.ch017

## INTRODUCTION

The number of elderly is increasing over the world. It is estimated that by the year 2020 the proportion of people aged 60 and over will be 25% worldwide. The ageing process in Europe is even at a higher level. By the year 2020, forecasts say that the percentage of people aged 60 and over will be about 50% in Europe (World, 2003), (UN, 2013).

The ageing of the society comes along with several specific problems. The increased frailty of the elderly, the increasing prevalence of diseases and the increasing resources used per patient have a major impact on the health systems. The ageing of the society comes along with several specific problems. The increased frailty of the elderly, the increasing prevalence of diseases and the increasing resources used per patient have a major impact on the healthcare systems. The awareness of the impact of the growing numbers of elderly has increased. The ageing society has been one of the key actions of the research programs worldwide and in Europe, UK in particular. Within those programs, much attention is paid to effective and efficient delivery of health and social care services to older people diagnosed with chronic diseases (CD) such as Dementia (incl. Alzheimer's disease) and Parkinson disease.

Monitoring different vital signs of patients with CD such as ECG (heart rate), SpO2, blood pressure for example – provides an important source of information to the doctor for defining treatment and planning and for the patients to manage their diseases. It is also an aid for prevention and early diagnosis. Recent advances in information technologies offer the possibility of a new generation of lightweight monitoring systems that a patient diagnosed with CD for example can wear while going about his/her daily business, or which can be carried around easily and used regularly. Such new systems and tools can now provide much more reliable data on multiple parameters, and transmit them to remote locations, so that medical professionals can make better decisions on treatment without having to meet the patients face-to-face. Visual information and remote monitoring of patient's behaviour can also be combined with different vital signs monitored using wireless medical devices for early diagnosis and thus limit the development of the symptoms of CD.

Furthermore, social networks have become a powerful tool for healthcare and helps patients to find remedies and seek advice from other patients with similar conditions or medical experts. For some individuals limited access to healthcare and information on the disease could lead to more severe consequences such as paralysis. Patients often look to the internet to find other people with similar illnesses to aid and advise them where their medical condition is concerned. Patients like these rely on online social media such as Facebook, Twitter, TuDiabetes and PatientsLikeMe Patientslikeme (2013) to find social support. The social networking sites are a powerful and cost effective communication tools.

In addition, modern ICT is increasingly used in healthcare aiming to improve and enhance medical services and reduce costs. In this context, cloud computing has become very appealing when managing the computation and storage resources. E-health clouds offer new possibilities, such as easy and ubiquitous access to medical data, and real-time transmission of heterogeneous data. However, they also bear new risks with respect to security and privacy aspects.

This book chapter discusses an integrated solution for reliable, secure and real-time e-health service delivery at homes and remote locations. It will cover state of the art technologies which can be deployed in a connected health environment such as embedded systems, social networking, data fusion and pattern recognition, cloud computing, security and knowledge management.

We aim to address the following issues required for the development of a complete connected healthcare system:

- Evaluate different embedded medical devices which can be used to acquire and process different vital signs such as ECG, temperature, blood pressure and acceleration signals;
- Analyse the extracted information from health social networking sites and its impact of CD management, treatment and prevention;
- Evaluate existing methods and present real-time solutions for remote heterogeneous data acquisition, fusion and processing and the deployment of secure cloud computing for big data processing, transmission and retrieval; and
- Evaluate knowledge management techniques used for intelligent data analysis and manipulation will be also addressed.

The authors present and discuss different software and hardware related issues to the design and implementation of a heterogeneous reconfigurable computing platform for connected health applications. The proposed solutions cover state of the art technologies which can be deployed in a connected health environment such as intelligent embedded systems, social networking and knowledge management, advanced signal, image and video processing, data fusion and pattern recognition, cloud computing, data security and privacy.

The structure of the remaining of this book chapter is as follows. Next section will present different challenges and an overview about the existing connected healthcare solutions in place. In the future research directions, we will highlight the main features of our proposed solutions. Finally concluding remarks will be included at the end of this chapter.

## STATE OF THE ART

In this section, a thorough and comprehensive review will be carried out on the following main pillars in the context of connected health environments:

- Embedded computing systems;
- Social networking and knowledge management;
- Data fusion and pattern recognition; and
- Cloud computing and security

### Embedded Computing Systems

The impact of world population ageing in healthcare costs has motivated an increasing effort in the development of Wearable Health-Monitoring Systems (WHMS) by both the research community and industry. Real-time monitoring of patient's health condition can significantly decrease these costs by providing feedback information to either physicians or users so that alerting events and alarms can be triggered for health threatening awareness.

WHMS usually consist of a number of sensors able to measure significant physiological parameters and signals such as blood pressure (BP), oxygen saturation ($SaO_2$), respiration, photoplethysmography (PPG) or electrocardiogram (ECG). Activity patterns obtained from 2D/3D accelerometers and other parameters conveying information on the patient's way of life can also be incorporated to provide context-based information. A central node is linked to these sensors providing connectivity to visualisation displays or transmission nodes for management at point-of-care. This latter connectivity shall be wirelessly provided [different alternatives do exist: Zigbee, bluetooth, 802.11g, etc., Pantelopoulos and Bourbakis (2010)] so that the user's daily activity is not interfered. On the other hand, links between sensors and the main node links can be wired depending on the specific application.

Pantelopoulos and Bourbakis (2010) presented a comprehensive survey on WHMS ranging from research prototypes to commercially available systems. An evaluation of the maturity state of the most relevant systems was also provided. It merely consists of an aggregate scoring of the different system capabilities such as wearability, real applicability, real-time properties, scalability or presence of decision support mechanisms. Each capability was weighted by a pooled "importance" coefficient obtained from different perspectives, namely, patient's, physician's and manufacturer's. The final maturity index consisted on 5 different levels (1=low, 2=medium-low, 3=medium, 4=high, 5=maximum). All the evaluated systems ranged in the 2-4 interval.

Considering research prototypes, those based on microcontroller boards or custom based platforms were evaluated in (Pantelopoulos and Bourbakis, 2010) as being in a medium-low stage of maturity. An example is the AMON (Advanced care and alert portable telemedical monitoring, Hao and Foster, 2008), developed within an EU IST FP5 funded project. The final prototype consists of a wrist-worn device which measures BP, Temperature, $SaO_2$, one-lead ECG and 2D acceleration and provides a GSM link to the telemedicine centre for signal analysis. This allowed the identification of health risk levels according to the world health organization thresholds (WHO). The LiveNet (Sung et al., 2005) mobile platform for long-term health monitoring provides real-time signal processing features and context classification from ECG, Electromyogram (EMG), 3D accelerations, and galvanic skin conductance (GSC). The foreseen applications included Parkinson long-term behavioural modelling, and epilepsy seizure detection.

The effort devoted to the development of smart textiles has leaded to final prototypes whose maturity level according to (Pantelopoulos and Bourbakis, 2010) ranges between medium (3) (Paradiso et al., 2005, Scilingo et al., 2005) and high (4) (Luprano et al., 2006, Di Rienzo et al., 2005, Pandian et al., 2008). Among them, different applications are targeted, from health monitoring in general (Pandian et al., 2008) and specific cases (elderly, chronic diseases) (Paradiso et al., 2005, Scilingo et al., 2005), to more ambitious applications such as prevention and early diagnosis of cardiovascular diseases (Luprano et al., 2006, Di Rienzo et al., 2005). Different signals are measured depending on the application (ECG, respiratory signal, BP, PPG, etc.). Moreover, signal processing and pattern recognition for feature extraction is also performed at different levels in some projects: The MyHeart project (Luprano et al., 2006) incorporated on-body signal processing algorithms to classify activity patterns into resting, walking, running, and going up/downstairs. ECG enhancement techniques were also implemented at body level. The WEALTHY project (Scilingo et al., 2005) and Smart Vest (Pandian et al., 2008) incorporated hardware removal of baseline noise and motion artifacts in the acquired signals.

In order to achieve multi-purpose reconfigurable WHMS, mote-based Body Area Networks (BAN) (Hao and Foster, 2008) are probably the best option. These so-called motes are wireless nodes responsible of collecting one or more types of physiological data and transmitting them to a central node. The wearable wireless BAN prototype described by Milenković et al. (2006) incorporates custom sensor platforms allowing measuring and preprocessing of different signals such as ECG, EMG, and acceleration. These sensors are further integrated on a commercially available platform. The system presented by Chung et al. (2008) integrated ECG and BP measurements with basic signal processing (simple feature extraction and if-then-rules) to extract suspicious patterns for diagnosis support. In they work, Milenković et al. (2006), discuss the lack of standardization in terms of platforms, transmission and wireless communications. Additionally, the authors propose to perform on-board signal processing to reduce the wireless transmission duty cycle and the power consumption. However, dealing with limited computing resources, real-time requirements, and memory space constitutes a challenging task (Pantelopoulos and Bourbakis, 2010).

Mote-based BANs such as (Shimmer, 2013) have attracted the research community interest in the recent years for the development of prototypes. These platforms can be configured to measure different signals and parameters such as 4-lead ECG, EMG, 3D acceleration, and angular velocity in multiple set-ups. They also provide different drivers and interfaces to signal processing platforms (Labview, Matlab) and smart mobile devices. Actually, incorporating daily-use devices to WHMS will decrease the final cost of the systems and increase their usability. Some specific platforms have also been developed. Microsoft HealthGear (Oliver and Flores-Mangas, 2006), provides $SaO_2$ and heart rate (HR) measurements and sends them to a cell phone to perform detection of sleep apnea episodes in both time and frequency domain. HealthToGo (Jin et al., 2009) is a cellphone based platform that performs real-time analysis of the ECG waveform in order to identify abnormal patterns. (Fensli et al, 2005) presented a proposal aimed at the detection of arrhythmias in a similar way. All of these prototypes use mobile devices to perform the signal processing tasks for feature extraction. The recent advances in smart phones and watches technology would additionally allow employing the embedded sensors for signal acquisition.

A final group of devices that is worth mentioning is composed of those which are commercially available for monitoring purposes. Specific health monitoring systems such as Lifeshirt® by Vivometrics (Heilman and Forges, 2007) and Bioharness™ (Zephyr Inc., 2013) provide remote access to ECG, respiration and activity data. These systems do not incorporate sophisticated feature extraction or decision support as is expected from the existing gap between commercially established products and research prototypes. Heart rate chest-belt sensors and wrist displays such as those from Polar (2013) have succeeded in sports applications with proprietary connectivity to fitness equipment (treadmills, bicycles, etc.). Latest releases provide connectivity with mobile devices so that the acquired data can be monitored and processed using Android or iOS applications. Activity monitors such as (Actigraph, 2013) have extensively been used for research purposes. First releases included wired raw data access for prospective analysis and specific software providing sleep reports. Latest ones do also incorporate wireless Bluetooth connectivity.

The preceding paragraphs provide a brief insight into some relevant so far proposed WHMS. The specificity of the customized design approaches can explain the lack of maturity (according to the evaluation by (Pantelopoulos and Bourbakis, 2010)) of these developments. Systems based on smart textiles present desirable wearability properties but are more limited in terms of flexibility and scalability. Mote-based BANs do overcome these problems, providing higher processing capability at the same time. If some of the measurement tasks were performed using smart phone or watch built-in sensors, BAN limited resources would be significantly released. Additionally, adopting daily use devices for health condition monitoring would pave the way for a higher impact of these systems. Nonetheless, the current research challenges in ubiquitous personalized healthcare demand context information to be included in complex signal models to derive physiological parameters of interest (Viswanathan et al., 2012).

To this end, computing and storage capabilities beyond those of sensor motes and mobile devices are required. In this context, cloud computing systems and dynamic resource management will play an important role.

## SOCIAL NETWORKING

Social networking sites have become very prevalent over the past decade and have stretched at a rapid percentage on the internet. More than one billion active users are using only facebook. It entices consideration through the competence of the user to create their own personalized profiles, to search long lost friends, to join special interest groups and also to converse with peers all over the world. Most of such types of social networking websites have become an efficient tool that fetches people with similar interests together to interact and discuss the same problems, feelings, thoughts and in some cases seek medical advice from one another (Sheth, 2010). Websites like Facebook, Twitter and Wikipedia can be used in a more health-specific manner to target health professionals and the public, is creating new, cost effective ways to embed a powerful tool into a healthcare system (Khorakhu et al. 2013). In addition, it is very useful tool for healthcare and helps patients to find remedies and seek advice from other patients with similar conditions or medical experts. The research conducted by (Scanfeld, 2010) exhibited that people start to share their health-related information or problems online. This result in a growing number of social networking sites directed towards health and well-being.

*Figure 1. Triple synergy of physical, cyber and social paradigm in eHealth framework*

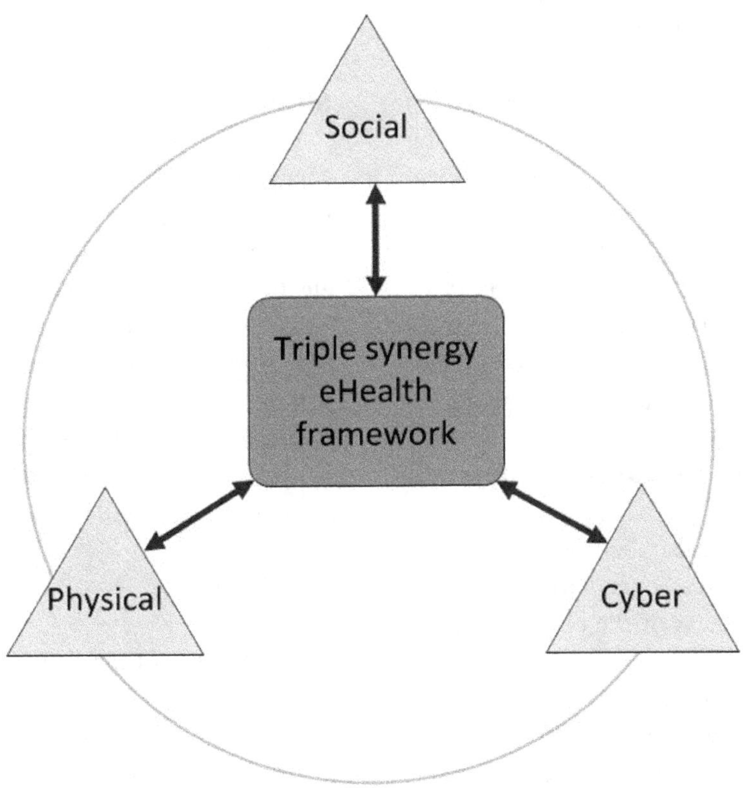

Recently a number of social applications allowing users to update their health status and health goals via online support groups have been proposed.

Personal devices such as laptops, smartphones and iPads can be used by people to monitor their own health-related behaviour wirelessly (Silva et al. 2011). The work by Afzal et al. (2012) integrated different social media websites such as Facebook, Youtube, Twitter as an input for decision support in healthcare information systems. Furthermore, the investigation in (Norval et al.,2011) proposed the use of social network like Facebook as a framework for telecare. (Griffin et al. 2009) presented the integration of paradigms in social networks into healthcare, i.e. information sharing, monitoring and message alerts. However, only the espousal of the architecture adapted with social networking technologies was proposed, rather than a social media platform. (Detmar et al. 2000) proposed a social network model for health monitoring. Compared to other work, the process has less automation, and did not exploit mobile devices, but did allow patients to control the access to their data. Based on a similar concept, (Ding et al 2012) and (Ayubi et al 2012) employed a monitoring unit, a smartphone and the Facebook platform for monitoring of physical activities. Based on the recent advances in technologies ranging from affordable smart devices to the accessibility of the Internet, along with the popularity of existing social networks, the usage of social media as an input to healthcare platform is already in progress.

## Triple Synergy of eHealth Framework

Triple synergy of physical, cyber and social media is the new and innovative concept to increase the reliability and robustness of the eHealth framework. The cyber-physical system constitutes on the computational and communication components closely interact with physical components. It enables better cyber-mediated observation and interaction with physical components.

## Physical-Cyber Platform

We've witnessed significant progress in technology that enhances human-computer interactions. Now we're experiencing increasingly intelligent interfaces which have demonstrated contextual use of knowledge to develop intelligent human–mobile-device interfaces (Sheth et al., 2013). We're also observing progress in how machines especially sensors and device, surroundings, and humans interact, enabled by advances in sensing the body, the mind, and place. Such recent research supports the ability to comprehend human actions, including human gestures and languages in increasingly diverse forms. The extending ability to provide any physical object an identity in the cyber world, will let machines leverage extensive knowledge about the object to complement what humans process. Some of the examples where health applications and tools that monitor a person physically and connect them to care provider is given below.

## MedApps

MedApps (MedApps 2013) provides a health information management platform that effectively connects patients to their healthcare providers and electronics medical records to enhance patient cars and drive down the related cost. The example of MedApps system is shown in Figure 2, where the patient data is collected by remote portable devices and sends it to MedApps server and compare with existing electronic medical record and generate alerts through emails or phone calls if needed.

## Cardionet

CardioNet (CardioNet, 2013) provides the next-generation ambulatory cardiac monitoring service with beat-to-beat, real time analysis, automatic arrhythmia detection and wireless ECG transmission. CardioNet prides a comprehensive suite

*Figure 2. MedApps health monitoring framework (MedApps 2013)*

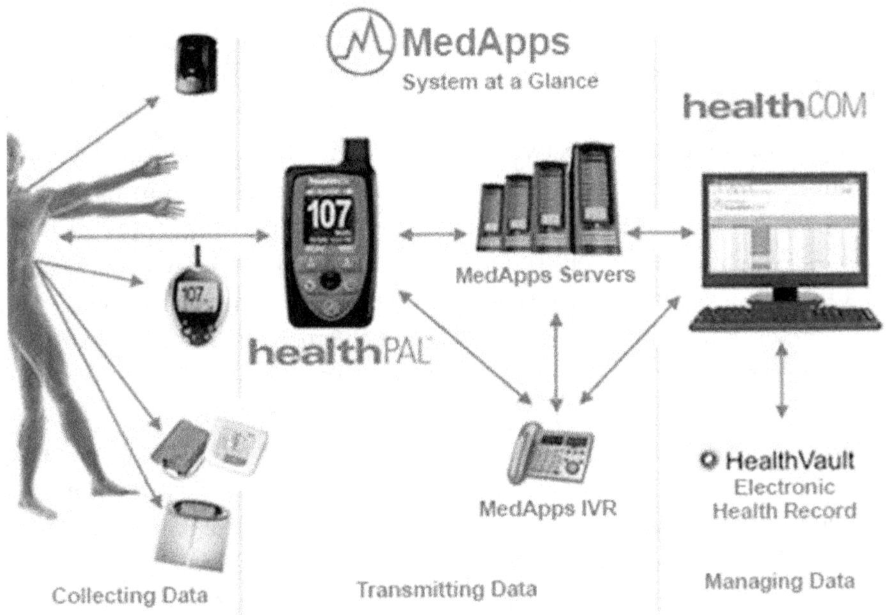


of post-symptom, looping, auto-trigger event monitors as part of its turn-key cardiac event monitoring services.

## LifeWatch

LifeWatch, (2013) provides ACT (Ambulatory Cardiac Telemetry), an automatically activated system that requires no patient intervention to either capture or transmit an arrhythmia when it occurs. Upon arrhythmia detection, the system automatically utilizes the integrated cellular phone to transmit the ECG waveform to LifeWatch monitoring sytem, where the ECG is analyzed. The patient's physician is notified of the arrhythmia based on pre-determined notification criteria prescribed by the patient's physician. Patients can be monitored for up to 30 days and all the data is available at the request of the physician during the service period and for 7 days following the end of service.

## Intelsense

Intelesens, (2013) offers a flexible Wireless Vital Signs Platform that can be customised to provide a range of monitoring products for in-hospital use and deployment at-home or on-the-move. It can be used as a short range or long range (cellular phone) monitor and specified with a variety of vital sign inputs and wireless systems. Highly miniaturized, light weight and with an extremely long battery life, the monitoring devices are small, unobtrusive and easily worn under clothes allowing patients freedom during monitoring.

## Cyber-Social Platform

In cyber-social world, people share their activities, knowledge, experience, opinions, and perceptions. The well-known social websites such as YouTube, Flickr, and Facebook. In such environments, the audio-video content is usually accompanied with metadata, tags, ratings, comments, information about the uploader and their social networks. Analysis of these "social media" shows a great potential in improving the performance of traditional multimedia information analysis/retrieval approaches by bridging the semantic gap between the "objective" multimedia content analysis and "subjective" users' needs and impressions. The integration of these aspects, however, is non-trivial and has created a vibrant, interdisciplinary field of research. There are only few social networks relating to health monitoring like:

### Patientslikeme

It is a free patient network where people can connect with others who have the same disease or condition and track and share their own experiences. When people share information on Patientslikeme, (2013), they generate data about the real-world nature of disease that helps researchers, pharmaceutical companies, regulators, providers and non-profits to develop more effective products, services and care.

### 23andMe

This social networking platform manages risk assessment and provides informed decisions based on gene sequencing (23andMe, 2013). It enables therapeutic developers to evaluate individualized responses to treatment at large scale, while providing research participants with a truly patient-centric study experience.

### MedHelp

It is one of the largest online health communities. It provides support for more than 300 different conditions, forums that connect consumers to doctors. (MedHelp, 2013) delivers unparalleled access to trusted information and advice tailored to consumers' personal health needs.

## Physical-Cyber-Social Platform

It is an emerging paradigm where physical, cyber, and social information interact with each other as shown in Figure 1. The remote sensors collect observation from the physical world. Data collected from physiological sensors analysed in the social context of similar people (Sheth 2013). The integration and interactions between physical, cyber, and social components need significant human involvement in the interpretation of physiological observations using their knowledge domain and social experiences.

Huge amount of information can be extracted from the social networks and medical sensors; hence there is a real need for knowledge management (KM) techniques which can improve the delivery of healthcare services (Nilakanta et al., 2009). A review on knowledge management in the healthcare industry was presented in (Nicolini et al., 2008, Sheffield, 2008) and has shown different challenges and techniques in this field. (Sheffield, 2008) states that KM is systemically more complex in healthcare because the three domain of knowledge creation, knowledge normalization and knowledge application. (Nicolini et al., 2008) has noted that KM research in healthcare over the years has focused on three overarching themes: "the nature of knowledge in the healthcare sector, the type of KM tools and initiatives that are suitable for the healthcare sector, and the barriers and enablers to adoption of KM practices". Classification and annotation techniques can be also used in KM based healthcare systems for automatic medical data classification and annotation which can help for treatment, diagnosis and disease management.

## Data Fusion and Pattern Recognition

With the advancement in ICT and circuit fabrication technologies sensory devices are becoming ubiquitous and smaller in size. ICT technologies have leverages these devices to transmit data over long distances and persist them for offline processing at the point of care. Fabrication technologies have significantly reduced their size and enabled them to add multiple sensors in a single device – today smartphones are equipped with accelerometer, gyroscope, proximity sensor (Scully et al, 2012), and further more sensors (*heart rate sensor, ECG sensors, and glucometer etc.*) can be connected through the Bluetooth protocol. Miniaturization of sensory devices has profound effect on healthcare industry, as it is becoming convenient for patient to use them without any hassle, most importantly a single device equipped with multiple sensors can be used for data acquisition considering multiple physiological and contextual parameters.

Fusing data from diverse sources (*clinical repositories, sensory devices*) is very important both for the patients and healthcare service providers. It can provide an insight view of patient's medical condition and can significantly elevate the efficacy of healthcare services (Craig et al., 2005). Clinical data accumulated at independent healthcare service providers can be fused for advance statistical analysis to develop a deeper clinical understanding of a particular disease. Medical data fusion for telemedicine is a distributed framework for processing clinical images and to facilitate knowledge sharing among physicians and researchers (Megalooikonomou et al., 2007). The proposed framework processes multiple clinical image repositories independently; whereas, distributed processing components synchronize their intermediate results. By utilizing dynamic recursive partitioning (DRP) the framework is able to identify region of interest in medical images (*tumor, lesions etc.*) that are discriminative among groups of subjects. The application of the proposed framework included identifying discriminative brain activation patterns in Alzheimer patients, and studying sexual morphological differentiation of the brain corpus callosum.

Clinical data analysis along with daily clinical observations can be used for medical risk analysis. Kyriacou et al. proposed an integrated system for assessing stroke risk (Kyriacou et al., 2007). The authors collected data from stroke patients by using non-invasive techniques. The collected data is then processed by using automated data analysis techniques and information rich features are extracted. Equipped with extracted information, patients are monitored for a period of 6 to 84 weeks. Statistical correlation techniques are applied to identify patients belonging to a high-risk category. Augmentation of clinical observations with processed clinical data assisted in early identification of critical parameters, thus assisting healthcare service provider to customize clinical services accordingly.

(Brzostowski et al., 2013) demonstrated the practicality of data driver models for e-Health applications. In their proposed model they utilized signals for heart rate, running speed and fatigue; combining expert knowledge with the sensory data – whereas conventional approaches of statistical analysis made use of data only. The authors propose a three tier application model. First tier transmits the data collected by wearable sensory devices, through body area network. Second tier is responsible for modelling and collective processing of transmitted data from all the sensory devices. The third tier works as a presentation layer for results, charts, and reports. The authors demonstrate the efficacy of their data driver model through endurance training for a runner. They utilise a mathematical model of cardiovascular system and fatigue during exercise, in order to evaluate optimized speed of a runner to achieve a particular goal, considering heart rate and level of fatigue.

Yan et al. propose a wireless sensor network based e-Health system to track elderly patients in smart-home environment (Yan et al., 2010). The proposed system integrates information from multiple sensory devices to find location of an elderly along with other contextual information gathered from pressure, fire and pulse sensor node to generate necessary alarm in case of an emergency. Moulton et al. highlight an important issue of data reliability in sensory data fusion for Personal Electronic Health Records (Bruce et al, 2009). They develop a prototype system to understand how the type, quality, installation, maintenance and calibration of the sensors can affect level of confidence practitioners have over the sensory data. Data from sensory devices having level of confidence is fused to make clinical decision. In sensory data processing for clinical purposes considering aforementioned parameters is very important. This is because usually not much consideration is given to these parameters in-home or ambulatory monitoring systems.

In the context of e-Health application situational aware plays an important role in making accurate recommendation and clinical decision. Advancements in sensing technology lead to context-aware devices (Buchmayr et al., 2011), which can assist in realization of effectual e-Health services and applications. (Wolf et al.,2008) proposed SOPRANO, an ambient assistive living platform, which utilizes environmental sensory data obtained from multiple sensors to process the contextual information and generate suitable recommendations / warnings. (Skubic et al., 2009) propose TigerPlace, an active retirement community project, designed specifically for smart-homes equipped with multiple sensory devices i.e., utilizes passive physiological sensor (*motion and bed sensors*) and event-driven video-sensor network. It fuses the output of sensory devices for behavioural activity analysis and to generate appropriate alerts and recommendations. Alarm Net (Wood et al. 2008) is an assistive living and residential monitoring environment for patients with diverse needs. It utilizes Body Area Network to record vital signs and activity information, and emplaced sensors to enable location tracking. Its back-end component provides analysis of the sensed data, whereas user-interface component is utilized by doctors, nurses and residents to query information.

The entire purpose of data fusion is to process data within the correct context e.g., activity information of a patient can be used to decide whether data from blood pressure sensor should be considered or not etc. Another important source of contextual information is social network. Social network analysis can play an important role in learning sentiments of a patient combined with daily routine to make correct and timely clinical recommendations. Fatima et al. proposed SmartCDSS: an integration of Social Media and Interaction Engine (SMIE) in healthcare for chronic disease patients (Fatima et al., 2013). In their proposed system the authors combined tweets, trajectory and email interaction analysis into vMR (*virtual medical record*). Augmented with ontological information (SNOMED CT), vMR assist health practitioners to understand the behaviour and lifestyle of patients for better decision making about their personalized treatment and clinical recommendation.

We are living through a transition phase of healthcare industry, where clinical services are being transformed into wellness services. The proliferation of Smartphone and wearable sensory devices are evidence to this transition phase. However, with the increasing number of sensory devices a normal person or patient can carry, the complexity of data fusion is also increasing. Data fusion methodologies must also take into account any contradiction which may arise among certain sub-group of sensory devices e.g., sensory devices dedicated to activity recognition may state that patient is doing exercise, on the contrary heart rate sensor shows normal heart rate activity. Another important challenge which is faced by data fusion methodologies is that sensory devices transmit data at different rate. For making clinical recommendation or decision it is very crucial that healthcare service provider has a synchronized and accurately correlated data from sensory devices. Even with these open challenges, sensory data fusion will continue to provide a single view of patient's medical condition assisting healthcare service provider to increase efficacy of treatment.

## Cloud Computing and Security

Modern ICT is increasingly utilised in healthcare aiming to improve and enhance medical services whilst reducing costs. In this context, cloud computing has become increasingly appealing in light of the vast and cost-effective computation and storage resources available in the cloud. E-health clouds offer new possibilities, such as ubiquitous access to medical data, and real-time transmission of multimedia data. However, they also bear new risks with respect to security and privacy aspects, which must be addressed for wide adoption of cloud-assisted/based e-health services.

## Ubiquitous Cloud Healthcare Services

Cloud-based ubiquitous healthcare services exploit the on-demand, location-independent and inexpensive computing and storage resources made available by the widely available Internet clouds. In such systems, the cloud platform is utilised to store the huge volume of data including user information, physiological data, Personal Health Records (PHRs), graphic data to processing and so on, in various databases such as those based on NoSQL (Sakr et al. 2011). The physiological data especially vital signs are collected in real time from the patents' body area networks via wireless biosensors (Benharref 2013) and other monitoring equipment, which can be implantable, wearable, or not (Yang et al. 2012). Computation-intensive tasks such as the visualisation of the monitoring results and massive multimedia data processing are offloaded to the cloud as well. Moreover, the service-oriented nature of clouds well suits the e-health services, which typically require high scalability and flexibility. To facilitate pervasive access to the services, mobile communication technologies including diverse wireless networks (3G/4G, WiFi, Bluetooth, ZigBee etc.) and user devices (smartphones, tablets etc.) are usually utilised. It is essential that all the involved subsystems are integrated carefully to provide a smooth, timely and pervasive service to the users, as shown in Figure 3.

For instance, (He, Fan & Li, 2013) described a city-wide health-monitoring system based on a private cloud platform. A six-layer deployment architecture was proposed, including Service interaction to provide a user interface, Service presentation for high concurrency capability and service interface, Session cache to store/cache user sessions, Cloud engine to coordinate the cloud components based on a message queue method, Medical data mining, and Cloud storage. In this system, users can view the graphical results via TVs as well as web browsers. Pilot testing results demonstrated that the proposed document-oriented system was advantageous compared with non-document-oriented alternative systems such as Amazon's Simple Storage Service or S3 (Amazon, 2013).

## Multimedia Cloud Healthcare Services

Gaining increasing popularity, cloud-based multimedia e-health applications exploit the computation and storage capabilities in clouds whilst benefiting from the advances in multimedia processing technologies. In particular, medical video transmission has been boosted by recent video compression standards such as H.264 Advanced Video Coding (AVC) (ITU-T & ISO/IEC 2010) and H.265 High Efficiency Video Coding

Figure 3. Ubiquitous Cloud healthcare services

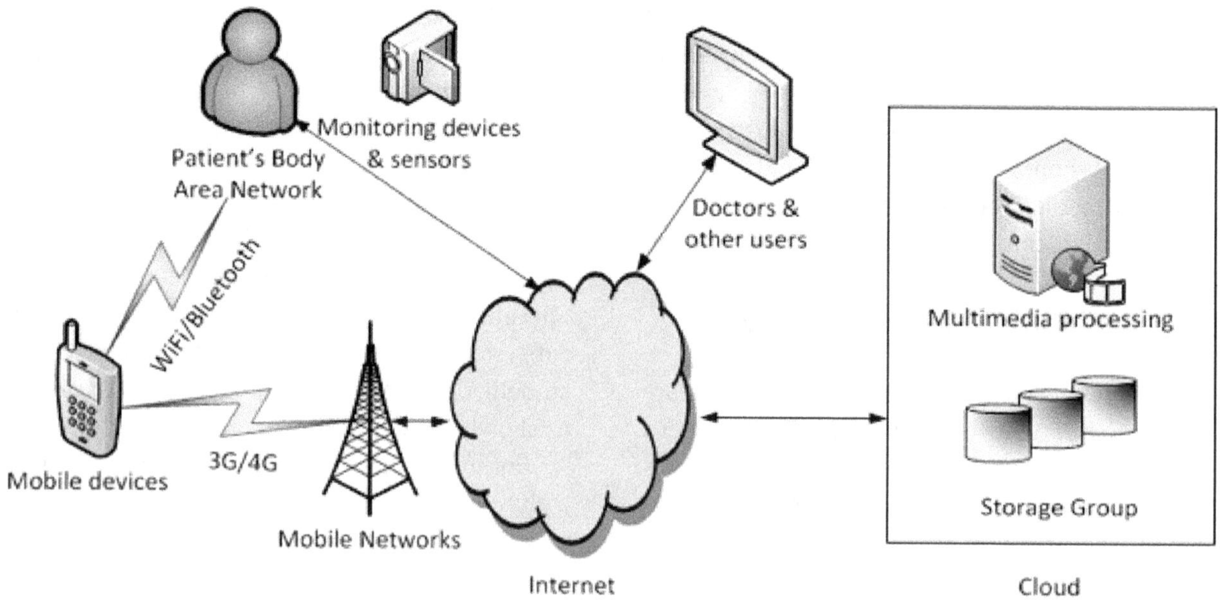


(HEVC) (ITU 2013). Reference software implementations of both AVC and HEVC standards are freely available and are widely used in the research community. Currently, H.264/AVC is the predominant video compression standard, and a number of implementations are existing. For instance, real-time, cross-platform AVC video streaming can be realised through VideoLAN's VLC player (VideoLAN, 2013). AVC is also employed by popular cloud-based streaming platforms such as Adobe Media Server (AMS) (Adobe, 2013) and Wowza (Wowza, 2013). For the future, it is expected that the H.265/HEVC standard will replace H.264 as the next-generation video coding standard, providing doubled compression efficiency for the same visual quality. However, real-time HEVC encoding is very challenging owning to the significantly increase computational complexity compared with H.264. Cloud-assisted HEVC processing is therefore a promising approach that should be explored. It is noted that HEVC is featured with built-in parallelisation facilities including the Tiles (rectangular regions of a picture), Wavefront Parallel Processing (WPP) and Dependent Slice Segments tools (Sullivan et al., 2012). These new facilities, in contrast to H.264, allow a more efficient integration of HEVC and clouds, with the latter support parallelisation inherently.

The advantages of HEVC over AVC for developing wireless ultrasound video telemedicine systems were investigated by (Panayides et al., 2012). The authors compared the compression efficiency of AVC and HEVC, and demonstrated the superiority of HEVC in terms of 37% reduction in bitrate requirement for equivalent clinical quality. The wireless transmission of AVC-encoded ultrasound video over a WiMAX network was also evaluated, and simulation results confirmed the feasibility of such a deployment. Due to the clinical nature of medical data, error resilience is essential in medical multimedia delivery, especially when wireless networks are involved (Panayides et al., 2011). The video streaming of HEVC content over loss-prone IP networks was reported in (James et al., 2012), and the system was empirically evaluated on a testbed.

Furthermore, (Wang et al., in press) discuss various mobile video cloud networks that can be further explored by cloud-assisted e-health video services over mobile networks. Moreover, SparkMed (Constantinescu, Kim & Feng, 2012) is a data integration framework that can dynamically integrate various e-health software and databases into a cloud-like peer-to-peer multimedia data store. A web-based transcoding facility was introduced to allow a seamless operation of hospital imaging software at any Internet-enabled devices such as smartphones. Image data are transcoded to lossless JPEG format with metadata provided in XML. For smooth navigation in the web browser-based display environment, SparkMed implemented local preliminary image processing at the end user's devices, and lossy FLV-based streaming of entire image stacks if required. For acceptably interactive performance, the system demands a "near-real-time" updating of the end user's device's data and visualisation content as it was manipulated at the cloud. Through empirical testing, it was found that users considered the system to be responsive when at least 5 frames/s frame rate was achieved for image streaming with a propagation time under 0.5 s.

## Security and Privacy in Cloud Healthcare Services

It is imperative that the shift of computational complexity (and potentially operation costs) in an e-health system to the cloud does not compromise the security of the system and the privacy of the clients. Security and privacy protection in cloud-based health systems is inherently tricky due to the combination of the semi-trusted cloud environment and the ever-existing malicious attacks to illegally acquire confidential medical and personal records. Highlighted here are a couple of top concerns including handling a range of potential attacks and risks originated from both outsiders and insiders, and allowing secure yet efficient access to the health data stored in the cloud at the same time.

The insider attacks are typically considered more difficult to be tackled and it was reported that insider attacks had cost the victimised institutions much more than what outsider counterparts had cost (Shaw, Ruby & Post 1998). Whilst outsider attacks could be handled in a rather trivial way such as through cryptographic mechanisms, insider attacks are typically significantly more difficult to deal with. To address insider attacks, a cloud-assisted mobile-Health monitoring system (CAM) was designed by Lin et al. (2013). CAM attempted to achieve a trade-off between privacy constrains and the operability of the system. The added difficulty of cloud environment for both data input and output was taken into account. An identity-based encryption scheme was designed in medical diagnostic branching programs to protect clients' privacy, and the decryption complexity was offloaded to the cloud. In addition, by applying a key private proxy re-encryption mechanism, computational load was shifted to the cloud from resource-constrained small companies for them to enter this market.

PHRs should be stored securely yet be accessed conveniently by the patients and authorised parties. MyPHRMachines (Van Gorp & Comuzzi 2012) is a cloud-based lifelong PHR system that aimed to achieve security and portability of health records. In this system, patients can upload their PHRs, remotely access their records via virtual machines (VMs), and share their remote VM sessions with selected trusted stakeholders, all in a secure manner as the design goals with various security techniques being investigated for different levels in the system. Two case uses including radiology image and sharing and personalised medicine were studied in a prototype. Furthermore, for fine-grained and scalable data access control to PHRs resident in a cloud, (Li et al., 2013) proposed a patient-centric framework and a set of mechanisms. Attribute-based encryption techniques were employed to encrypt the patients PHRs for secure sharing and to handle efficient and on-demand user revocation, and multiple security domains were introduced to reduce security key management complexity, among other considerations. The system's security, scalability, and efficiency were evaluated through analytical and experimental results.

Moreover, in practice, cloud-assisted e-Health systems also need to be compliant with relevant standards, regulations and laws in healthcare. For example, the USA Health Insurance Portability and Accountability Act (HIPAA) should apply to US e-healthcare providers who employ cloud computing technologies. It is reported that Amazon Web Services (AWS), ClearData Networks and other cloud e-health providers have developed HIPAA-compliant services. In addition, to facilitate secure interoperation of different, often heterogeneous cloud-based e-health systems, standardisation work should be intensified. It is expected that more cloud healthcare specific standards, together with national and international regulations and recommendations, will emerge in the near future.

## FUTURE RESEARCH DIRECTIONS

The review of existing technologies and systems in connected health applications reveals that most of the approaches can be further improved by looking at new intelligent embedded devices which can handle and interpret the huge amount of medical data coming from different medical sensors and other sources. Our future research directions, which are also aligned with the current trends and research challenges in the area, focus on the development and implementation of a reconfigurable supporting connected health environment for people with CD using reconfigurable hardware in the form of field programmable gate arrays (FPGAs). The research aims at developing a real-time embedded healthcare system for remote management and treatment of people with CD. The proposed environment is innovative and consists of new advanced technologies at both the system and component levels. Appropriate embedded processing platforms and interactive- internet services will be developed where robust intelligent data fusion algorithms can be deployed for data analysis. The main component of the system is an auto-adaptive self-calibrating platform deployed for remote heterogeneous data acquisition and processing. It is a reconfigurable platform which adapts itself depending on the environment changes and parameters. It has advanced on-board processing and communication capabilities which facilitate the wireless communication with different sensors.

Accurate measurement will be carried out at both the sensor and embedded monitoring platform. Advanced filtering, visualisation, processing and analysis techniques and algorithms will be prototyped and embedded in the wireless medical biosensors and the real-time monitoring platform. The system will process heterogeneous data acquired from different medical biosensors, ambient and vision sensors. The system will be used for real-time multi-parametric monitoring of people with CD and will deploy cloud computing for secure data transmission and retrieval. We aim to build wireless medical devices where clinical knowledge can be combined with intelligent algorithms used for data analysis which will provide more accurate decisions that help for early detection and prevention.

Our solution can focuses on remote management and treatment of patients at home but can be also deployed in mobile environments such mobile hospitals and ambulances. The current and future status of the patient will be assessed based on the acquisition of heterogeneous data, videos for behavioural analysis, and robust accurate methods for modelling and prediction.

We will also look at the power of consumption of the devices used and we aim to use advanced low power wearable medical devices for the acquisition of different vital signs. Human-computer interfaces, interactive web and internet services including social networks will be deployed in the system to visualise and analysis heterogeneous data. Intelligent systems, knowledge management techniques and advanced data mining techniques will be investigated for efficient storage of data, modelling and prediction of the current and future patient' status. The system will process and interpret different vital signs for accurate alerting and signalling of risks and for supporting healthcare professionals in their decision making. Novel and robust pattern recognition algorithms to analyse the correlation between the multi-parametric data will be investigated. New modelling and prediction algorithms will be deployed for diagnosing worsening of conditions and prompting early intervention. New advanced encryption and security algorithms and architectures will be developed and implemented for clinical data and other patient's related data transmission and storage in a cloud environment.

## CONCLUSION

The number of elderly and people diagnosed specifically with chronic diseases is increasing dramatically in all regions in the world. This has a huge impact on the cost, quality and delivery of healthcare services which are changing from the traditional approach to the connected model. We have discussed in this chapter the recent advances in connected health technologies and applications. We have proposed a reconfigurable supporting connected health framework for people diagnosed with chronic diseases using a reconfigurable hardware and intelligent data interpretation and analysis. In addition, a thorough review on the existing information and communications technologies and challenges in the area of connected health including embedded medical devices, sensors, social networking, knowledge management, data fusion and cloud computing is presented in this book chapter. Finally, future directions and ongoing research in the area of connected health are presented. Our current and future research priorities and problem were discussed and an integrated complete solution which deploys embedded intelligent computing, data fusion, knowledge management, social networking and cloud computing is presented. We anticipate that the proposed solution would have an impact on the medical and scientific communities as it would provide automatically and in real-time a full objective assessment on the current and future status of the patient, something that is difficult to achieve.

## ACKNOWLEDGMENT

The authors would like to thank the anonymous reviewers and the editor for their insightful comments and suggestions.

## REFERENCES

*23andMe*. (2013). Retrieved from https://www.23andme.com/

*Actigraph*. (2013). Available from http://www.actigraphcorp.com

Adobe. (2013). *Adobe media server family*. Available at http://www.adobe.com/uk/products/adobe-media-server-family.html

Afzal, M. Hussain M. Khan W. Lee S. and Ahmad H. (2012). Social media canonicalization in healthcare: Smart cdss as an exemplary application. *IEEE 14th Intl. Conf. on e-Health Networking, Applications and Services (HealthCom)*, Oct 2012, pp. 419–422.

*Amazon Simple Storage Service (S3) Documentation*. (2013). Available at http://aws.amazon.com/documentation/s3/

Ayubi, S., & Parmanto, B., & Person, A. (2012). Persuasive social network for physical Activity. In *Proceedings of IEEE Int. Conf. on Engineering in Medicine and Biology Society (EMBC)* (pp. 2153–2157). IEEE.

Benharref, A. (2013). *Novel Cloud and SOA Based Framework for E-health Monitoring Using Wireless Biosensors. IEEE Journal of Biomedical and Health Informatics.*

Bruce, M., Chaczko, Z., & Karatovic, M. (2009). Data Fusion and Aggregation Methods for Pre-Processing Ambulatory Monitoring and Remote Sensor Data for Upload to Personal Electronic Health Records. *International Journal of Digital Content Technology and its Applications, 3*(4), 120-127.

Brzostowski, K., Drapala, J., & Swiatek, J. (2013). Data-Driven Models for eHealth Applications. *International Journal of Computer Science and Artificial Intelligence*, *3*(1), 1–9. doi:10.5963/IJCSAI0301001

Buchmayr, M., & Kurschl, W. (2011). A survey on situation-aware ambient intelligence systems. *Journal of Ambient Intelligence and Humanized Computing*, *2*(3), 175–183. doi:10.1007/s12652-011-0055-1

*CardioNet*. (2013). Retrieved from https://www.cardionet.com/

Chung, W.-Y., Lee, S.-C., & Toh, S.-H. (2008). WSN based mobile u-healthcare system with ecg, blood pressure measurement function. In *Proceedings of IEEE-EMBS 2008. 30th Annual International Conference of the Engineering in Medicine and Biology Society*, (pp. 1533–1536). IEEE.

Constantinescu, L., Kim, J., & Feng, D. D. (2012). SparkMed: A framework for dynamic integration of multimedia medical data into distributed m-Health systems. *IEEE Transactions on Information Technology in Biomedicine*, *16*(1), 40–52. doi:10.1109/TITB.2011.2174064 PMID:22049371

Craig, J., & Patterson, V. (2005). Introduction to the practice of telemedicine. *Journal of Telemedicine and Telecare*, *11*(1), 3–9. doi:10.1258/1357633053430494 PMID:15829036

Detmar, S., Aaronson, N., Wever, L., Muller, M., & Schornagel, J. (2000). How are you feeling? Who wants to know? Patients and oncologists preferences for discussing health-related quality-of-life issues. *Journal of Clinical Oncology*, *18*(18), 3295–3301. PMID:10986063

Di Rienzo, M., Rizzo, F., Parati, G., Brambilla, G., Ferratini, M., & Castiglioni, P. (2005). Magic system: A new textile-based wearable device for biological signal monitoring. applicability in daily life and clinical setting. In *Proceedings of IEEE-EMBS 2005: 27th Annual International Conference of the Engineering in Medicine and Biology Society*, (pp. 7167–7169). IEEE.

Ding, D., Ayubi, S., Hiremath, S., & Parmanto, B. (2012). Physical activity monitoring and sharing platform for manual wheelchair users. In Proceedings of IEEE Intl. Conf. Engineering in Medicine and Biology Society (EMBC) (pp. 5833–5836). IEEE.

Fatima, I., Halder, S., Saleem, M. A., Batool, R., Fahim, M., Lee, Y., & Lee, S. (2013). Smart CDSS: integration of Social Media and Interaction Engine (SMIE) in healthcare for chronic disease patients. *Multimedia Tools and Applications*, 1–21.

Fensli, R., Gunnarson, E., & Gundersen, T. (2005). A wearable ECG-recording system for continuous arrhythmia monitoring in a wireless tele-home-care situation. In *Proceedings of 18th IEEE Symposium on Computer-Based Medical Systems,* (pp. 407–412). IEEE.

Griffin, L., & de Leastar, E. (2009). Social networking healthcare. In *Proceedings of 6th Intl. Workshop on Wearable Micro and Nano Technologies for Personalized Health* (pHealth), (pp. 75–78). pHealth.

Hao, Y., & Foster, R. (2008). Wireless body sensor networks for health-monitoring applications. *Physiological Measurement*, *29*(11), R27–R56. doi:10.1088/0967-3334/29/11/R01 PMID:18843167

He, C., Fan, X., & Li, Y. (2013). Toward ubiquitous healthcare services with a novel efficient cloud platform. *IEEE Transactions on Bio-Medical Engineering*, *60*(1), 230–234. doi:10.1109/TBME.2012.2222404 PMID:23060318

Heilman, K. J., & Porges, S. W. (2007). Accuracy of the lifeshirt® (vivometrics) in the detection of cardiac rhythms. *Biological Psychology*, *75*(3), 300–305. doi:10.1016/j.biopsycho.2007.04.001 PMID:17540493

*Intelsense.* (2013). Retrieved from http://intellisense.io/

ITU. (2013, April). *High efficiency video coding.* ITU-T H.265.

ITU-T, & ISO/IEC. (2010). *Advanced video coding.* ITU-T Rec. H.264 and ISO/IEC 14496-10.

Jin, Z., Oresko, J., Huang, S., & Cheng, A. (2009). Hearttogo: A personalized medicine technology for cardiovascular disease prevention and detection. In *Proceedings of Life Science Systems and Applications Workshop,* (pp. 80–83). IEEE.

Khorakhu, C., & Bhatti, S. (2013). Remote Health Monitoring Using Online Social Media Systems. In *Proceedings of 6th Joint Wireless and Mobile Networking Conference.* Dubai, UAE: IEEE.

Kshetri, N. (2010, October). Cloud Computing in Developing Economies. *IEEE Computer,* 47–55.

Kyriacou, E. C., Pattichis, C. S., Karaolis, M. A., Loizou, C. P., Christodoulou, C. I., & Pattichis, M. S. et al. (2007). An integrated system for assessing stroke risk. *IEEE Engineering in Medicine and Biology Magazine*, *26*(5), 43–50. doi:10.1109/EMB.2007.901794 PMID:17941322

Li, M., Yu, S., Zheng, Y., Ren, K., & Lou, W. (2013). Scalable and Secure Sharing of Personal Health Records in Cloud Computing Using Attribute-Based Encryption. *IEEE Transactions on Parallel and Distributed Systems*, *24*(1), 131–143. doi:10.1109/TPDS.2012.97

*LifeWatch.* (2013). Retrieved from http://www.lifewatch.com/

Lin, H., Shao, J., Zhang, C., & Fang, Y. (2013). CAM: Cloud-Assisted Privacy Preserving Mobile Health Monitoring. *IEEE Transactions on Information Forensics and Security*, *8*(6), 985–997. doi:10.1109/TIFS.2013.2255593

Luprano, J., Sola, J., Dasen, S., Koller, J.-M., & Chetelat, O. (2006). Combination of body sensor networks and on-body signal processing algorithms: the practical case of myheart project. In *Proceedings of International Workshop on Wearable and Implantable Body Sensor Networks,* (pp. 76–79). BSN.

Martín-Martínez, D., Casaseca-de-la Higuera, P., Alberola-López, S., Andrés-de Llano, J., López-Villalobos, J. A., Ardura-Fernández, J., & Alberola-López, C. (2012). Nonlinear analysis of actigraphic signals for the assessment of the attention-deficit/hyperactivity disorder (adhd). *Medical Engineering & Physics*, *34*(9), 1317–1329. doi:10.1016/j.medengphy.2011.12.023 PMID:22297088

*MedApp*. (2013). Retrieved from https://health-com.medapps.net/Login.aspx

*MedHelp*. (2013). Retrieved from http://www.medhelp.org/

Megalooikonomou, V., & Kontos, D. (2007). Medical Data Fusion for Telemedicine. *IEEE Engineering in Medicine and Biology Magazine, 26*(5), 36-42.

Milenković, A., Otto, C., & Jovanov, E. (2006). Wireless sensor networks for personal health monitoring: Issues and an implementation. *Computer Communications*, *29*(13–14), 2521–2533. doi:10.1016/j.comcom.2006.02.011

Mirota, D. J., Wang, H., Taylor, R. H., Ishii, M., Gallia, G. L., & Hager, G. D. (2012). A system for video-based navigation for endoscopic endonasal skull base surgery. *IEEE Transactions on Medical Imaging*, *31*(4), 963–976. doi:10.1109/TMI.2011.2176500 PMID:22113772

Nicolini, D., Powell, J., Conville, P., & Martinez-Solano, L. (2008). Managing knowledge in the healthcare sector. A review. *International Journal of Management Reviews*, *10*, 245–263. doi:10.1111/j.1468-2370.2007.00219.x

Nightingale, J., Wang, Q., & Grecos, C. (2012). HEVStream: a framework for streaming and evaluation of high efficiency video coding (HEVC) content in loss-prone networks. *IEEE Transactions on Consumer Electronics*, *58*(2), 404–412. doi:10.1109/TCE.2012.6227440

Nilakanta, S., Miller, L., Peer, A., & Bojja, V. M. (2009). Contribution of Knowledge and Knowledge Management Capability on Business Processes among Healthcare Organizations. In *Proceedings of System Sciences*. IEEE.

Norval, C., Arnott, J., Hine, N., & Hanson, V. (2011). Purposeful social media as support platform: Communication frameworks for older adults requiring care. In *Proceedings of 5th International Conference on Pervasive Computing Technologies for Healthcare (PervasiveHealth)*, (pp. 492–494). Academic Press.

Oliver, N., & Flores-Mangas, F. (2006). Healthgear: A real-time wearable system for monitoring and analyzing physiological signals. In *Proceedings of International Workshop on Wearable and Implantable Body Sensor Networks,* (pp. 1-4). BSN.

Panayides, A., Pattichis, M. S., Pattichis, C. S., & Pitsillides, A. (2011). A tutorial for emerging wireless medical video transmission systems. *IEEE Antennas and Propagation Magazine*, *53*(2), 202–213. doi:10.1109/MAP.2011.5949369

Pandian, P., Mohanavelu, K., Safeer, K., Kotresh, T., Shakunthala, D., Gopal, P., & Padaki, V. (2008). Smart vest: Wearable multi-parameter remote physiological monitoring system. *Medical Engineering & Physics*, *30*(4), 466–477. doi:10.1016/j.medengphy.2007.05.014 PMID:17869159

Pantelopoulos, A., & Bourbakis, N. (2010). A survey on wearable sensor-based systems for health monitoring and prognosis. *IEEE Transactions on Systems, Man and Cybernetics. Part C, Applications and Reviews*, *40*(1), 1–12. doi:10.1109/TSMCC.2009.2032660

Paradiso, R., Loriga, G., & Taccini, N. (2005). A wearable healthcare system based on knitted integrated sensors. *IEEE Transactions on Information Technology in Biomedicine*, *9*(3), 337–344. doi:10.1109/TITB.2005.854512 PMID:16167687

*Patientlikeme.* (2013). Retrieved from http://www.patientslikeme.com/

*Polar UK.* (2013). Available http://www.polar.com/uk-en

Sakr, S., Liu, A., Batista, D. M., & Alomari, M. (2011). A Survey of Large Scale Data Management Approaches in Cloud Environments. *IEEE Communications Surveys & Tutorials, 13*(3), 311–336. doi:10.1109/SURV.2011.032211.00087

Scanfeld, D., Scanfeld, V., & Larson, E. (2010). Dissemination of health information through social networks: Twitter and antibiotics. *American Journal of Infection Control, 38*(3), 182–188. doi:10.1016/j.ajic.2009.11.004 PMID:20347636

Scilingo, E., Gemignani, A., Paradiso, R., Taccini, N., Ghelarducci, B., & De Rossi, D. (2005). Performance evaluation of sensing fabrics for monitoring physiological and biomechanical variables. *IEEE Transactions on Information Technology in Biomedicine, 9*(3), 345–352. doi:10.1109/TITB.2005.854506 PMID:16167688

Scully, C. G., Lee, J., Meyer, J., Gorbach, A. M., Granquist-Fraser, D., Mendelson, Y., & Chon, K. H. (2012). Physiological parameter monitoring from optical recordings with a mobile phone. *IEEE Transactions on* Biomedical Engineering, *59*(2), 303–306.

Shaw, E., Ruby, K., and Post, J. (1998). The insider threat to information systems: the psychology of the dangerous insider. *Security Awareness Bulletin, 2*(98), 1–10.

Sheffield, J. (2008). Inquiry in health knowledge management. *Journal of Knowledge Management, 12*, 160–172. doi:10.1108/13673270810884327

Sheth, A. (2010). Computing for Human Experience: Semantics-Empowered Sensors, Services, and Social Computing on the Ubiquitous Web. *IEEE Internet Computing, 14*(1), 88–91. doi:10.1109/MIC.2010.4

Sheth, A., Anantharam, P., & Henson, C. (2013). Physical-Cyber-Social Computing: An Early 21st Century Approach. IEEE Intelligent Systems, 78-82.

*Shimmer*. (2013). Available: http://www.shimmersensing.com/

Silva, B. B., Lopes, I., Rodrigues, J., & Ray, P. (2011). SapoFitness: A mobile health application for dietary evaluation. In *Proceedings of 13th IEEE Intl. Conf. on e-Health Networking Applications and Services (HealthCom)*, (pp. 375–380). IEEE.

Skubic, M., Alexander, G., Popescu, M., Rantz, M., & Keller, J. (2009). A smart home application to eldercare: Current status and lessons learned. *Technology and Healthcare, 17*(3), 183–201. PMID:19641257

Sullivan, G. J., Ohm, J., Han, W.-J., & Wiegand, T. (2012). Overview of the high efficiency video coding (HEVC) standard. *IEEE Transactions on Circuits and Systems for Video Technology, 22*(12), 1649–1668. doi:10.1109/TCSVT.2012.2221191

Sung, M., Marci, C., & Pentland, A. (2005). Wearable feedback systems for rehabilitation. *Journal of Neuroengineering and Rehabilitation, 2*, 17. doi:10.1186/1743-0003-2-17 PMID:15987514

UN. (2013). *Department of Economic and Social Affairs: Population Division: Population database*. UN.

Van Gorp, P., & Comuzzi, M. (2013). *Lifelong Personal Health Data and Application Software via Virtual Machines in the Cloud. IEEE Journal of Biomedical and Health Informatics.*

Video LAN. (2013). *VLC media player*. Available at http://www.videolan.org/vlc/index.html

Viswanathan, H., Chen, B., & Pompili, D. (2012). Research challenges in computation, communication, and context awareness for ubiquitous healthcare. *IEEE Communications Magazine, 50*(5), 92–99. doi:10.1109/MCOM.2012.6194388

Wang, Q., Nightingale, J., Wang, R., Ramzan, N., Grecos, C., & Wang, X. et al. (in press). Mobile Video Cloud Networks. In J. Rodrigues, K. Lin, & J. Lloret (Eds.), *Mobile Computing over Cloud: Technologies, Services, and Applications*. IGI Global. doi:10.4018/978-1-4666-4781-7.ch009

Wolf, P., Schmidt, A., & Klein, M. (2008). *SOPRANO-An extensible, open AAL platform for elderly people based on semantical contracts*. Paper presented at the 3rd Workshop on Artificial Intelligence Techniques for Ambient Intelligence (AITAmI'08), 18th European Conference on Artificial Intelligence (ECAI 08). Patras, Greece.

Wood, A., Stankovic, J., Virone, G., Selavo, L., He, Z., & Cao, Q. et al. (2008). Context-aware wireless sensor networks for assisted living and residential monitoring. *IEEE Network*, *22*(4), 26–33. doi:10.1109/MNET.2008.4579768

World, W. P. P. (2003). The 2002 Revision, Highlights (Report No.: ESA/P/WP. 180). New York: United Nations Population Division.

*Wowza*. (2013). Available at http://www.wowza.com/

Yan, H., Huo, H., Xu, Y., & Gidlund, M. (2010). Wireless sensor network based E-health system implementation and experimental results. *IEEE Transactions on* Consumer Electronics, *56*(4), 2288–2295.

Yang, C., Tsai, C., Member, S., Cheng, K., & Chen, S. (2012). Low-Invasive Implantable Devices of Low-Power Consumption Using High-Efficiency Antennas for Cloud Healthcare. *IEEE Journal on Emerging and Selected Topics in Circuits and Systems*, *2*(1), 14–23. doi:10.1109/JETCAS.2012.2187469

*Zephyr Inc*. (2013). Available: http://www.zephyranywhere.com/

## KEY TERMS AND DEFINITIONS

**Cloud Security:** Cloud security issues such as data protection, privacy, trust/identity management, authentication/authorisation/accounting in a cloud and inter-clouds.

**Cloud-Based Video Applications:** Video applications that utilise the resources provided by a cloud.

**Connected Health:** The convergence of medical, security and communication devices. Systems which can be used for remote monitoring.

**Data Fusion:** The process of integration of multiple data acquired from different medical sensors, social networks and other information sources.

**Knowledge Management:** Comprises a range of strategies and practices used in the organisation, representation, and distribution, of medical data.

**Mobile Cloud Computing:** Cloud computing for mobile users.

**Reconfigurable Hardware:** Type of hardware which can be customised once or as much as needed, usually in the form of field programmable gate arrays.

**Social Networking:** Platforms to build social networks or social relations among people who, in our case, share experiences, interests, activities, or backgrounds, in healthcare.

# Compilation of References


*23andMe*. (2013). Retrieved from https://www.23andme.com/

Abbasi, A., Hossain, L., Uddin, S., & Rasmussen, K. J. R. (2011). Evolutionary dynamics of scientific collaboration networks: multi-levels and cross-time analysis. *Scientometrics*, *89*(2), 687–710. doi:10.1007/s11192-011-0463-1

Abbasi, A., Uddin, S., & Hossain, L. (2012). Socio-economic analysis of patient-centric networks: effects of patients and hospitals' characteristics and network structure on hospitalization costs. *The European Journal of Health Economics*, *13*(3), 267–276. doi:10.1007/s10198-011-0303-5 PMID:21347691

Abidi, S. R. (2008). A Conceptual Framework for Ontology Based Automating and Merging of Clinical Pathways of Comorbidities. *K4HelP, 5626*, 55-66.

Abidi, S. R. (2011). *Ontology-based knowledge modeling to provide decision support for comorbid diseases*. Paper presented at the 19th European Conference in Artificial Intelligence. Retrieved from http://www.scopus.com/inward/record.url?eid=2-s2.0-79952016090&partnerID=40&md5=d6e8e7441e3e9118fa395e5fc0b77b95

Abidi, S. S. R. (2001). Knowledge management in healthcare: towards 'knowledge-driven' decision-support services. *International Journal of Medical Informatics*, *63*(1-2), 5–18. doi:10.1016/S1386-5056(01)00167-8 PMID:11518661

ABS. (2011). *Population Projections, Australia, 2006 to 2101*. Canberra: Australian Bureau of Statistics.

ABS. (2013). *Australian Demographics Statistics, Mar 2013*. Canberra: Australian Bureau of Statistics.

*Actigraph*. (2013). Available from http://www.actigraphcorp.com

Adam Mahmood, M. O., Burn, J. M., Gemoets, L. A., & Jacquez, C. (2000). Variables affecting information technology end-user satisfaction: a meta-analysis of the empirical literature. *International Journal of Human-Computer Studies*, *52*(4), 751–771. doi:10.1006/ijhc.1999.0353

Adobe. (2013). *Adobe media server family*. Available at http://www.adobe.com/uk/products/adobe-media-server-family.html

Afzal, M. Hussain M. Khan W. Lee S. and Ahmad H. (2012). Social media canonicalization in healthcare: Smart cdss as an exemplary application. *IEEE 14th Intl. Conf. on e-Health Networking, Applications and Services (HealthCom)*, Oct 2012, pp. 419–422.

Ahmedani, B. K., Harold, R. D., Fitton, V. A., & Shifflet Gibson, E. D. (2011, October). What Adolescents Can Tell Us: Technology and the Future of Social Work Education. *Social Work Education*, *30*(7), 830–846. doi:10.1080/02615479.2010.504767

Ahuja, M., Galletta, D., & Carley, K. (2003). Individual centrality and performance in virtual R&D groups: An empirical study. *Management Science*, *49*(1), 21–38. doi:10.1287/mnsc.49.1.21.12756

AIHW. (2010). *Residential aged care in Australia 2008-09: a statistical overview Aged care statistics series no. 31 (Vol. AGE 62)*. Canberra: Australian Institute of Health and Welfare.

AIHW. (2012). *Health expenditure Australia 2010-11 Health and welfare expenditure series no. 47 (Vol. HWE 56)*. Canberra: Australian Institute of Health and Welfare.

AIHW. (2013a). *Australian trends in life expectancy*. Canberra: Australian Institute of Health and Welfare.

AIHW. (2013b). *Life expectancy*. Canberra: Australian Institute of Health and Welfare.

*AI Topics*. (2014). Retrieved February 28, 2014 from http://aitopics.org/

Ajzen, I. (1985). From Intentions to Actions: A Theory of Planned Behavior. In J. Kuhl, & J. Beckmann (Eds.), *Action Control* (pp. 11–39). Springer. doi:10.1007/978-3-642-69746-3_2

Ajzen, I. (1989). Attitude, structure, influence and role expectations on shopping center patronage intentions. *Journal of the Academy of Marketing Science*, *24*(3), 208–218.

Ajzen, I. (1991). The theory of planned behavior. *Organizational Behavior and Human Decision Processes*, *50*(2), 179–211. doi:10.1016/0749-5978(91)90020-T

Akerstedt, T., & Nilsson, P. M. (2003). Sleep as restitution: an introduction. *Journal of Internal Medicine*, *254*(1), 6–12. doi:10.1046/j.1365-2796.2003.01195.x PMID:12823638

Al-adwane, A., & Smedley, J. (2012). Implementing e-learning in the Jordanian Higher Education System: Factors affecting impact. *International Journal of Education and Development using Information and Communication Technology*, *8*(1), 121-135.

Albirini, A. (2006). Teachers' Attitudes toward Information and Communication Technology: The case of Syrian EFL Teachers. *Computers & Education*, *47*(4), 373–398. doi:10.1016/j.compedu.2004.10.013

Albu, J., Sohler, N., Matti-Orozco, B., Sill, J., Baxter, D., Burke, G., & Young, E. (2013). Expansion of electronic health record-based screening, prevention, and management of diabetes in New York City. *Preventing Chronic Disease*, *10*, E13. doi:10.5888/pcd10.120148 PMID:23369766

Alizadehsani, et al. (2013). A data mining approach for diagnosis of coronary artery disease. *Computer Methods and Programs in Biomedicine*, *111*(1), 52–61. doi:10.1016/j.cmpb.2013.03.004 PMID:23537611

Almond, H., Cummings, E., & Turner, P. (2013). Australia's personally controlled electronic health record and primary healthcare: Generating a framework for implementation and evaluation. *Studies in Health Technology and Informatics*, *188*, 1–6. PMID:23823280

Alonso Díaz, L., & Blázquez Entonado, F. (2009). Are the Functions of Teachers in e-Learning and Face-to-Face Learning Environments Really Different? *Journal of Educational Technology & Society*, *12*(4), 331–343.

Alonso, F., Caraca-Valente, P. J., Gonzalez, A. L., & Montes, C. (2002). Combining expert knowledge and data mining in a medical diagnosis domain. *Expert Systems with Applications*, *23*(4), 367–375. doi:10.1016/S0957-4174(02)00072-6

Alshawi, M. (2007). *Rethinking IT in construction and engineering: Organisational readiness*. Psychology Press.

Alzougool, B., Chang, S., & Gray, K. (2008). Towards a comprehensive understanding of health information needs. *Electronic Journal of Health Informatics*, *3*(2), e15.

*Amazon Simple Storage Service (S3) Documentation*. (2013). Available at http://aws.amazon.com/documentation/s3/

American Nurses Association. (2008). Nursing informatics: Scope and standards of practice. Author.

Ammenwerth, E., Iller, C., & Mahler, C. (2006). IT-adoption and the interaction of task, technology and individuals: a fit framework and a case study. *BMC Medical Informatics and Decision Making*, *6*(1), 3. doi:10.1186/1472-6947-6-3 PMID:16401336

Andrews, J. (2013). Seniors on the move: As media technology has advanced, so have programs for seniors' improved well-being. Assisted Living, 11(5).

Anselma, L., Bottrighi, A., Molino, G., Montani, S., Terenziani, P., & Torchio, M. (2011). Supporting knowledge-based decision making in the medical context: The glare approach. *International Journal of Knowledge-Based Organizations*, *1*(1), 42–60. doi:10.4018/ijkbo.2011010103

Anselma, L., Bottrighi, A., Montani, S., & Terenziani, P. (2013). Extending bcdm to cope with proposals and evaluations of updates. *IEEE Transactions on Knowledge and Data Engineering*, *25*(3), 556–570. doi:10.1109/TKDE.2011.170

Anselma, L., Terenziani, P., Montani, S., & Bottrighi, A. (2006). Towards a comprehensive treatment of repetitions, periodicity and temporal constraints in clinical guidelines. *Artificial Intelligence in Medicine*, *38*(2), 171–195. doi:10.1016/j.artmed.2006.03.007 PMID:16766167

Anttiroiko, A. & Kallio, O. (1999). *Johdon tietojärjestelmät kunnallishallinnossa. [Management software in municipal administration]*. Tampere: Tampereen yliopisto.

Anttonen, A., & Sipilä, J. (1996). European Social Care Services: Is It Possible To Identify Models? *Journal of European Social Policy*, *6*(2), 87–100. doi:10.1177/095892879600600201

Aral, K. D., Guvenir, H. A., Sabuncuoglu, I., & Akar, A. R. (2012). A prescription fraud detection model. *Computer Methods and Programs in Biomedicine*, *106*(1), 37–46. doi:10.1016/j.cmpb.2011.09.003 PMID:22088866

Arbuthnott, A., & Sharpe, D. (2009). The effect of physician-patient collaboration on patient adherence in non-psychiatric medicine. *Patient Education and Counseling*, *77*(1), 60–67. doi:10.1016/j.pec.2009.03.022 PMID:19395222

Arts, D. G., Bosman, R. J., de Jonge, E., Joore, J. C., & de Keizer, N. F. (2003). Training in data definitions improves quality of intensive care data. *Critical Care (London, England)*, *7*(2), 179–184. doi:10.1186/cc1886 PMID:12720565

Arts, D. G., De Keizer, N. F., & Scheffer, G. J. (2002). Defining and improving data quality in medical registries: a literature review, case study, and generic framework. *Journal of the American Medical Informatics Association*, *9*(6), 600–611. doi:10.1197/jamia.M1087 PMID:12386111

Arts, D., de Keizer, N., Scheffer, G. J., & de Jonge, E. (2002). Quality of data collected for severity of illness scores in the Dutch National Intensive Care Evaluation (NICE) registry. *Intensive Care Medicine*, *28*(5), 656–659. doi:10.1007/s00134-002-1272-z PMID:12029418

Asada, H. H., Shaltis, P., Reisner, A., Sokwoo, R., & Hutchinson, R. C. (2003). Mobile monitoring with wearable photoplethysmographic biosensors. *Engineering in Medicine and Biology Magazine, IEEE*, *22*(3), 28–40. doi:10.1109/MEMB.2003.1213624 PMID:12845817

Ash, J., Kilo, C. M., Shapiro, M., Wasserman, J., McMullen, C., & Hersh, W. (2011). *Roadmap for Provision of Safer Healthcare Information Systems: Preventing e-Iatrogenesis*. Institute of Medicine.

Askeland, G. A., & Payne, M. (1999). Authors and audiences: towards a sociology of case recording. *European Journal of Social Work*, *2*(1), 55–65. doi:10.1080/13691459908413805

Askim, J., Fimreite, A. L., Moseley, A., & Holm Pedersen, L. (2011). One-stop shops for social welfare: the adaptation of an organizational form in three countries. *Public Administration*, *89*(4), 1451–1468. doi:10.1111/j.1467-9299.2011.01933.x

Australian e-health standards. (2010). *Electronic Health Record Interoperability*. Available at http://www.e-health.standards.org.au/IT014SubjectAreas/EHRInteroperability.aspx

Australian Institute of Health and Welfare (AIHW). (2012). *Residential aged care in Australia 2010-11: a statistical overview, Aged care statistics series no. 36, Cat. No. AGE 68*. Canberra: AIHW.

Australian Institute of Health and Welfare 2005. *National Community Services Information Strategic Plan 2005-09*. Retrieved April 12, 2011, from http://www.aihw.gov.au/publication-detail/?id=6442467798

Australian Institute of Health and Welfare. (2013). In National Health Priority Areas. Retrieved May 1, 2013, from http://www.aihw.gov.au/national-health-priority-areas/

Australian Medical Workforce Advisory Committee. (2000). *The Specialist Thoracic Medicine Workforce In Australia*. Retrieved 31 March 2008, from http://www5.health.nsw.gov.au/amwac/amwac/pdf/thoracic_medicine_2000.1.pdf

Avison, D., Lau, F., Myers, M., & Nielsen, P. A. (1999). Action Research. *Communications of the ACM*, *42*(1), 94–97. doi:10.1145/291469.291479

Ayubi, S., & Parmanto, B., & Person, A. (2012). Persuasive social network for physical Activity. In *Proceedings of IEEE Int. Conf. on Engineering in Medicine and Biology Society (EMBC)* (pp. 2153–2157). IEEE.

Azaouagh, A., & Stausberg, J. (2008). Frequency of hospital-acquired pneumonia--comparison between electronic and paper-based patient records. *Pneumologie (Stuttgart, Germany)*, *62*(5), 273–278. doi:10.1055/s-2008-1038099 PMID:18270924

Bacheldor, B. (2006, October). RFID Fills Security Gap at Psychiatric Ward. *RFID Journal.*

Bacheldor, B. (2007, August). RFID documents surgery at Huntsville hospital. *RFID Journal.*

Bagozzi, R., & Yi, Y. (1988). On the evaluation of structural equation models. *Journal of the Academy of Marketing Science*, *16*(1), 74–94. doi:10.1007/BF02723327

Bailey, C., & Clarke, M. (2001). Managing knowledge for personal and organizational benefit. *Journal of Knowledge Management*, *5*(1), 58. doi:10.1108/13673270110384400

Baldwin, G., & Larkin, M. (2008, January). Where did we put that wheelchair?. *Technology, HealthLeaders*, 33-34.

Ballantyne, D. (2000). Internal relationship marketing: A strategy for knowledge renewal. *International Journal of Bank Marketing*, *18*(6), 274. doi:10.1108/02652320010358698

Barchini, G., Álvarez, M., & Herrera, S. (2006). Sistemas de información: Nuevos escenarios basados en ontologías/ information systems: New ontology-based scenarios. *Journal of Information Systems and Technology Management*, *3*(1), 2–18. doi:10.4301/S1807-17752006000100001

Barcy, W. R., & Barcy, R. T. (2008). The Relationship of Computer Attitudes to Reported Use and Observed Behavioural Proficiency. *Journal of Technology in Human Services*, *26*(1), 19–44. doi:10.1300/J017v26n01_02

Baron, R. M., & Kenny, D. A. (1986). The moderator-mediator variable distinction in social psychological research: Conceptual, strategic, and statistical considerations. *Journal of Personality and Social Psychology*, *51*(6), 1173–1182. doi:10.1037/0022-3514.51.6.1173 PMID:3806354

Barr, H., Freeth, D., Hammick, M., Koppel, I., & Reeves, S. (2002). *Evaluating interprofessional education: a United Kingdom review of health and social care*. London, UK: Centre for the Advancement of Interprofessional Education.

Bavelas, A. (1950). Communication patterns in task-oriented groups. *The Journal of the Acoustical Society of America*, *22*, 725–730. doi:10.1121/1.1906679

Baxter, G., & Sommerville, I. (2011). Socio-technical systems: From design methods to systems engineering. *Interacting with Computers*, *23*(1), 4–17. doi:10.1016/j.intcom.2010.07.003

Beauchamp, M. (1965). An improved index of centrality. *Behavioral Science*, *10*(2), 161–163. doi:10.1002/bs.3830100205 PMID:14284290

Bellazzi, R., Ferrazzi, F., & Sacchi, L. (2011). Predictive data mining in clinical medicine: a focus on selected methods and applications. *WIREs Data Mining and Knowledge Discovery*, *1*(5), 416–430. doi:10.1002/widm.23

Bellazzi, R., & Zupan, B. (2008). Predictive data mining in clinical medicine: Current issues and guidelines. *International Journal of Medical Informatics*, *77*(2), 81–97. doi:10.1016/j.ijmedinf.2006.11.006 PMID:17188928

Benharref, A. (2013). *Novel Cloud and SOA Based Framework for E-health Monitoring Using Wireless Biosensors. IEEE Journal of Biomedical and Health Informatics.*

Bennett, C. C., Doub, T. W., & Selove, R. (2012). EHRs connect research and practice: Where predictive modeling, artificial intelligence, and clinical decision support intersect. *Health Policy and Technology*, *1*(2), 105–114. doi:10.1016/j.hlpt.2012.03.001

Benzie, D. (1995). IFIP Working group 3.5: Using computers to support young learners. In J.D. Tinsley & T.J. van Weert (Eds.), *World Conference on Computers in Education VI: WCCE' 95 Liberating the Learner* (pp. 35-42). Chapman & Hall.

Berdichevsky, D., & Neuenschwander, E. (1999). Toward an Ethics of Persuasive Technology. *Communications of the ACM*, *42*(5).

Bergeron, F., & Raymond, L. (1992). Evaluation of EIS from a managerial perspective1. *Information Systems Journal*, *2*(1), 45–60. doi:10.1111/j.1365-2575.1992.tb00066.x

Bergersen, B. (2004). User satisfaction and influencing issues. *Network and System Administration Research Surveys*, *1*, 5–26.

Bergrath, S., Ro¨rtgen, D., Rossaint, R., Beckers, S. K., Fischermann, H., & Brokmann, J. C. et al. (2011). Technical and organisational feasibility of a multifunctional telemedicine system in an emergency medical service - an observational study. *Journal of Telemedicine and Telecare*, *17*(7), 371–377. doi:10.1258/jtt.2011.110203 PMID:21933897

Berman, Y., Eaglestein, A. S., & Phillips, D. (1995). Policy Impact on Information Technology Programming in the Social Services. *Knowledge and Policy*, *8*(1), 23–32. doi:10.1007/BF02698554

Bernat, J. L. (2013). Ethical and quality pitfalls in electronic health records. *Neurology, 80*(11), 1057-61 doi: 10.1212/WNL.0b013e318287288c.

Bertea, P. (2009). Measuring students' attitude towards e-learning: A case study. In *Proceedings of 5th International Scientific Conference*. Elearning and Software for Education.

Bian, J., Topaloglu, U., & Yu, F. (2012). Towards large-scale twitter mining for drug-related adverse events. In *Proceedings of the International Workshop on Smart Health and Wellbeing*, (pp. 25-32). Hawaii, HI: IEEE. doi:10.1145/2389707.2389713

Biljon, J. v., & Kotz, P. (2007). *Modelling the factors that influence mobile phone adoption*. Paper presented at the 2007 annual research conference of the South African institute of computer scientists and information technologists on IT research in developing countries. New York, NY.

Billipp, S. H. (2001). The psychosocial impact of interactive computer use within a vulnerable elderly population: A report on a randomized prospective trial in a home health care setting. *Public Health Nursing (Boston, Mass.)*, *18*(2), 138–145. doi:10.1046/j.1525-1446.2001.00138.x PMID:11285108

Binney, D. (2000). The knowledge management spectrum-understanding the KM landscape. *Journal of Knowledge Management*, *5*(1), 21–32.

Blair, D. C. (2002). Knowledge Management: Hype, Hope or Help? *Journal of the American Society for Information Science and Technology*, *53*(12), 1019. doi:10.1002/asi.10113

Blaschke, C. M., Freddolino, P. P., & Mullen, E. E. (2009). Ageing and Technology: A Review of the Research Literature. *British Journal of Social Work*, *39*(4), 641–656. doi:10.1093/bjsw/bcp025

Bliernel, M., & Hassanein, K. (2004). E-health: applying business process reengineering principles to healthcare in Canada. *International Journal of Electronic Business*, *2*(6), 625–643. doi:10.1504/IJEB.2004.006129

Blobel, B. (2005). Advances in secure and architectural EHR approaches. *International Journal of Medical Informatics*, *75*(3-4), 185–190. Epub 2005 Aug 19 doi:10.1016/j.ijmedinf.2005.07.017 PMID:16112891

Bolton, L. B., Gassert, C. A., & Cipriano, P. F. (2008). Technology solutions can make nursing care safer and more efficient. *Journal of Healthcare Information Management*, *22*(4), 24–30. PMID:19267016

Bonacich, P. (1991). Simultaneous group and individual centralities. *Social Networks*, *13*(2), 155–168. doi:10.1016/0378-8733(91)90018-O

Borgman, M., Kemppainen, T., Mäntysaari, M., Pohjola, A. & Vuorensyrjä, M. (2005). *Sosiaalialan osaamis-, työvoima- ja koulutustarpeiden ennakointihanke.* [*Foresight of know-how, workforce and educational needs of social care*]. Helsinki: Sosiaali- ja terveysministeriö.

Bottrighi, A., Giordano, L., Molino, G., Montani, S., Terenziani, P., & Torchio, M. (2010). Adopting model checking techniques for clinical guidelines verification. *Artificial Intelligence in Medicine*, *48*(1), 1–19. doi:10.1016/j.artmed.2009.09.003 PMID:19864118

Boyd, D. (2008). Facebook's Privacy Trainwreck. *Convergence: The International Journal of Research into New Media Technologies*, *14*(1), 13–20. doi:10.1177/1354856507084416

Brand, N., & Kolk, H. V. D. (1995). *Workflow Analysis and Design*. Kluwer.

Brandtzæg, P. B., Lüders, M., & Skjetne, J. H. (2010). Too many Facebook "friends"? Content sharing and sociability versus the need for privacy in social network sites. *International Journal of Human-Computer Interaction, 26*(11-12), 1006–1030. doi:10.1080/10447318.2010.516719

Brank, J., Grobelnik, M., & D., M. (2005). *A survey of ontology evaluation techniques*. Paper presented at the 8th Int. Multi-Conf. Information Society. New York, NY.

Brass, D. (1981). Structural relationships, job characteristics, and worker satisfaction and performance. *Administrative Science Quarterly, 26*(3), 331–348. doi:10.2307/2392511

Brass, D. (1985). Technology and the structuring of jobs: Employee satisfaction, performance, and influence. *Organizational Behavior and Human Decision Processes, 35*(2), 216–240. doi:10.1016/0749-5978(85)90036-6

*BraveHeart*. (2014). Retrieved February 28, 2014 from http://braveheartveterans.org/

Brewster, C., Alani, H., Dasmahapatra, S., & Wilks, Y. (2004). *Data Driven Ontology Evaluation*. Paper presented at the International Conference on Language Resources and Evaluation. Retrieved from http://eprints.soton.ac.uk/259062/

Britt, H., Miller, G., & Bayrarn, C. (2007). The quality of data on general practice - A discussion of BEACH reliability and validity. *Australian Family Physician, 36*(1-2), 36–40. PMID:17252082

Brosnan, M. J. (1998). The impact of computer anxiety and self-efficacy upon performance. *Journal of Computer Assisted Learning, 14*(3), 223–234. doi:10.1046/j.1365-2729.1998.143059.x

Brossette, S. E., Hymel P. A. (2008). Data mining and infection control. *Clinics in Laboratory Medicine, 28*(1), 119–126.

Bruce, M., Chaczko, Z., & Karatovic, M. (2009). Data Fusion and Aggregation Methods for Pre-Processing Ambulatory Monitoring and Remote Sensor Data for Upload to Personal Electronic Health Records. *International Journal of Digital Content Technology and its Applications, 3*(4), 120-127.

Brüggemann, S., & Grüning, F. (2009). Using ontologies providing domain knowledge for data quality management. *Studies in Computational Intelligence, 221*, 187–203. doi:10.1007/978-3-642-02184-8_13

Brzostowski, K., Drapala, J., & Swiatek, J. (2013). Data-Driven Models for eHealth Applications. *International Journal of Computer Science and Artificial Intelligence, 3*(1), 1–9. doi:10.5963/IJCSAI0301001

Buabeng-Andoh, C. (2012). Factors influencing teachers'adoption and integration of information and communication technology into teaching: A review of the literature. *International Journal of Education and Development using Information and Communication Technology, 8*(1), 136-155.

Buchanan, D. (1998). Representing process: the contribution of a re-engineering frame. *International Journal of Operations & Production Management, 18*(12), 1163–1188. doi:10.1108/01443579810236610

Buchanan, T. (2003). Internet-based questionnaire assessment: Appropriate use in clinical contexts. *Cognitive Behaviour Therapy, 32*(3), 100–109. doi:10.1080/16506070310000957 PMID:16291542

Buchmayr, M., & Kurschl, W. (2011). A survey on situation-aware ambient intelligence systems. *Journal of Ambient Intelligence and Humanized Computing, 2*(3), 175–183. doi:10.1007/s12652-011-0055-1

Bullock, D. (2004). Moving from theory to practice: An examination of the factors that pre-service teachers encounter as they attempt to gain experience teaching with technology during field placement experiences. *Journal of Technology and Teacher Education, 12*(2), 221–237.

Buranarach, M., Chalortham, N., Chatvorawit, P., Thein, Y., & Supnithi, T. (2009). *An Ontology-based Framework for Development of Clinical Reminder System to Support Chronic Disease Healthcare*. Retrieved from http://text.hlt.nectec.or.th/ontology/sites/default/files/reminder_isbme09_cr_0.pdf

Burgess, H. (2004). Redesigning the Curriculum for Social Work Education: Complexity, Conformity, Chaos, Creativity, Collaboration? *Social Work Education*, *23*(2), 163–183. doi:10.1080/0261547042000209189

Burns, L. R., & Muller, R. W. (2008). Hospital-Physician Collaboration: Landscape of Economic Integration and Impact on Clinical Integration. *The Milbank Quarterly*, *86*(3), 375–434. doi:10.1111/j.1468-0009.2008.00527.x PMID:18798884

Burnum, J. F. (1989). The misinformation era: The fall of the Medical Record. *Annals of Internal Medicine*, *110*, 482–484. doi:10.7326/0003-4819-110-6-482 PMID:2919852

Burton, J., & van den Broek, D. (2009). Accountable and Countable: Information Managements Systems and the Bureaucratization of Social Work. *British Journal of Social Work*, *39*(7), 1326–1342. doi:10.1093/bjsw/bcn027

Cainelli, G., Maggioni, M. A., Uberti, T. E., & De Felice, A. (2010). *The strength of strong ties: Co-authorship and productivity among Italian economists*. University of Padova.

Calongne, C. M. (2001). Designing for web site usability. *Journal of Computing Sciences in Colleges*, *16*(3).

Cao, L. (2010). Domain-driven data mining: challenges and prospects. *IEEE Transactions on Knowledge and Data Engineering*, *22*(6), 755–769. doi:10.1109/TKDE.2010.32

Cao, L., Yu, S. P., Zhang, C., & Zhao, Y. (2010). *Domain driven data mining*. Springer. doi:10.1007/978-1-4419-5737-5

*CardioNet*. (2013). Retrieved from https://www.cardionet.com/

Cardozo, R. N. (1965). An experimental study of customer effort, expectation, and satisfaction. *JMR, Journal of Marketing Research*, 244–249. doi:10.2307/3150182

Carlbring, P., Brunt, S., Bohman, S., Austin, D., Richards, J., Öst, L.-G., & Andersson, G. (2007). Internet vs. paper and pencil administration of questionnaires commonly used in panic/agoraphobia research. *Computers in Human Behavior*, *23*(3), 1421–1434. doi:10.1016/j.chb.2005.05.002

Carrilio, T. E. (2007). Using Client Information Systems in Practice Settings: Factors Affecting Social Workers´ Use of Information Systems. *Journal of Technology in Human Services*, *25*(4), 41–62. doi:10.1300/J017v25n04_03

Cartwright, C., Sankaran, S., & Kelly, J. (2008). *Developing a New Leadership Framework for Not-For-Profit Health and Community Care Organisations in Australia*. Lismore, Australia: Southern Cross University.

Cases, et al. (2013). Improving data and knowledge management to better integrate health care and research. *Journal of Internal Medicine*, *274*(4), 321–328. doi:10.1111/joim.12105 PMID:23808970

Cavoukian, A. (2008). *RFID and Privacy - Guidance for Health Care Providers- A report*. January, Canada: Information Privacy Commissioner of Ontario and Hewlett Packard Company.

*CEN. ISO 13606 standard. The EN 13606 Association*. (2009-2011). Retrieved September 29, 2013 from www.en13606.org

Cha, M., Haddadi, H., Benevenuto, F., & Gummandi, K. P. (2010). Measuring User Influence in Twitter: The Million Follower Fallacy. In *Proceedings of the 4th International AAAI Conference on Weblogs and Social Media (ICWSM)*, (pp. 10-17). Washington, DC: ICWSM. doi:10.1.1.167.192

Chae, Y., Kim, H., Tark, H., Park, H., & Ho, S. (2003). Analysis of healthcare quality indicator using data mining and decision support system. *Expert Systems with Applications*, *24*(2), 167–172. doi:10.1016/S0957-4174(02)00139-2

*Chatbots* . (2014). Retrieved February 28, 2014 from http://www.chatbots.org/

Chau, P. Y., & Hu, P. J.-H. (2002). Investigating healthcare professionals' decisions to accept telemedicine technology: an empirical test of competing theories. *Information & Management, 39*(4), 297–311. doi:10.1016/S0378-7206(01)00098-2

Chen, W. L., Zhang, S. D., & Gao, X. (2009). *Anchoring the Consistency Dimension of Data Quality Using Ontology in Data Integration.* IEEE.

Chen, C. C., Wu, J., Su, Y. S., & Yang, S. C. (2008). Key drivers for the continued use of RFID technology in the emergency room. *Management Research News, 31*(4), 273–288. doi:10.1108/01409170810851348

Chen, F. H. (2009). Modeling the effect of information quality on risk behavior change and the transmission of infectious diseases. *Mathematical Biosciences, 217*(2), 125–133. doi:10.1016/j.mbs.2008.11.005 PMID:19059272

Chen, H. Y., Chuang, C. H., Yang, Y. J., & Wu, T. P. (2011). Exploring the risk factors of preterm birth using data mining. *Expert Systems with Applications, 38*(5), 5384–5387. doi:10.1016/j.eswa.2010.10.017

Chen, Hsinchun, Chiang, Roger H L, & Storey, Veda C. (2012). Business intelligence and analytics: From big data to big impact. *Management Information Systems Quarterly, 36*(4), 1165–1188.

Chen, Y. S., Cheng, C. H., Lai, C. J., Hsu, C. Y., & Syu, H. J. (2012). Identifying patients in target customer segments using a two-stage clustering-classification approach: A hospital-based assessment. *Computers in Biology and Medicine, 42*(2), 213–221. doi:10.1016/j.compbiomed.2011.11.010 PMID:22177941

Chervin, R. D. (2000). The multiple sleep latency test and Epworth sleepiness scale in the assessment of daytime sleepiness. *Journal of Sleep Research, 9*(4), 399–400. doi:10.1046/j.1365-2869.2000.0227a.x PMID:11123526

Chi, C. L., Street, W. N., & Katz, D. A. (2010). A decision support system for cost-effective diagnosis. *Artificial Intelligence in Medicine, 50*(3), 149–161. doi:10.1016/j.artmed.2010.08.001 PMID:20933375

Chi, C. L., Street, W. N., & Ward, M. M. (2008). Building a hospital referral expert system with a prediction and optimization-based decision support system algorithm. *Journal of Biomedical Informatics, 41*(2), 371–386. doi:10.1016/j.jbi.2007.10.002 PMID:18054523

Chin, W. W. (1998b). *The partial least squares approach for structural equation modeling*. Academic Press.

Chin, W., Marcolin, B., & Newsted, P. (1996). *A partial least squares latent variable modeling approach for measuring interaction effects: results from a Monte Carlo simulation study and voice mail emotion/adoption study*. Academic Press.

Chin, W. W. (1998a). Commentary: Issues and opinion on structural equation modeling. *Management Information Systems Quarterly*, vii–xvi.

Chodorow, S. (1996). Educators must take the electronic revolution seriously. *Academic Medicine, 71*, 221–226. doi:10.1097/00001888-199603000-00009 PMID:8607916

Cho, I., Park, I., Kim, E., Lee, E., & Bates, D. W. (2013). Using EHR data to predict hospital-acquired pressure ulcers: A prospective study of a bayesian network model. *International Journal of Medical Informatics, 82*(11), 1059–1067. doi:10.1016/j.ijmedinf.2013.06.012 PMID:23891086

Chong, C. S. (2005, June). Critical factors in the successful implementation of Knowledge Management. *Journal of Knowledge Management*, 21–42.

Choquet, R., Qouiyd, S., Ouagne, D., Pasche, E., Daniel, C., Boussaïd, O., et al. (2010). *The information quality triangle: A methodology to assess clinical information quality.* Paper presented at the 13th World Congress on Medical and Health Informatics, Medinfo 2010. Cape Town, South Africa.

Choules, A. P. (2007). The use of e-learning in medical education: a review of the current situation. *Postgraduate Medical Journal, 83*, 212–216. doi:10.1136/pgmj.2006.054189 PMID:17403945

Chumley-Jones, H. S., Dobbie, A., & Alford, C. L. (2002). Web-based learning: sound educational method or hype? A review of the evaluation literature. *Academic Medicine*, *77*(10), 86–93. doi:10.1097/00001888-200210001-00028 PMID:12377715

Chung, W.-Y., Lee, S.-C., & Toh, S.-H. (2008). WSN based mobile u-healthcare system with ecg, blood pressure measurement function. In *Proceedings of IEEE-EMBS 2008. 30th Annual International Conference of the Engineering in Medicine and Biology Society*, (pp. 1533–1536). IEEE.

Cios, K., & Moore, G. W. (2002). Uniqueness of medical data mining. *Artificial Intelligence in Medicine*, *26*(1-2), 1–24. doi:10.1016/S0933-3657(02)00049-0 PMID:12234714

CoA. (2011). *Don't fall for it. Falls can be prevented!* Canberra: Commonwealth of Australia.

Cohn, B., & Marriott, M. (1958). Networks and centres in the integration of Indian civilization. *Journal of Social Research*, *1*(1), 1–9.

Collins, J. (2005, July). India adopts 865-867 MHz for RFID. *RFID Journal*.

Collins, S. C., Bhatti, J. Z., Dexter, S. L., & Rabbitt, P. M. (1992). Elderly people in a new world: attitudes to advanced communications technologies. In H. Boumqa, & J. A. M. Graafmans (Eds.), *Gerontechnology* (p. 35). Amsterdam: IOS Press.

Colten, Harvey R, & Alterogt, MBruce M. (2006). *Sleep disorders and sleep deprivation: An unmet public health problem.* Retrieved from http://books.nap.edu/catalog.php?record_id=11617#toc

Comondore, V. R., Devereaux, P. J., Zhou, Q., Stone, S. B., Busse, J. W., & Ravindran, N. C. et al. (2009). Quality of care in for-profit and not-for-profit nursing homes: systematic review and meta-analysis. *BMJ (Clinical Research Ed.)*, *339*, b2732. doi:10.1136/bmj.b2732 PMID:19654184

Congress, E. P. (2012, Fall). Continuing Education: Lifelong Learning for Social Work Practitioners and Educators. *Journal of Social Work Education*, *48*(3), 397–401. doi:10.5175/JSWE.2012.201200085

Conrath, D. W., & Mignen, O. P. (1990). What is being done to measure user satisfaction with EDP/MIS. *Information & Management*, *19*(1), 7–19. doi:10.1016/0378-7206(90)90010-F

Conrick, Moya. (2006). *Health informatics: transforming healthcare with technology*. Melbourne: Thomson Social Science Press.

Constantinescu, L., Kim, J., & Feng, D. D. (2012). SparkMed: A framework for dynamic integration of multimedia medical data into distributed m-Health systems. *IEEE Transactions on Information Technology in Biomedicine*, *16*(1), 40–52. doi:10.1109/TITB.2011.2174064 PMID:22049371

Cook-Craig, P. G., & Sabah, Y. (2009). The Role of Virtual Communities of Practice in Supporting Collaborative Learning among Social Workers. *British Journal of Social Work*, *39*(4), 725–739. doi:10.1093/bjsw/bcp048

Cornwall, A., & Jewkes, R. (1995). What is participatory research? *Social Science & Medicine*, *41*(12), 1667–1676. doi:10.1016/0277-9536(95)00127-S PMID:8746866

Cowan, M., Shapiro, M., Hays, R., Afifi, A., Vazirani, S., Ward, C., & Ettner, S. (2006). The effect of a multidisciplinary hospitalist/physician and advanced practice nurse collaboration on hospital costs. *The Journal of Nursing Administration*, *36*(2), 79–85. doi:10.1097/00005110-200602000-00006 PMID:16528149

Cox, J. (2008). RFID proving to be Rx for hospitals. *Network World*, *25*(33), 24.

Craig, J., & Patterson, V. (2005). Introduction to the practice of telemedicine. *Journal of Telemedicine and Telecare*, *11*(1), 3–9. doi:10.1258/1357633053430494 PMID:15829036

Cross, R., & Cummings, J. (2004). Tie and network correlates of individual performance in knowledge-intensive work. *Academy of Management Journal*, *47*(6), 928–937. doi:10.2307/20159632

Cruz, A. M. (2013). Evaluating record history of medical devices using association discovery and clustering techniques. *Expert Systems with Applications*, *40*(13), 5292–5305. doi:10.1016/j.eswa.2013.03.034

Cunningham, F. C., Ranmuthugala, G., Plumb, J., Georgiou, A., Westbrook, J. I., & Braithwaite, J. (2012). Health professional networks as a vector for improving healthcare quality and safety: a systematic review. *BMJ Quality & Safety*, *21*(3), 239–249. doi:10.1136/bmjqs-2011-000187 PMID:22129933

Cunningham-Myrie, C., Reid, M., & Forrester, T. E. (2008). A comparative study of the quality and availability of health information used to facilitate cost burden analysis of diabetes and hypertension in the Caribbean. *The West Indian Medical Journal*, *57*(4), 383–392. PMID:19566021

Cyert, R., & March, J. (1963). *A behavioural theory of the 4rm. Englewood Cli8s*. Prentice-Hall.

Czaja, S. J., & Lee, C. C. (2001). The Internet and older adults: Design challenges and opportunities. In N. Charness, & D. C. Parks (Eds.), *Communication, and aging: Opportunities and challenges for the future* (pp. 60–78). New York: Springer.

Da Silva, S. F., Ribeiro, M. X., Batista Neto, J. D. E. S., Traina-Jr, C., & Traina, A. J. M. (2011). Improving the ranking quality of medical image retrieval using a genetic feature selection method. *Decision Support Systems*, *51*(4), 810–820. doi:10.1016/j.dss.2011.01.015

Davenport, T. H., & Prusak, L. (2000). Working Knowledge: How Organisations Manage What They Know. Harvard Business School Press.

Davis, F. (1989, September). Perceived Usefulness, Perceived Ease Of Use, and User Acceptance of Information Technology. *Management Information Systems Quarterly*.

Davis, F. D., Bagozzi, R. P., & Warshaw, P. R. (1989). User acceptance of computer technology: a comparison of two theoretical models. *Management Science*, *35*(8), 982–1003. doi:10.1287/mnsc.35.8.982

Davis, F. D. Jr. (1986). *A technology acceptance model for empirically testing new end-user information systems: Theory and results*. Massachusetts Institute of Technology.

De Clerq, E. (2008). Problem-oriented patient record model as a conceptual foundation for a multi-professional electronic patient record. *International Journal of Medical Informatics*, *77*(9), 565–575. doi:10.1016/j.ijmedinf.2007.11.002 PMID:18248847

De Couvreur, L., Dejonghe, W., Detand, J., & Goossens, R. H. M. (2013). The role of subjective well-being in co-designing open-design assistive devices. *International Journal of Design*, *7*(3), 57–70.

De Keizer, N. F., & Ammenwerth, E. (2008). The quality of evidence in health informatics: How did the quality of healthcare IT evaluation publications develop from 1982 to 2005? *International Journal of Medical Informatics*, *77*(1), 41–49. doi:10.1016/j.ijmedinf.2006.11.009 PMID:17208040

de Lusignan, S., Khunti, K., Belsey, J., Hattersley, A., van Vlymen, J., & Gallagher, H. et al. (2010). A method of identifying and correcting miscoding, misclassification and misdiagnosis in diabetes: a pilot and validation study of routinely collected data. *Diabetic Medicine*, *27*, 203–209. doi:10.1111/j.1464-5491.2009.02917.x PMID:20546265

Delen, D., Fuller, C., McCann, C., & Ray, D. (2009). Analysis of healthcare coverage: A data mining approach. *Expert Systems with Applications*, *36*(2), 995–1003. doi:10.1016/j.eswa.2007.10.041

Delone, W. H., & Mclean, E. R. (2004). Measuring e-commerce success: applying the DeLone & McLean information systems success model. *International Journal of Electronic Commerce*, *9*(1), 31–47.

Dement, W. C. (2008). History of sleep medicine. *Sleep Medicine Clinics*, *3*, 147–156. doi:10.1016/j.jsmc.2008.01.003

Demiris, G., Rantz, M., Aud, M., Marek, K., Tyrer, H., Skubic, M., & Hussam, A. (2004). Older adults' attitudes towards and perceptions of "smart home" technologies: a pilot study. *Medical Informatics and the Internet in Medicine*, *29*(2), 87–94. doi:10.1080/14639230410001684387 PMID:15370989

Department of Health and Ageing (Australian Government) (DoHA). (2012). Living Longer: Living Better. DoHA.

Department of Health and Aging. (2008). *National E-Health Strategy*. Retrieved May 15, 2011, from http://www.health.gov.au/internet/main/publishing.nsf/content/national+Ehealth+strategy

Desmet, P. M. A., & Hekkert, P. (2009). Special issue editorial: Design & emotion. *International Journal of Design*, *3*(2), 1–6.

Despont-Gros, C., Mueller, H., & Lovis, C. (2005). Evaluating user interactions with clinical information systems: a model based on human–computer interaction models. *Journal of Biomedical Informatics*, *38*(3), 244–255. doi:10.1016/j.jbi.2004.12.004 PMID:15896698

Detmar, S., Aaronson, N., Wever, L., Muller, M., & Schornagel, J. (2000). How are you feeling? Who wants to know? Patients and oncologists preferences for discussing health-related quality-of-life issues. *Journal of Clinical Oncology*, *18*(18), 3295–3301. PMID:10986063

Devillers, R., Bedard, Y., Jeansoulin, R., & Moulin, B. (2007). Towards spatial data quality information analysis tools for experts assessing the fitness for use of spatial data. *International Journal of Geographical Information Science*, *21*(3), 261–282. doi:10.1080/13658810600911879

Dey, A. K., & Guzman, E. d. (2006). *From awareness to connectedness: the design and deployment of presence displays.* Paper presented at the SIGCHI Conference on Human Factors in Computing Systems. Montreal, Canada.

Di Rienzo, M., Rizzo, F., Parati, G., Brambilla, G., Ferratini, M., & Castiglioni, P. (2005). Magic system: A new textile-based wearable device for biological signal monitoring. applicability in daily life and clinical setting. In *Proceedings of IEEE-EMBS 2005: 27th Annual International Conference of the Engineering in Medicine and Biology Society*, (pp. 7167–7169). IEEE.

Ding, D., Ayubi, S., Hiremath, S., & Parmanto, B. (2012). Physical activity monitoring and sharing platform for manual wheelchair users. In Proceedings of IEEE Intl. Conf. Engineering in Medicine and Biology Society (EMBC) (pp. 5833–5836). IEEE.

Dumbrell, D., & Steele, R. (2012). What are the Characteristics of Highly Disseminated Public Health-related Tweets? In *Proceedings of the 24th Australian Computer-Human Interaction Conference*, (pp. 115-118). Melbourne, Australia: IEEE.

Dumbrell, D., & Steele, R. (2013). Twitter and health in the Australian context: What types of information are health-related organizations tweeting? In *Proceedings of System Sciences (HICSS), 2013 46th Hawaii International Conference* (pp. 2666-2675). IEEE.

Ecole supérieure de l'éducation nationale de l'enseignement supérieur et de la recherché. (2012). *ENT-Espace Numérique de Travail.* Retrieved November 24, 2013 from http://www.esen.education.fr/index.php?id=79&a=102&cHash=fa2c3c0948

Economics, D. A. (2011). *Re-awakening Australia: The economic cost of sleep disorders in Australia, 2010.* Australia: Sleep Health Foundation.

Edwards, H. R., & Hoefer, R. (2011). Are Social Work Advocacy Groups Using Web 2.0 Effectively? *Journal of Policy Practice*, *9*(3), 220–239.

Eisenhardt, K. (1989). Building theories from case study research. *Academy of Management Review*, *14*(4), 532-550

Eisenhardt, K., & Graebner, M. E. (2007). Theory building from cases: Opportunities and Challenges. *Academy of Management Journal*, *50*(1), 25–32. doi:10.5465/AMJ.2007.24160888

Ellis, R. D., & Allaire, J. C. (1999). Modeling computer interest in older adults: The role of age, education, computer knowledge, and computer anxiety. *Human Factors: The Journal of the Human Factors and Ergonomics Society*, *41*(3), 345–355. doi:10.1518/001872099779610996 PMID:10665203

El-Masri, S., & Saddik, B. (2012). An Emergency System to Improve Ambulance Dispatching, Ambulance Diversion and Clinical Handover Communicationâ-A Proposed Model. *Journal of Medical Systems*, *36*(6), 3917–3923. doi:10.1007/s10916-012-9863-x PMID:22673893

El-Sappagh, S. H., & El-Masri, S. (2013). A distributed clinical decision support system architecture. *Journal of King Saud University-Computer and Information Sciences*, *26*(1), 69–78. doi:10.1016/j.jksuci.2013.03.005

Ernest, K., Lamei, C., Mohamed, S., Shakshuk, M., Badreldin, I., & ElBabli, I. (2011, 21-24 Feb. 2011). *A ZigBee-based telecardiology system for remote healthcare service delivery.* Paper presented at the Biomedical Engineering (MECBME). New York, NY.

Esposito, M. (2008b). *An ontological and non-monotonic rule-based approach to label medical images*. Los Alamitos, CA: IEEE Computer Soc.

Esposito, M. (2008a). Congenital Heart Disease: An ontology-based approach for the examination of the cardiovascular system. In I. Lovrek (Ed.), *Knowledge - Based Intelligent Information and Engineering Systems* (Vol. 5177, pp. 509–516). doi:10.1007/978-3-540-85563-7_65

European Union. (1993). *Growth, Competitiveness, Employment, The Challenge and Ways forward into 21st Century*. Retrieved April 12, 2011, from http://aei.pitt.edu/1139/

Euzenat, J. (2007). *Semantic Precision and Recall for Ontology Alignment Evaluation*. Paper presented at the Twentieth International Joint Conference on Artificial Intelligence (IJCAI-07). New York, NY.

Fan, L., & Suh, Y. H. (2014). Why do users switch to an advanced technology? An empirical study based on Expectation-Disconfirmation Theory. *Information & Management*, *51*, 240–248. doi:10.1016/j.im.2013.12.004

Fares, A. (2007). *ICT Infrastructure, Applications, Society, and Education*. Nairobi: Strathmore University.

Fasola, J., & Matarić, M. (2013). Socially Assistive Robot Exercise Coach: Motivating Older Adults to Engage in Physical Exercise. *Springer Tracts in Advanced Robotics*, *88*, 463–479. doi:10.1007/978-3-319-00065-7_32

Fatima, I., Halder, S., Saleem, M. A., Batool, R., Fahim, M., Lee, Y., & Lee, S. (2013). Smart CDSS: integration of Social Media and Interaction Engine (SMIE) in healthcare for chronic disease patients. *Multimedia Tools and Applications*, 1–21.

Faust, K. (1997). Centrality in affiliation networks. *Social Networks*, *19*(2), 157–191. doi:10.1016/S0378-8733(96)00300-0

Fayyad, U., Piatetsky-Shapiro, G., & Smyth, P. (1996). From Data Mining to Knowledge Discovery in Databases. *AI Magazine*, *17*(3), 37–54.

Feil-Seifer, D., & Matarić, M. (2011). Ethical Principles for Socially Assistive Robotics. *IEEE Robotics & Automation Magazine*, *18*(1), 24-31.

Fensli, R., Gunnarson, E., & Gundersen, T. (2005). A wearable ECG-recording system for continuous arrhythmia monitoring in a wireless tele-home-care situation. In *Proceedings of 18th IEEE Symposium on Computer-Based Medical Systems,* (pp. 407–412). IEEE.

Ferguson, H. (2008). Liquid Social Work: Welfare Interventions as Mobile Practices. *British Journal of Social Work*, *38*(3), 561–579. doi:10.1093/bjsw/bcl367

Fethi, A. (2010). L'Environnement Numérique de Travail (ENT). *Bulletin de l'Université*, *24*, 22.

Fink, A., & Beck, J. C. (2013). Developing and Evaluating a Website to Guide Older Adults in Their Health Information Searches A Mixed-Methods Approach. *Journal of Applied Gerontology*, *32*(4). PMID:24652883

Finn, J., & Kerman, B. (2004). The Use of Online Social Support by Foster Families. *Journal of Family Social Work*, *8*(4), 67–85. doi:10.1300/J039v08n04_04

Fishbein, M., & Ajzen, I. (1975). *Belief, Attitude, Intention, and Behavior: An Introduction to Theory and Research*. Boston: Addison-Wesley.

Fisher, J. A., & Monahan, T. (2008). Tracking the social dimensions of RFID systems in hospitals. *International Journal of Medical Informatics*, *77*(3), 176–183. doi:10.1016/j.ijmedinf.2007.04.010 PMID:17544841

Fitch, D. (2005). The Diffusion of Information Technology in Human Services: Implications for Social Work Education. *Journal of Teaching in Social Work*, *25*(1/2), 191–204. doi:10.1300/J067v25n01_12

Fitch, D. (2006). Examination of the Child Protective Services Decision-Making Context with Implications for Decision Support System Design. *Journal of Social Service Research*, *32*(4), 117–134. doi:10.1300/J079v32n04_07

Flemons, W., Douglas, N. J., Kuna, S. T., Rodenstein, D. O., & Wheatley, J. (2004). Access to diagnosis and treatment of patients with suspected sleep apnea. *American Journal of Respiratory and Critical Care Medicine*, *169*, 668–672. doi:10.1164/rccm.200308-1124PP PMID:15003950

Foster, K. A., & Stiffman, A. R. (2009). Child Welfare Workers´ Adoption of Decision Support Technology. *Journal of Technology in Human Services*, *27*(2), 106–126. doi:10.1080/15228830902749039 PMID:20198123

Fox, J., Johns, N., & Rahmanzadeh, A. (1998). Disseminating medical knowledge: the proforma approach. *Artificial Intelligence in Medicine*, *14*(1-2), 157–182. doi:10.1016/S0933-3657(98)00021-9 PMID:9779888

Frank, O., & Strauss, D. (1986). Markov graphs. *Journal of the American Statistical Association*, *81*(395), 832–842. doi:10.1080/01621459.1986.10478342

Fraunholz, B. (2001). Project Management in the German Trade Sector – A (preliminary) framework for computer assisted management of Projects in Small and Medium Sized Enterprises. In *Proceedings of Australasian Conference on Information Systems*. Academic Press.

Freddolino, P. P., & Han, A. S. (2011). Direct Service Applications of Videoconferencing Technologies: Case Examples from Korea and the United States. *Journal of Technology in Human Services*, *16*(2/3), 19–33.

Freeman, L. (1978). Centrality in social networks: Conceptual clarification. *Social Networks*, *1*(3), 215–239. doi:10.1016/0378-8733(78)90021-7

Freeman, L., Roeder, D., & Mulholland, R. (1979). Centrality in Social Networks: II. Experimental Results. *Social Networks*, *2*(80), 119–141. doi:10.1016/0378-8733(79)90002-9

Fridsma, D. B. (2001). Special Issue on Workflow Management and Clinical Guidelines. *Journal of the American Medical Informatics Association*, *22*(1).

Fuchsberger, V., Sellner, W., Moser, C., & Tscheligi, M. (2012). Benefits and hurdles for older adults in intergenerational online interactions. In *Computers Helping People with Special Needs* (pp. 697–704). Springer Berlin Heidelberg. doi:10.1007/978-3-642-31522-0_104

Gaboury, I., Bujold, M., Boon, H., & Moher, D. (2009). Interprofessional collaboration within Canadian integrative healthcare clinics: Key components. *Social Science & Medicine*, *69*(5), 707–715. doi:10.1016/j.socscimed.2009.05.048 PMID:19608320

Gangemi, A., Catenacci, C., Ciaramita, M., & Lehmann, J. (2006). *Modelling ontology evaluation and validation*. Paper presented at the 3rd European Conference on the Semantic Web: Research and Applications. New York, NY.

Garets, D., & Davis, M. (2006, January 26). *Electronic medical records vs. electronic health records: yes, there is a difference*. HIMSS Analytics. Retrieved 2013, September 28, from: http://www.himssanalytics.org/docs/wp_emr_ehr.pdf

Garret, P. M. (2005). Social work's 'electronic turn': notes on the deployment of information and communication technologies in social work with children and families. *Critical Social Policy*, *25*(4), 529–553. doi:10.1177/0261018305057044

Garrett, P., & Seidman, J. (2011). US Department of Health & Human Services. *EMR vs EHR – What is the Difference?* Retrieved 2013, September 28, from: http://www.healthit.gov/buzz-blog/electronic-health-and-medical-records/emr-vs-ehr-difference/

Garrett, P., & Seidman, P. (2011). *EMR vs EHR – What is the Difference?*. Retrieved August 10, 2013, from http://www.healthit.gov/buzz-blog/electronic-health-and-medical-records/emr-vs-ehr-difference/

Garrison, D., & Anderson, T. (2003). *E-learning in the 21st Century*. London: Routledge Falmer. doi:10.4324/9780203166093

Gatto, S. L., & Tak, S. H. (2008). Computer, internet, and e-mail use among older adults: Benefits and barriers. *Educational Gerontology*, *34*(9), 800–811. doi:10.1080/03601270802243697

Gaver, W., Bowers, J., Boucher, A., Gellerson, H., Pennington, S., Schmidt, A., et al. (2004). The Drift Table: Designing for ludic engagement. In *Proc. CHI'04 Design Expo*. New York: ACM Press.

Gedzelman, S., Simonet, M., Bernhard, D., Diallo, G., & Palmer, P. (2005). Building an ontology of cardiovascular diseases for concept-based information retrieval. In *Proceedings of Computers in Cardiology 2005,* (Vol. 32, pp. 255-258). New York: IEEE.

Gelderman, M. (1998). The relation between user satisfaction, usage of information systems and performance. *Information & Management, 34*(1), 11–18. doi:10.1016/S0378-7206(98)00044-5

*Gerijoy*. (2014). Retrieved February 28, 2014 from http://www.gerijoy.com/

Ghazavi, S. N., & Liao, T. W. (2008). Medical data mining by fuzzy modeling with selected features. *Artificial Intelligence in Medicine, 43*(3), 195–206. doi:10.1016/j.artmed.2008.04.004 PMID:18534831

Gibbons, P. (2007). Health Level Seven EHR Interoperability Work Group. *Coming to terms: Scoping Interoperability for Health Care.* Retrieved 2013, October 2, from: http://www.hln.com/assets/pdf/Coming-to-Terms-February-2007.pdf

Gibbons, A., & Fairweather, P. (2000). Computer-based instruction. In S. Tobias, & J. Fletcher (Eds.), *Training & Retraining: A Handbook for Business* (pp. 410–442). Macmillan Reference.

Gijsen, R., Hoeymans, N., & Schellevis, F. G. (2001). Causes and consequences of comorbidity: a review. *Journal of Clinical Epidemiology, 54*(7), 661–674. doi:10.1016/S0895-4356(00)00363-2 PMID:11438406

Gilbert, M., & Ddembe, W. (2008). A Flexible Approach for User Evaluation of Biomedical Ontologies. *International Journal of Computing and ICT Research,* 2(2), 62–74.

Gil, D., & Johnsson, M. (2010). Using support vector machines in diagnoses of urological dysfunctions. *Expert Systems with Applications, 37*(6), 4713–4718. doi:10.1016/j.eswa.2009.12.055

Gillies, A. (2000a). Assessing and improving the quality of information for health evaluation and promotion. *Methods of Information in Medicine, 39*(3), 4. PMID:10992745

Gillingham, P. (2011, September). Computer-based Information Systems and Human Service Organisations: Emerging Problems and Future Possibilities. *Australian Social Work, 64*(3), 299–312. doi:10.1080/0312407X.2010.524705

Glaser, B., & Strauss, A. (1967). *The Discovery of Grounded Theory: Strategies for Qualitative Research.* Chicago, IL: Aldine Publishing Company.

Godinez, V. (2007). *RFID tracks hospitals devices: System improves heart facility's care, 29th April.* Dallas, TX: Dallas Morning News.

GOI. (2002). National Health Policy. Government of India, NIC, India.

Goldwater, J.C., Kwon, N.J., Nathanson, A., Muckle, A.E., Brown, A., &Cornejo, K. (2013). Open source electronic health records and chronic disease management. *Journal of American Medical Informatics Association.* doi: 11367amiajnl-2013-001672

González, M., Buiza, C., Etxeberria, I., Yanguas, J., Ortiz, A., & Carretero, M. et al. (2007). *The Effect of an Avatar in Natural Interaction. IOS Press Ebooks* (Vol. 20). Challenges for Assistive Technology.

Gordon, C., & Christensen, J. P. (1995). *Health telematics for clinical guidelines and protocols.* IOS Press.

Graber, M. L., & Mathew, A. (2008). Performance of a Web-Based Clinical Diagnosis Support System for Internists. *Journal of General Internal Medicine, 23*(Supplement 1), 37–40. doi:10.1007/s11606-007-0271-8 PMID:18095042

Gravelle, H., & Siciliani, L. (2008). Optimal quality, waits and charges in health insurance. *Journal of Health Economics, 27*(3), 663–674. doi:10.1016/j.jhealeco.2007.08.004 PMID:18191254

Graves, J., & Corcoran, S. (1989). The study of nursing informatics. *Image*, *21*(4), 227–231. PMID:2807330

Grealy, C., Olver, K., Connell, J., Power, J., Bramich, M., & Yeomans, J. (2008). *Comprehensive scoping study on the use of assistive technology by frail older people living in the community*. Canberra: Commonwealth Department of Health and Ageing.

Grebel, H., & Steyaert, J. (1995). Social Informatics: beyond technology. A research project in schools of social work in the European Community. *International Social Work*, *38*(2), 151–164. doi:10.1177/002087289503800205

Greene, J. (2005, September). Is your Hospital Ready for Radio Frequency Identification? Above Board Technology. *Trustee*, 30–32. PMID:16196403

Gregori, D., Petrinco, M., Bo, S., Rosato, R., Pagano, E., Berchialla, P., & Merletti, F. (2011). Using data mining techniques in monitoring diabetes care. The simpler the better? *Journal of Medical Systems*, *35*(2), 277–281. doi:10.1007/s10916-009-9363-9 PMID:20703563

Greig, M., & Skehill, C. (2008). Increasing Staff and Student Capacity to Use the Communication Facility in Queen's Online in Order to Support Learning and Teaching on a BSW Programme. *Social Work Education*, *27*(6), 634–646. doi:10.1080/02615470802201705

Griffin, L., & de Leastar, E. (2009). Social networking healthcare. In *Proceedings of 6th Intl. Workshop on Wearable Micro and Nano Technologies for Personalized Health* (pHealth), (pp. 75–78). pHealth.

Gruber, T. (2009). Ontology. In L. Liu, & M. Tamer Özsu (Eds.), Encyclopedia of Database Systems (pp. 1963-1965). Springer US.

Guardado, M., & Shi, L. (2007). ESL students' experiences of online peer feedback. *Computers and Composition*, *24*(4), 443–461. doi:10.1016/j.compcom.2007.03.002

Guenther, K. (2004). Know the fundamentals and good design will follow. *Online*, *28*(1), 54–56.

Guerrero, et al. (2012). Self-Organising Maps: A new way to screen the level of satisfaction of dialysis patients. *Expert Systems with Applications*, *39*(10), 8793–8798. doi:10.1016/j.eswa.2012.02.001

Gunasekaran, A., & Ichimura, T. (1997). Business Process Reengineering: Modelling and Analysis. *International Journal of Production Economics*, *50*, 65–68. doi:10.1016/S0925-5273(97)00031-5

Gupta, A., Ludäscher, B., Grethe, J. S., & Martone, M. E. (2003). Towards a formalization of disease-specific ontologies for neuroinformatics. *Neural Networks*, *16*(9), 1277–1292. doi:10.1016/j.neunet.2003.07.008 PMID:14622884

Gürsel, G., Zayim, N., Gülkesen, K. H., Arifoğlu, A., & Saka, O. (2014). A new approach in the evaluation of hospital information systems. *Turk J Electr Eng Co*, *22*(1), 214–222. doi:10.3906/elk-1110-15

H&HN. (2004, May). Beyond Bar Codes, Technology, Inbox. *Hospitals and Health Networks Magazine*, 26.

H&HN. (2005, June). Behind the Hype, Technology, Inbox. *Hospitals and Health Networks Magazine*, 22-24.

Habib, J. L. (2010). EHRs, meaningful use, and a model EMR. *Drug Benefit Trends*, *22*(4), 99–101.

Hadzic, M., & Chang, E. (2005, Dec 11 2005). *Ontology-based multi-agent systems support human disease study and control*. Paper presented at the International Conference on Self Organization and Adaptation of Multi-Agent and Grid Systems (SOAS). Glasgow, UK.

Haggie, K., & Kingston, J. (2003). Choosing your knowledge management strategy. *Journal of Knowledge Management Practice*, 1 – 20.

Haggie, J. K., & Kingston, J. (2003, June). Choosing a knowledge management strategy. *Journal of Knowledge Management*, 33–56.

Halewood, N., & Kenny, C. (2008). Young people and ICTs in Developing Countries. *Information Technology for Development Journal, 14*.

Halilovic, S., & Cicic, M. (2013). Antecedents of information systems user behaviour–extended expectation-confirmation model. *Behaviour & Information Technology*, *32*(4), 359–370. doi:10.1080/0144929X.2011.554575

Hall, R. (2003). *"Knowledge Management in the New Business Environment", A report prepared for the Australian Business Foundation, ACCIRT*. University of Sydney.

Hall, C., Parton, N., Peckover, S., & White, S. (2010). Child-Centric Information and Communication Technology (ICT) and the Fragmentation of Child Welfare Practice in England. *Journal of Social Policy*, *39*(3), 393–413. doi:10.1017/S0047279410000012

Hall, R. (2003). *Knowledge Management in the New Business Environment (A report prepared for the Australian Business Foundation)*. Sydney: ACIRRT, University of Sydney.

Hämäläinen, P., Reponen, J., & Winblad, I. (2008). eHealth of Finland. In *Checkpoint 2008*. Jyväskylä: Gummerus. Retrieved February 10, 2014, from http://www.julkari.fi/bitstream/handle/10024/79888/f5ca5a36-f2c6-4e94-ae95-a7b439b1169b.pdf?sequence=1

Hamilton, W. T., Round, A. P., Sharp, D., & Peters, T. J. (2003). The quality of record keeping in primary care: a comparison of computerised, paper and hybrid systems. *The British Journal of General Practice*, *53*(497), 929–933, discussion 933. PMID:14960216

Hammer, M. (1990). Reengineering Work: Don't automate, obliterate. *Harvard Business Review*, *68*(4), 104–113.

Hand, D. J. (1998). Data mining: statistics and more? *American Statistical Association*, *52*, 112–118.

Hanson, E., & Magnusson, L. (2011). The role of ICT support services to promote ageing in place: The ACTION service. *Eurohealth*, *17*(2-3), 24–26.

Hanson, E., Magnusson, L., Arvidsson, H., Claesson, A., Keady, J., & Nolan, M. (2007). Working together with persons with early stage dementia and their family members to design a user-friendly technology based support service. *Dementia (London)*, *6*(3), 411–434. doi:10.1177/1471301207081572

Hanson, V. L. (2010). Influencing technology adoption by older adults. *Interacting with Computers*, *22*(6), 502–509. doi:10.1016/j.intcom.2010.09.001

Hao, Y., & Foster, R. (2008). Wireless body sensor networks for health-monitoring applications. *Physiological Measurement*, *29*(11), R27–R56. doi:10.1088/0967-3334/29/11/R01 PMID:18843167

Hardey, M., & Loader, B. (2009). The Information of Welfare: Older People and the Role of Digital Services. *British Journal of Social Work*, *39*(4), 657–669. doi:10.1093/bjsw/bcp024

Harkin, J., & Huber, J. (2004). Eternal youths: How the baby boomers are having their time again. *Demos (Mexico City, Mexico)*.

Harrison, J. H. (2008). Introduction to the mining of clinical data. *Clinics in Laboratory Medicine*, *28*(1), 1–7. doi:10.1016/j.cll.2007.10.001 PMID:18194715

Harrop, P. (2006). Rapid Adoption of RFID in Healthcare. *RFID in Healthcare 2006-2016, idtechex*.

Hart, C. (2003). *Doing a Literature Review*. London: SAGE Publications Ltd.

Hassenzahl, M., Eckoldt, K., Diefenbach, S., Laschke, M., Lenz, E., & Kim, J. (2013). Designing moments of meaning and pleasure. Experience design and happiness. *International Journal of Design*, *7*(3), 21–31.

Hassenzahl, M., Heidecker, S., Eckoldt, K., Diefenbach, S., & Hillmann, U. (2012). All You Need is Love: Current Strategies of Mediating Intimate Relationships through Technology. *ACM Transactions on Computer-Human Interaction*, *19*(4), 30. doi:10.1145/2395131.2395137

Hauskrecht, M., Batal, I., Valko, M., Visweswaran, S., Cooper, G. F., & Clermont, G. (2013). Outlier detection for patient monitoring and alerting. *Journal of Biomedical Informatics*, *46*(1), 47–55. doi:10.1016/j.jbi.2012.08.004 PMID:22944172

Haux, R. (2010). Medical informatics: Past, present, future. *International Journal of Medical Informatics*, *79*(9). doi:10.1016/j.ijmedinf.2010.06.003 PMID:20615752

Hayes, D., & Devaney, J. (2004). Accessing Social Work Case Files for Research Purposes. *Qualitative Social Work*, *3*(3), 313–333. doi:10.1177/1473325004045667

Haynes, R. B., Sackett, D. L., Guyatt, G. H., & Tugwell, P. (2006). Clinical epidemiology: How to do clinical practice research (3rd ed.). Philadelphia: Lippincott Williams & Wilkins

Hayrinen, K., Saranto, K., & Nykanen, P. (2008). Definition, structure, content, use and impacts of electronic health records: A review of the research literature. *International Journal of Medical Informatics*, *77*, 291–304. doi:10.1016/j.ijmedinf.2007.09.001 PMID:17951106

Heaivilin, N., Gerbert, B., Page, J. E., & Gibbs, J. L. (2011). Public Health Surveillance of Dental Pain via Twitter. *Journal of Dental Research*, *90*(9), 1047–1051. doi:10.1177/0022034511415273 PMID:21768306

Healthcare Industry. (n.d.). In *Wikipedia*. Retrieved Sep 17, 2013, from http://en.wikipedia.org/wiki/Health_care_industry

He, C., Fan, X., & Li, Y. (2013). Toward ubiquitous healthcare services with a novel efficient cloud platform. *IEEE Transactions on Bio-Medical Engineering*, *60*(1), 230–234. doi:10.1109/TBME.2012.2222404 PMID:23060318

Heerink, M., Krose, B., Evers, V., & Wielinga, B. (2006). The Influence of a Robot's Social Abilities on Acceptance by Elderly Users. In *Proceedings of 15th IEEE International Symposium on Robot and Human Interactive Communication*. IEEE.

Heerink, M., Krose, B., Evers, V., & Wielinga, B. (2009). Measuring acceptance of an assistive social robot: a suggested toolkit. In *Proceedings of 18th IEEE International Symposium on Robot and Human Interactive Communication*. IEEE.

Heilman, K. J., & Porges, S. W. (2007). Accuracy of the lifeshirt® (vivometrics) in the detection of cardiac rhythms. *Biological Psychology*, *75*(3), 300–305. doi:10.1016/j.biopsycho.2007.04.001 PMID:17540493

Heinssen, R. K., Glass, C. R., & Knight, L. A. (1987). Assessing computer anxiety: Development and validation of the Computer Anxiety Rating Scale. *Computers in Human Behavior, 3*(1), 49-59. doi: 10.1016/0747-5632(87)90010-0

Henkemans, O. A. B., Caine, K. E., Rogers, W. A., Fisk, A. D., & Ruyter, B. d. (2007). *Medical Monitoring for Independent Living: User-Centered Design of Smart Home Technologies for Older Adults.* Paper presented at the Med-e-Tel conference for eHealth, telemedicine and health information and communication technologies. Luxembourg.

Henman, P., & Adler, M. (2003). Information technology and the governance of social security. *Critical Social Policy*, *23*(2), 139–164. doi:10.1177/0261018303023002002

Heo, J. a. K., J. and Won, Y. (2012). Exploring the Relationship Between Internet Use and Leisure Satisfaction Among Older Adults. *Activities, Adaptation and Aging*, *35*(1), 43–54. doi:10.1080/01924788.2010.545975

Hersh, W. R., Cimino, J., Payne, P. R.O., Embi, P., Logan, J., Weiner, M., Bernstam, E. V., Lehmann, H., Hripcsak, G., Hartzog, T., & Saltz, J. (2013). Recommendations for the use of operational Electronic Health Record data in comparative effectiveness research. *eGEMs, 1*(1), Article 14. DOI: 10.13063/2327-9214.1018

HFM. (2006, August). RFID tracks ED overcrowding, Technology. *Health Facilities Management*, 8.

Hillmer, M. P., Wodchis, W. P., Gill, S. S., Anderson, G. M., & Rochon, P. A. (2005). Nursing home profit status and quality of care: Is there any evidence of an association? *Medical Care Research and Review*, *62*(2), 139–166. doi:10.1177/1077558704273769 PMID:15750174

Hirakis, O., & Karakounos, S. (2006). Goals and benefits of knowledge management in healthcare. In A. A. Lazakidou (Ed.), *Handbook of Research on Informatics in Healthcare and Biomedicine* (pp. 193–200). Idea Group Reference. doi:10.4018/978-1-59140-982-3.ch025

Holden, R. J., & Karsh, B.-T. (2010). The technology acceptance model: its past and its future in health care. *Journal of Biomedical Informatics*, *43*(1), 159–172. doi:10.1016/j.jbi.2009.07.002 PMID:19615467

Hoog, W. d., Keller, I., & Stappers, P. J. (2004). *Gustbowl: technology supporting affective communication through routine ritual interactions.* Paper presented at the CHI '04 Extended Abstracts on Human Factors in Computing Systems. Vienna, Austria.

Horton, W. (2001). *Evaluating E-learning*. Alexandria, VA: American Society for Training and Development.

Hoskins, R. (2006). *InfoLogix Announces HealthTrax RFID Asset Tracking Software for Hospital Mobile Assets Management*. Retrieved March 30, 2006 from http://www.bbwexchange.com/pubs/2006/02/11/page1395-98309.asp

Hossain, L., Wu, A., & Chung, K. (2006). *Actor centrality correlates to project based coordination*. Academic Press.

Hovmand, P. S., Jonson-Reid, M., & Drake, B. (2007). Mapping Service Networks. *Journal of Technology in Human Services*, *25*(4), 1–21. doi:10.1300/J017v25n04_01

Hrastinski, S. (2008). Asynchronous and synchronous e-learning. *EDUCAUSE Quarterly*, *31*(4), 51–55.

Hripcsak, G., & Albers, D. J. (2012). Next-generation phenotyping of electronic health records. *Journal of the American Medical Informatics Association*, *0*, 1–5. doi: doi:10.1136/amiajnl-2012-001145 PMID:22955496

Huaman, M. A., Araujo-Castillo, R. V., Soto, G., Neyra, J. M., Quispe, J. A., & Fernandez, M. F. et al. (2009). Impact of two interventions on timeliness and data quality of an electronic disease surveillance system in a resource limited setting (Peru): a prospective evaluation. *BMC Medical Informatics and Decision Making*, 9. PMID:19183479

Hume, C., Clarke, P., & Hume, M. (2012). The role of knowledge management in the large non profit firm: building a framework for KM success. *International Journal of Organisational Behaviour*, *17*(3), 82–104.

Hume, C., & Hume, M. (2008). The strategic role of knowledge management in nonprofit organizations. *International Journal of Nonprofit and Voluntary Sector Marketing*, *13*(2), 129–140.

Hume, C., Pope, N., & Hume, M. (2012). KM 100: Introductory knowledge management for not-for-profit organizations. *International Journal of Organisational Behaviour*, *17*(2), 56.

Humphreys, L., Gill, P., & Krishnamurthy, B. (2010). How much is too much? Privacy issues on Twitter. In Proceedings of Conference of International Communication Association. Singapore: Academic Press.

Hung, M.-C., & Jen, W.-Y. (2012). The Adoption of Mobile Health Management Services: An Empirical Study. *Journal of Medical Systems*, *36*(3), 1381–1388. doi:10.1007/s10916-010-9600-2 PMID:20878452

Hung, S. Y., Hung, W. H., Tsai, C. A., & Jiang, S. C. (2010). Critical factors of hospital adoption on CRM system: Organizational and information system perspectives. *Decision Support Systems*, *48*(4), 592–603. doi:10.1016/j.dss.2009.11.009

Huntington, A., & Sudbery, J. (2005). Virtual Classrooms: Experiences of European Collaborative Teaching and Learning. *Social Work education*, *24*(3), 363–371. doi:10.1080/02615470500050677

Hunt, J. S., Siemienczuk, J., Pape, G., Rozenfeld, Y., MacKay, J., LeBlanc, B. H., & Touchette, D. (2008). A randomized controlled trial of team-based care: impact of physician-pharmacist collaboration on uncontrolled hypertension. *Journal of General Internal Medicine*, *23*(12), 1966–1972. doi:10.1007/s11606-008-0791-x PMID:18815843

Iahad, A, N., Rahim, A., Zairah, N., & Oye, N. (2012). Acceptance and usage of ICT by university academicians using UTAUT model: A case study of University of Port Harcourt, Nigeria. *Journal of Emerging Trends in Computing and Information Sciences*, *3*(1), 81–89.

ICD-10. (2010). *International Classification of ICD*. Available at: http://www.who.int/classifications/icd/en/

ICD-9-CM. (2011). International Classification of Diseases, Ninth Revision, Clinical Modification. Available at http://www.cdc.gov/nchs/icd/icd9cm.htm#ftp

Ince, D., & Griffiths, A. (2011). A Chronicling System for Children's Social Work: Learning from the ICS Failure. *British Journal of Social Work*, *41*, 1497–1513. doi:10.1093/bjsw/bcr016

Indulska, M., Recker, J., Rosemann, M., & Greene, P. (2009). Business process modelling: Current issues and future Challenges. In P. Van Eck, J. Gordijn, & R. Wierings (Eds.), CAiSE 2009, (LNCS) (vol. 5565, pp. 501–514). Berlin: Springer. doi:10.1007/978-3-642-02144-2_39

Institute of Medicine (IOM). (2012). *Health IT and Patient Safety: Building Safer Systems for Better Care*. Washington, DC: The National Academies Press.

Institute of Medicine, Committee on Quality Health Care in America. (2001). Crossing the quality chasm: A new health system for the 21st century. National Academy Press.

*Intelsense* . (2013). Retrieved from http://intellisense.io/

International Health Terminology Standards Development Organisation. (n.d.). *Snomed Clinical Terms*. Retrieved October 2013, from IHTSDO website: http://www.ihtsdo.org/snomed-ct/

*International Medical Informatics Association (IMIA)*. (2014). Retrieved February 10, 2014, from http://www.imia-medinfo.org/new2/

International Medical Informatics Association. (2010). *IMIA Education Recommendations 2010*. Retrieved February 10, 2014, from http://www.schattauer.de/en/magazine/subject-areas/journals-a-z/methods/contents/archive/issue/1053/manuscript/12538.html

ISO 18308 Conformance. (n.d.). *OpenEHR Foundation*. Retrieved September 29, 2013 from http://www.openehr.org

Iso-Markku, P. & Kurhila, J. (1999). *Sosiaalialan tietotekniikkakartoitus 1999. [Social services ICT review 1999]*. Helsinki: Osaavien keskusten verkosto.

ITU. (2013, April). *High efficiency video coding*. ITU-T H.265.

ITU-T, & ISO/IEC. (2010). *Advanced video coding*. ITU-T Rec. H.264 and ISO/IEC 14496-10.

Ivanova, I., Morales, J., de By, R. A., Beshe, T. S., & Gebresilassie, M. A. (2013). Searching for spatial data resources by fitness for use. *Journal of Spatial Science*, *58*(1), 15–28. doi:10.1080/14498596.2012.759087

Ives, B., Olson, M. H., & Baroudi, J. J. (1983). The measurement of user information satisfaction. *Communications of the ACM*, *26*(10), 785–793. doi:10.1145/358413.358430

Jacquelinet, C., Burgun, A., Delamarre, D., Strang, N., Boutin, B., & Le Beux, P. (2001). Building an ontology for end-stage diseases and organ failure in the context of transplantation and dialysis. In V. L. Patel, R. Rogers, & R. Haux (Eds.), *Medinfo 2001: Proceedings of the 10th World Congress on Medical Informatics, Pts 1 and 2* (Vol. 84, pp. 297-297). Amsterdam: I O S Press.

Jacquelinet, C., Burgun, A., Delamarre, D., Strang, N., Djabbour, S., Boutin, B., et al. (2003). Developing the ontological foundations of a terminological system for end-stage diseases, organ failure, dialysis and transplantation. *International Journal of Medical Informatics, 70*(2-3), 317-328. doi: 10.1016/S1386-5056(03)00046-7

Jafarpour, B., & Abidi, S. S. (2013). Merging Disease-Specific Clinical Guidelines to Handle Comorbidities in a Clinical Decision Support Setting. In *Proceedings of 14th Conference on Artificial Intelligence in Medicine* (vol. 7885, pp. 28-32). Murcia, Spain: Springer.

James, M., Chui, M., Brown, B., Bughin, J., Dobbs, R., Roxburgh, C., & Byers, A. H. (2011, May). Big data: The next frontier for innovation, competition, and productivity. *Harvard Business Review*, 59–69.

Jang, K. (2013). An Understanding of Optimal Knowledge Management for Social Work Practice: Based on a Process-Oriented Conceptualisation of Knowledge Integration. *British Journal of Social Work*, *43*, 1364–1383. doi:10.1093/bjsw/bcs053

Jansà, M., Vidal, M., Viaplana, J., Levy, I., Conget, I., Gomis, R., et al. (2006). Telecare in a structured therapeutic education programme addressed to patients with type 1 diabetes and poor metabolic control. *Diabetes Research and Clinical Practice, 74*(1), 26-32. doi: 10.1016/j.diabres.2006.03.005

Jansen-Vullers, M.H., & Reijers, H.A. (2005). Business Process Redesign in HealthCare: Towards a structured approach. *INFOR - Journal of the Canadian Operational Research Society*, *43*(4), 321-339.

Jansen, W., & Hooven, H.M. v.d., Jägers, M., & Steenbakkers, J. (2002). The added value of e-learning. *Informing Science*.

Janz, B. D., & Prasarnphanich, P. (2003). Understanding the antecedents of effectiveness knowledge management: The importance of a knowledge-center culture. *Decision Sciences*, *34*(2), 351–384. doi:10.1111/1540-5915.02328

Jara, A. J., Blaya, F. J., Zamora, M. A., & Skarmeta, A. F. G. (2009). *An Ontology and Rule Based Intelligent Information System to Detect and Predict Myocardial Diseases*. New York: IEEE.

Jen, W.-Y., & Chao, C.-C. (2008). Measuring mobile patient safety information system success: An empirical study. *International Journal of Medical Informatics*, *77*(10), 689-697. doi: 10.1016/j.ijmedinf.2008.03.003

Jensen, C. (2008). Worlds of welfare services and transfers. *Journal of European Social Policy*, *18*(2), 151–162. doi:10.1177/0958928707087591

Jensen, P. (1978). Miten atk palvelee sosiaalitointa? (How does IT serve social services?). *Sosiaaliturva*, *66*(22), 935–938.

Jensen, P. B., & Jensen, L, J, Brunak, S. (2012). Mining electronic health records: towards better research applications and clinical care. *Nature Reviews. Transactional Genetics*, *13*(6), 395–405.

Jeong, S., & Keatinge, D. (2004). Innovative leadership and management in a nursing home. *Journal of Nursing Management*, *12*, 445–451. doi:10.1111/j.1365-2834.2004.00451.x PMID:15509274

Jeon, Y. H., Merlyn, T., & Chenoweth, L. (2010). Leadership and management in the aged care sector: a narrative synthesis. *Australasian Journal on Ageing*, *29*(2), 54–60. doi:10.1111/j.1741-6612.2010.00426.x PMID:20553534

*Jeopardy*. (2014). Retrieved February 28, 2014 from http://www.youtube.com/watch?v=vsUDWSEp_6o

Jin, Z., Oresko, J., Huang, S., & Cheng, A. (2009). Hearttogo: A personalized medicine technology for cardiovascular disease prevention and detection. In *Proceedings of Life Science Systems and Applications Workshop*, (pp. 80–83). IEEE.

Joellenbeck, L. M., Russell, P. K., & Guze, S. B. (Eds.), *Strategies to Protect the Health of Deployed US Forces* (pp. 79–82). Washington, DC: National Academy Press.

Jo, H. S., Hwang, M. S., & Lee, H. (2010). Market segmentation of health information use on the Internet in Korea. *International Journal of Medical Informatics*, *79*(10), 707–715. doi:10.1016/j.ijmedinf.2010.07.006 PMID:20810307

Johnson, C. E., Hurtubise, L. C., & Castrop, J. et al. (2004). Learning management systems: technology to measure the medical knowledge competency of the ACGME. *Medical Education*, *38*, 599–608. doi:10.1111/j.1365-2929.2004.01792.x PMID:15189256

Johnson, J. A. (2005). Ascertaining the validity of individual protocols from Web-based personality inventories. *Journal of Research in Personality*, *39*(1), 103–129. doi:10.1016/j.jrp.2004.09.009

Jones, A. (2012). Teacher perceptions and use of ICT in unfamiliar classroom situations. In *Proceedings of International Conference on Information Communication Technologies in Education*, (pp. 314-322). Academic Press.

Jones, N. B., Herschel, R. T., & Moesel, D. D. (2003). Using knowledge champions to facilitate knowledge management. *Journal of Knowledge Management*, *7*(1), 49. doi:10.1108/13673270310463617

Jovanov, E., O'Donnel, A., Morgan, A., Priddy, B., & Hormigo, R. (2002). *Prolonged telemetric monitoring of heart rate variability using wireless intelligent sensors and a mobile gateway*. Paper presented at the Engineering in Medicine and Biology, 2002. 24th Annual Conference and the Annual Fall Meeting of the Biomedical Engineering Society EMBS/BMES Conference. New York, NY.

Judd, R. G., & Johnston, L. B. (2012, Spring). Ethical Consequences of Using Social Network Sites for Students in Professional Social Work Programs. *Journal of Social Work Values & Ethics*, *9*(1), 5–12.

Kaarakainen, M. (2009). Hajauttaminen valtion ja kuntien välisissä suhteissa 1945 - 2015. Valtiollisesta järjestelmästä kohden kuntaverkostojen perusterveydenhuoltoa. [Decentralization in state and municipal relationships from 1945 to 2015. From national primary health care towards municipality networks]. *Social Sciences*, 153.

Kahn, M. (2008, June). RFID in hospitals could pose risks. *PC Magazine Online*, 25.

Kahn, B. K., Strong, D. M., & Wang, R. Y. (2002). Information quality benchmarks: product and service performance. *Communications of the ACM*, *45*(4), 8. doi:10.1145/505248.506007

Kahn, M. G., Batson, D., & Schilling, L. M. (2012). Data model considerations for clinical effectiveness researchers. *Medical Care*, *50*(Suppl), S60–S67. doi:10.1097/MLR.0b013e318259bff4 PMID:22692260

Kahn, M. G., Raebel, M. A., Glanz, J. M., Riedlinger, K., & Steiner, J. F. (2012). A pragmatic framework for single-site and multisite data quality assessment in electronic health record-based clinical research. *Medical Care*, *50*, S21–S29. doi:10.1097/MLR.0b013e318257dd67 PMID:22692254

Kakilehto, T., Salo, S., & Larmas, M. (2009). Data mining of clinical oral health documents for analysis of the longevity of different restorative materials in Finland. *International Journal of Medical Informatics*, *78*(12), e68–e74. doi:10.1016/j.ijmedinf.2009.04.004 PMID:19428290

Kalra, D. (2006). Electronic Health Standards. *IMIA Yearbook of Medical Informatics*, *45*(Suppl1), S136–S144.

Kandula, S., Zeng-Treitler, Q., Chen, L., Salomon, W. L., & Bray, B. E. (2011). A bootstrapping algorithm to improve cohort identification using structured data. *Journal of Biomedical Informatics*, *44*(1), S63–S68. doi:10.1016/j.jbi.2011.10.013 PMID:22079803

Kane, R. (2003). Definition, Measurement, and Correlates of Quality of Life in Nursing Homes: Toward a Reasonable Practice, Research, and Policy Agenda. *The Gerontologist*, *43*, 28–36. doi:10.1093/geront/43.suppl_2.28 PMID:12711722

Kapp, S. A., & Stipp, K. F. (2010). Trolling the Useful Data in an Automated Information Management System: Experiences of Kansas City Community Mental Health Managers. *Administration in Social Work*, *34*(2), 135–147. doi:10.1080/03643101003608927

Kautto, M. (2002). Investing in services in West European welfare states. *Journal of European Social Policy*, *12*(1), 53–65. doi:10.1177/0952872002012001636

Keegan Eamon, M., Wu, C.-F., Moroney, G., & Gundari, M. (2013). Teaching the Importance and Use of Web-Based Services to Assist Clients in Obtaining Public Benefits. *Journal of Teaching in Social Work*, 2(33), 143–158. doi:10.1080/08841233.2013.777011

Keegan, D. (2004). *The impact of new technologies on distance learning students*. Distance Education International.

Keikhosrokiani, P., Mustaffa, N., Zakaria, N., & Sarwar, M. I. (2012). A Proposal to Design a Location-Based Mobile Cardiac Emergency System (LMCES). *Studies in Health Technology and Informatics*, *182*, 83–92. PMID:23138083

Keirnan, A., & Pedell, S. (2014). *Developing a Personal Alarm Pendadant for Older Adults at Home* (White Paper). Swinburne University of Technology.

Kerr, K., Norris, A., & Stockdale, R. (2007). *Data quality, information and decision making: A healthcare case study.* Paper presented at the 18th Australasian Conference on Information Systems. Toowoomba, Australia.

Kersaint, G., Horton, B., Stohl, H., & Garofalo, J. (2003). Technology beliefs and practices of mathematics education faculty. *Journal of Technology and Teacher Education, 11*(4), 549–577.

Kerslake, A. (1998). Computerisation of the *Looking After Children* Records: Issues of Implementation. *Children & Society, 12*(3), 236–237.

Kevin, H., & Yuan-Ting, Z. (2003). Implementation of a WAP-based telemedicine system for patient monitoring. *IEEE Transactions on* Information Technology in Biomedicine, *7*(2), 101–107.

Keymolen, E., & Broeders, D. (2013). Innocence Lost: Care and Control in Dutch Digital Youth Care. *British Journal of Social Work, 43*, 41–63. doi:10.1093/bjsw/bcr169

Khalifa, M., & Liu, V. (2004). The state of research on information system satisfaction.[JITTA]. *Journal of Information Technology Theory and Application, 5*(4), 4.

Khorakhu, C., & Bhatti, S. (2013). Remote Health Monitoring Using Online Social Media Systems. In *Proceedings of 6th Joint Wireless and Mobile Networking Conference.* Dubai, UAE: IEEE.

Kim, K. O. (2012). *The Emotional Responses of Older Adults to New Technology.* (PhD Thesis). University of Illinois at Urbana-Champaign, Urbana-Champaign, IL.

Kiragga, A. N., Castelnuovo, B., Schaefer, P., Muwonge, T., & Easterbrook, P. J. (2011). Quality of data collection in a large HIV observational clinic database in sub-Saharan Africa: Implications for clinical research and audit of care. *Journal of the International AIDS Society, 14*(1). doi:10.1186/1758-2652-14-3 PMID:21251327

Kirkendall, E. S., Goldenhar, L. M., Simon, J. L., Wheeler, D. S., & Andrew Spooner, S. (2013). Transitioning from a computerized provider order entry and paper documentation system to an electronic health record: Expectations and experiences of hospital staff. *International Journal of Medical Informatics, 82*(11), 1037–1045. doi:10.1016/j.ijmedinf.2013.08.005 PMID:24041453

Kirkpatrick, D. (1998). *Evaluating Training Programs* (2nd ed.). San Francisco: Berrett-Koehler.

Knaus, W. E., Draper, W. D. P., & Zimmerman, J. E. (1986). An evaluation of outcome from intensive care in major medical centers. *Annals of Internal Medicine, 104*(3), 410–418. doi:10.7326/0003-4819-104-3-410 PMID:3946981

Kokko, S. (2009). Integrated primary health care: Finnish solutions and experiences. *International Journal of Integrated Care*, (9). Retrieved July 27, 2010, from http://www.ijic.org

Kolodner, J. (1993). Case-Based Reasoning. Morgan Kaufmann Publishers.

Koppel, R., Metlay, J. P., & Cohen, A. (2005). Role of Computerized Physician Order Entry Systems in Facilitating Medication Errors. *Journal of the American Medical Association, 293*(10), 1197–1203. doi:10.1001/jama.293.10.1197 PMID:15755942

Korhonen, I., Parkka, J., & Van Gils, M. (2003). Health monitoring in the home of the future. *IEEE Engineering in Medicine and Biology Magazine, 22*(3), 66–73. doi:10.1109/MEMB.2003.1213628 PMID:12845821

Korpi, K. (1985). Yhtenäinen asiakastietokanta sosiaalitoimelle? [Uniform client data base for social services?]. *Sosiaaliturva, 73*(10), 465–467.

Kramer, N. R., Cook, T. E., & Carlisle, C. C., Corwin, R. W., & Millman, R. P. (1999). The role of the primary care physician in recognizing obstructive sleep apnea. *Archives of Internal Medicine, 159*(9), 965–968. doi:10.1001/archinte.159.9.965 PMID:10326938

Krishnakumar, R., & Rajesh Kumar, M. (2011). Attitude of teachers' of higher education towards e-learning. *Journal of Education and Practice*, *2*(4), 48–53.

Kshetri, N. (2010, October). Cloud Computing in Developing Economies. *IEEE Computer,* 47–55.

Kudyakov, R., Bowen, J., Ewen, E., West, S. l., Daoud, Y., Fleming, N., & Masica, A. (2012). Electronic health record use to classify patients with newly diagnosed versus preexisting type 2 diabetes: infrastructure for comparative effectiveness research and population health management. *Population Health Management*, *15*(1), 3–11. doi:10.1089/pop.2010.0084 PMID:21877923

Kuhn, T. A. (1970). *The Structure of Scientific Revolutions*. Chicago: University of Chicago Press.

Kumar, M., Ghani, R., & Mei, Z. S. (2010). Data mining to predict and prevent errors in health insurance claims processing. In *Proceedings of the 16th ACM SIGKDD International Conference on Knowledge Discovery and Data Mining* (pp. 65-74). ACM.

Kum, H., Duncan, D. F., & Stewart, C. J. (2009). Supporting self-evaluation in local government via Knowledge Discovery and Data Mining. *Government Information Quarterly*, *26*(2), 295–304. doi:10.1016/j.giq.2008.12.009

Kunkel, B., & Yowell, T. (2001). *e*-Tools and Organization Transformation Techniques for Collaborative Case Management. *Journal of Technology in Human Services*, *18*(1/2), 117–134. doi:10.1300/J017v18n01_10

Kuo, Y. T., Lonie, A., Sonenberg, L., & Paizis, K. (2007). Domain Ontology Driven Data Mining. In *Proceedings of the 2007 international Workshop on Domain Driven Data Mining* (pp 11-17). Academic Press.

Kuusisto-Niemi, S. & Saranto, K. (2009). Sosiaali- ja terveydenhuollon tiedonhallinta - Paradigma tieteenalan perustana. [Health and Human Services Informatics – the Paradigm as the Foundation of the Discipline]. *Finnish Journal of eHealth and eWelfare*, *1*(1), 19-23. Retrieved October 21, 2010, from http://ojs.tsv.fi/index.php/stty/article/view/1734

Kuusisto-Niemi, S., & Saranto, K. (2008). Sosiaali- ja terveydenhuollon tietohallinto oppiaineena ja tieteenalana: kehityskulkuja ja näköaloja. [Health and Human Services Informatics as a subject and a discipline: progression and views]. In Sosiaali- ja terveydenhuollon tietotekniikan ja tiedonhallinnan tutkimuspäivät: Tutkimuspaperit 2008 (pp. 60-65). Retrieved May 12, 2011, from http://stty.org/joomla/index.php?option=com_content&view=category&layout=blog&id=44&Itemid=79

Kwak, H., Lee, C., Park, H., & Moon, S. (2010). What is Twitter, a Social Network or a News Media? In *Proceedings of the 19th International Conference on World Wide Web*, (pp. 591-600). Academic Press.

Kyriacou, E. C., Pattichis, C. S., Karaolis, M. A., Loizou, C. P., Christodoulou, C. I., & Pattichis, M. S. et al. (2007). An integrated system for assessing stroke risk. *IEEE Engineering in Medicine and Biology Magazine*, *26*(5), 43–50. doi:10.1109/EMB.2007.901794 PMID:17941322

Lacks, P., & Morin, C. M. (1992). Recent advances in the assessment and treatment of insomnia. *Journal of Consulting and Clinical Psychology*, *60*(4), 586–594. doi:10.1037/0022-006X.60.4.586 PMID:1506506

Lain, S. J., Roberts, C. L., Hadfield, R. M., Bell, J. C., & Morris, J. M. (2008). How accurate is the reporting of obstetric haemorrhage in hospital discharge data? A validation study. *Australian and New Zealand Journal of Obstetrics and Gynaecology*, *48*(5), 481–484. doi:10.1111/j.1479-828X.2008.00910.x PMID:19032664

LaMendola, W. (2010). Social Work and Social Presence in an Online World. *Journal of Technology in Human Services*, *28*(1), 108–119. doi:10.1080/15228831003759562

Landon, B. E., Keating, N. L., Barnett, M. L., Onnela, J.-P., Paul, S., & O'Malley, A. J. et al. (2012). Variation in patient-sharing networks of physicians across the United States. *Journal of the American Medical Association*, *308*(3), 265–273. doi:10.1001/jama.2012.7615 PMID:22797644

Landon, B. E., Onnela, J.-P., Keating, N. L., Barnett, M. L., Paul, S., & O'Malley, A. J. et al. (2013). Using Administrative Data to Identify Naturally Occurring Networks of Physicians. *Medical Care*. doi:10.1097/MLR.0b013e3182977991 PMID:23807593

Landt, J. (2001, October). *Shrouds of Time: The history of RFID*. Association for Automatic Identification and Mobility.

Larsen, A. K., Sanders, R., Astray, A. A., & Hole, G. O. (2008). E-teacher Challenges and Competencies in International Comparative Social Work Courses. *Social Work Education*, *27*(6), 623–633. doi:10.1080/02615470802201671

Laurillard, D. (2004). E-Learning in higher education. In P. Ashwin (Ed.), *Changing higher education*. London: Routledge Falmer.

Lavrac, N., Bohanec, M., Pur, A., Cestnik, B., Debeljak, M., & Kobler, A. (2007). Data mining and visualization for decision support and modeling of public health-care resources. *Journal of Biomedical Informatics*, *40*(4), 438–447. doi:10.1016/j.jbi.2006.10.003 PMID:17157076

Lazarou, C., Karaolis, M., Matalas, A. L., & Panagiotakos, D. B. (2012). Dietary patterns analysis using data mining method. An application to data from the CYKIDS study. *Computer Methods and Programs in Biomedicine*, *108*(2), 706–714. doi:10.1016/j.cmpb.2011.12.011 PMID:22296977

Leavitt, H. (1949). *Some effects of certain communication patterns on group performance*. Boston: MIT Press.

Leavitt, H. (1951). Some effects of certain communication patterns on group performance. *Journal of Abnormal and Social Psychology*, *46*(1), 38–50. doi:10.1037/h0057189 PMID:14813886

Lee, C. S., Wang, M. H., Acampora, G., Loia, V., & Hsu, C. Y. (2009). *Ontology-based Intelligent Fuzzy Agent for Diabetes Application*. New York: IEEE.

Lee, C. P., & Shim, J. P. (2007). An exploratory study of radio frequency identification (RFID) adoption in the healthcare industry. *European Journal of Information Systems*, *16*, 712–772. doi:10.1057/palgrave.ejis.3000716

Lee, J. W., & Giraud-Carrier, C. (2013). Results on mining NHANES data: A case study in evidence-based medicine. *Computers in Biology and Medicine*, *43*(5), 493–503. doi:10.1016/j.compbiomed.2013.02.018 PMID:23566395

Lee, M. C. (2010). Explaining and predicting users' continuance intention toward e-learning: An extension of the expectation–confirmation model. *Computers & Education*, *54*(2), 506–516. doi:10.1016/j.compedu.2009.09.002

Lee, T. T., Liu, C. Y., Kuo, Y. H., Mills, M. E., Fong, J. G., & Hung, C. (2011). Application of data mining to the identification of critical factors in patient falls using a web-based reporting system. *International Journal of Medical Informatics*, *80*(2), 141–150. doi:10.1016/j.ijmedinf.2010.10.009 PMID:21115393

Lee, W., & Shih, B. (2009). Application of neural networks to recognize profitable customers for dental services marketing-a case of dental clinics in Taiwan. *Expert Systems with Applications*, *36*(1), 199–208. doi:10.1016/j.eswa.2007.09.028

Lee, W., Shih, B., & Chung, Y. S. (2008). The exploration of consumers' behavior in choosing hospital by the application of neural network. *Expert Systems with Applications*, *34*(2), 806–816. doi:10.1016/j.eswa.2006.10.020

Lehman, T. M., Guld, M. O., Deselaers, T., Keysers, D., Schubert, H., & Spitzer, K. et al. (2005). Automatic categorization of medical images for content-based retrieval and data mining. *Computerized Medical Imaging and Graphics*, *29*(2-3), 143–155. doi:10.1016/j.compmedimag.2004.09.010 PMID:15755534

Lehtinen, V., Näsänen, J., & Sarvas, R. (2009). A little silly and empty-headed: Older adults' understandings of social networking sites. In *Proceedings of the 23rd British HCI Group Annual Conference on People and Computers: Celebrating People and Technology* (pp. 45-54). British Computer Society.

Lettieri, E., Borga, F., & Savoldelli, A. (2004). Knowledge Management in Nonprofit Organizations. *Journal of Knowledge Management*, *8*(6), 16. doi:10.1108/13673270410567602

Leung, W. C. (2002). Competency based medical training[review]. *BMJ (Clinical Research Ed.)*, *325*, 693–696. doi:10.1136/bmj.325.7366.693 PMID:12351364

Leung, Z. S. (2009). Knowledge Management in Social Work: Types and Processes of Knowledge Sharing in Social Service Organizations. *British Journal of Social Work*, *39*(4), 693–709. doi:10.1093/bjsw/bcp034

Liao, S. H., Chu, P. H., & Hsiao, P. Y. (2012). Data mining techniques and applications – A decade review from 2000 to 2011. *Expert Systems with Applications*, *39*(12), 11303–11311. doi:10.1016/j.eswa.2012.02.063

Liaw, S., Taggart, J., Dennis, S., & Yeo, A. (2011). *Data quality and fitness for purpose of routinely collected data –A general practice case study from an electronic Practice-Based Research Network (ePBRN)*. Paper presented at the AMIA 2011 Annual Symposium Improving Health: Informatics and IT Changing the World. New York, NY.

Liaw, S. T., Rahimi, A., Ray, P., Taggart, J., Dennis, S., & de Lusignan, S. et al. (2013). Towards an ontology for data quality in integrated chronic disease management: A realist review of the literature. *International Journal of Medical Informatics*, *82*(2), 139. doi:10.1016/j.ijmedinf.2012.12.007 PMID:23122633

Liaw, S., Chen, H., Maneze, D., Taggart, J., Dennis, S., & Vagholkar, S. et al. (2011). Health reform: is current electronic information fit for purpose? *Emergency Medicine Australasia*. PMID:22313561

Libman, E., Fichten, C. S., Bailes, S., & Amsel, R. (2000). Sleep Questionnaire Versus Sleep Diary: Which Measure Is Better? *International Journal of Rehabilitation and Health*, *5*(3), 205–209. doi:10.1023/A:1012955423123

Li, E. Y. (1997). Perceived importance of information system success factors: a meta analysis of group differences. *Information & Management*, *32*(1), 15–28. doi:10.1016/S0378-7206(97)00005-0

*Lifenaut*. (2014). Retrieved February 28, 2014 from https://www.lifenaut.com/bina48/

*LifeWatch*. (2013). Retrieved from http://www.lifewatch.com/

Li, H. C., & Ko, W. M. (2007). *Automated food ontology construction mechanism for diabetes diet care*. New York: IEEE. doi:10.1109/ICMLC.2007.4370653

Li, M., Yu, S., Zheng, Y., Ren, K., & Lou, W. (2013). Scalable and Secure Sharing of Personal Health Records in Cloud Computing Using Attribute-Based Encryption. *IEEE Transactions on Parallel and Distributed Systems*, *24*(1), 131–143. doi:10.1109/TPDS.2012.97

Lima, L., Novais, P., Costa, R., Cruz, J., & Neves, J. (2010). Decision Making Based on Quality-of-Information a Clinical Guideline for Chronic Obstructive Pulmonary Disease Scenario. In A. de Leon F. de Carvalho, S. Rodríguez-González, J. De Paz Santana & J. Rodríguez (Eds.), Distributed Computing and Artificial Intelligence (Vol. 79, pp. 417-424). Springer.

Lin, H., Shao, J., Zhang, C., & Fang, Y. (2013). CAM: Cloud-Assisted Privacy Preserving Mobile Health Monitoring. *IEEE Transactions on Information Forensics and Security*, *8*(6), 985–997. doi:10.1109/TIFS.2013.2255593

Link, T. M., & Marz, R. (2006). Computer literacy and attitudes towards e-learning among first medical students. *BMC Medical Education*, *6*(34). PMID:16784524

Li, S.-H., Cheng, K.-A., Lu, W.-H., & Lin, T.-C. (2011). Developing an Active Emergency Medical Service System Based on WiMAX Technology. *Journal of Medical Systems*, *36*(5), 3177–3193. doi:10.1007/s10916-011-9809-8 PMID:22109672

Liszka, K. J., Mackin, M. A., Lichter, M. J., York, D. W., Dilip, P., & Rosenbaum, D. S. (2004). Keeping a beat on the heart. *IEEE Pervasive Computing*, *3*(4), 42–49. doi:10.1109/MPRV.2004.10

Littlejohn, A. (2003). Issues in reusing online resources. In A. Littlejohn (Ed.), *Reusing online resources: A Sustainable Approach to eLearning* (pp. 1–6). London: Creative Print and Design.

Li, Z. (2010). *An ontology-driven concept-based information retrieveal approach for Web documents*. Edmonton, Canada: University of Alberta.

Loader, B. D., Hardey, M., & Keeble, L. (2008). Health informatics for older people: a review of ICT facilitated integrated care for older people. *International Journal of Social Welfare*, *17*(1), 46–53. doi:10.1111/j.1468-2397.2007.00489.x

*Loebner*. (2014). Retrieved February 28, 2014 from http://loebner.net/Prizef/loebner-prize.html

Lopez-Lorca, A. A., Miller, T., Pedell, S., Sterling, L., & Curumsing, M. K. (2014). (Manuscript submitted for publication). *Modelling People's Emotions for Socio-technical Systems.*

López-Vallverdú, J. A., Riaño, D., & Collado, A. (2012). Rule-Based Combination of Comorbid Treatments for Chronic Diseases Applied to Hypertension, Diabetes Mellitus and Heart Failure. *ProHealth/KR4HC, 7738*, 30-41.

Los, R. K., van Ginneken, A. M., Roukema, J., Moll, H. A., & van der Lei, J. (2005).. . *Medical Informatics and the Internet in Medicine*, *30*(4), 267–276. doi:10.1080/14639230500367563 PMID:16531353

Lucas, P., & Ten Teije, S. M. (2008). *Computer-based Medical Guidelines and Protocols: A Primer and Current Trends*. IOS Press.

Lunnas, H. & Kuusisto-Niemi, S. (1991). *Sosiaalitoimen ohjelmistoselvitys 1991* [*Report on social services software 1991*]. Helsinki: Kunnallishallinnon tietotekniikkaneuvottelukunta.

Luostarinen, H., & Väliverronen, E. (1991). *Tekstinsyöjät. Yhteiskuntatieteellisen kirjallisuuden lukutaidosta. [Text Eaters. About the social science literature literacy.]*. Tampere: Vastapaino.

Luprano, J., Sola, J., Dasen, S., Koller, J.-M., & Chetelat, O. (2006). Combination of body sensor networks and on-body signal processing algorithms: the practical case of myheart project. In *Proceedings of International Workshop on Wearable and Implantable Body Sensor Networks,* (pp. 76–79). BSN.

Lyytinen, K., & Hirschheim, R. (1988). Information systems failures—a survey and classification of the empirical literature. In *Oxford surveys in information technology* (pp. 257–309). Oxford University Press, Inc.

Mabotuwana, T., & Warren, J. (2009). An ontology-based approach to enhance querying capabilities of general practice medicine for better management of hypertension. *Artificial Intelligence in Medicine*, *47*(2), 87–103. doi:10.1016/j.artmed.2009.07.001 PMID:19709865

Macaulay, A. C. (2007). Promoting Participatory Research by Family Physicians. *Annals of Family Medicine*, *5*(6), 557–560. doi:10.1370/afm.755 PMID:18025494

Madden, M., & Smith, A. (2010). *Pew Research Center. Reputation Management and Social Media*. Retrieved from http://pewinternet.org/~/media//Files/Reports/2010/PIP_Reputation_Management_with_topline.pdf

Maillart, L.M., Kamrani, A., Norman B.A., Rajgopal, J., & Hawrylak, P.J. (2010). Optimizing RFID tag-inventorying algorithms. *IEEE Transactions,* (42), 690-702.

Manthorpe, J., Kharicha, K., Goodman, C., Harari, D., Swift, C., & Iliffe, S. (2010). Smarter Working in Social and Health Care: Professional Perspectives on a New Technology for Risk Appraisal with Older People. *British Journal of Social Work*, *40*(6), 1829–1846. doi:10.1093/bjsw/bcp100

Maragoudakis, M., Lymberopoulos, D., Fakotakis, N., & Spiropoulos, K. (2008). A Hierarchical, Ontology-Driven Bayesian Concept for Ubiquitous Medical Environments-A Case Study for Pulmonary Diseases. In *Proceedings of 2008 30th Annual International Conference of the Ieee Engineering in Medicine and Biology Society,* (pp. 3807-3810). New York: IEEE.

Marcano-Cedeno, A., Chausa, P., Garcia, A., Caceres, C., Tormos, J. M., & Gomez, E. J. (2013). Data mining applied to the cognitive rehabilitation of patients with acquired brain injury. *Expert Systems with Applications*, *40*(4), 1054–1060. doi:10.1016/j.eswa.2012.08.034

Marchewka, J. T., Liu, C., & Kostiwa, K. (2007). An application of the UTAUT model for understanding student perceptions using course management software. *Communications of the IIMA*, *7*(2), 93–104.

Marshall, J. (2014). Agent-Based Modelling of Emotional Goals in Digital Media Design Projects. *IJPOP special issue on Emotions and People-Oriented Programming*, *3*(1), 44-59.

Martín-Martínez, D., Casaseca-de-la Higuera, P., Alberola-López, S., Andrés-de Llano, J., López-Villalobos, J. A., Ardura-Fernández, J., & Alberola-López, C. (2012). Nonlinear analysis of actigraphic signals for the assessment of the attention-deficit/hyperactivity disorder (adhd). *Medical Engineering & Physics*, *34*(9), 1317–1329. doi:10.1016/j.medengphy.2011.12.023 PMID:22297088

Martinsons, M., & Hosley, S. (1993). Planning a strategic information system for a market-oriented non-profit organization. *Journal of Systems Management*, *44*(2), 14.

Masrom, M., & Hussein, R. (2008). *User Acceptance of Information Technology:Understanding Theories and Models: Venton Publishing (M)*. Sdn. Bhd.

Maylahn, C., Fleming, D., & Birkhead, G. (2013). Health departments in a brave new world. *Preventing Chronic Disease*, *10*, E41. doi:10.5888/pcd10.130003 PMID:23517584

McGarry, K., Garfield, S., & Wermter, S. (2007). Auto-extraction, representation and integration of a diabetes ontology using Bayesian networks. In P. Kokol, V. Podgorelec, D. MiceticTurk, M. Zorman & M. Verlic (Eds.), In *Proceedings of Twentieth IEEE International Symposium on Computer-Based Medical Systems,* (pp. 612-617). IEEE.

McGuinness, D. L., & van Harmelen, F. (2004). *OWL Web Ontology Language*. Retrieved from W3C Recommendation: http://www.w3.org/TR/owl-features/

McJunkin, M. C. (1995). Precision and recall in title keyword searches. *Information Technology and Libraries*, *14*(3), 161–171.

Mcneil, K., Gordon, P. M., & Brna, K. E. (2012). Epilepsy in the Twitter Era: A Need to Re-tweet the Way we Think about Seizures. *Epilepsy & Behavior*, *23*(2), 127–130. doi:10.1016/j.yebeh.2011.10.020 PMID:22134096

McNutt, J.G. (2000). Coming Perspectives in the Development of Electronic Advocacy for Social Policy Practice. *Critical Social Work, 1*(1). Retrieved May 12, 2011, from http://www.uwindsor.ca/criticalsocialwork/coming-perspectives-in-the-development-of-electronic-advocacy-for-social-policy-practice-0

McNutt, J. (1996). National Information Infrastructure Policy and the Future of the American Welfare State: Implications for the Social Welfare Policy Curriculum. *Journal of Social Work Education*, *32*(3), 375–388.

*MedApp*. (2013). Retrieved from https://healthcom.medapps.net/Login.aspx

*MedHelp*. (2013). Retrieved from http://www.medhelp.org/

*Medicare and Medicaid EHR Incentive Programs*. (2013). Available at http://www.healthit.gov/providers-professionals/ehr-incentive-programs

Megalooikonomou, V., & Kontos, D. (2007). Medical Data Fusion for Telemedicine. *IEEE Engineering in Medicine and Biology Magazine, 26*(5), 36-42.

Mehrjerdi, Y. Z. (2008). RFID enabled systems: a brief review. *Assembly Automation*, *28*(3), 235–245. doi:10.1108/01445150810889493

Melander-Wikman, A., Faltholm, Y., & Gard, G. (2008). Safety vs. privacy: elderly persons' experiences of a mobile safety alarm. *Health & Social Care in the Community*, *16*(4), 337–346. doi:10.1111/j.1365-2524.2007.00743.x PMID:18613909

Meltzer, D., Chung, J., Khalili, P., Marlow, E., Arora, V., Schumock, G., & Burt, R. (2010). Exploring the use of social network methods in designing healthcare quality improvement teams. *Social Science & Medicine*, *71*(6), 1119–1130. doi:10.1016/j.socscimed.2010.05.012 PMID:20674116

Meng, X. H., Huang, Y. X., Rao, D. P., Zhang, Q., & Liu, Q. (2013). Comparison of three data mining models for predicting diabetes or prediabetes by risk factors. *The Kaohsiung Journal of Medical Sciences*, *29*(2), 93–99. doi:10.1016/j.kjms.2012.08.016 PMID:23347811

Menon, G. M., & Miller-Cribbs, J. (2002). Online Social Work Practice: Issues and Guidelines for the Profession. *Administration in Social Work*, *3*(2), 104–116.

Meyer, D., Marx, T., & Ball-Seiter, V. (2011). Social isolation and telecommunication in the nursing home: A pilot study. *Gerontechnology (Valkenswaard), 10*(1), 51–58. doi:10.4017/gt.2011.10.01.004.00

Michalowski, M., Wilk, S., Michalowski, W., Farion, K., Lin, D., & Mohapatra, S. (2013). Using Constraint Logic Programming to Implement Iterative Actions and Numerical Measures during Mitigation of Concurrently Applied Clinical Practice Guidelines. In *Proceedings of 14th Conference on Artificial Intelligence in Medicine* (vol. 7885, pp. 17-22). Murcia, Spain: Springer.

Miguel, K. D. S., & Lewin, G. (2008). Personal emergency alarms: what impact do they have on older people's lives? *Australasian Journal on Ageing, 27*(2), 103–105. doi:10.1111/j.1741-6612.2008.00286.x PMID:18713202

Milenković, A., Otto, C., & Jovanov, E. (2006). Wireless sensor networks for personal health monitoring: Issues and an implementation. *Computer Communications, 29*(13–14), 2521–2533. doi:10.1016/j.comcom.2006.02.011

Miles, M. B., & Huberman, A. M. (1994). *An Expanded Sourcebook:Qualitative Data Analysis* (2nd ed.). Sage Publications International.

Miles, M. B., & Huberman, A. M. (1994). *Qualitative data analysis* (2nd ed.). Sage.

Miller, T., Pedell, S., Mendoza, A., Keirnan, A., Sterling, L., & Lopez-Lorca, A. A. (2014). *Emotionally-driven models for people-oriented requirements engineering: the case study of emergency alarm systems.* (Under review).

Miller, T., Pedell, S., Sterling, L., & Lu, B. (2011). Engaging Stakeholders with Agent-Oriented Requirements Modelling. In D. Weyns, & M.-P. Gleizes (Eds.), *Agent-Oriented Software Engineering XI* (Vol. 6788, pp. 62–78). Springer. doi:10.1007/978-3-642-22636-6_4

Min, H., Manion, F. J., Goralczyk, E., Wong, Y. N., Ross, E., & Beck, J. R. (2009). Integration of prostate cancer clinical data using an ontology. *Journal of Biomedical Informatics, 42*(6), 1035–1045. doi:10.1016/j.jbi.2009.05.007 PMID:19497389

Ministry of Social Affairs and Health. (2011). *Development project for social services underway.* Retrieved May 14, 2011, from http://www.stm.fi/en/pressreleases/pressrelease/view/1287485

Mirota, D. J., Wang, H., Taylor, R. H., Ishii, M., Gallia, G. L., & Hager, G. D. (2012). A system for video-based navigation for endoscopic endonasal skull base surgery. *IEEE Transactions on Medical Imaging, 31*(4), 963–976. doi:10.1109/TMI.2011.2176500 PMID:22113772

Mishna, F., Bogo, M., Root, J., Sawyer, J.-L., & Khoury-Kassabri, M. (2012). "It just crept in": The Digital Age and Implications for Social Work Practice. *Journal of Clinical Social Work, 40*, 277–286. doi:10.1007/s10615-012-0383-4

Mitchell, et al. (2011). 50 Years of Informatics Research on Decision Support: What's Next. *Methods of Information in Medicine, 50*, 525–535. doi:10.3414/ME11-06-0004 PMID:22146915

Mitchell, J., & Westerduin, F. (2008). Emergency department information system diagnosis: how accurate is it? *Emergency Medicine Journal, 25*(11), 784. doi:10.1136/emj.2007.050104 PMID:18955631

Monnickendam, M., Savaya, R., & Waysman, M. (2004). Equity Perceptions as a Determinant of Computer User Satisfaction in Human Services. *Journal of Social Service Research, 31*(2), 41–50. doi:10.1300/J079v31n02_03

Montani, S., & Terenziani, P. (2006). Exploiting decision theory concepts within clinical guideline systems: Toward a general approach. *International Journal of Intelligent Systems, 21*(6), 585–599. doi:10.1002/int.20149

Moody, D. L., & Shanks, G. G. (2003). Improving the quality of data models: empirical validation of a quality management framework. *Information Systems, 28*(6), 619–650. doi:10.1016/S0306-4379(02)00043-1

Moon, S. S., & DeWeaver, K. L. (2005). Electronic Advocacy and Social Welfare Policy Education. *Journal of Teaching in Social Work, 25*(1/2), 57–68. doi:10.1300/J067v25n01_04

Moon, S. S., Kang, S. Y., Jitpitaklert, W., & Kim, S. B. (2012). Decision tree models for characterizing smoking patterns of older adults. *Expert Systems with Applications, 39*(1), 445–451. doi:10.1016/j.eswa.2011.07.035

Moro, M. L., & Morsillo, F. (2004). Can hospital discharge diagnoses be used for surveillance of surgical-site infections? *The Journal of Hospital Infection, 56*(3), 239–241. doi:10.1016/j.jhin.2003.12.022 PMID:15003675

Mullen, B., & Eduardo, J. (1991). Effects of communication network structure: Components of positional centrality* 1. *Social Networks*, *13*(2), 169–185. doi:10.1016/0378-8733(91)90019-P

Murphy, L., Parnass, P., Mitchell, D. L., Hallett, R., Cayley, P., & Seagram, S. (2009). Client Satisfaction and Outcome Comparisons of Online and Face-to-face Counselling Methods. *British Journal of Social Work*, *39*(4), 627–640. doi:10.1093/bjsw/bcp041

Murray, P., & Carter, L. (2005). Improving marketing intelligence through learning systems and knowledge communities in not-for-profit workplaces. *Journal of Workplace Learning*, *17*(7), 421–435. doi:10.1108/13665620510620016

Musen, M., Goldstein, M. K., Tu, S., Martins, S., Nyulas, C., Jung, H., & Kum, P. (2011). *GLINDA Interaction Ontology*. Retrieved from GLINDA: GuideLine INteraction Detection Arch.: http://glinda-project.stanford.edu/guidelineinteractionontology.html

Mynatt, E. D., Rowan, J., Craighill, S., & Jacobs, A. (2001). *Digital family portraits: supporting peace of mind for extended family members*. Paper presented at the SIGCHI Conference on Human Factors in Computing Systems. Seattle, WA.

Naccarato, T. (2010). Child Welfare Informatics: A proposed subspecialty for social work. *Children and Youth Services Review*, *32*(12), 1729–1734. doi:10.1016/j.childyouth.2010.07.016

Nagy, A. (2005). The Impact of E-Learning. In P. A. Bruck, A. Buchholz, Z. Karssen, & A. Zerfass (Eds.), *E-Content: Technologies and Perspectives for the European Market* (pp. 79–96). Berlin: Springer-Verlag. doi:10.1007/3-540-26387-X_4

Nagy, P., George, I., Bernstein, W., Caban, J., Klein, R., Mezrich, R., & Park, A. (2006). Radio Frequency Identification Systems Technology in the Surgical Setting. *Surgical Innovation*, *13*(1), 61–67. doi:10.1177/155335060601300110 PMID:16708157

Nahar, J., Imam, T., Tickle, K. S., & Chen, Y. P. (2013). Association rule mining to detect factors which contribute to heart disease in males and females. *Expert Systems with Applications*, *40*(4), 1086–1093. doi:10.1016/j.eswa.2012.08.028

Nahas, H. A., & Deogun, J. S. (2007). Radio Frequency Identification Applications in Smart Hospitals. In *Proceedings of the Twentieth IEEE International Symposium on Computer-Based Medical Systems (CBMS'07)*. IEEE.

Nair, B. R., & Finucane, P. M. (2003). Reforming medical education to enhance the management of chronic disease. *The Medical Journal of Australia*, *179*, 257–259. PMID:12924974

Najaftorkaman, M., Ghapanchi, A. H., Talaei-Khoei, A., & Ray, P. (2013). Recent research areas and grand challenges in Electronic Health Record: A Literature survey approach. *The International Technology Management Review*, *3*(1), 12–21. doi:10.2991/itmr.2013.3.1.2

*NAO*. (2014). Retrieved February 25th 2014 from http://www.aldebaran-robotics.com/en/

National Institute for Health and Welfare THL. (2010). *Facts about Social Welfare and Health Care in Finland 2010*. Helsinki: National Institute for Health and Welfare.

Netting, F. E., & Williams, F. G. (1996). Case manager-physician collaboration: Implications for professional identity, roles, and relationships. *Health & Social Work*, *21*(3), 216–224. PMID:8854126

Nevo, D., & Wade, M. (2005). *Why Good Technologies Disappoint*. Academic Press.

Ngyuen, L. H. (2007). Child Welfare Informatics: A New Definition for an Established Practice. *Social Work*, *52*(4), 361–363. doi:10.1093/sw/52.4.361 PMID:18232246

Nicolini, D., Powell, J., Conville, P., & Martinez-Solano, L. (2008). Managing knowledge in the healthcare sector. A review. *International Journal of Management Reviews*, *10*, 245–263. doi:10.1111/j.1468-2370.2007.00219.x

Nightingale, J., Wang, Q., & Grecos, C. (2012). HEVStream: a framework for streaming and evaluation of high efficiency video coding (HEVC) content in loss-prone networks. *IEEE Transactions on Consumer Electronics*, *58*(2), 404–412. doi:10.1109/TCE.2012.6227440

Nilakanta, S., Miller, L., Peer, A., & Bojja, V. M. (2009). Contribution of Knowledge and Knowledge Management Capability on Business Processes among Healthcare Organizations. In *Proceedings of System Sciences*. IEEE.

Nimmagadda, S. L., Nimmagadda, S. K., & Dreher, H. (2008). Ontology based data warehouse modeling and managing ecology of human body for disease and drug prescription management. In *Proceedings of 2008 2nd IEEE International Conference on Digital Ecosystems and Technologies* (pp. 465-473). IEEE.

Nonaka, I., & Takeuchi, H. (1995). The Knowledge Creating Company. Oxford University Press.

Norval, C., Arnott, J., Hine, N., & Hanson, V. (2011). Purposeful social media as support platform: Communication frameworks for older adults requiring care. In *Proceedings of 5th International Conference on Pervasive Computing Technologies for Healthcare (PervasiveHealth)*, (pp. 492–494). Academic Press.

Nunnally, J. C. (2010). *Psychometric theory*. India: McGraw-Hill Education.

O'Connor, M.C. (2005, August). Efficiencies Drive RFID adoption. *RFID Journal*.

O'Connor, M.C. (2006, November). Toronto area hospital kicks off asset tracking pilot. *RFID Journal*.

O'Sullivan, H., & McKimm, J. (2011). Doctor as professional and doctor as leader: same attributes, attitudes and values? *British Journal of Hospital Medicine*, *72*, 463–466. doi:10.12968/hmed.2011.72.8.463 PMID:21841592

O'Donoghue, J., Herbert, J., O'Reilly, P., & Sammon, D. (2009). Towards Improved Information Quality: The Integration of Body Area Network Data within Electronic Health Records. In M. Mokhtari, I. Khalil, J. Bauchet, D. Zhang, & C. Nugent (Eds.), *Ambient Assistive Health and Wellness Management in the Heart of the City* (Vol. 5597, pp. 299–302). doi:10.1007/978-3-642-02868-7_46

Office of the National Coordinator for Health Information Technology (ONC). (2013). *Health IT Policy Committee: Recommendations to the National Coordinator for Health IT*. Retrieved September 12, 2013 from http://www.healthit.gov/policy-researchers-implementers/health-it-policy-committee-recommendations-national-coordinator-heal

Oliver, N., & Flores-Mangas, F. (2006). Healthgear: A real-time wearable system for monitoring and analyzing physiological signals. In *Proceedings of International Workshop on Wearable and Implantable Body Sensor Networks*, (pp. 1-4). BSN.

Oliver, S., & Kandadi, K. R. (2006). How to develop knowledge culture in organizations? A multiple case study of large distributed organizations. *Journal of Knowledge Management*, *10*(4), 6–24. doi:10.1108/13673270610679336

Omurtag, K., Jimenez, P. T., Ratts, V., Odem, R., & Cooper, A. R. (2012). The ART of Social Networking: how SART Member Clinics are Connecting with Patients Online. *Fertility and Sterility*, *97*(1), 88–94. doi:10.1016/j.fertnstert.2011.10.001 PMID:22088209

Orentlicher, D. (2010). Prescription data mining and the protection of patients' interests. *The Journal of Law, Medicine & Ethics*, *38*(1), 74–84. doi:10.1111/j.1748-720X.2010.00468.x PMID:20446986

Orme, A. M., Yao, H., & Etzkorn, L. H. (2007). Indicating ontology data quality, stability, and completeness throughout ontology evolution. *Journal of Software Maintenance and Evolution-Research and Practice*, *19*(1), 49–75. doi:10.1002/smr.341

Ou-Yang, C., Agustianty, S., & Wang, H. C. (2013). Developing a data mining approach to investigate association between physician prescription and patient outcome – A study on re-hospitalization in Stevens–Johnson Syndrome. *Computer Methods and Programs in Biomedicine*, *112*(1), 84–91. doi:10.1016/j.cmpb.2013.07.004 PMID:23910224

Ozok, A. A., Gurses, A., Wu, H., Nelson, M., Moen, D., & Wei, J. (2009). Usability and User Acceptance for Personal Health Records: A Perspective from Healthcare Citizens. In A. A. Ozok, & P. Zaphiris (Eds.), *Online Communities and Social Computing* (Vol. 5621, pp. 690–699). Springer. doi:10.1007/978-3-642-02774-1_74

Ozuah, P. O. (2002). Undergraduate medical education: thoughts on future challenges. *BMC Medical Education*, *2*, 8–10. doi:10.1186/1472-6920-2-8 PMID:12149136

Paay, J., Sterling, L., Vetere, F., Howard, S., & Boettcher, A. (2009). Engineering the social:The role of shared artifacts. *International Journal of Human-Computer Studies*, *67*(5), 437–454. doi:10.1016/j.ijhcs.2008.12.002

Page L. (2007, May). Hospitals tune into RFID – Testing gives way to implementation. *Material Management in Health Care*, 18-20.

Page, L. (2007, August). Hospitals tap into RFID to track patients and equipment, Upfront, News and Trends. *Health Facilities Management*, 5–6.

Palmer, E., & Eveline, J. (2012). Sustaining low pay in aged care work. *Gender, Work and Organization*, *19*, 254–275.

Panayides, A., Pattichis, M. S., Pattichis, C. S., & Pitsillides, A. (2011). A tutorial for emerging wireless medical video transmission systems. *IEEE Antennas and Propagation Magazine*, *53*(2), 202–213. doi:10.1109/MAP.2011.5949369

Pandian, P., Mohanavelu, K., Safeer, K., Kotresh, T., Shakunthala, D., Gopal, P., & Padaki, V. (2008). Smart vest: Wearable multi-parameter remote physiological monitoring system. *Medical Engineering & Physics*, *30*(4), 466–477. doi:10.1016/j.medengphy.2007.05.014 PMID:17869159

Pannarale, P., Catalano, D., De Caro, G., Grillo, G., Leo, P., & Pappada, G. et al. (2012). GIDL: A rule based expert system for GenBank Intelligent Data Loading into the Molecular Biodiversity Database. *BMC Bioinformatics*, *13*(Suppl 4), S4. doi:10.1186/1471-2105-13-S4-S4 PMID:22536971

Pantelopoulos, A., & Bourbakis, N. (2010). A survey on wearable sensor-based systems for health monitoring and prognosis. *IEEE Transactions on Systems, Man and Cybernetics. Part C, Applications and Reviews*, *40*(1), 1–12. doi:10.1109/TSMCC.2009.2032660

Pappu, M., Singhal, R., & Zoghi, B. (2004). *RFID in hospitals: Issues and Solutions.* A report from the Consortium for the Accelerated Deployment of RFID in Distribution.

Paradiso, R., Loriga, G., & Taccini, N. (2005). A wearable healthcare system based on knitted integrated sensors. *IEEE Transactions on Information Technology in Biomedicine*, *9*(3), 337–344. doi:10.1109/TITB.2005.854512 PMID:16167687

Parhizi, S., Steege, L. S., & Pasupathy, K. S. (2013). Mining the relationships between psychosocial factors and fatigue dimensions among registered nurses. *International Journal of Industrial Ergonomics*, *43*(1), 82–90. doi:10.1016/j.ergon.2012.11.010

Park, Y. J. (2013). Digital literacy and privacy behavior online. *Communication Research*, *40*(2), 215–236. doi:10.1177/0093650211418338

*Paro*. (2014). Retrieved February 28, 2014 from http://www.parorobots.com/

Parton, N. (2009). Challenges to practice and knowledge in child welfare social work: From the 'social' to the 'informational'? *Children and Youth Services Review*, *31*(7), 715–721. doi:10.1016/j.childyouth.2009.01.008

Patel, et al. (2009). The coming of age of artificial intelligence in medicine. *Artificial Intelligence in Medicine*, *46*(1), 5–17. doi:10.1016/j.artmed.2008.07.017 PMID:18790621

Pathak, J., Kiefer, R. C., Bielinski, S. J., & Chute, C. G. (2012). Mining the human phenome using semantic web technologies: a case study for Type 2 Diabetes. In Proceedings of*AMIA ... Annual Symposium Proceedings*, (pp. 699–708). AMIA. PMID:23304343

Pathak, J., Kiefer, R. C., & Chute, C. G. (2012). Using semantic web technologies for cohort identification from electronic health records for clinical research. *AMIA Summits Transl Sci Proc*, *2012*, 10–19. PMID:22779040

*Patientlikeme* . (2013). Retrieved from http://www.patientslikeme.com/

Patlak, M. (2005). *Tips to help you detect common sleep disorders*. Retrieved 31 March 2008, from http://www.acpinternist.org/archives/2005/03/sleep.htm#pool

Patton, M. Q. (2002). *Qualitative research and evaluation methods*. Thousand Oaks, CA: Sage Publications, Inc..

Patton, Q. M. (1990). *Qualitative Evaluation and Research Methods* (2nd ed.). Sage Publications.

Päykkönen, K. & Pohjola, A. (2007). *Selvitys sosiaalialan tiedonhallinnan nykytilasta Suomessa.* [*Account of the present state of social services knowledge management in Finland*]. Retrieved May 13, 2011, from http://www.sosiaaliportti.fi/fi-FI/tikesos/aineistot/selvitykset/

PC. (2008). *Trends in Aged Care Services: some implications* (Commission Research Paper). Canberra: Productivity Commission.

Peckover, S., Hall, C., & White, S. (2009). From Policy to Practice: The Implementation and Negotiation of Technologies in Everyday Child Welfare. *Children & Society*, *23*(2), 136–148. doi:10.1111/j.1099-0860.2008.00143.x

Pedell, S., Miller, T., Sterling, L., Vetere, F., & Howard, S. (2014). (forthcoming). Tools for participation: Intergenerational technology design for the home. *International Journal of Design*.

Pedell, S., Sterling, L., Keirnan, A., & Dobson, G. (2013). *Emotions around emergency alarm use: A field study with older adults (Report for Smart Services CRC)*. Swinburne University of Technology.

Peeters, P. H. (2000). Design criteria for an automatic safety-alarm system for elderly. *Technology and health Care, 8*(2), 81-91.

Peleg, M., Boxwala, A. A., & Ogunyemi, O. (2000). Glif3: the evolution of a guideline representation format. *Proc AMIA Symp*, 645–649. PMID:11079963

Pelgrum, W. J. (2001). Obstacles to the integration of ICT in education: results from a worldwide educational assessment. *Computers & Education*, *37*, 163–178. doi:10.1016/S0360-1315(01)00045-8

Pérez-Rey, D., Maojo, V., García-Remesal, M., Alonso-Calvo, R., Billhardt, H., Martín-Sánchez, F., & Sousa, A. (2006). ONTOFUSION: Ontology-based integration of genomic and clinical databases. *Computers in Biology and Medicine*, *36*(7-8), 712–730. doi:10.1016/j.compbiomed.2005.02.004 PMID:16144697

Perron, B. E., Taylor, H. O., Glass, J. E., & Margerum-Leys, J. (2010). Information and Communication Technologies in Social Work. *Administration in Social Work*, *11*(1), 67–81. PMID:21691444

Petter, S. (2008). Managing user expectations on software projects: Lessons from the trenches. *International Journal of Project Management*, *26*(7), 700–712. doi:10.1016/j.ijproman.2008.05.014

Petter, S., DeLone, W., & McLean, E. R. (2013). Information Systems Success: The Quest for the Independent Variables. *Journal of Management Information Systems*, *29*(4), 7–62. doi:10.2753/MIS0742-1222290401

Pfeffer, J. (1980). A partial test of the social information processing model of job attitudes. *Human Relations*, *33*(7), 457. doi:10.1177/001872678003300702

Pfeil, U., Zaphiris, P., & Wilson, S. (2009). Older adults' perceptions and experiences of online social support. *Interacting with Computers*, *21*(3), 159–172. doi:10.1016/j.intcom.2008.12.001

Phelps, C., & Michea, Y. F. (2003). Learning management systems' evaluation focuses on technology not learning. In *Proceedings of AMIA Annual Symposium*. AMIA.

Pilemalm, S., & Timpka, T. (2008). Third generation participatory design in health informatics—Making user participation applicable to large-scale information system projects. *Journal of Biomedical Informatics*, *41*(2), 327–339. doi:10.1016/j.jbi.2007.09.004 PMID:17981514

Pinnington, A. (2011). Leadership Development: Applying the same leadership theories and development practices to different contexts? *Leadership*, *7*, 335. doi:10.1177/1742715011407388

Pinto, H. S. (2004). Ontologies: How can They be Built? *Knowledge and Information Systems*, *6*(4), 441–464. doi:10.1007/s10115-003-0138-1

Pithouse, A., Broadhurst, K., Hall, C., Peckover, S., Wastell, D., & White, S. (2012). Trust, risk and the (mis)management of contingency and discretion through new information technologies in children's services. *Journal of Social Work*, *12*(2), 158–178. doi:10.1177/1468017310382151

Pithouse, A., Hall, C., Peckover, S., & White, S. (2009). A Tale of Two CAFs: The Impact of the Electronic Common Assessment Framework. *British Journal of Social Work*, *39*(4), 599–612. doi:10.1093/bjsw/bcp020

Pitts, F. (1965). A graph theoretic approach to historical geography. *The Professional Geographer*, *17*(5), 15–20. doi:10.1111/j.0033-0124.1965.015_m.x

Pleace, N. (2011). Workless People and Surveillant Mashups. Social policy and data sharing in the UK. *Information Communication and Society*, *10*(6), 943–960. doi:10.1080/13691180701751171

Poblete, B., Garcia, R., Mendoza, G.M. & Jaimes, A. (2011). Do All Birds Tweet the Same? Characterizing Twitter Around the World. In *Proceedings of the 20th ACM International Conference on Information and Knowledge Management*, (pp. 1025-1030). New York, NY: ACM.

Pohjola, A., Kääriäinen, A., & Kuusisto-Niemi, S. (Eds.). (2010). Sosiaalityö, tieto ja teknologia. [Social work, information and technology]. Jyväskylä: PS-kustannus.

*Polar UK*. (2013). Available http://www.polar.com/uk-en

Pollack, N. (2005). Intelligent Technology for an Aging Population: The Use of AI to Assist Elders with Cognitive Impairment. *AI Magazine*, *26*(2).

Pollard, J. K., Rohman, S., & Fry, M. E. (2001). *A Web-based mobile medical monitoring system.* Paper presented at the Intelligent Data Acquisition and Advanced Computing Systems: Technology and Applications. New York, NY.

Preece, A., Missier, P., Ernbury, S., Jin, B., & Greenwood, M. (2008). An ontology-based approach to handling information quality in e-Science. *Concurrency and Computation*, *20*(3), 253–264. doi:10.1002/cpe.1195

Prochaska, J. J., Pechmann, C., Kim, R., & Leonhardt, J. M. (2011). Twitter=Quitter? An Analysis of Twitter Quit Smoking Social Networks. *Tobacco Control*, *21*(4), 447–449. doi:10.1136/tc.2010.042507 PMID:21730101

Productivity Commision. (2010). Contribution of the Not-for-Profit Sector (Research Report). Canberra: Author.

Productivity Commission. (2011). *Caring for Older Australians, Report No. 53, Final Inquiry Report*. Canberra: Author.

Project Management Institute. (2008). *A Guide to the Project Management Body of Knowledge: PMBOK® Guide*. Project Management Institute.

*Protégé Ontology Library*. (2014). Retrieved February 28, 2014 from http://protegewiki.stanford.edu/wiki/Protege_Ontology_Library

Proynova, R., Paech, B., Koch, S. H., Wicht, A., & Wetter, T. (2011). *Investigating the influence of personal values on requirements for health care information systems.* Paper presented at the Proceedings of the 3rd Workshop on Software Engineering in Health Care. Waikiki, HI.

Pullin, G. (2009). *Design meets disability*. MIT Press.

Quaglini, S., Stefanelli, M., Lanzola, G., Caporusso, V., & Panzarasa, S. (2001). Flexible guideline-based patient care. *Artificial Intelligence in Medicine*, *22*(1), 65–80. doi:10.1016/S0933-3657(00)00100-7 PMID:11259884

Quan, H., Li, B., Saunders, L. D., Parsons, G. A., Nilsson, C. I., & Alibhai, A. et al. (2008). Assessing validity of ICD-9-CM and ICD-10 administrative data in recording clinical conditions in a unique dually coded database. *Health Services Research*, *43*(4), 1424–1441. doi:10.1111/j.1475-6773.2007.00822.x PMID:18756617

Queensland Government Chief Information Office. (2008). *Current information standards, guidelines and reviews*. Retrieved from http://www.qgcio.qld.gov.au/02_infostand/standards.htm

Queensland Government Chief Information Office. (2010). *2009 Queensland Household Survey - Computer and Internet Use*. Retrieved 7 February 2011, from http://www.qgcio.qld.gov.au/SiteCollectionDocuments/Resources/householdsurvey2009.pdf

Queensland Government. (2001). *Information Standard No 42A: Information privacy for the Queensland Department of Health.* http://www.qgcio.qld.gov.au/02_infostand/standards/is42a.pdf

Rafferty, J., & Waldman, J. (2006). Fit for Virtual Social Work Practice? *Journal of Technology in Human Services*, *24*(2/3), 1–22. doi:10.1300/J017v24n02_01

Rahman, R. M., & Hasan, F. R. M. (2011). Using and comparing different decision tree classification techniques for mining ICDDR,B Hospital Surveillance data. *Expert Systems with Applications*, *38*(9), 11421–11436. doi:10.1016/j.eswa.2011.03.015

Rashty, D. (2003). *Traditional learning vs. e-learning*. Retrieved August 02, 2013 from http://www.researchtrail.com/articles/Traditional_Learning_vs_eLearning.pdf

Raymond, L. (1985). Organizational characteristics and MIS success in the context of small business. *Management Information Systems Quarterly*, *9*(1), 37–52.

Redman, T. (2005). Measuring data accuracy. In W. Rea (Ed.), *Information Quality* (p. 21). Armonk, NY: ME Sharpe Inc.

Reid, R. J., Coleman, K., Johnson, E. A., Fishman, P. A., Hsu, C., & Soman, M. P. et al. (2010). The group health medical home at year two: cost savings, higher patient satisfaction, and less burnout for providers. *Health Affairs*, *29*(5), 835–843. doi:10.1377/hlthaff.2010.0158 PMID:20439869

Reuss, E., Menozzi, M., Büchi, M., Koller, J., & Krueger, H. (2004). Information access at the point of care: what can we learn for designing a mobile CPR system? *International Journal of Medical Informatics*, *73*(4), 363–369. doi:10.1016/j.ijmedinf.2004.02.003 PMID:15135755

Reynolds, A. (2009). *The Myer Foundation 2020: A Vision for Aged Care in Australia*. Fitzroy, Australia: Outcomes Review, Brotherhood of St Laurence.

RFID Journal. (2005, August). A summary of RFID standards. *RFID Journal*.

Riaño, D., & Collado, A. (2013). Model-Based Combination of Treatments for the Management of Chronic Comorbid Patients. In *Proceedings of 14th Conference on Artificial Intelligence in Medicine* (vol. 7885, pp. 11-16). Murcia, Spain: Springer.

Richardson, M., Zorn, T., & Weaver, C. K. (2011). Older people and new communication technologies: Narratives from the literature. In C. T. Salmon (Ed.), *Communication yearbook 35* (pp. 121–152). Routledge Taylor & Francis Group.

Riege, A. (2005). Three dozen knowledge sharing barriers managers must consider. *Journal of Knowledge Management*, *9*(3), 18–35. doi:10.1108/13673270510602746

Roark, D. C., & Miguel, K. (2006). Bar coding's replacement? *Nursing Management*, *37*(2), 29–31. doi:10.1097/00006247-200602000-00009 PMID:16452888

*Robert & Frank*. (2012). Retrieved February 28, 2014 from http://www.imdb.com/title/tt1990314/news

Robert Wood Johnson Foundation and Partnership for Solutions. (2004, September). *Chronic Conditions: Making the Case for Ongoing Care*. Johns Hopkins University.

Robins, G., Pattison, P., Kalish, Y., & Lusher, D. (2007). An introduction to exponential random graph (p*) models for social networks. *Social Networks, 29*(2), 173-191. DOI: 10.1016/j.socnet.2006.08.002

*Robot Astronaut*. (2013). Retrieved February 28, 2014 from http://www2.toyota.co.jp/en/news/13/09/0905.pdf

*Robot-Era*. (2014). Retrieved February 28, 2014 from http://www.robot-era.eu/robotera/

*Robots+Avatars*. (2014). Retrieved February 28, 2014 from http://www.robotsandavatars.net/

Rock, B. (1999). The New Confidentiality for the 21st Century in a Managed Care Environment. *Social Work*, *44*(3), 253–262. doi:10.1093/sw/44.3.253 PMID:10348698

Roham, M., & Gabrielyan, A, R., Archer, N. P. (2012). Predicting the impact of hospital health information technology adoption on patient satisfaction. *Artificial Intelligence in Medicine*, *56*(2), 123–135. doi:10.1016/j.artmed.2012.08.001 PMID:22964161

Rosemann, M. (2006). Potential Pitfalls in process modelling- Part 1. *Business Process Management Journal, 12*(2), 249-254.

Ross, P. E. (2004). Managing care through the air [remote health monitoring]. *IEEE Spectrum, 41*(12), 26-31.

Rubin, D. L., Lewis, S. E., Mungall, C. J., Misra, S., Westerfield, M., & Ashburner, M. et al. (2006). National Center for Biomedical Ontology: advancing biomedicine through structured organization of scientific knowledge. *OMICS: A Journal of Integrative Biology*, *10*(2), 185–198. doi:10.1089/omi.2006.10.185 PMID:16901225

Ruch, P. (2010). Section Editor for the IMIA Yearbook Section on Decision Support Systems. Findings from the yearbook 2010 section on decision support systems. *IMIA Yearbook of Medical Information*, *2010*, 55–57.

Ruiz, J. G., Mintzer, M. J., & Leipzig, R. M. (2006). The Impact of E-Learning in Medical Education. *Academic Medicine*, *81*(3), 207–212. doi:10.1097/00001888-200603000-00002 PMID:16501260

Russell, H. (2011). Later Life ICT Learners Ageing Well. *International Journal of Ageing and Later Life*, *6*(2), 103–127. doi:10.3384/ijal.1652-8670.1162103

Russell, T. L. (2001). *The no significant difference phenomenon* (5th ed.). Montgomery, AL: International Distance Education Certification Center.

Ryker, R., Nath, R., & Henson, J. (1997). Determinants of computer user expectations and their relationships with user satisfaction: an empirical study. *Information Processing & Management*, *33*(4), 529–537. doi:10.1016/S0306-4573(97)00016-2

Saadé, R. G. (2007). Dimensions of perceived usefulness: Toward enhanced assessment. *Decision Sciences Journal of Innovative Education*, *5*(2), 289–310. doi:10.1111/j.1540-4609.2007.00142.x

Saba, V. K., & McCormick, K. A. (Eds.). (2001). *Essentials of Computers for Nurses: Informatics for the New Millennium*. McCraw-Hill Companies.

Safran, C., Jones, P. C., Rind, D., Bush, B., Cytryn, K. N., & Patel, V. L. (1998). Electronic communication and collaboration in a health care practice. *Artificial Intelligence in Medicine*, *12*(2), 137–151. doi:10.1016/S0933-3657(97)00047-X PMID:9520221

Sakr, S., Liu, A., Batista, D. M., & Alomari, M. (2011). A Survey of Large Scale Data Management Approaches in Cloud Environments. *IEEE Communications Surveys & Tutorials*, *13*(3), 311–336. doi:10.1109/SURV.2011.032211.00087

Salancik, G., & Pfeffer, J. (1978). A social information processing approach to job attitudes and task design. *Administrative Science Quarterly*, *23*(2), 224–253. doi:10.2307/2392563 PMID:10307892

Salipante, P., & Aram, J. D. (2003). Managers as knowledgeable generators: The nature of practitioner-scholar research in the non-profit sector. *Nonprofit Management & Leadership*, *14*(2), 129–150. doi:10.1002/nml.26

Sánchez-Garzón, I., Fernández-Olivares, J., Onaindia, E., Milla, G., Jordán, J., & Castejón, P. (2013). A Multi-agent Planning Approach for the Generation of Personalized Treatment Plans of Comorbid Patients. *14th Conference on Artificial Intelligence in Medicine, 7885*, 23-27.

Sankaran, S., Cartwright, C., Kelly, J., Shaw, K., & Soar, J. (2010). Leadership of non-profit organisations in the aged care sector in Australia. In *Proceedings of the 54th Meeting of the International Society for the Systems Sciences*. Academic Press.

Santos, R. S., Malheiros, S. M. F., Cavalheiro, S., & Parente de Oliveira, J. M. (2013). A data mining system for providing analytical information on brain tumors to public health decision makers. *Computer Methods and Programs in Biomedicine*, *109*(3), 269–282. doi:10.1016/j.cmpb.2012.10.010 PMID:23122302

Saranto, K., & Kuusisto-Niemi, S. (2012). Tiedonhallinnan koulutusohjelma arvioitavana – kokemuksia kansainvälisestä akkreditoinnista. (Health and Human Services Informatics Master´s Degree Program in Evaluation – Experiences from the international accreditation). *Finnish Journal of eHealth and eWelfare*, *4*(2), 140-144. Retrieved February 12, 2014, from http://ojs.tsv.fi/index.php/stty/article/view/6558/5375

Scanfeld, D., Scanfeld, V., & Larson, E. (2010). Dissemination of health information through social networks: Twitter and antibiotics. *American Journal of Infection Control*, *38*(3), 182–188. doi:10.1016/j.ajic.2009.11.004 PMID:20347636

Scilingo, E., Gemignani, A., Paradiso, R., Taccini, N., Ghelarducci, B., & De Rossi, D. (2005). Performance evaluation of sensing fabrics for monitoring physiological and biomechanical variables. *IEEE Transactions on Information Technology in Biomedicine*, *9*(3), 345–352. doi:10.1109/TITB.2005.854506 PMID:16167688

Scottish Government. (2011). *eHealth Programme*. Retrieved May 12, 2011, from http://www.ehealth.scot.nhs.uk/

Scully, C. G., Lee, J., Meyer, J., Gorbach, A. M., Granquist-Fraser, D., Mendelson, Y., & Chon, K. H. (2012). Physiological parameter monitoring from optical recordings with a mobile phone. *IEEE Transactions on* Biomedical Engineering, *59*(2), 303–306.

Sebastian, Y., & Then, P. H. H. (2011). Domain-driven KDD for mining functionally novel rules and linking disjoint medical hypotheses. *Knowledge-Based Systems*, *24*(5), 609–620. doi:10.1016/j.knosys.2011.01.008

Seddon, P. B. (1997). A respecification and extension of the DeLone and McLean model of IS success. *Information Systems Research*, *8*(3), 240–253. doi:10.1287/isre.8.3.240

Self-Organizing Map. (n.d.). In *Wikipedia*. Retrieved Sep 10, 2013, from http://en.wikipedia.org/wiki/Self-organizing_map

Selwyn, N., Gorard, S., Furlong, J., & Madden, L. (2003). Older adults' use of information and communications technology in everyday life. *Ageing and Society*, *23*, 561–582. doi:10.1017/S0144686X03001302

Semenova, T. (2004). Discovering patterns of medical practice in large administrative health databases. *Data & Knowledge Engineering*, *51*(2), 149–160. doi:10.1016/j.datak.2004.02.001

Senge, P. M. (1990). *The Fifth Dimension - The Art and Patience of The Learning Organisation*. New York: Doubleday.

Senge, P. M., Roberts, C., Ross, R. B., Smith, B. J., & Kleinter, A. (1994). *The Fifth Discipline Field Book: Strategies and Tools for Building a Learning Organisation*. New York: Doubleday.

Shahar, Y., Musen, M., & Tu, S. W. (1996). Eon: A component-based approach to. *Journal of the American Medical*, 367-388.

Shahar, Y., Miksch, S., & Johnson, P. D. (1998). The Asgaard project: a task-specific framework for the application. *Artificial Intelligence in Medicine*, 29–51. doi:10.1016/S0933-3657(98)00015-3 PMID:9779882

Shahian, D. M., Wolf, R. E., Iezzoni, L. I., Kirle, L., & Normand, S. L. T. (2010). Variability in the measurement of hospital-wide mortality rates. *The New England Journal of Medicine*, *363*(26), 2530–2539. doi:10.1056/NEJMsa1006396 PMID:21175315

Shah, N. (2012). Welfare and technology in the network society – Concerns for the future of welfare. *Futures*, *44*, 659–665. doi:10.1016/j.futures.2012.04.004

Shanmugam, R. (2012). Booming medical tourism and economic indices. *International Journal of Research in Nursing*, *3*(2), 38–47. doi:10.3844/ijrnsp.2012.38.47

Shapira, N., Barak, A., & Gal, I. (2007). Promoting older adults' well-being through Internet training and use. *Aging & Mental Health*, *11*(5), 477–484. doi:10.1080/13607860601086546 PMID:17882585

Sharp, H., Rogers, Y., & Preece, J. (2007). *Interaction design: Beyond human-computer interaction* (2nd ed.). Chichester, UK: John Wiley and Sons Limited.

Shaw, E., Ruby, K., and Post, J. (1998). The insider threat to information systems: the psychology of the dangerous insider. *Security Awareness Bulletin*, *2*(98), 1–10.

Shaw, I., Bell, M., Sinclair, I., Sloper, P., Mitchell, W., & Dyson, P. et al. (2009). An Exemplary Scheme? An Evaluation of the Integrated Children's System. *British Journal of Social Work*, *39*(4), 613–626. doi:10.1093/bjsw/bcp040

Sheffield, J. (2008). Inquiry in health knowledge management. *Journal of Knowledge Management*, *12*, 160–172. doi:10.1108/13673270810884327

Shepertycky, M. R., Banno, K., & Kryger, M. H. (2005). Differences between men and women in the clinical presentation of patients diagnosed with Obstructive Sleep Apnea Syndrome. *Sleep*, *28*(3), 309–314. PMID:16173651

Sheppard, V. B., Williams, K. P., Harrison, T. M., Jennings, Y., Lucas, W., Stephen, J., . . . Taylor, K. L. (2009). Development of decision-support intervention for Black women with breast cancer. *Psycho-Oncology*.

Sheth, A., Anantharam, P., & Henson, C. (2013). Physical-Cyber-Social Computing: An Early 21st Century Approach. IEEE Intelligent Systems, 78-82.

Sheth, A. (2010). Computing for Human Experience: Semantics-Empowered Sensors, Services, and Social Computing on the Ubiquitous Web. *IEEE Internet Computing*, *14*(1), 88–91. doi:10.1109/MIC.2010.4

Shiffman, R. N., Karras, B. T., Agrawal, A., Chen, R., Marenco, L. N., & Nath, S. (2000). Model formulation: Gem: A proposal for a more comprehensive guideline document model using xml. *Journal of the American Medical Informatics Association*, *7*(5), 488–498. doi:10.1136/jamia.2000.0070488 PMID:10984468

Shimada, K., Wang, R., Hirasawa, K., & Furuzuki, T. (2008). Medical association rule mining using genetic network programming. *Electronics and Communications in Japan*, *91*(2), 46–54. doi:10.1002/ecj.10022

*Shimmer*. (2013). Available: http://www.shimmersensing.com/

Shippy, R., Cantor, M., & Brennan, M. (2004). Social networks of aging gay men. *Journal of Men's Studies*, *13*(1), 107–120. doi:10.3149/jms.1301.107

Shortlife, E. H., & Cimino, J. J. (2006). Biomedical informatics: Computer applications in health care and biomedicine (3rd ed.). New York: Springer.

Shortliffe, E. H. (1993). The adolescence of AI in medicine: will the field come of age in the 90s? *Artificial Intelligence in Medicine*, *5*(2), 93–106. doi:10.1016/0933-3657(93)90011-Q PMID:8358494

Siliquini, R. (2011). Surfing the internet for health information: an italian survey on use and population choices. *BMC Medical Informatics and Decision Making*, (11), 21. doi:10.1186/1472-6947-11-21 PMID:21470435

Sillence, E., Briggs, P., Fishwick, L., & Harris, P. (2004). Trust and Mistrust of Online Health Sites. In *Proceedings of the SIGCHI Conference on Human Factors In Computing Systems*, (pp. 663-670). New York, NY: ACM.

Silva, B. B., Lopes, I., Rodrigues, J., & Ray, P. (2011). SapoFitness: A mobile health application for dietary evaluation. In *Proceedings of 13th IEEE Intl. Conf. on e-Health Networking Applications and Services (HealthCom)*, (pp. 375–380). IEEE.

Simpson, G. (2007). Hospitals need RFID injection. *ZdNet Asia Communications*.

Sinha, P. K., Sunder, G., Bendale, P., Mantri, M. D., & Dande, A. C. (2013). *Electronic Health Record. Standards, Coding Systems, Frameworks, and Infrastructure. Wiley*. IEEE Press.

Sittig, D. F., Wright, A., Osheroff, J. A., Middleton, B., Teich, J. M., & Ash, J. S., Campbell, Emily M., Bates, D. W. (2008). Grand challenges in clinical decision support. *Journal of Biomedical Informatics*, *41*(2), 387–392. doi:10.1016/j.jbi.2007.09.003 PMID:18029232

Škrinjar, R., & Trkman, P. (2013). Increasing process orientation with business process management: Critical practices'. *International Journal of Information Management*, *33*(1), 48–60. doi:10.1016/j.ijinfomgt.2012.05.011

Skubic, M., Alexander, G., Popescu, M., Rantz, M., & Keller, J. (2009). A smart home application to eldercare: Current status and lessons learned. *Technology and Healthcare*, *17*(3), 183–201. PMID:19641257

Smith, H., Rogers, Y., & Brady, M. (2003). *Managing one's social network: Does age make a difference*. Academic Press.

Smith, R. (2004). *Guidelines for Authors of Learning Objects*. Retrieved November 26, 2013 from http://archive2.nmc.org/guidelines/NMC%20LO%20Guidelines.pdf

Smith, S., Lang, C., Sullivan, K., & Warren, J. (2004). Two new tools for assessing patients' knowledge and beliefs about Obstructive Sleep Apnea and Continuous Positive Airway Pressure therapy. *Sleep Medicine*, *5*(4), 359–367. doi:10.1016/j.sleep.2003.12.007 PMID:15222992

Snijders, T. A. B., Pattison, P. E., Robins, G. L., & Handcock, M. S. (2006). New specifications for exponential random graph models. *Sociological Methodology*, *36*(1), 99–153. doi:10.1111/j.1467-9531.2006.00176.x

Snyder, K. D., Paulson, P., & McGrath, P. (2005). Improving processes in a small health care network: A value mapping case study. *Business Process Management Journal*, *2*(1), 87-99.

SocialMediaNews.com.au. (2014). Social Media Statistics Australia – December 2013. In *December 2013 Statistics*. Retrieved January 13, 2014, from http://www.socialmedianews.com.au/social-media-statistics-australia-december-2013/

Sokwoo, R., Boo-Ho, Y., Kuowei, C., & Asada, H. H. (1998). *The ring sensor: A new ambulatory wearable sensor for twenty-four hour patient monitoring*. Paper presented at the Engineering in Medicine and Biology Society. New York, NY.

Sommers, L. S., Marton, K. I., Barbaccia, J. C., & Randolph, J. (2000). Physician, nurse, and social worker collaboration in primary care for chronically ill seniors. *Archives of Internal Medicine*, *160*(12), 1825–1833. doi:10.1001/archinte.160.12.1825 PMID:10871977

Soroush, L., Hafeez-Baig, A., & Gururajan, R. (2010). *Clinicians' perception of using digital stethoscopes in telehealth platform: Queensland telehealth preliminary study*. Paper presented at the 21st Australasian Conference on Information Systems. Brisbane, Australia. Retrieved from http://aisel.aisnet.org/acis2010/43/

Sosiaali- ja terveysministeriö. (1996). *Sosiaali- ja terveydenhuollon tietotekniikan hyödyntämisstrategia*. [*Ministry of Social Affairs and Health. The utilization strategy for social affairs and health*]. Helsinki: Sosiaali- ja terveysministeriö.

*Sosiaalialan tiedonhallinnan tutkimusohjelma*. (2009). Retrieved February 14, 2014, from http://www.sosiaaliportti.fi/File/fd89a662-d7e8-4053-b56d-45ea45ecc8db/Tiedonhallinnan+ohjelma.pdf

*Sosiaalihuollon tiedonhallinta*. (2014). Retrieved February 10, 2014, from http://www.thl.fi/fi_FI/web/fi/aiheet/tietopaketit/sosiaalihuollon_tiedonhallinta

Sosiaaliportti. (2014). *Sosiaaliportti - The Social Gateway*. Retrieved February 14, 2014, from http://www.sosiaaliportti.fi/en-GB/

Sosiaalitoimen atk-toimikunta. (1981). *Sosiaalitoimen atk-selvitys* [*National Working Group for ICT in Social Services. Account on social services ICT*]. Helsinki: Suomen Kaupunkiliitto, Suomen Kunnallisliitto.

Sosiaalitoimen atk-toimikunta. (1986). *Sosiaalihuollon tietojenkäsittelyn kehittäminen* [*National Working Group for ICT in Social Services. Development of ICT in social services*]. Helsinki: Suomen Kaupunkiliitto, Suomen Kunnallisliitto.

Sosiaalitoimen atk-toimikunta. (1993). *Sosiaalitoimen järjestelmien peruskäsitteet*. [*National Working Group for ICT in Social Services. The core data set of social services ICT*]. Helsinki: Kunnallishallinnon tietotekniikkaneuvottelukunta.

Sparrowe, R., Liden, R., Wayne, S., & Kraimer, M. (2001). Social networks and the performance of individuals and groups. *Academy of Management Journal*, *44*(2), 316–325. doi:10.2307/3069458

Spasic, I., & Ananiadou, S. (2005). A flexible measure of contextual similarity for biomedical terms. *Pacific Symposium on Biocomputing. Pacific Symposium on Biocomputing*, 197–208. PMID:15759626

Srinivasan, U., & Arunasalam, B. (2013). Leveraging Big Data Analytics to reduce Healthcare Costs. *IT Professional*, *15*(6), 21–28. doi:10.1109/MITP.2013.55

Standing, C., & Cripps, H. (2013). Critical Success Factors in the Implementation of Electronic Health Records: A Two-Case Comparison. *Systems Research and Behavioral Science*. doi:10.1002/sres.2209

Stanford, V. (2002). Using pervasive computing to deliver elder care. *Pervasive Computing, IEEE*, *1*(1), 10–13. doi:10.1109/MPRV.2002.993139

Stantic, B., Terenziani, P., Governatori, G., Bottrighi, A., & Sattar, A. (2012). An implicit approach to deal with periodically repeated medical data. *Artificial Intelligence in Medicine*, *55*(3), 149–162. doi:10.1016/j.artmed.2012.03.002 PMID:22503730

Staples, D. S., Wong, I., & Seddon, P. B. (2002). Having expectations of information systems benefits that match received benefits: does it really matter? *Information & Management*, *40*(2), 115–131. doi:10.1016/S0378-7206(01)00138-0

Steele, R. (2011). Social media, mobile devices and sensors: categorizing new techniques for health communication. In *Proceedings of the 5th International Conference on Sensing Technology*, (pp. 187-192). Palmerston North, New Zealand: IEEE.

Steele, R., & Lo, A. (2009). Future personal health records as a foundation for computational health. In Proceedings of Computational Science and Its Applications – ICCSA 2009 (pp. 719-733). Springer.

Steele, R., Lo, A., Secombe, C., & Wong, Y. K. (2009). Elderly persons' perception and acceptance of using wireless sensor networks to assist healthcare. *International Journal of Medical Informatics*, *78*(12), 788–801. doi:10.1016/j.ijmedinf.2009.08.001 PMID:19717335

Steele, R., Min, K., & Lo, A. (2012). Personal health record architectures: Technology infrastructure implications and dependencies. *Journal of the American Society for Information Science and Technology*, *63*(6), 1079–1091. doi:10.1002/asi.22635

Steers, W. D. (2013). The Electronic Medical Record: How Not to Communicate. *The Journal of Urology*, *190*(5), 1636–1637. doi:10.1016/j.juro.2013.08.003 PMID:23933460

Sterling, L. S., & Taveter, K. (2009). *The art of agent-oriented modeling*. Massachusetts Institute of Technology.

Steyaert, J., & Gould, N. (2009). Social Work and the Changing Face of the Digital Divide. *British Journal of Social Work*, *39*(4), 740–753. doi:10.1093/bjsw/bcp022

Stillman, L., & McGrath, J. (2008). Is it Web 2.0 or is it Better Information and Knowledge That We Need? *Australian Social Work*, *61*(4), 421–428. doi:10.1080/03124070802441889

Stranieri, A., Zeleznikow, J., Gawler, M., & Lewis, B. (1999). A hybrid rule – neural approach for the automation of legal reasoning in the discretionary domain of family law in Australia. *Artificial Intelligence and Law*, *7*(2-3).

Stvilia, B., Mon, L., & Yi, Y. J. (2009). A Model for Online Consumer Health Information Quality. *Journal of the American Society for Information Science and Technology*, *60*(9), 1781–1791. doi:10.1002/asi.21115

Sullivan, G. J., Ohm, J., Han, W.-J., & Wiegand, T. (2012). Overview of the high efficiency video coding (HEVC) standard. *IEEE Transactions on Circuits and Systems for Video Technology*, *22*(12), 1649–1668. doi:10.1109/TCSVT.2012.2221191

Sullivan, S. J., Schneiders, A. G., Cheang, C., Kitto, E., Lee, H., & Redhead, J. et al. (2012). 'What's Happening?' A Content Analysis of Concussion-related Traffic on Twitter. *British Journal of Sports Medicine*, *46*(4), 258–263. doi:10.1136/bjsm.2010.080341 PMID:21406451

Sung, M., Marci, C., & Pentland, A. (2005). Wearable feedback systems for rehabilitation. *Journal of Neuroengineering and Rehabilitation*, *2*, 17. doi:10.1186/1743-0003-2-17 PMID:15987514

Szajna, B., & Scamell, R. W. (1993). The effects of information system user expectations on their performance and perceptions. *Management Information Systems Quarterly*, 493–516. doi:10.2307/249589

Szymanski, D. M., & Henard, D. H. (2001). Customer satisfaction: a meta-analysis of the empirical evidence. *Journal of the Academy of Marketing Science*, *29*(1), 16–35. doi:10.1177/0092070301291002

Taimiaho, A. (1987). Henkilörekisterilaki voimaan vuoden alusta. (Data security act into operation from the beginning of the year). *Sosiaaliturva*, *75*(22), 1252–1254.

Tai, Y. M., & Chiu, H. W. (2009). Comorbidity study of ADHD: Applying association rule mining (ARM) to National Health Insurance Database of Taiwan. *International Journal of Medical Informatics*, *78*(12), e75–e83. doi:10.1016/j.ijmedinf.2009.09.005 PMID:19853501

Tan, P. N., Steinbach, M., & Kumar, V. (2005). *Introduction to data mining*. Pearson Addison-Wesley.

Tartarisco, G., Baldus, G., Corda, D., Raso, R., Arnao, A., & Ferro, M. et al. (2012). Personal Health System architecture for stress monitoring and support to clinical decisions. *Computer Communications*, *35*(11), 1296–1305. doi:10.1016/j.comcom.2011.11.015

Tavangarian, D., Leypold, M., Nölting, K., & Röser, M. (2004). Is e-learning the Solution for Individual Learning?. *Journal of e-Learning*.

Taylor, M. J., Wade, S., & England, D. (2003). Informing IT system web site design through normalisation. *Internet Research: Electronic Networking Applications and Policy*, *13*(5), 342–355. doi:10.1108/10662240310501621

*Tele-Presence Robots*. (2014). Retrieved February 28, 2014 from http://telepresencerobots.com/

Tenhunen, E., Hämäläinen, P., Kärki, J., & Väinälä, A. (2006). Sosiaaliala ja sosiaali- ja terveydenhuollon tietoteknologiakehitys. [Field of social welfare and the ICT development of social and health care]. In Sosiaali- ja terveydenhuollon tietotekniikan ja tiedonhallinnan tutkimuspäivät: Tutkimuspaperit 2006 (pp. 96-101). Retrieved May 13, 2011, from http://stty.org/joomla/index.php?option=com_content&view=category&layout=blog&id=44&Itemid=79

Tenorio, J. M., Hummel, A. D., Cohrs, F. M., Sdepanian, V. L., Pisa, I. T., & Marin, H. D. F. (2011). Artificial intelligence techniques applied to the development of a decision–support system for diagnosing celiac disease. *International Journal of Medical Informatics*, *80*(11), 793–802. doi:10.1016/j.ijmedinf.2011.08.001 PMID:21917512

Terenziani, P., Bottrighi, A., Torchio, M., Molino, G., Anselma, L., & Correndo, G. (2003). Applying artificial intelligence to clinical guidelines: the glare approach. AI*IA, 2829, 536-547.

Terenziani, P., Molino, G., & Torchio, M. (2001). A modular approach for representing and executing clinical guidelines. *Artificial Intelligence in Medicine*, *23*(3), 249–276. doi:10.1016/S0933-3657(01)00087-2 PMID:11704440

Terenziani, P., Montani, S., Bottrighi, A., Molino, G., Torchio, M., & Correndo, G. (2004). A context-adaptable approach to clinical guidelines. *Studies in Health Technology and Informatics*, 169–173. PMID:15360797

Thackeray, R., Neiger, B. L., Smith, A. K., & Van Wagenen, S. B. (2012). Adoption and use of social media among public health departments. *BMC Public Health*, *12*(1), 242. doi:10.1186/1471-2458-12-242 PMID:22449137

The Department of Health. (2011). *Defining the electronic social care record* (final version 7.2). Retrieved April 13, 2011, from http://www.dh.gov.uk/en/Managingyourorganisation/Informationpolicy/Informationforsocialcare/DH_4073714

The National Alliance for Health Information Technology. (2008). *Report to the Office of the National Coordinator for Health Information Technology on Defining Key Health Information Technology Terms*. Retrieved September 12, 2013 at http://hitechanswers.wpengine.netdna-cdn.com/wp-content/uploads/2013/05/NAHIT-Definitions2008.pdf

Thioune, R.M.C. (2003). *Information and communication technologies for development in Africa: Opportunities and challenges for community development*. Retrieved October 28, 2013 from http://www.idrc.ca

Thomas, K. (2008, May 30). Radio wrist tags that make for smoother operations: A technology for tracing consumer goods may help save lives and keep track of hospital equipment. *Financial Times*, p. 12.

Ting, S. L., Kwok, S. K., Tsang, A. H. C., & Lee, W. B. (2011). A hybrid knowledge-based approach to supporting the medical prescription for general practitioners: Real case in a Hong Kong medical center. *Knowledge-Based Systems*, *24*(3), 444–456. doi:10.1016/j.knosys.2010.12.011

Topalis, P., Dialynas, E., Mitraka, E., Deligianni, E., Siden-Kiamos, I., & Louis, C. (2011). A set of ontologies to drive tools for the control of vector-borne diseases. *Journal of Biomedical Informatics*, *44*(1), 42–47. doi:10.1016/j.jbi.2010.03.012 PMID:20363364

Tregeagle, S., & Darcy, M. (2008). Child Welfare and Information and Communication Technology: Today's Challenge. *British Journal of Social Work*, *38*(8), 1481–1498. doi:10.1093/bjsw/bcm048

Treleaven, L., & Sykes, C. (2005). Loss of organizational knowledge: From supporting clients to serving head office. *Journal of Organizational Change Management*, *18*(4), 353–368. doi:10.1108/09534810510607056

Tsai, C.-T., & Chang, P.-L. (2005). An integration framework of innovation assessment for the knowledge-intensive service industry. *International Journal of Technology Management*, *30*(1-2), 85-104.

Tu, Y.-J., Zhou, W., & Piramuthu, S. (2009). Identifying RFID-embedded objects in pervasive healthcare applications. *Decision Support Systems*, *46*(2), 586–593. doi:10.1016/j.dss.2008.10.001

Uddin, M. S., & Hossain, L. (2009). *Exploring physical, mental and psychological health for elders through their personal networks*. Paper presented at the e-Health Networking, Applications and Services. Sydney, Australia.

Uddin, M., & Hossain, L. (2009). Towards coordination preparedness of soft-target organisation. Electronic Government, 54-64.

Uddin, S., & Hossain, L. (2012). Effects of Physician Collaboration Network on Hospital Outcomes. In *Proceedings of Australasian Workshop on Health Informatics and Knowledge Management*. Academic Press.

Uddin, S., Chung, K. S. K., & Piraveenan, M. (2012). *Capturing Actor-level Dynamics of Longitudinal Networks*. Paper presented at the Advances in Social Networks Analysis and Mining (ASONAM). New York, NY.

Uddin, S., Murshed, S. T. H., & Hossain, L. (2011). Power-law behaviour in complex organizational communication network during crisis. *Physica A: Statistical Mechanics and its Applications, 390*(15), 2845-2853.

Uddin, S., Piraveenan, M., Chung, K., & Hossain, L. (2013). *Topological Analysis of Longitudinal Networks*. Paper presented at the Hawaii International Conference on System Sciences (HICSS-46). Hawaii, HI.

Uddin, M. S., & Hossain, L. (2011). Social Networks Enabled Coordination Model for Cost Management of Patient Hospital Admissions. *Journal for Healthcare Quality*, *33*(5), 37–48. doi:10.1111/j.1945-1474.2010.00118.x PMID:23845132

Uddin, S., Hamra, J., & Hossain, L. (2013a). Exploring communication networks to understand organizational crisis using exponential random graph models. *Computational & Mathematical Organization Theory*, *19*(1), 25–41. doi:10.1007/s10588-011-9104-8

Uddin, S., Hamra, J., & Hossain, L. (2013b). Mapping and modeling of physician collaboration network. *Statistics in Medicine*, *32*(20), 3539–3551. doi:10.1002/sim.5770 PMID:23468249

Uddin, S., & Hossain, L. (2011). Disaster coordination preparedness of soft target organisations. *Disasters*, *35*(3), 623–638. doi:10.1111/j.1467-7717.2011.01229.x PMID:21272059

Uddin, S., & Hossain, L. (2013). Dyad and Triad Census Analysis of Crisis Communication Network. *Social Networking*, *2*(1), 32–41. doi:10.4236/sn.2013.21004

Uddin, S., Hossain, L., Abbasi, A., & Rasmussen, K. (2012). Trend and efficiency analysis of co-authorship network. *Scientometrics*, *90*(2), 687–699. doi:10.1007/s11192-011-0511-x

Uddin, S., Hossain, L., Hamra, J., & Alam, A. (2013). A study of physician collaborations through social network and exponential random graph. *BMC Health Services Research*, *13*(1), 234–247. doi:10.1186/1472-6963-13-234 PMID:23803165

Uddin, S., Hossain, L., & Kelaher, M. (2012). Effect of physician collaboration network on hospitalization cost and readmission rate. *European Journal of Public Health*, *22*(5), 629–633. doi:10.1093/eurpub/ckr153 PMID:22037593

Uddin, S., Hossain, L., & Rasmussen, K. (2013). Network Effects on Scientific Collaborations. *PLoS ONE*, *8*(2), e57546. doi:10.1371/journal.pone.0057546 PMID:23469021

Uddin, S., & Jacobson, M. J. (2013). Dynamics of email communications among university students throughout a semester. *Computers & Education*, *64*, 95–103. doi:10.1016/j.compedu.2013.01.014

Uddin, S., Thompson, K., Schwendimann, B., & Piraveenan, M. (2014). The impact of study load on the dynamics of longitudinal email communications among students. *Computers & Education*, *72*, 209–219. doi:10.1016/j.compedu.2013.11.007

UN. (2013). *Department of Economic and Social Affairs: Population Division: Population database*. UN.

University of British Columbia Institute of Health Promotion Research. (1996). *Guidelines and categories for classifying participatory research projects in health*. Retrieved from http://www.lgreen.net/guidelines.html

Unnithan, C., Smith, R., & Fraunholz, B. (2009). Maximising the Benefits of Radio Frequency Identification Technology (RFID) Integration in Clinical Contexts: A Linear Conduit. In *Proceedings of HIC'09 Conference*. Canberra: Health Informatics Society of Australia.

*US eMERGE network The Electronic Medical Records and Genomics (eMERGE) Network*. (n.d.). Retrieved from http://emerge.mc.vanderbilt.edu/

*USC-ICT*. (2014). Retrieved February 28, 2014 from http://ict.usc.edu/

Väestötietojärjestelmä. (2014). *Kuntien asukasluvut aakkosjärjestyksessä 31.8.2013*. [Population Information System. Inhabitants in the municipalities, August 31, 2013.]. Retrieved February 10, 2014, from http://vrk.fi/default.aspx?docid=7675&site=3&id=0

Valencia-Garcia, R., Fernandez-Breis, J. T., Ruiz-Martinez, J. M., Garcia-Sanchez, F., & Martinez-Bejar, R. (2008). A knowledge acquisition methodology to ontology construction for information retrieval from medical documents. *Expert Systems: International Journal of Knowledge Engineering and Neural Networks*, *25*(3), 314–334. doi:10.1111/j.1468-0394.2008.00464.x

Valtiovarainministeriö. (1995). *Suomi tietoyhteiskunnaksi. [Ministry of Finance. Finland - towards an information society, A National Outline]*. Helsinki: Valtiovarainministeriö.

Van Gorp, P., & Comuzzi, M. (2013). *Lifelong Personal Health Data and Application Software via Virtual Machines in the Cloud. IEEE Journal of Biomedical and Health Informatics*.

Varady, P., Benyo, Z., & Benyo, B. (2002). An open architecture patient monitoring system using standard technologies. *IEEE Transactions on* Information Technology in Biomedicine, *6*(1), 95–98.

Varshney, U. (2003). Location management for mobile commerce applications in wireless Internet environment. *ACM Transactions on Internet Technology*, *3*(3), 236–255. doi:10.1145/857166.857169

Varshney, U. (2007). Pervasive Healthcare and Wireless Health Monitoring. *Mobile Networks and Applications*, *12*(2-3), 113–127. doi:10.1007/s11036-007-0017-1

Vasconcelos, J., Seixas, P., Kimble, C., & Lemos, P. (2005). Knowledge management in non-government organisations: A partnership for the future. In *Proceedings of the 7th International Conference on Enterprise Information Systems* (ICEIS 2005). ICEIS.

Vencatachellum, I., & Munusami, V. (2006). *Barriers to effective corporate e-learning in Mauritius*. Retrieved August 04, 2013 from http://www.ufhrd.co.uk/wordpress/wp-content/uploads/2008/06/1-1_vencatachellum_munusami.pdf

Venkatesh, V., Morris, M. G., Davis, G. B., & Davis, F. D. (2003). User Acceptance of Information Technology: Toward a Unified View. *Management Information Systems Quarterly*, *27*(3).

Venturato, L., & Drew, L. (2010). Beyond'doing': Supporting clinical leadership and nursing practice in aged care through innovative models of care. *Contemporary Nurse*, *35*(2), 157–170. doi:10.5172/conu.2010.35.2.157 PMID:20950197

Vergados, D., Alevizos, A., Mariolis, A., & Caragiozidis, M. (2008). *Intelligent services for assisting independent living of elderly people at home*. Paper presented at the 1st international conference on Pervasive Technologies Related to Assistive Environments. Athens, Greece.

Verma, A., Kasabov, N., Rush, A., & Song, Q. (2008, 2008). *Ontology based personalized modeling for chronic disease risk analysis: an integrated approach*. Paper presented at the 15th International Conference on Advances in Neuro-Information Processing. New York, NY.

Verma, A., Fiasché, M., Cuzzola, M., Iacopino, P., Morabito, P., & Kasabov, N. (2009). Ontology based personalized modeling for type 2 diabetes risk analysis: An Investigated Approach. In C. S. Leung, M. Lee, & J. H. Chan (Eds.), *ICONIP 2009, Part II* (pp. 360–366). Berlin: Springer-Verlag.

Vestal, W. (2005). Making sense of KM costs. *KM World*, *14*(7), 8–11.

Vetere, F., Davis, H., Gibbs, M., & Howard, S. (2009). The Magic Box and Collage: Responding to the challenge of distributed intergenerational play. *International Journal of Human-Computer Studies*, *67*(2), 165–178. doi:10.1016/j.ijhcs.2008.09.004

Vicente, J., Garcia-Gomez, J. M., Vidal, C., Marti-Bonmati, L., Arco, A. D., & Robles, M. (2004). SOC: A Distributed Decision Support Architecture for Clinical Diagnosis. *Biological and Medical Data Analysis. Lecture Notes in Computer Science*, *3337*, 96–104. doi:10.1007/978-3-540-30547-7_11

Vichitvanichphong, S., Kerr, D. T.-K. A., & Amir, H. G. (2013). *Analysis of Research in Adoption of Assistive Technologies for Aged Care*. Paper presented at the 24th Australasian Conference on Information Systems. Melbourne, Australia.

Vichitvanichphong, S., Kerr, D., Talaei-Khoei, A., & Ghapanchi, A. (2013). Analysis of Research in Adoption of Assistive Technologies for Aged Care. In *Proceedings of 24th Australasian Conference on Information Systems*. Melbourne: Academic Press.

Video LAN. (2013). *VLC media player*. Available at http://www.videolan.org/vlc/index.html

Viswanathan, H., Chen, B., & Pompili, D. (2012). Research challenges in computation, communication, and context awareness for ubiquitous healthcare. *IEEE Communications Magazine*, *50*(5), 92–99. doi:10.1109/MCOM.2012.6194388

Vital, J., Couceiro, M., Rodrigues, N., Figueiredo, C., & Ferreira, N. (2013). Fostering the NAO platform as an elderly care robot. In *Proceedings of IEEE 2nd International Conference on Serious Games and Applications for Health* (SeGAH). IEEE.

Wagner, N., Hassanein, K., & Head, M. (2010). Computer use by older adults: A multi-disciplinary review. *Computers in Human Behavior*, *26*(5), 870–882. doi:10.1016/j.chb.2010.03.029

Wan Ismail, W. K., Chan, P. H. K., Buhari, N., & Muzaini, A. (2012). *Acceptance of Smartphone in Enhancing Patient-Caregivers Relationship* (Vol. 7). Academic Press.

Wand, Y., & Wang, Y. (1996). Anchoring Data Quality Dimensions in Ontological Foundations. *Communications of the ACM*, *36*(11), 86–95. doi:10.1145/240455.240479

Wang, M. H., Lee, C. S., Li, H. C., & Ko, W. M. (2007). *Ontology-based fuzzy inference agent for diabetes classification*. New York: IEEE. doi:10.1109/NAFIPS.2007.383815

Wang, Q., Nightingale, J., Wang, R., Ramzan, N., Grecos, C., & Wang, X. et al. (in press). Mobile Video Cloud Networks. In J. Rodrigues, K. Lin, & J. Lloret (Eds.), *Mobile Computing over Cloud: Technologies, Services, and Applications*. IGI Global. doi:10.4018/978-1-4666-4781-7.ch009

Wang, R. (1998). A product perspective on total data quality management. *Communications of the ACM*, *41*(2), 58–65. doi:10.1145/269012.269022

Wang, R., Strong, D., & Guarascio, L. (1996). Beyond accuracy: What data quality means to data consumers. *Journal of Management Information Systems*, *12*(4), 5–33.

Wasserman, S., & Faust, K. (2003). *Social network analysis: Methods and applications*. Cambridge: Cambridge University Press.

Wasserman, S., & Pattison, P. (1996). Logit models and logistic regressions for social networks: I. An introduction to Markov graphs and P. *Psychometrika*, *61*(3), 401–425. doi:10.1007/BF02294547

Wastell, D., White, S., Broadhurst, K., Peckover, S., & Pithouse, A. (2010). Children's services in the iron cage of performance management: Street-level bureaucracy and the spectre of Švejkism. *International Journal of Social Welfare*, *19*(3), 310–320. doi:10.1111/j.1468-2397.2009.00716.x

Waterman, H., Marshall, M., Noble, J., Davies, H., Wakshe, K., Sheaff, R., & Elwyn, G. (2007). The role of action research in the investigation and diffusion of innovations in health care: The Pride Project. *Qualitative Health Research*, *17*(3), 373–381. doi:10.1177/1049732306298976 PMID:17301345

Waycott, J., Pedell, S., Vetere, F., Ozanne, E., Kulik, L., Gruner, A., & Downs, J. (2012). *Actively Engaging Older Adults in the Development and Evaluation of Tablet Technology*. Paper presented at the 24th Australian Computer-Human Interaction Conference (OzCHI' 12). Melbourne, Australia.

Webster, D., Needell, B., & Wildfire, J. (2002). Data are Your Friends: Child Welfare Agency Self-Evaluation in Los Angeles County with the Family to Family Initiative. *Children and Youth Services Review*, *24*(6/7), 471–484. doi:10.1016/S0190-7409(02)00197-4

Weerakkody, V., & Currie, W. (2003). Integrating business process reengineering with information systems development: issues & implications. In *Business Process Management* (pp. 302–320). Springer Berlin Heidelberg. doi:10.1007/3-540-44895-0_21

Wei, J., Lin, S., Weng, C., & Wu, H. (2012). A case study of applying LRFM model in market segmentation of a children's dental clinic. *Expert Systems with Applications*, *39*(5), 5529–5533. doi:10.1016/j.eswa.2011.11.066

Weiner, J. P., Fowles, J., & Chan, K. S. (2012). New paradigms for measuring clinical performance using electronic health records. *International Journal for Quality in Health Care*, *24*(3), 200–205. doi:10.1093/intqhc/mzs011 PMID:22490301

Weiskopf, N. G., Hripcsak, G., Swaminathan, S., & Weng, C. (2013). Defining and measuring completeness of electronic health records for secondary use. *Journal of Biomedical Informatics*, *46*, 830–836. doi:10.1016/j.jbi.2013.06.010 PMID:23820016

Weiskopf, N. G., & Weng, C. (2013). Methods and dimensions of electronic health record data quality assessment: enabling reuse for clinical research. *Journal of the American Medical Informatics Association*, *20*(1), 144–151. doi:10.1136/amiajnl-2011-000681 PMID:22733976

Wenger, E. C., & Snyder, W. M. (2000). Communities of practice: The organizational frontier. *Harvard Business Review*, *78*(1), 139–145. PMID:11184968

Wessels, B., Walsh, S., & Adam, E. (2008). Mediating Voices: Community Participation in the Design of E-Enabled Community Care Services. *The Information Society*, *24*(1), 30–39. doi:10.1080/01972240701774683

West, D., & Heath, D. (2011). Theoretical pathways to the future: Globalization, ICT and social work theory and practice. *Journal of Social Work*, *11*(2), 209–221. doi:10.1177/1468017310386835

Wetter, T., & Paech, B. (2010). *What if "business process" is the wrong metaphor? Exploring the potential of Value Based Requirements Engineering for clinical software.* Paper presented at the 13th International Congress on Medical Informatics. Cape Town, South Africa.

White, G. W., Suchowierska, M., & Campbell, M. (2004). Developing and systematically implementing participatory action research. *Archives of Physical Medicine and Rehabilitation*, *85*(Supplement 2), 3–12. doi:10.1016/j.apmr.2003.08.109 PMID:15083417

White, S., Hall, C., & Peckover, S. (2009). The Descriptive Tyranny of the Common Assessment Framework: Technologies of Categorization and Professional Practice in Child Welfare. *British Journal of Social Work*, *39*(7), 1197–1217. doi:10.1093/bjsw/bcn053

White, S., Wastell, D., Broadhurst, K., & Hall, C. (2010). When policy o'erlaps itself: The 'tragic tale' of the Integrated Children's System. *Critical Social Policy*, *30*(3), 405–429. doi:10.1177/0261018310367675

Whittemore, R., & Knalf, K. (2005). Methodological issues in nursing research: The integrative review: updated methodology. *Journal of Advanced Nursing*, *52*(2), 546–553. doi:10.1111/j.1365-2648.2005.03621.x PMID:16268861

WHO Collaborating Centre for Drug Statistics Methodology. (n.d.). *Anatomical Therapeutic Chemical classification system*. Retrieved October 2013, from WHOCC website: http://www.whocc.no/atc

WHO. (2012). Legal frameworks for e-health. Global observatory for ehealth series – Vol.5.

Wicks, A.M., & Visich, J.K., & Suhong, L. (2006). Radio Frequency Identification Applications in Hospital Environments. *Hospital Topics*, *84*(3), 3–8. doi:10.3200/HTPS.84.3.3-9 PMID:16913301

Wiig, K. M. (1997). Integrating intellectual capital and knowledge management. *Long Range Planning*, *30*(3), 399–405. doi:10.1016/S0024-6301(97)90256-9

Wilde, M. H., & Garvin, S. (2007). A concept analysis of self-management. *Journal of Advanced Nursing*, *57*(3), 339–350. doi:10.1111/j.1365-2648.2006.04089.x PMID:17233653

Wilk, S., Michalowski, M., Michalowski, W., Farion, K., Hing, M. M., & Mohapatra, S. (2013). Mitigation of adverse interactions in pairs of clinical practice guidelines using constraint logic programming. *Journal of Biomedical Informatics*, *46*(2), 341–353. doi:10.1016/j.jbi.2013.01.002 PMID:23376273

Willems, D. (2000). Managing one's body using self-management techniques: practicing autonomy. *Theoretical Medicine and Bioethics*, *21*(1), 23–38. doi:10.1023/A:1009995018677 PMID:10927967

Williams, T. R. (2000). Guidelines for designing and evaluating the display of information on the web. *Technical Communication*, *47*(3), 383–397.

Winfrey, E. C. (1999). Kirkpatrick's Four Levels of Evaluation. In B. Hoffman (Ed.), *Encyclopedia of Educational Technology*. Retrieved November 26, 2013, fromhttp://www.4cleanair.org/Kirkpatrick.pdf

Wolf, P., Schmidt, A., & Klein, M. (2008). *SOPRANO-An extensible, open AAL platform for elderly people based on semantical contracts*. Paper presented at the 3rd Workshop on Artificial Intelligence Techniques for Ambient Intelligence (AITAmI'08), 18th European Conference on Artificial Intelligence (ECAI 08). Patras, Greece.

Wong, Y. C., Fung, J. Y. C., Law, C. K., Lam, J. C. Y., & Lee, V. W. P. (2009). Tackling the Digital Divide. *British Journal of Social Work*, *39*(4), 745–767. doi:10.1093/bjsw/bcp026

Wood, A., Stankovic, J., Virone, G., Selavo, L., He, Z., & Cao, Q. et al. (2008). Context-aware wireless sensor networks for assisted living and residential monitoring. *IEEE Network*, *22*(4), 26–33. doi:10.1109/MNET.2008.4579768

Woodrow, J. E. (1992). The influence of programming traininig on the computer literacy and attitudes of preservice teachers. *Journal of Research on Computing in Education*, *25*(2), 200–219.

World, W. P. P. (2003). The 2002 Revision, Highlights (Report No.: ESA/P/WP. 180). New York: United Nations Population Division.

*Wowza*. (2013). Available at http://www.wowza.com/

Wuensch, K., Aziz, S., Ozan, E., Kishore, M., & Tabrizi, M. H. (2008). Pedagogical characteristics of online and face-to-face classes. *International Journal on E-Learning*, *3*(7), 523–532.

Wu, I.-L., Li, J.-Y., & Fu, C.-Y. (2011). The adoption of mobile healthcare by hospital's professionals: An integrative perspective. *Decision Support Systems*, *51*(3), 587–596. doi:10.1016/j.dss.2011.03.003

Wu, J.-H., Wang, S.-C., & Lin, L.-M. (2007). Mobile computing acceptance factors in the healthcare industry: A structural equation model. *International Journal of Medical Informatics*, *76*(1), 66–77. doi:10.1016/j.ijmedinf.2006.06.006 PMID:16901749

Yang, C. C., Lin, W. T., Chen, H. M., & Shi, Y. H. (2009). Improving scheduling of emergency physicians using data mining analysis. *Expert Systems with Applications*, *36*(2), 3378–3387. doi:10.1016/j.eswa.2008.02.069

Yang, C., Tsai, C., Member, S., Cheng, K., & Chen, S. (2012). Low-Invasive Implantable Devices of Low-Power Consumption Using High-Efficiency Antennas for Cloud Healthcare. *IEEE Journal on Emerging and Selected Topics in Circuits and Systems*, *2*(1), 14–23. doi:10.1109/JETCAS.2012.2187469

Yan, H., Huo, H., Xu, Y., & Gidlund, M. (2010). Wireless sensor network based E-health system implementation and experimental results. *IEEE Transactions on* Consumer Electronics, *56*(4), 2288–2295.

Yan, H., Jiang, Y., & Zheng, J., Fu, B., Xiao, S., & Peng, C. (2004). The internet-based knowledge acquisition and management method to construct large-scale distributed medical expert systems. *Computer Methods and Programs in Biomedicine*, *74*(1), 1–10. doi:10.1016/S0169-2607(03)00076-2 PMID:14992822

Yan, Q., Yan, H., Han, F., Wei, X., & Zhu, T. (2009). SVM-based decision support system for clinic aided tracheal intubation predication with multiple features. *Expert Systems with Applications*, *36*(3), 6588–6592. doi:10.1016/j.eswa.2008.07.076

Yao, H., Orme, A., & Etzkorn, L. H. (2005). Cohesion metrics for ontology design and application. *Journal of Computer Science, 1*(1), 107–113. doi:10.3844/jcssp.2005.107.113

Yao, L., Zhang, Y., Li, Y., Sanseau, P., & Agarwal, P. (2011). Electronic health records: Implications for drug discovery. *Drug Discovery Today, 16*(13/14), 594–599. doi:10.1016/j.drudis.2011.05.009 PMID:21624499

Yeh, J. Y., Wu, T. H., & Tsao, C. W. (2011). Using data mining techniques to predict hospitalization of hemodialysis patients. *Decision Support Systems, 50*(2), 439–448. doi:10.1016/j.dss.2010.11.001

Yen, B., Hu, P. J.-H., & Wang, M. (2007). Toward an analytical approach for effective Web site design: A framework for modeling, evaluation and enhancement. *Electronic Commerce Research and Applications, 6*(2), 159–170. doi:10.1016/j.elerap.2006.11.004

Yi, M. Y., Jackson, J. D., Park, J. S., & Probst, J. C. (2006). Understanding information technology acceptance by individual professionals: Toward an integrative view. *Information & Management, 43*(3), 350–363. doi:10.1016/j.im.2005.08.006

Yi, Y. (1990). A critical review of consumer satisfaction. *Revista de Marina (Valparaiso, Chile), 4*(1), 68–123.

Youn, E. (2007). The Relationship Between Technology Content in a Masters of Social Work Curriculum and Technology Use in Social Work Practice: A Qualitative Research Study. *Journal of Technology in Human Services, 25*(1), 45–58. doi:10.1300/J017v25n01_03

Young, L., Tu, S. W., Tennakoon, L., Vismer, D., Astakhov, V., Gupta, A., et al. (2009). Ontology Driven Data Integration for Autism Research. In *Proceedings of 2009 22nd IEEE International Symposium on Computer-Based Medical Systems* (pp. 54-60). New York: IEEE.

Young, T., Peppard, P. E., & Gottlieb, D. J. (2002). Epidemiology of Obstructive Sleep Apnea: A population health perspective. *American Journal of Respiratory and Critical Care Medicine, 165*(9), 1217–1239. doi:10.1164/rccm.2109080 PMID:11991871

Yu, F. Y., & Liu, Y. H. (2009). Creating a psychologically safe online space for a student generated questions learning activity via different identity revelation modes. *British Journal of Educational Technology, 40*(6), 1109–1123. doi:10.1111/j.1467-8535.2008.00905.x

Yu, J., Ha, I., Choi, M., & Rho, J. (2005). Extending the TAM for a t-commerce. *Information & Management, 42*(7), 965–976. doi:10.1016/j.im.2004.11.001

Zayed, N., Awad, A. B., El-Akel, W., Doss, W., Awad, T., Radwan, A., & Mabrouk, M. (2013). The assessment of data mining for the prediction of therapeutic outcome in 3719 Egyptian patients with chronic hepatitis C. *Clinics and Research in Hepatology and Gastroenterology, 37*(3), 254–261. doi:10.1016/j.clinre.2012.09.005 PMID:23141214

*Zephyr Inc.* (2013). Available: http://www.zephyranywhere.com/

Zhang, D., Zhao, J. L., Zhou, L., & Nunamaker, J. F. Jr. (2004). Can e-learning replace classroom learning? *Communications of the ACM, 47*(5), 75–79. doi:10.1145/986213.986216

Zhao, D., & Weng, C. (2011). Combining PubMed knowledge and EHR data to develop a weighted Bayesian network for pancreatic cancer prediction. *Journal of Biomedical Informatics, 44*(5), 859–868. doi:10.1016/j.jbi.2011.05.004 PMID:21642013

Zickuhr, K., & Madden, M. (2012). Older adults and internet use. *Pew Internet & American Life Project.* Retrieved from http://pewinternet.org/Reports/2012/Older-adults-and-internet-use.aspx

Zikmund, W. G. (2003). Business research methods (7th ed.). Mason, OH: Thomson South-Western.

Zuber-Skerritt, O. (2001). *Action Learning and action research: paradigm, praxis and programs. Effective change management using action research and action learning: Concepts, frameworks, process and applications.* Lismore, Australia: Southern Cross University Press.

Zuehlke, P., Li, J. H., Talaei-Khoei, A., & Ray, P. (2009). A functional specification for mobile eHealth (mHealth) systems. In *Proceedings of E-Health Networking, Applications and Services.* IEEE.

# About the Contributors

**Madjid Tavana** is a professor of Business Systems and Analytics and the Lindback Distinguished Chair of Information Systems and Decision Sciences at La Salle University, where he served as Chairman of the Management Department and Director of the Center for Technology and Management. He is a Distinguished Research Fellow at the Kennedy Space Center, Johnson Space Center, Naval Research Laboratory at Stennis Space Center, and Air Force Research Laboratory. He was recently honored with the prestigious Space Act Award by NASA. He holds a MBA, PMIS, and PhD in Management Information Systems and received his Post-Doctoral Diploma in Strategic Information Systems from the Wharton School at the University of Pennsylvania. He is the Editor-in-Chief of *Decision Analytics, International Journal of Applied Decision Sciences, International Journal of Management and Decision Making, International Journal of Strategic Decision Sciences,* and *International Journal of Enterprise Information Systems.* He has published several books and over one hundred and fifty research papers in academic journals such as *Information Sciences, Decision Sciences, Information Systems, Interfaces, Annals of Operations Research, Advances in Space Research, Omega, Information and Management, Knowledge-Based Systems, International Journal of Production Research, Expert Systems with Applications, European Journal of Operational Research, Journal of the Operational Research Society, Computers and Operations Research, Energy Economics, Applied Soft Computing,* and *Energy Policy.*

**Amir Hossein Ghapanchi** is a tenured faculty member at the School of Information and Communication Technology, Griffith University, Australia. Prior to that he has worked at the University of Technology Sydney and the University of New South Wales (UNSW). He obtained his PhD in Information Systems from the University of New South Wales (UNSW), Australia. Dr Ghapanchi has also been an active member of the Institute for Integrated Intelligent Systems (IIIS) and Asia-Pacific ubiquitous Healthcare Research Centre (APuHC). He has been involved in a research initiative called 'Assistive eHealth Technologies for Aged Care.' He has also been involved in an ongoing Randomised Controlled Trial of robots for aged care in 53 sites in six countries including Australia, as part of the €2.36 Million EU project Victoryahome led by the Norwegian Centre for Integrated Care and Telemedicine (NST). Dr Ghapanchi is a section editor for the *Australasian Journal of Information System*, and an associate editor for the *International Journal of Enterprise Information Systems*, and *International Journal of Strategic Decision Sciences.* He has published over 50 referred publications including 40 journal articles in prestigious information systems and management journals such as *Information and Organization, Journal of the Association for Information Science and Technology (JASIST), Electronic Markets, Journal of Medical Internet Research, Journal of Computer and System Sciences, International Journal of Project Management, Journal of Systems and Software*, and *International Journal of Information Management.* He has been in receipt of several internal/external research and L&T grants.

**Amir Talaei-Khoei** is a faculty member at the University of Technology, Sydney (UTS), where he coordinates an international initiative for Adoption of Assistive Technologies in Aged Care involving several universities, research institutes, and industrial partners. Since 2008, he has been an active member of the Asia-Pacific ubiquitous Healthcare Research Centre (APuHC). He has recently joined the Lab for Agile Information Systems in which he collaborates with his colleagues at UTS to build industrial partnerships for innovative technological solutions applicable in complex healthcare systems. He is also a member of the Centre for Human Centred Technology Design at UTS where he works on the use of interactive technologies such as games for aged care. Dr Talaei-Khoei is a member of the editorial boards for Australasian Journal of Information Systems and Health Informatics. He presently serves as an executive in the Australian Association of Information Systems (AAIS). Dr Talaei-Khoei's research interests lie in the area of health informatics ranging from theoretical applications of agent-based contextual awareness in complex and wicked healthcare problems to adoption and management of technologies in healthcare and aged care settings. He received his PhD from the University of New South Wales (UNSW) in Australia and holds a MSc of Information Technology from the Royal Institute of Technology (KTH) in Sweden.

* * *

**Abbes Amira** is a professor in visual communication at the University of the West of Scotland (UWS), Scotland. He also holds a position of Professor of Computer Engineering at Qatar University, Qatar. Prior to joining UWS, he took academic positions at the University of Ulster-UK, Qatar University-Qatar, Brunel University-UK, and Queen's University Belfast-UK. He received his PhD from Queen's University Belfast in 2001. He has been awarded a number of grants from the government and the industry and has published around 200 publications in the area of reconfigurable computing and image processing during his career to date. He has been invited to give talks at many universities and international conferences and being chair, program committee for a number of conferences. He is also one of the 2008 VARIAN prize recipients. He holds two visiting professor positions at the University of Nancy, France, and the University of Tunn Hussein Onn, Malaysia. He is a Fellow of IET, Senior Member of the IEEE and Senior Member of ACM.

**Ahmad Suhaimi Baharudin** graduated with a specialization in computer science from Indiana state, in 1987. He continued his MBA at the Universiti Sains Malaysia, followed by a PhD in Technology Management. He is a senior lecturer in Universiti Sains Malaysia and supervising several PhD and master students. He has a wide knowledge in finance, and he is teaching Msc IT Technopreneurship students on Financial Planning and Management for several years. He has special interest towards finance as exhibited through his working experience. His specializations consist of Service Science and Innnovation, Human Computer Interaction (HCI), Management of Information Systems (MIS), Information Technology (IT) Operations and Management, Technopreneurship. He has published in several journals.

**Iman Barazandeh** received his MS degree in computer engineering in 2009, and he is currently completing his another MS program (IT engineering) in the School of Industrial Engineering at the Iran University of Science and Technology (IUST), Tehran. Presently, he is faculty member of the department of Electrical and Computer Engineering in Islamic Azad University, Mahshahr branch. He has contributed several research papers to national and international journals and conferences and entrepreneurship communities. He is a member of a number of national conference program committees and has carried out a number of projects in collaboration with the university. His current research interests are knowledge discovery and data mining, biomedical informatics, distributed systems and decision making theory. He is also interested in both the technical and business sides of entrepreneurship and startups.

**Jacqueline Blake** is an Associate Lecturer at the University of the Sunshine Coast. Her research interests are in the development and evaluation of decision support systems for healthcare, Evaluation of social policies, and the implementation of sustainability programs. Jacqueline Blake has published in journals such as *Knowledge Based Systems, and book chapters, business-to-business communication, e-health and community capacity building*. Jacqui has completed a PhD by designing and building a web-application which would support the diagnosis by physicians of sleep disorders. Her research masters was completed investigating business-to-business communication within supply chains of the Australian wood product and timber industry. Jacqui's research interests are focused on optimising and evaluating organisational processes and eHealth.

**Pablo Casaseca-de-la-Higuera** is a Lecturer in Image Processing with the School of Computing at the University of the West of Scotland (UWS). Before joining UWS, he worked for the aerospace industry (2000-2003) and took different academic positions at the ETSI Telecomunicación, University of Valladolid (Spain), where he is still linked to the Laboratory of Image Processing (LPI). His research interests include statistical modelling and nonlinear methods for signal and image processing, with a special focus on bioengineering. He is a reviewer of several scientific journals and main conferences, and has co-authored more than 40 journal and conference papers.

**Michele Ceruti**, born 1979, MD, is a resident student of the Postgraduate School of Public Health of the University of Turin. Member of the Italian Society of Health Technology Assessment, he is part of national and international working groups for telemedicine projects. He is currently involved in research studies in the fields of e-health, Connecting Health, Health Impact Assessment, as well as in local feasibility studies assessing electronic health record systems use for clinical governance purposes. Since 2011, he has been involved in United Europe cross-border healthcare projects, especially for elderly patient needs. He is currently exploring risk and operative models and solutions with Patient Organizations and Non Governmental Organizations about the issue of continuity of care for European citizens receiving cross-border care in the European Union.

**Samir Diouny** is a lecturer of linguistics and Chairman of the English Department at Chouaib Doukkali University (CDU) in El Jadida, Morocco. He received his PhD in Neurolinguistics from Hassan II University - Mohamedia in 2005. He was a Fulbright grantee on two occasions, once to read for a PhD (University of Texas at Austin, USA from 1998-2000) and the second as a Post-doctoral researcher (The Boston Medical School, USA in 2007). In 2011, he was a visiting lecturer at Toulouse University le Mirail in France. His research interests include the use of ICT in language teaching and learning, language impairment in adults, and linguistics aspects of schizophrenia. He has published in IMIA Yearbook of Medical Informatics and in journals such as *Assistive Technology*.

**Dan Dumbrell** is a PhD Candidate under the Discipline of Health Informatics at the University of Sydney. With a background in Exercise and Sport Science and Health Informatics, his main focus with his current research is the study of emerging technologies (i.e. social media) and their effects on public health information dissemination. Publications include studies on the interactions and methods of health information on Twitter, as well as the role of the various entities involved in health communication through this media. Dan has worked as a research assistant on the Connecting Older Adults Project, which addressed the effect of social media technologies on socially isolated older adults.

**Bardo Fraunholz** is an academic in Information and Business Analytics with Deakin University, Australia. He holds a Professional Business Degree in Information Systems and Accounting (University of Trier, Germany) and GradDip in Legal studies specialising in IT, Media, and Corporate Law from London (UK). He has lectured at the University of Koblenz, Germany, in enterprise modelling, project management, small business and knowledge management. He spent several years in the ICT sector managing/consulting with a number of projects involving mobile applications, SMEs, and e-learning. His research interests are in mobile applications, e-learning technologies, and environment sustainability.

**Silvio Geninatti**, born 1956, practiced clinical activity as a psychologist from 1985 to 1995. Since 1990, he addressed his professional interests towards information technology, data mining and medical statistics. In 1999, he completed a Masters course in Epidemiology, and in 2009, he earned a Degree in Statistics. Since 2009, he has managed Statistics and Epidemiological Services in the Local Health Unit #2 of Torino. At the moment he cooperates with Sacro Cuore Catholic University and Turin University for Statistics teaching activities. Since 2011, he has been a Member of the Technical Scientific Committee of CSI Piedmont, the Information System Consortium to which Piedmont's Public Administration entrusts the management and implementation of its ICT services, where he is carrying on activities to develop tools for online reuse of EHR for the management of health systems.

**M. R. Gholamian** is an Assistant Professor at the School of Industrial Engineering at the Iran University of Science and Technology (IUST), Tehran. He received his MS degree in Industrial Engineering from Isfahan University of Technology (IUT), Isfahan, and in 1998, he obtained a PhD in Industrial Engineering from Amirkabir University of Technology (AUT), Tehran, in 2005 for the work in the field of Hybrid Intelligent Decision Making Systems. Presently, he is a faculty member of IT Group in the School of Industrial Engineering and is actively engaged in conducting Academic, Research, and Development Programs in the field of Industrial Engineering and Information Technology. He has contributed more than 122 research papers to many national and international journals and conferences. Besides this, he has published 4 books by reputed publishers. His research interests include Data Mining, Soft Computing, and Decision Theory.

**Christos Grecos**, SMIEEE, SMSPIE, is a professor in Visual Communication Standards and the Head of the School of Computing at the University of the West of Scotland. Before coming to Scotland he has worked at the universities of Central Lancashire and Loughborough. He has more than 120 publications and has obtained significant funding for his research from the Engineering and Physical Sciences

Research Councils (UK), Technology Strategy Board (UK), European Regional Development Fund, and Scottish Funding Council. He is also in the international and technical programme committees of many prestigious conferences. His main areas of expertise are image and video compression algorithms and standards.

**Güney Gürsel** was born in 1972 in İzmir, Turkey. He graduated from the Military Academy in 1994, as a systems engineer. He earned his MSc degree in the Information Systems field in 2003 at the Middle East Technical University (METU) and his PhD in the Medical Informatics field in 2012 again at METU. He is working in the Department of Medical Informatics at the Gülhane Military Medical Academy, as a medical informatics specialist. He speaks advanced English. He is working in the fields of Healthcare Information Systems (HCIS), Evaluation of HCIS, end user expectations from HCIS, Fuzzy logic application in HCIS, and Interoperability in HCIS. He is married and has two kids.

**Craig Hume** has over 30 years of experience in information technology analytics and project management. He has recently completed his PhD in the role of knowledge management in non profit organisations through Griffith University QLD. He has a solid track record of publications and is seen as an expert in the field of knowledge management and knowledge hubs.

**Margee Hume** specialises in service experience mapping and innovation and IT service management. Her focus is on sustainable work communities research . She is the Campus Academic Co-ordinator for Research Development at Springfield Campus USQ and is a leader on the Collaborative Research Network: Digital futures. She is a member of the Australian Centre for Sustainable Business Development and the Australian Digital Futures Institute.

**Paul Johnston** is a Joint Managing Partner of South-South Capital Partners (SSCP), a boutique consulting firm, focused on the Sustainability, Healthcare and Infrastructure industries, specializing in Latin American and Asian market entry outcomes, through delivery of the agreed Partner Transaction (PACT). Paul gained his MBA in Technology Commercialisation and New Venture Creation from the University of Queensland. Since this time, he has acted in multiple sales and marketing director roles. Paul is currently acting in parallel for Care Systems, an Aged Care IT provider entering Asia and e-cofueling, an innovative biofuels transport technology, and entering Latin America.

**Pantea Keikhosrokiani** is currently a PhD student and teaching assistant in School of Computer Sciences at the Universiti Sains Malaysia. Prior to this, she finished her masters in Information Technology (Technopreneurship) from the same university. She obtained her bachelors degree in Electrical Engineering Electronics from Iran. She worked as an electrical design engineer at Fara Tahghigh Sepahan Consulting Engineers, Isfahan, Iran for a few years. Pantea has some publications in the area of mobile healthcare and User Based Studies including Human Computer Interactions, mobile commerce, and location-based services. She is interested in mobile healthcare systems, mobile-commerce, location-based services and applications, and Technopreneurship and innovation.

**Don Kerr** is an Associate Professor of Informatics at the University of the Sunshine Coast. His research interests include the development and evaluation of decision support systems for healthcare and agricultural applications. He has published over 100 peer reviewed papers in Information systems and management journals and conferences over the past 20 years, including in journals such as *Decision Support Systems, Expert systems with Applications, Knowledge Based Systems,* and *Agricultural Systems*. He has supervised eight PhD students to completion (5 as principal and 3 as associate) and is presently supervising five PhD students.

**Sirpa Kuusisto-Niemi** works as Senior Lecturer in Health and Human Services Informatics at the University of Eastern Finland in the Department of Health and Social Management, and in 2000 launched the first Masters degree programme in Health and Human Services Informatics in Finland. Her main research interests are social services and social work informatics, data structures, and terminological research. She teaches also in continuing education courses in data protection and ICT development at the University of Eastern Finland. She has been involved actively in national activities for IT development in social services since 1993. Her former tasks include social services ICT development issues in the National R&D Centre for Welfare and Health, international consultancy tasks in social care ICT, an expert membership in child custody at the County Administrative Court, and social work.

**Ihssane Lembachar** is a resident physician at the Medical Informatics Laboratory of the Medical School of Casablanca, Morocco. In 2010, she received her doctorate in Medicine from the Medical School of Casablanca and in 2011, she earned her degree in Statistics Applied to Medicine from the University of Paris VI, France. She is currently undertaking a Master's degree in Engineering Expertise and Information Systems in Healthcare from the faculty of Medicine of Marseille. Her research interests are in information and communication technology, e-learning, telemedicine, and health IT systems. Ihssane Lembachar has published in journals such as Sante Publique.

**Lundy Lewis** is a Professor of Computer Information Technology at Southern New Hampshire University in the USA. He holds an endowed chair – The Christos and Mary Papoutsy Distinguished Chair in Ethics and Social Responsibility – through which he performs research and development on the use of technology to address social concerns. Dr. Lewis is interested in how technologies can be used to address important social issues of the present and the future, e.g. taking care of the elderly, desensitization of anxieties, and sparking learning in under-privileged students. His lifelong scholarly activity has revolved around the application of Artificial Intelligence methods to practical business problems and to building prototype systems e.g. using AI in business intelligence, situational reasoning, computer networks, video games, avatars, and robots. He holds 35 US patents involving technology and has been a Principal Investigator on several multi-year projects for the US Department of Defense and the Australian Research Council. He has published three books on computer networks and has published numerous journal articles and conference papers on the application of AI methods to real-world problems.

**Siaw-Teng Liaw** is a Professor of General Practice at the University of NSW and Director of the South Western Sydney Local Health District General Practice Unit, which is based in Fairfield Hospital. Professor Liaw's R&D program revolves around primary and integrated care informatics and clinical decision support, focused on quality of routinely collected data in Electronic Health Records, information governance, chronic disease management, and quality use of medicines in a cross-cultural health context. He has experience and expertise in the use of mixed methods to examine complex interventions, including cluster randomised trials, pre-and-post studies, national surveys, and a range of qualitative methods.

**Antonio A. Lopez-Lorca** is a Research Fellow in the Faculty of Science, Engineering, and Technology at Swinburne University of Technology. He received his PhD in 2012, from the University of Wollongong, Australia. Antonio has studied ways of applying semantic web techniques to agent-oriented models to validate them prior to software development. In his current position, he continues to use agent-oriented models to study how to incorporate users' emotions into software development. Alex's expertise in this area is fundamentally around analysing and modelling people-oriented systems. The majority of these projects focus on socio-technical systems, such as aged care support systems and mental health online programs, in which people's emotions are particularly important.

**Chunbo Luo** is a lecturer in networks at the University of the West of Scotland (UWS). He received BEng and MEng degrees in Electronic Engineering from the University of Electronic Science and Technology of China (UESTC), China, in 2005 and 2007 respectively. He received a PhD degree from the University of Reading, UK in 2011. He is with the Centre of Audio-Visual Communications and Networks (AVCN) at UWS, and he is a member of IEEE. His research interests include wireless communication, signal processing, wireless sensor networks, and Unmanned Aerial Vehicle (UAV) networks.

**Tim Miller** is a Senior Lecturer in the Department of Computing and Information Systems at the University of Melbourne. He obtained his PhD from the University of Queensland in April 2005, where he explored the link between requirements verification and software testing. After receiving his PhD, Tim spent four years as a postdoctoral researcher and software engineer in the Agent ART group at the University of Liverpool, UK. After this, he took up his current post. Tim's primary research interests lie in the areas of software verification and testing, software engineering for people-oriented systems, agent-oriented software engineering, and human-agent interaction.

**Gianpaolo Molino** has degrees in Medicine and Surgery, Gastroenterology, Occupational Medicine, and Internal Medicine. He is a lecturer in Medical Patology and Clinical Metodology. He was an associate professor of Internal Medicine at Torino University from 1980-1990; then, he was Chief of a Division of Internal Medicine, Center for Medical Informatics in the Department of Internal Medicine and a Consultant in Clinical Informatics at the Azienda Ospedaliera San Giovanni Battista di Torino. His main research topics include hepatobiliary transports, cortico-hypophyseal function, compartmental models, expert systems, dynamic tests for liver function, optimization of jaundice diagnosis, medical e-learning, and medical informatics. He has authored more than 500 published papers.

**Norlia Mustaffa** graduated from Indiana State University, USA completing both her Bachelors and Masters degrees. Currently, she is a senior lecturer in School of Computer Sciences at the Universiti Sains Malaysia supervising several PhD and masters students. She is teaching Msc IT Technopreneurship students on Business Organizations and Environments for a few years. Her specializations are in the area of System Analysis and Design, Information Systems, and Business Process Engineering. Her other area of interest includes Information Retrieval, Database Security, E-Learning, and Business related Information Systems. Her research interest is mainly in the area of Information Systems. She has outstanding publications.

**Mohammed Bennani Othmani** is the Head of Casablanca Medical Informatics Laboratory at the Medical School of Casablanca, Morocco. He has earned a Master's Degree in Medical Informatics at the Faculty of Medicine of Rennes, France. He is the vice Dean for Academic Affairs, University Hospital activities, and student life at the Medical School of Casablanca and the President of the Moroccan Society of Medical Informatics and Health. His research interests include the use of Information and Communication Technology in Medical Education, e-learning, and telemedicine. He has published in IMIA Yearbook of Medical Informatics and in journals such as Assistive Technology.

**Sonja Pedell** has been a Senior Lecturer in the Department of Communication and Digital Media Design at Swinburne University of Technology since January 2012. She has completed her PhD in Interaction Design in 2008 at the University of Melbourne, Australia. Her research interests are user-centred design methods, scenario-based and mobile design, agent-based modelling, domestic technology development, and the design of engaging novel technologies for various user groups, in particular for the ageing population. Sonja holds a Masters of Psychology from the Technical University of Berlin (Germany) and was employed as an Interaction Designer, Usability Consultant and Product Manager in industry for several years.

**Zeeshan Pervez** is a lecturer in Web Technology at the University of the West of Scotland. He received a PhD degree from Kyung Hee University South Korea in 2013. His research interests are mainly cloud computing, data security and privacy, privacy-aware computation and encrypted data search. He has been involved in a number of research projects funded by the Ministry of Knowledge Economy (MKE), South Korea and Microsoft Asia. For his research on privacy-aware data sharing in the public cloud he received 3rd Best Paper award from IEEE Seoul Section in year 2010.

**Luca Piovesan** obtained his Bachelors Degree in Computer Science at the University of Turin in 2010 and Masters Degree in Computer Science at the University of Turin in 2012, with a thesis entitled "A CSP Based Approach to Plan Adaptation in Domains with Numeric Fluents." Since 2013, he has been a PhD Student in Computer Science at the Doctoral School of Sciences and Innovative Technologies at the Department of Computer Science at the University of Turin, Turin, Italy. He is working on the project titled "Intelligent techniques in medical informatics," which aims at developing intelligent techniques to support physicians in the treatment of patients through clinical guidelines. His research interests are artificial intelligence (in particular, knowledge representation, ontologies, and reasoning), medical informatics (in the field of computer-interpretable clinical guidelines), decision support systems, planning, and temporal database.

**Alireza Rahimi** is a PhD candidate at the School of Public Health and Community Medicine at the University of New South Wales, Australia. He holds a MSc in Library and Information Science. As a senior lecturer, he founded the Health Information Technology Research Center at Isfahan University of Medical Science, Isfahan, Iran and has served in a number of medical library and information systems projects. His main research interests included data quality in clinical information systems, design ontological based approaches, IT human resource management, information organization, and automated library software. He has published in several high ranking information systems journals (English and Persian) and peer reviewed journals in the field of health and medical informatics.

**Naeem Ramzan,** FHEA, MIEEE, MIET, received an MS in Telecom from Brest, France and a PhD in Electronics Engineering form Queen Mary University of London in 2004 and 2008 respectively. From 2008 to 2012, he worked on EU projects aceMedia, PetaMedia, SARACEN, and CUBRIK in Queen Mary University of London. Currently, he is a lecturer in Visual Communication at the University of the West of Scotland. His research interest includes image and video coding, scalable video coding, multimedia search and retrieval, multimedia transmission over wireless, and P2P networks. He has been a co-chair of special session in ACM MIR 2010, (WIAMIS) 2009, WIAMIS 2010 and WIAMIS 2011, and the co-organiser and co-chair of ACM Multimedia workshop SAP 2010, SBNMA 2011, UXeLate 2012. He has published more than 60 research publications, and served as Guest Editor of a special issue of the Elsevier Journal Signal Processing: Image Communication and IEEE COMSOC E-Letter.

**Pradeep Kumar Ray** is a Professor of Information Systems, Technology, and Management at the University of New South Wales (UNSW), Australia. He is the founding Chair of the Asia Pacific ubiquitous Health Care research Centre (APuHC) at UNSW since 2007. He is the Chair of the IEEE eHealth Technical Committee and the founder of IEEE Healthcom that is now the forum of discussions for the IEEE/ITU-D/WHO initiatives on eHealth and mHealth (see Research Program 3 at www.apuhc.unsw.edu.au). Pradeep has been leading several international initiatives, such as the WHO Research on the Assessment of eHealth for Health Care Delivery (involving India, China, Vietnam and Philippines).

**Sari Rissanen** is currently working as a part-time Professor in Social Work, especially Welfare Services, and as part-time lecturer in health and social management at the University of Eastern Finland. She holds a PhD in Social Policy and a Licentiate in Health Management Sciences. Her multidisciplinary research group has addressed various elderly care management and organizational issues from multi-agency perspectives (e.g., clients, employees, entrepreneurs or relatives). The research focuses on the role of private care, mergers and quality of home care and home help and wellbeing of the elderly, among other things. Currently, she is a partner in the EU-funded Innovating Care for People with Multiple Chronic Conditions in Europe (ICARE4EU) – project, which is coordinated by the Netherlands Institute for Health Services Research.

**Kaija Saranto** works as a Professor in Health and Human Services Informatics at the University of Eastern Finland, Department of Health and Social Management, and in 2000, launched the first Masters degree programme in Health and Human Services Informatics in Finland, following the international development in the field. Dr. Saranto has a number of memberships in both academic and expert groups focusing on ICT use in society. Her research interests include the role of classifications in EHRs, as well as educational and organizational issues in information system implementation. She is currently leading a research group focusing on patient safety. She is the past president of the Finnish Health Informatics Association under IMIA and Acendio. Dr. Saranto also acts as the Deputy Director of the Finnish Centre for Evidence-Based Health Care, affiliated with the Joanna Briggs Institute established in 2010.

**Zineb Serhier** is an Associate Professor of Medical Informatics at the Faculty of Medicine and Pharmacy of Casablanca. She has earned a Master's degree in Public Health at the Institute of Public Health, Epidemiology and Development in Bordeaux and in Engineering Expertise and Information Systems in Healthcare from the Faculty of Medicine of Marseille. She has published in journals such as: *Diagnostic Molecular Pathology, American Journal of Health Promotion, Journal of Obstetrics & Gynaecology, Rheumatology International, Eastern Mediterranean Health Journal,* and *Sante Publique.*

**Roberta Siliquini** born 1966, specialized in "Hygiene and Preventive Medicine." Since 1995, she carried out her professional activities within the Department of Public Health and Pediatric Sciences (formerly the Institute of Hygiene) at the University of Turin. Full Professor of Public Health, since 2007, she is the Director of the Postgraduate School of Hygiene and Preventive Medicine of Turin University (and was confirmed in 2014). In 2009, she was appointed as Vice Dean of the Faculty with responsibility for the relations with external companies and with advanced Masters courses. Involved with particular interest in the Research Area of Health Impact Assessment and Health Management, she is the project leader of studies assessing the behaviors of Italian citizen towards use of the Internet for health purposes, particularly for those categories of users who are most vulnerable.

**Jeffrey Soar** has 20+ years experience in eHealth and informatics for ageing and aged-care. He has a successful track record in health informatics and enabled technology publications with over 150 publications. Dr Soar is the founder and current Board Member of Aged Care and Healthy Ageing within the Health Informatics Society of Australia (HISA). He has been a HISA national board member and is the founder and organiser of the national Aged Care Informatics Conference (ACIC) which is entering its ninth annual event.

**Uma Srinivasan** is a Lead Scientist at Capital Markets Cooperative Research Centre and CMC Insurance Solutions, Sydney. Her experience in designing large software solutions for hospitals and health departments has shaped her research focus on technologies and solutions that enable efficient and high quality healthcare. Her current research interests are in the area of pattern analysis, data mining and social network analytics that can be applied to understanding and predicting provider behaviour and health outcomes for patients. She has several international publications that include a book on Multimedia Semantics, several book chapters, papers in leading international journals, and conference proceedings. She has contributed to several international standards bodies that include multimedia standards such as MPEG-7, and health information standards such as HL-7. Uma holds a PhD in computer science from the University of New South Wales, Australia, and serves as an Adjunct Associate Professor at the University of Western Sydney, Australia.

**Robert Steele** is the Head of Discipline and Chair of the Discipline of Health Informatics at The University of Sydney and the Director of the Health Informatics, Computation, and Innovation Lab. He is the author of over 120 peer-reviewed articles in the areas of Internet and mobile technologies, and health informatics and his professional service includes the role of Vice Chair of ACM SIGMOBILE 2009-2013. His research focuses on how emerging technologies can provide transformative benefits and innovative solutions in various application domains. He has been the lead Chief Investigator on numerous Australian Research Council grants and other externally funded research projects.

**Leon Sterling** is Pro Vice Chancellor (Digital Frontiers) at Swinburne University of Technology in Melbourne. Leon received a BSc (Hons) from the University of Melbourne and a PhD in Pure Mathematics from the Australian National University. He has worked at universities in the UK, Israel, the US, and Australia. His teaching and research specialties are software engineering, artificial intelligence, and logic programming. Prior to this role Leon was a Professor of Software Innovation and Engineering and the Director of e-Research at the University of Melbourne and Dean of Information and Communication Technologies at Swinburne. He was the President of the Australian Council of Deans of ICT.

**Jane Taggart** is a Research Fellow at the University of NSW Centre for Primary Health Care and Equity. Her research is focused on clinical informatics and linked data for improving data quality, chronic disease management (particularly related to diabetes), health outcomes, and integrated primary health care. Jane has research experience and expertise in mixed methods, a randomised controlled trial of an intervention examining the impact of teamwork on chronic care, systematic reviews around health literacy, and program evaluations. She currently manages and is an investigator on the electronic Practice Based Research Network program which is located in a disadvantaged and Culturally and Linguistically Diverse health neighbourhood.

**Paolo Terenziani** has been a Full Professor in DISIT at the Università del Piemonte Orientale, Alessandria, Italy since October 2000. Paolo Terenziani's research activity covers different areas of Computer Science: Artificial Intelligence (Knowledge Representation, Formal Ontologies, Temporal Reasoning), Databases (Temporal Relational Databases, Semantics), and Medical Informatics. As regards Medical Informatics, since 1997, he has been involved with Azienda Ospedaliera S. Giovanni Battista in Turin in a long-term project for the development of GLARE, a semi-automatic manager of clinical guidelines. Paolo Terenziani published more than 100 papers about these topics in refereed international journals and conference proceedings.

**Shahadat Uddin** is a lecturer in the Project Management Program and Complex Systems Research Centre at the University of Sydney. He conducts research in the area of complex healthcare coordination and collaboration networks, health informatics, and data analysis and modelling. His research addresses interdisciplinary issues related to understanding the impact of network structure and dynamics on group performance and coordination outcomes in complex, dynamic and distributed environments. Dr Uddin has published in several international health-related journals including *Statistics in Medicine, BMC Health Services Research Journal, European Journal of Public Health, European Journal of Health Economic,* and *Journal for Healthcare Quality*. He completed his PhD at the University of Sydney, Australia in 2012. Dr. Uddin was awarded the *Certificate for Research Excellence 2010* by the University of Sydney in recognition of his outstanding research achievement during the course of his PhD studies.

**Chandana Unnithan** is an academic in the field of Information and Business Analytics and currently teaches project management at Deakin University, Australia. She holds degrees in Arts, Commerce, Computer Sciences, and an MBA and a Masters in Business Computing (MbusComp) from Australia. She has held varied positions in the ICT industry, ranging from Business Analyst, Project Manager, and Knowledge Manager with multinationals such as IBM and TATA. Her doctoral research focused on RFID adoption in hospitals with a socio-technical perspective. Her research is in Health Informatics, Electronic Governance, Social Media Informatics, and Women in ICT. She has published in journals such as the *International Journal of ANT and Technology Innovation (IJANTTI) and International Journal of e-adoption (IJED).*

**Qi Wang** is a senior lecturer with the School of Computing at the University of the West of Scotland (UWS), UK. He is the Principal Investigator of the EPSRC project "Enabler for Next-Generation Mobile Video Applications" and several industry-sponsored projects. His research interests include mobile/wireless networks, video networking, and cloud computing. He has published over 50 peer-reviewed papers in these areas with over 500 peer citations. He is a winner of two IEEE ICCE Best Paper Awards (2012 and 2014) and a finalist of the IEE 3G2003 Best Paper Award. He is a recipient of a UWS 2013 STAR Award (Highly Commended) for Outstanding Research and Knowledge Exchange and an ORS Award by the Higher Education Funding Council for England (HEFCE). He is a Regional Editor for the international journal of Recent Advances in Communications and Networking Technology by Bentham Science.

**Xinheng Wang** is a professor in networks at the University of the West of Scotland. He has attracted a number of research grants including two EPSRC projects "A Universal PAN Architecture for Monitoring Multiple Chronic Conditions" and "Distributed and Iterative Processing for Wireless Sensor Networks with Multiple Local Fusion Centres", several TSB/KTP projects, and other nationally/internationally funded projects with overall the research grants exceeding one million pounds. Nearly 100 papers have been published, including the Best Student Paper Award for "Smartphone-Based 3D In-Building Localization and Navigation Service" on the 10$^{th}$ International Conference on Mobile and Ubiquitous Multimedia. Under his supervision, eight research students have been completed their study over the last five years. He is actively engaged with industry, and acting as a member of BSI (British Standards Institution) Committee in ICT, Electronics and Healthcare.

**Jon Whitty** (PM) has extensive organisational consulting experience in project management, complex project delivery, lessons learnt evolutionary networks and the resilient organization. He has expertise in data capture methodology and practice and has a strong track record in project management research. Jon is well regarded in the industry and is the leader of project management research and teaching. He has received several citations for excellence in project management.

**Hairong Yu** is a Senior Research Fellow at the University of NSW Centre for Primary Health Care and Equity. She has experience and expertise in establishing a service-oriented platform which supports cutting-edge collaborative eHealth, applying large data sets with electronic health records for basic, translational, and clinical research. Her research focuses on utilizing knowledge engineering in the medical domain. She currently cooperates and is an investigator on the electronic Practice Based Research Network program which is located in a disadvantaged and Culturally and Linguistically Diverse health neighbourhood.

**Nasriah Zakaria** graduated in Biomedical Engineering (Cum Laude) from Rensselaer Polytechnic Institute, Troy, New York, USA (1997 & 2002) completing both her Bachelors and Masters degrees. Her PhD was in Information Science and Technology from Syracuse University, Syracuse, New York, USA (2006). She is a senior lecturer and program chairman of the information system group in the School of Computer Sciences at the Universiti Sains Malaysia. Currently, she is as Assistant Professor in the Medical Informatics and E-learning Unit (MIELU), Medical Education Department, College of Medicine at King Saud University, Riyadh. She is supervising several PhD and masters students. Her research interests are Information Privacy in Various contexts (Hospital Information Systems, Social Networking Sites, e-health), E-health developments (including m-health) and User Based Studies including Human Computer Interactions (usability and Sociability), IT Adoptions, User based studies for e-learning, and Information Literacy.

# Index

## A



## B



## C



## D



## E



## F



## H

## T



## U



## W

www.ingramcontent.com/pod-product-compliance
Lightning Source LLC
LaVergne TN
LVHW060400300926
849162LV00006B/1309